Thieme

Challenging Cases in Musculoskeletal Imaging

Juergen Freyschmidt, MD
Professor
Reference Center for Osteoradiology
Zentralklinikum Bremen Mitte
University Teaching Hospital of the University of Göttingen
Bremen, Germany

1438 illustrations

Thieme
Stuttgart • New York • Delhi • Rio de Janeiro

Library of Congress Cataloging-in-Publication Data

Freyschmidt, J. (Jürgen), author.
[Schwierige Diagnosen in der Skelettradiologie. English]
Challenging cases in musculoskeletal imaging / Juergen Freyschmidt ; translator, Terry C. Telger.
p. ; cm.
This book is an authorized translation of the German edition published and copyrighted 2013 by Georg Thieme Verlag, Stuttgart. Title of the German edition: Schwierige Diagnosen in der Skelettradiologie.
Includes bibliographical references and index.
ISBN 978-3-13-176401-0 (hardback : alk. paper) – ISBN 978-3-13-176411-9 (eISBN)
I. Title.
[DNLM: 1. Bone Diseases–diagnosis–Case Reports. 2. Diagnostic Imaging–Case Reports. 3. Fractures, Bone–diagnosis–Case Reports. WE 225]
RC925.7
616.7'07548–dc23
2014048126

This book is an authorized translation of the German edition published and copyrighted 2013 by Georg Thieme Verlag, Stuttgart. Title of the German edition: Schwierige Diagnosen in der Skelettradiologie

Translator: Terry C. Telger, Fort Worth, TX, USA

Illustrator: Roland Geyer Weilerswist, Germany

Important note: Medicine is an ever-changing science undergoing continual development. Research and clinical experience are continually expanding our knowledge, in particular our knowledge of proper treatment and drug therapy. Insofar as this book mentions any dosage or application, readers may rest assured that the authors, editors, and publishers have made every effort to ensure that such references are in accordance with **the state of knowledge at the time of production of the book.**

Nevertheless, this does not involve, imply, or express any guarantee or responsibility on the part of the publishers in respect to any dosage instructions and forms of applications stated in the book. **Every user is requested to examine carefully** the manufacturers' leaflets accompanying each drug and to check, if necessary in consultation with a physician or specialist, whether the dosage schedules mentioned therein or the contraindications stated by the manufacturers differ from the statements made in the present book. Such examination is particularly important with drugs that are either rarely used or have been newly released on the market. Every dosage schedule or every form of application used is entirely at the user's own risk and responsibility. The authors and publishers request every user to report to the publishers any discrepancies or inaccuracies noticed. If errors in this work are found after publication, errata will be posted at www.thieme.com on the product description page.

Some of the product names, patents, and registered designs referred to in this book are in fact registered trademarks or proprietary names even though specific reference to this fact is not always made in the text. Therefore, the appearance of a name without designation as proprietary is not to be construed as a representation by the publisher that it is in the public domain.

Thieme Publishers Stuttgart
Rüdigerstrasse 14, 70469 Stuttgart, Germany
+49 [0]711 8931 421, customerservice@thieme.de

Thieme Publishers New York
333 Seventh Avenue, New York, NY 10001 USA
+1 800 782 3488, customerservice@thieme.com

Thieme Publishers Delhi
A-12, Second Floor, Sector-2, Noida-201301
Uttar Pradesh, India
+91 120 45 566 00, customerservice@thieme.in

Thieme Publishers Rio, Thieme Publicações Ltda.
Argentina Building 16th floor, Ala A, 228 Praia do Botafogo
Rio de Janeiro 22250-040 Brazil
+55 21 3736-3631

Cover design: Thieme Publishing Group
Typesetting by DiTech Process Solutions Pvt. Ltd., India

Printed in China by Everbest Printing Ltd 5 4 3 2 1

ISBN 9783131764010

Also available as an e-book:
eISBN 9783131764119

MIX
Paper from responsible sources
FSC® C021256

For my wife Dr. Gisela Freyschmidt, dermatologist

Contents

Preface

Long years of experience in the daily practice of radiology and observations in the training of radiologists have shown that factual knowledge alone is not always enough to make a clinically useful diagnosis. Often more can be gained by taking a systematic approach to image analysis and piecing together available facts. Based on my observations in daily conferences and refresher courses, I have repeatedly found that even less experienced readers with relatively little factual knowledge could solve difficult or challenging cases simply by taking a systematic approach to image analysis and then interpreting their findings in the light of clinical data. By contrast, "old hands" at radiology can diagnose most cases at a glance owing to their extensive experience, but this "shooting from the hip" will often miss the mark when it comes to more challenging diagnoses. Thus, having made several blunders in the past, I have made it a practice to recheck a seemingly obvious diagnosis for its logical plausibility and correctness.

In writing this book, I hope to show how even challenging cases can be diagnosed by following a systematic approach to image interpretation, and how many cases that initially presented as difficult can be turned into ones that only "seemed" difficult.

Juergen Freyschmidt, MD

Acknowledgment to Prof. Helmut Ostertag, MD

Every abnormal finding in diagnostic imaging is based on an underlying structural pathoanatomic change that must be identified before an accurate diagnosis can be made.

For many years I have collaborated with the Hannover pathologist Prof. Helmut Ostertag, MD, whose comprehensive general and specialized knowledge in osteopathology has unveiled many of the secrets of musculoskeletal diseases, helping me to understand and interpret even complex diseases and disorders.

I thank him sincerely for all the time that he sacrificed in reviewing the manuscript for this book. As a dilettante in macroscopy and histology, I needed his help to make sure that the pathoanatomic details of the cases in this book conformed to reality.

Juergen Freyschmidt, MD

Abbreviations List

ADC	apparent diffusion coefficient
ARA	American Rheumatism Association
ARCO	Association for Research of Circulation Osseus
ASAS	Ankolysing Spondylitis Assessment Study
BPOP	bizarre parosteal osteochondromatous proliferation
CNO	chronic nonbacterial osteitis or osteomyelitis
CPPD	calcium pyrophosphate dehydrate deposition disease
CRMO	chronic recurrent multifocal osteomyelitis
CRP	C-reactive protein
CSF	cerebrospinal fluid
CT	computed tomography
CUP	cancer of unknown primary
DISH	diffuse idiopathic skeletal hyperostosis
DSA	digital subtraction angiography
EPI	echo planar imaging
FDG	fluorodeoxyglucose
FLAIR	fluid attenuated inversion recovery
FS	fat suppression
HRCT	high-resolution computed tomography
MPR	multiplanar reconstruction
MRA	magnetic resonance angiography
MRI	magnetic resonance imaging
NSAID	nonsteroidal anti-inflammatory drug
PAO	pustular arthro-osteitis
PDW	proton density weighted
PEO	pustular enthesio-osteitis
PET	positron emission tomography
PPP	pustulosis palmoplantaris
PVNS	pigmented villonodular synovitis
RAP	regional acceleratory phenomenon
SAPHO	synovitis, acne, pustulosis, hyperostosis, osteitis (syndrome)
SCCH	sternocostoclavicular hyperostosis
SPAIR	spectral presatuation inversion recovery
SPECT	single-photon emission computed tomography
SPIR	spectral attenuated inversion recovery
STIR	short tau inversion recovery
STT	scapho-trapezio-trapezoid
SUV	standard uptake value
TIRM	turbo-inversion recovery magnitude
TSE	turbo spin echo
WHO	World Health Organization

1 From Symptom to Diagnosis

Orthopedics and trauma surgery, rheumatology, the vast field of oncology and, to a degree, even biopsy-based pathology must rely heavily on skeletal imaging. Radiologists must be well versed in these areas to ensure that their services will continue to be relevant. What, then, do these specialties require in terms of a good diagnosis? And how should a "good diagnosis" be defined?

First and foremost, a radiologic diagnosis must be useful. It must alter the treatment strategy for a patient. On the other hand, it does not necessarily have to be definitive; it does not have to be the final diagnosis like that supplied by histology, clinical chemistry, molecular biology, or the clinical course. Above all it must be logical and well founded and it must reflect due diligence. That is the only justifiable aspect of a radiologic diagnosis—not its absolute correctness, which may draw even highly specialized experts into a dispute that no judge could resolve.

Every radiologist must provide two essential services:

- Selecting the correct imaging modality
- Image interpretation

1.1 Selecting the Correct Imaging Modality

The following imaging modalities should be available and selectively utilized at centers where skeletal examinations are performed:

- Plain radiography
- CT (computed tomography)
- Bone scintigraphy including SPECT (single-photon emission computed tomography)
- MRI (magnetic resonance imaging)
- PET (positron emission tomography) and PET-CT fusion
- Ultrasound

The patients who are seen in the everyday practice of skeletal radiology fall into one of three scenarios:

1. A patient undergoes initial imaging for the investigation of a clinical problem. The patient has had no previous imaging studies, and ideally the radiologist is challenged to tailor the imaging study to the specific problem, using his or her skills and experience.
2. A patient is referred for the further investigation of findings noted in one or more previous imaging studies. In this situation the radiologist must select the study that can supply the fastest and most accurate, clinically useful diagnosis.
3. A patient with an established diagnosis presents for follow-up imaging.

1.1.1 Available Imaging Studies

What, then, are the most suitable and rewarding imaging studies for a particular problem? Which of the procedures listed above will yield the desired information most rapidly and accurately while causing the least amount of patient compromise?

To answer these questions, it is helpful to review briefly the capabilities and limitations of the imaging modalities listed above.

Plain Radiography

Plain radiography creates an image based on differences in the X-ray absorption characteristics of different tissues. Thus, bone tissue or any bony or calcified structures are portrayed in high contrast while most soft tissues are imaged in low contrast, unless contrast medium is used. The main disadvantage of plain radiography in skeletal studies is the presence of summation effects, since radiographs give only a superimposed, two-dimensional view of three-dimensional body structures. Thus, from a modern-day perspective (and based on current requirements), plain radiography is unsuitable for detecting focal lesions (1.5–2 cm in diameter) in body regions that are sensitive to projection effects such as the thoracic and lumbar spine, sacrum, and skull base. On the other hand, there are systemic bone diseases with more or less fine structural changes (e.g., osteopathies such as osteoporosis, hyperparathyroidism, osteomalacia, Paget disease) in which summation effects are diagnostically useful and may detect structural changes that would often be missed in sectional imaging procedures.

Plain radiography is inherently unsuitable for the evaluation of soft-tissue structures such as bone marrow, muscle, tendons, ligaments, cartilage, etc. A major advantage of skeletal plain radiography, which has been in use for over a century, is that valid pattern-recognition algorithms and engrams (cognitive links) have been established that permit the fast and accurate detection of abnormalities. This capability is useful, for example, in the analysis of osteolytic areas by Lodwick grading and for recognizing ossification patterns in a tumor matrix, such as the "ground-glass" pattern for woven bone (see Case 139) and the "popcorn" pattern for cartilaginous matrix (see Case 108).

Computed Tomography

CT basically works like plain radiography by converting tissue X-ray absorption values into an image. The advantage of CT is that it can generate sectional, nonsuperimposed images of body structures with a contrast resolution many times higher than that of conventional radiographs. As a sectional modality, it is particularly useful for providing nonsuperimposed views of the axial skeleton and of complex processes in the appendicular skeleton. It can also provide limited views of soft-tissue structures like muscle, fat, and hematomas. Scanning after the administration of intravenous contrast medium can significantly expand the ability of CT to define soft-tissue structures, especially when the proper window setting is used. CT densitometry permits the accurate identification of fat, fluid, and other media based on their attenuation values. Modern multidetector-row scanners can produce three-dimensional images that are essential for the accurate localization of structures and lesions. From a physical standpoint, the indications for CT are the same as those for plain radiographs, aside from its sectional imaging capabilities. Also, owing to the establishment of pattern-recognition algorithms and engrams with high diagnostic specificity, CT, which is slightly less than 40 years old, has features in common with plain radiography in skeletal examinations and offers numerous advantages over the "younger" modalities of MRI and PET-CT.

Bone Scintigraphy

Bone scintigraphy with Tc-99 m (technetium-99 m methylene diphosphonate) is an imaging technique based on radioactive tracer uptake in bones and adjacent soft tissues. The amount of tracer uptake is dependent on local bone metabolism, local perfusion, and regional tracer affinity, so that planar "bone scans" with a gamma camera supply information on global, regional, and focal bone metabolism. This is helpful in determining, for example, whether a systemic process with increased bone turnover, such as hyperparathyroidism (see Case 15 and ▸ Fig. 6.30 **g** in Case 111), is present as opposed to a focal or a multifocal process representing a bone metastasis. Bone scans can reliably determine whether a sclerotic lesion is active or not, which may be particularly helpful in oncologic evaluations (see Case 145 and Case 149). Bone scintigraphy, then, is a functional imaging study. Today there is no radiologic technique that can supply such precise information on bone metabolism with "one look" and with a relatively simple protocol. In patients thought to have smaller and less active lesions, another sectional imaging technique, SPECT, is of great value in many cases owing to its ability to provide non-superimposed three-dimensional views.

Unfortunately, bone scintigraphy is not widely practiced today despite the fact that it is widely available and supplies functional information not obtainable with CT or MRI. In recent years we have been able to define more than 20 tracer distribution patterns which are highly specific for certain skeletal diseases and refute the common argument against bone scans, namely that "they are not specific enough."[1] The radiation safety aspects of bone scintigraphy will not be explored here, but suffice it to say that radiation exposure is relatively low and such risk is greatly outweighed by the benefits of the study for sick patients.

Magnetic Resonance Imaging

MRI, in which the relaxation times and proton content of body tissues are measured, is a sectional imaging modality that has fundamental physical differences from the X-ray absorption modalities. It is the method of first choice for imaging soft-tissue structures (bone marrow, muscle, tendons, fascia, neurovascular bundles, cartilage, synovial membrane, intra-articular fluid) and currently has a relatively broad role in skeletal investigations. Yet the initial euphoria that this modality could handle all skeletal imaging tasks without X-rays has been tempered by the results of clinical imaging studies. Meanwhile, sound and appropriate indications for MRI have been crystalizing, especially in the diagnosis of articular, bone-marrow and muscular diseases and in the staging of skeletal tumors. It should be noted that bony structures (especially healthy cortical bone) appear as signal voids on MR images and thus can be identified only indirectly; this may lead to problems of differential diagnosis. The same applies to processes that are associated with more or less subtle ossifications or calcifications, which are clearly demonstrable by CT.

The information content of MRI can be increased by dynamic contrast-enhanced imaging (e.g., to assess the perfusion of a lesion) and by diffusion-weighted imaging. But these techniques cannot in themselves provide reliable information on general and local bone metabolism in the strict sense, and unlike bone scintigraphy they cannot answer the question of whether a sclerotic lesion, for example, is active. Unlike plain radiographs, CT scans, and bone scans, MRI still does not have well-established pattern recognition algorithms and engrams (e.g., Lodwick grades, ground-glass appearance, systemic sclerosing diseases), apart from joint trauma, which could guide the radiologist quickly and confidently to a correct diagnosis. Moreover, there is still no good, comprehensive catalog of normal variants like that available for the more conventional modalities.

Not infrequently, problems in the availability of MRI can distort its range of indications. This means that other imaging studies are ordered (e.g., radiographs of the spine and sacroiliac joints for suspected early spondyloarthritis) even though it is known that early enthesitic changes are not detectable on plain radiographs. Or perhaps a pelvic radiograph is ordered for suspected early osteonecrosis of the femoral head, even though ARCO stage I or II disease (ARCO = Association for Research of Circulation Osseous) can be detected only by MRI. At the same time, more or less useless MRIs are being scheduled for, say, lumbago without neurologic deficits and are depriving patients who could truly benefit from an early MRI examination.

Note

A very important rule for MRI protocols: If scanning is performed with contrast medium, the sequences before and after contrast administration should be identical (e.g., T1 weighting before and after contrast injection). Otherwise, possible enhancement cannot be evaluated. Unfortunately this technical principle is often violated in clinical practice. For example, a T1-weighted (T1w) sequence is performed before contrast administration but a fat-suppressed T1w sequence or water-sensitive sequence is performed afterward.

Positron Emission Tomography (and PET-CT)

PET, like bone scintigraphy, is a functional imaging modality. Today, over 90% of all PET scans employ the glucose analog ^{18}F-FDG (^{18}F-2-fluoro-2-deoxyglucose), tagged with the fluorine radioisotope ^{18}F. The method is based on the imaging of a circumscribed change in specific cellular functions, such as the intensity of glucose metabolism as determined by ^{18}F-FDG PET. Increased glucose metabolism is a relatively nonspecific indicator, however, which is seen in inflammatory processes as well as neoplasms and tumorlike lesions. The standard uptake value (SUV) provides a semiquantitative indicator of tumor metabolism (see below).

PET can be combined with simultaneous CT imaging in two interconnected scanners to produce a system known as PET-CT. This integrated system can generate a PET-CT fusion image without having to change the patient position, respiratory position, slice thickness, etc. Increasingly, PET-CT is becoming an established tool in oncologic musculoskeletal studies, as in the diagnosis of lymphoma and plasmacytoma[2,3] and skeletal metastases. In a recent meta-analysis of 23 studies, however, Liu et al[4] found that MRI was superior to ^{18}F-FDG PET and bone scintigraphy for detecting skeletal metastases in breast cancer patients (pooled sensitivity on a per-patient basis: 97.1% for MRI, 83.3% for PET, and 87.0% for bone scintigraphy; pooled sensitivity on a per-lesion basis: 97% for MRI, 94.5% for PET, and 88.1% for bone scintigraphy).

As for the diagnosis of primary bone tumors,[5,6] to date there have been only scattered publications, based largely on case reports, which do not provide conclusive information (see below). But given the generally low incidence of bone tumors, it is still too early to expect definitive answers.

FDG-PET can be very useful for monitoring bone tumors during treatment, since by its very nature it is accurate in assessing tumor viability. The SUV for FDG provides a semiquantitative measure of metabolic tumor activity. Because tumor metabolism is usually heterogeneous, the SUV in a region of interest (ROI) within the tumor provides an excellent index for evaluating tumor metabolism. Hawkins et al[7] investigated the maximum SUV before and after neoadjuvant chemotherapy for the Ewing sarcoma family of tumors. Patients with an SUV of less than 2 after therapy tended to have an excellent response (10% or less viable tumor) with a 4-year disease-free survival. Hawkins et al[8] found similar results for osteosarcoma.

Gaston et al[9] obtained somewhat different results in their recent study: the change in maximum SUV between baseline examination and post-treatment scanning was not significantly associated with histologic response for either osteosarcoma or Ewing sarcoma. The metabolic tumor volume and the percentage of injected ^{18}F-FDG dose were different in the osteosarcoma and Ewing sarcoma response subgroups. A 50% reduction in metabolic tumor volume was found to be significantly associated with a good histologic response in osteosarcoma but not in Ewing sarcoma. When the cut-off value for Ewing sarcoma was increased to a 90% reduction in metabolic tumor volume, a good correlation was found with histologic response.

These essentially positive results of FDG-PET scans cannot be applied directly to the problem of benign/malignant differentiation (see above). Aoki et al[5] found no significant difference between the SUVs of osteosarcoma and giant cell tumor or between fibrous dysplasia and chondrosarcoma; this is not surprising (see above). Feldman et al,[6] on the other hand, studied 29 cartilage tumors (11 enchondromas, 6 osteochondromas, 11 chondrosarcomas) and found that ^{18}FDG-PET, using a maximum SUV cut-off of 2.0, could discriminate between malignant and benign lesions with a sensitivity of 90.9%, a specificity of 100%, and an accuracy of 96.6%. On closer analysis, the patients in their study comprised a very heterogeneous group. Bredella et al[10] evaluated FDG-PET in differentiating benign from malignant compression fractures (33 patients with 43 fractures). In a total of 14 malignant and 29 benign compression fractures, five cases with a benign fracture were falsely classified as malignant (false-positive). Three of those patients had undergone prior treatment with bone-marrow stimulating agents. There were two false-negative results. Sensitivity, specificity, and accuracy were in the range of approximately 70 to 90%. In our view these results are not too significant when we consider that the patients participating in the study had multiple fractures that most likely had the same cause. Moreover, only nine of the cases were histologically confirmed, and the tumor entities underlying the malignant fractures were extremely heterogeneous. The authors state that the difference between the SUV values for benign and malignant fractures was statistically significant (1.9 ± 0.97 and 3.9 ± 1.52, respectively). Shin et al[11] found basically the same results in a similar population, although they performed all examinations with PET-CT and obtained measurements separately for the cortex and bone marrow.

Thus, we find no real consensus in the current literature on the efficacy of FDG-PET in diagnosing bone tumors, aside from initially positive results in the follow-up of Ewing sarcoma and osteosarcoma during treatment. This is to be expected, since this modality is relatively recent and the spectrum of primary and secondary bone tumors is very broad with respect to tumor dynamics and tumor biology. One critical note on the above follow-up studies is that none has yet compared PET with traditional modalities such as MRI, CT, scintigraphy, and plain radiography.

1.1.2 Imaging Strategies

Initial Imaging Study

Given the specific characteristics of the imaging modalities described above, it is important to ask which one should be used for the initial investigation of a given clinical problem in a patient not previously imaged. See scenario 1. In ▶ Table 1.1 we have attempted to match various disease groups and entities with the imaging modality that years of personal experience has shown to provide the fastest and surest route to a correct diagnosis—one that will direct the referring colleague in selecting further clinical and laboratory tests and then planning appropriate treatment. That is the only diagnosis of any real value. A simple description of findings that does not supply a working diagnosis is of no use to the referring clinician. Nor is it enough to report "no evidence of malignancy," especially if the clinical presentation does not raise the problem of benign/malignant differentiation, as in patients with stress-related disorders.

Note

Basic guidelines for selecting an imaging modality:

- Imaging bony structures: plain radiography, CT
- Imaging soft-tissue structures (muscle, tendons, cartilage, synovial membrane, "foreign tissue" in bone, etc.): ultrasound, otherwise MRI
- Evaluating the activity of a lesion: whole-body bone scintigraphy

Supplemental Imaging Study

Recommendations on selecting a suitable imaging modality to supplement a previous imaging study (scenario 2) are derived from the specificity of the modality in question. With some restrictions, the following rule applies:

Note

When selecting an imaging modality for the further investigation of a lesion detected by a different modality, never select a modality that is less sensitive or less specific than the previous study.

For example, if bone scintigraphy has detected small focal lesions in the spine, it would be wrong to order radiographs in two

Table 1.1 Recommendations on selecting a modality for an initial imaging study

Clinical suspicion	Recommended primary imaging study
Oncologic radiology	
Bone metastases	Whole-body bone scintigraphy; if available whole-body MRI; positive findings warrant further investigation of appendicular skeleton by radiography, axial skeleton by CT
Multiple myeloma	Whole-body MRI or whole-body CT; if available PET-CT; for larger lesions found in the appendicular skeleton radiographs to determine fracture risk
Langerhans cell histiocytosis	Whole-body MRI in children; adults may require whole-body CT or bone scintigraphy (see Case 24 and Case 92)
Symptomatic bone tumor	Radiographs in two planes for appendicular skeleton; CT for diagnostic problem (cartilaginous or bony matrix?); if signs of malignancy are present → staging MRI, then open biopsy; primary CT for axial skeleton (see also WHO algorithm, ▶ Fig. 1.1)
Asymptomatic bone tumor (detected incidentally on radiographs)	In appendicular skeleton: no further investigation is needed if appearance is benign (fibrous metaphyseal defect, fibro-osseous lesion of proximal femur, fibrous dysplasia, ganglion, osteochondroma)
Stress-related skeletal changes	
Stress fracture (fatigue fracture)	Radiography of presumed location; if negative and there is high index of clinical suspicion → repeat radiographs in 2 weeks; with low clinical probability and negative radiographs → MRI or bone scintigraphy; with positive bone scan and atypical or equivocal MRI → CT (algorithm in ▶ Fig. 1.2; see also Case 129)
Insufficiency fracture	Radiography and bone scintigraphy (see also under Osteomalacia in this table)
Entheseal stress (e.g., greater tuberosity, crest of greater and lesser tuberosity, calcaneus)	Radiography; if negative → MRI or possibly CT for suspected bursitis or calcaneal tendinitis (see Case 75, Case 77, Case 102, Case 103, Case 104, and Case 113)
Perfusion disorders of bone and bone marrow	
Osteonecrosis with a long history	Radiography; if negative → MRI; if equivocal → CT to confirm fragmentation
Osteonecrosis with a shorter history (less than ca. 3–4 weeks)	MRI
Systemic osteonecrosis (e.g., vasculitic, steroid-induced, hemoglobinopathies, pancreatitic)	MRI; CT may be used to check for possible fragmentation
Bone marrow necrosis (e.g., fresh bone marrow infarction in pancreatitis, hypercorticism, etc.)	MRI
Reflex sympathetic dystrophy in the strict sense	Radiography; if negative and there are strong clinical signs → MRI; if not available → multiphase bone scan of the affected region (e.g., hands)
Transient edema	MRI (see Case 76)
Transient osteoporosis	MRI; if positive → radiography (see Case 76)
Skeletal hyperostoses[a]	
Tumor, inflammation, reactive process in circumscribed sclerosis	Whole-body bone scan; if positive → CT (see Case 31, Case 40, Case 47, Case 107, Case 145, and Case 149)
Osteopoikilosis, osteopathia striata with multifocal lesions	Radiography of the hands as a test region (see Case 31)
Melorheostosis with enosseous or cortical sclerosis with "flowing candle wax" density	Radiography of the whole affected limb, and of the whole side of the body if necessary; or, with spinal location, radiography of the whole spine (see Case 17, Case 88, and Case 99)
Osteopetrosis and other congenital generalized hyperostoses	Representative skeletal radiograph with single-plane views
Osteomyelosclerosis syndrome	Radiography of the spine and pelvis, lateral radiograph of the skull, single-plane radiograph of the whole limb on one side of the body
DISH	Radiography of the spine and pelvis (see Case 28)

Table 1.1 (continued) Recommendations on selecting a modality for an initial imaging study

Clinical suspicion	Recommended primary imaging study
Metabolic skeletal diseases	
Osteoporosis	Lateral radiograph of the thoracic and lumbar spine with DXA or QCT
Osteomalacia	Whole-body bone scan; if scan shows hot spots suspicious for insufficiency fracture → radiographs of the appendicular skeleton; CT of the ribs, bony thorax, and pelvis (see Case 62)
Primary and secondary hyperparathyroidism	Hand radiographs (subperiosteal resorption!), bone scintigraphy (superscan, look for brown tumors); special views may be added as required (see Case 15 Case 42, ▶ Fig. 5.27 in Case 90, Case 111, and ▶ Fig. 6.46 in Case 121)
Pseudohyperparathyroidism	Hand radiographs (shortening of metacarpal bones)
Renal osteopathy	Hand radiographs (subperiosteal resorption, carpal pseudocysts in amyloidosis); radiographs of the axial skeleton (rugger jersey spine) and pelvis (insufficiency fractures; see Case 42)
Adynamic bone disease in renal osteopathy	Radiographs of the spine and bony thorax (look for fractures)
Fluorosis	Radiography of the spine and pelvis (white bone with coarse porosity, periosteal and ligament ossifications); whole-body bone scan; if scan shows abnormalities in appendicular skeleton → radiography to check for insufficiency fractures
MPS (RES) diseases and sarcoidosis	
Gaucher disease[b]	Whole-body MRI (bone marrow displacement, necrosis), lateral thoracic and lumbar spine (fractures, sclerosis), AP thigh (Erlenmeyer flask deformity)
Lipoid granulomatosis (Erdheim–Chester disease)	Whole-body bone scintigraphy; radiography of scintigraphic abnormalities, usually about the knee joints and in the pelvis; whole-body MRI (organ involvement such as CNS or retroperitoneum) (see ▶ Fig. 7.29 in Case 145)
Systemic mastocytosis[c]	MRI of the spine and proximal long bones (bone marrow infiltration); if necessary, radiography of the affected regions (osteoporosis and/or sclerosis)
Sarcoidosis	Whole-body bone scan; if necessary, radiography or CT of the affected regions (sclerosis, destruction); always obtain radiographs of the hands and feet (see Case 122)
Phacomatoses	
Neurofibromatosis type 1	Radiography of the skull (sphenoid dysplasia); with suggestive clinical presentation → radiography of the spine (scoliosis), pelvis (asymmetry, hip dysplasia), and long bones (narrowing, bowing, pseudarthrosis)
Tuberous sclerosis	Lateral radiographs of the lumbar spine, pelvis, and skull (focal sclerotic areas)
Gorlin–Goltz syndrome	Radiographs of the jaw and long bones (cysts)
Polycystic lipomembranous osteodysplasia with sclerosing leukoencephalopathy (Nasu–Hakola disease)	Radiographs of the hands and feet, AP radiographs of the upper and lower limbs (look for pseudocysts); CT in selected cases for densitometry of some pseudocysts, which consist entirely of mature fatty tissue (see Case 119)
Proteus syndrome	CT or MRI of hypertrophic skeletal regions to detect fatty tissue and pathologic vessels
Vascular malformations	
Extra- or intraosseous drainage anomaly (e.g., tibia)	Dynamic MRI or CT
Arteriovenous malformation	Radiography of the affected skeletal region (vascular prints), dynamic MRI; if necessary, DSA
Venous malformation	Radiography of the affected skeletal region (vascular prints), MRI; if necessary, direct venography and spiral CT (see Case 154)
Lymphatic malformation	MRI

(Continued)

Table 1.1 (continued) Recommendations on selecting a modality for an initial imaging study

Clinical suspicion	Recommended primary imaging study
Inflammatory bone diseases	
Acute extra-axial osteomyelitis in children (see ▶ Fig. 1.3)	Ultrasound (periosteal abscess), MRI (bone–soft tissue edema equivalent and/or abscess); radiographs if needed
Acute extra-axial osteomyelitis in adults (see ▶ Fig. 1.3)	Radiography of the affected limb; if positive → aspiration biopsy; if negative → MRI or bone scintigraphy, supplemented if necessary by inflammation scintigraphy; CT is best for detecting sequestra
Chronic extra-axial osteomyelitis	Radiography; CT (for detecting sequestra); MRI with contrast (medullary spread, recurrent abscess; see Case 109)
Acute and chronic spondylitis	MRI; CT if required (bone status)
CNO (if recurrent and multifocal: CRMO)	Whole-body bone scintigraphy; radiography; possible CT investigation of suspicious regions; primary MRI is also appropriate (see Case 82 and Case 153)
Paget disease	Radiography of appendicular skeleton; radiography or CT of skull and spine; whole-body bone scan (number and size of lesions; if doubt exists, extensive uptake always suggests Paget disease; see Case 9, Case 12, Case 14, Case 46, Case 51, Case 83, Case 107, and Case 140)
Joint diseases (▶ Fig. 1.4)	
Rheumatoid arthritis, early stage (symptoms: 6 weeks to 2 months)	MRI of the hands and symptomatic joints; for an experienced examiner → ultrasound
Rheumatoid arthritis, intermediate stage (symptomatic for 2–3 months) and late stage	Radiographs of the hands, feet, symptomatic joints, and craniovertebral joints
Systemic sclerosis	Radiography of the hands (diffuse osteoporosis, acro-osteolysis, interstitial calcinosis)
Systemic lupus erythematosus	MRI if necrosis is suspected; otherwise radiography of symptomatic regions (deformities, etc.)
Enthesiopathies (early changes) (spondyloarthritides: ankylosing spondylitis, Reiter syndrome, intestinal arthropathies, psoriatic spondyloarthritis, juvenile spondyloarthritis)	MRI of the spine, sacroiliac joints, and symptomatic entheses (e.g., pelvis, Achilles tendons); with atypical pattern, supplement with CT (simultaneous destruction and proliferation; see Case 39, Case 40, and Case 97
With a longer history	Radiography of the spine and sacroiliac joints; CT if required (see Case 48, Case 49, and Case 145)
With psoriasis and pustulosis palmoplantaris and anterior chest wall symptoms	CT of the sternocostoclavicular region (see Case 40 and Case 97)
Infectious (septic) arthritis	MRI; percutaneous aspiration if required; radiographs for follow-up
Degenerative arthritis	Radiography of the affected joint; MRI if required (edema equivalent, cartilage status; see Case 121)
Joint trauma	Radiography, MRI
Chondrocalcinosis	Radiographs of the hands (metacarpophalangeal joints, scapholunar dissociation, cartilage calcifications) and symptomatic joints; CT if required (see Case 41, ▶ Fig. 6.61 in Case 127, and Case 155)
Hemochromatosis	Radiographs of the hands (metacarpophalangeal joints) and symptomatic joints (see Case 155)
Gout	Radiographs of the feet and symptomatic joints (see ▶ Fig. 3.43 **a–c** in Case 41, ▶ Fig. 6.62 in Case 127, and Case 136)
Ochronosis	Radiography of the spine (disk and annular calcifications)
Neurogenic arthropathy	Radiographs of symptomatic joints
Diabetic osteoarthropathy	Radiographs of the feet (destruction of tarsals and metatarsals, periosteal calcifications); if infection is suspected → CT/MRI
Hemophilic joint disease	MRI and radiography of the symptomatic joint

Table 1.1 (continued) Recommendations on selecting a modality for an initial imaging study

Clinical suspicion	Recommended primary imaging study
Joint tumors	MRI; radiographs if required (calcifications; Case 71 and Case 72)

[a]Patient is referred with clinical suspicion or suspicious radiographs.
[b]Gaucher disease is actually a storage disease and is listed here for pragmatic reasons.
[c]Systemic mastocytosis is classified among the myoproliferative diseases and is listed here for pragmatic reasons.
Abbreviations:
AP = anteroposterior
CNO = chronic nonbacterial osteomyelitis
CNS = central nervous system
CRMO = chronic recurrent multifocal osteomyelitis
DISH = diffuse idiopathic skeletal hyperostosis
DSA = digital subtraction angiography
DXA = dual X-ray absorptiometry
MPS = mononuclear phagocyte system
QCT = quantitative CT
RES = reticuloendothelial system

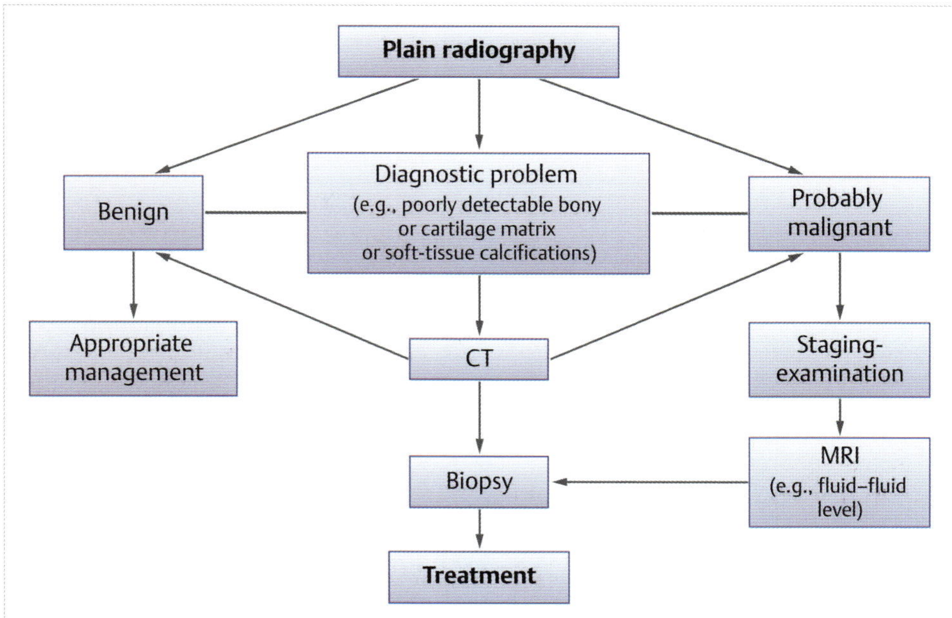

Fig. 1.1 Diagnostic algorithm for a suspected bone tumor.[15]

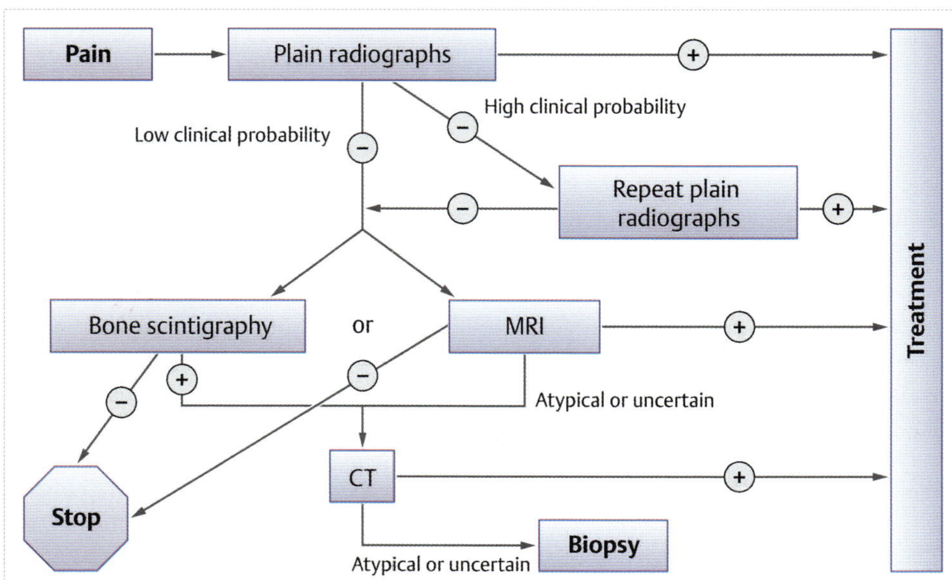

Fig. 1.2 Diagnostic algorithm for a presumed stress fracture.

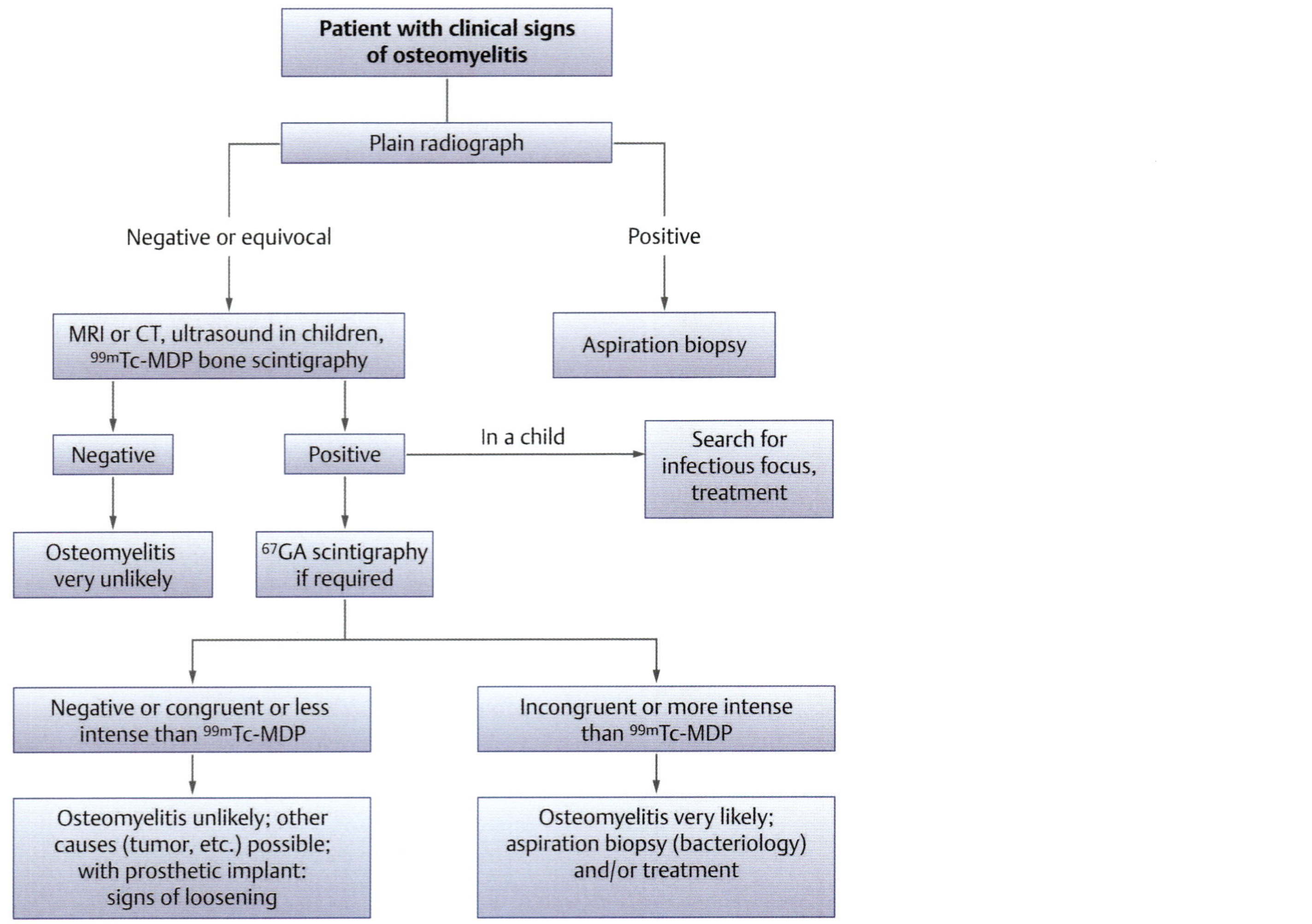

Fig. 1.3 Diagnostic algorithm for suspected osteomyelitis.

planes for further investigation of the lesions because plain radiographs usually cannot detect osteolytic or mixed osteolytic-osteoblastic lesions (e.g., metastases from breast cancer) smaller than 1.5–2 cm due to their low sensitivity. Since it is reasonable to expect that scintigraphic abnormalities are true bone metastases rather than metastases confined to bone marrow—that is, metastases that have already interacted with the bone—further investigation by CT (not MRI) would be indicated owing to the higher specificity of CT for an osseous process.

A more detailed look at scenario 2:

- If plain radiographs show an indeterminate lesion that appears to involve bony structures, CT should be ordered next to provide a nonsuperimposed view in the "bone mode." We do not recommend changing the physical mode in this situation (e.g., from measuring absorption differences to measuring proton content and relaxation times) because this would address entirely different questions (see above). But if radiographs suggest that the lesion originates from soft tissues (e.g., tumor involvement of the medullary cavity), MRI is recommended (see Case 8, Case 9, Case 10, Case 12, Case 14, Case 16, Case 30, Case 34, Case 45, Case 48, Case 49, Case 58, Case 94, ▸ Fig. 6.21 in Case 107, Case 118, Case 119, ▸ Fig. 7.12 in Case 135, Case 139, Case 142, and Case 145).
- If MRI was performed first and could not answer questions relating specifically to bone structure or ossifications, it should be supplemented with a modality that can directly image the bone: plain radiography or CT. CT should be chosen whenever nonsuperimposed views are required. As a sectional modality, it provides image slices that can "unmask" a detail of interest (see Case 7, Case 17, Case 19, Case 20, Case 22, Case 29, Case 30, Case 36, Case 39, Case 60, Case 63, Case 64, Case 74, Case 101, Case 104, Case 107, Case 113, Case 127, Case 129, Case 131, Case 136, Case 145, Case 146, and Case 149).
- If the initial study was PET or PET-CT (the latter may be nondiagnostic due to less-than-optimal image quality of the CT component), dedicated spiral CT is recommended for the further investigation of a bony process (see ▸ Fig. 4.50 in Case 77). If the goal is to investigate a soft-tissue lesion revealed by PET-CT, MRI will provide an effective adjunct. With a negative PET scan (screening for metastases, suspected plasmacytoma), the recommended course of action is clinical follow-up, depending on the patient's symptoms.
- If the goal is to determine the activity of a lesion detected by other methods (especially important in oncologic radiology), the next recommended study is bone scintigraphy. For example, a sclerotic lesion that is negative on bone scans (osteoma, old fibrous dysplasia, old lipoma, old infarction, healed reactive inflammatory process, etc.) is more likely to be old and harmless than a lesion that shows uptake (e.g., sclerosing metastasis, bone-forming tumor, etc.). When uptake is found, bone scintigraphy can advance the differential diagnosis by

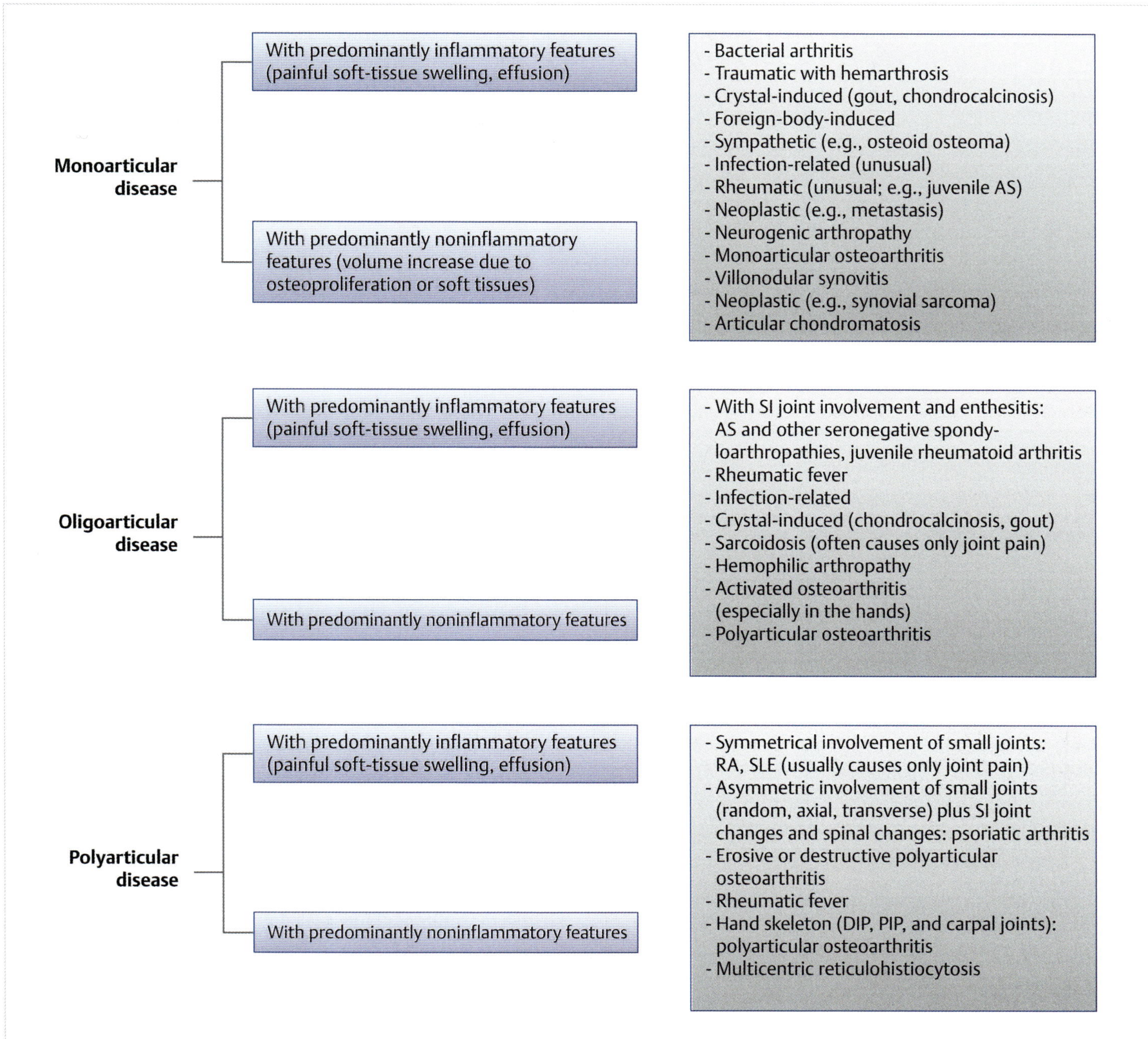

Fig. 1.4 Guidelines for diagnosing joint diseases.
AS = ankylosing spondylitis
DIP joints = distal interphalangeal joints
PIP joints = proximal interphalangeal joints
RA = rheumatoid arthritis
SI joint =sacroiliac joint
SLE = systemic lupus erythematosus

determining whether the lesion is solitary (e.g., fibrous dysplasia, which is often multifocal, versus lipoma, which is usually solitary; metastasis, which is usually multiple, versus a bone-forming tumor like osteoid osteoma, which is almost always solitary; see also Case 12, Case 31, Case 32, Case 47, Case 50, Case 73, Case 74, Case 78, Case 102, Case 107, and Case 133).

- If the initial study was bone scintigraphy showing one or more sites of focal uptake, the next study should be one that directly images the bone, depending on the site(s) of involvement. The options, are plain radiography and CT (see Case 20), since scintigraphy demonstrates the *activity* of a bony process. In many cases, however, the distribution pattern on scintigraphy will in itself suggest the correct diagnosis (see ▶ Fig. 4.22 in Case 62, ▶ Fig. 5.8 **h, i** in Case 82, Case 83, ▶ Fig. 5.13 in Case 84, and Case 103).
- If initial CT scans showed one or more lesions originating from soft tissue, the recommended supplemental study is MRI. Of course, this modality is also used to investigate a bone tumor detected by CT or by supplemental CT after plain radiography, as it can detect tumor spread into adjacent soft tissues and supply valuable additional information (see Case 45, Case 54, Case 57, Case 70, Case 86, Case 106, Case 111, and ▶ Fig. 7.12 in Case 135).

Finally a word about costs: the use of one or more necessary imaging modalities can be very expensive. But such costs must be weighed against the benefits for properly selected patients. A frequent benefit from a financial standpoint is that a proper imaging work-up can eliminate many unnecessary invasive procedures (e.g., open biopsy) and prevent diagnostic errors. Moreover, when we consider the relatively low incidence of nontraumatic skeletal lesions, which form the major portion of our topic, the costs are almost negligible when compared with other costs incurred in the health care industry (approximately 0.1% or less).

Follow-up Imaging

Whenever possible, the follow-up imaging of patients with an established diagnosis (scenario 3) should employ the same modality and should follow a consistent protocol. This is essential to allow a meaningful comparison of images.

1.2 Image Interpretation

Before any remarkable image details are interpreted, they must be described. This does not require a lengthy narrative but may be done concisely in a "key-word" format. The description of findings should nevertheless be exacting and, above all, should avoid potentially misleading language. For example, a lucent area on a radiograph or CT scan should be described as such and should not be called a "cystic" or "cystlike" osteolysis, as this could bias further conclusions that may be drawn in the light of other findings. Another example is "bone marrow edema," a term that is frequently overused in MRI reporting (see below).

> **Note**
>
> Image analysis requires a detailed knowledge of the normal radiologic anatomy of the musculoskeletal system and its principal variants.

1.2.1 Pathoanatomic Background

When a finding is classified as definitely abnormal, the first essential question should address its possible pathoanatomic background, because each of the known basic entities (see below) is associated with a more or less specific pathoanatomic change. For example, a tumor or inflammatory process is associated with destruction, necrosis with fragmentation, and a reparative process with new bone formation. An effort should also be made to determine whether a finding may be only an epiphenomenon (e.g., hemorrhage, callus) that accompanies an underlying process. In assigning findings to a pathoanatomic substrate, it is always important to consider the capabilities for tissue discrimination (fat, fluid, etc.) that are available with the modality being used. Unfortunately, this capability is often forgotten in the case of CT (see Case 58).

In the process of image interpretation, it is dangerous to use terms that describe either a disease entity in the strict sense or a sign with a variegated background. This principle will be explained more fully based on the two examples mentioned above:

Example: Rounded Lucency

In many cases a rounded lucency seen on a radiograph or CT scan is described as a "cyst" or a "cystic or cystlike lucency," even though it is more often caused by a solid destructive lesion. This wording may steer case deliberations still further in the wrong direction, implying that the finding may be innocent. The term "cyst" is reserved exclusively for a fluid-filled cavity such as a juvenile bone cyst, a subchondral synovial cyst, or an aneurysmal bone cyst. The fluid content should first be established by CT or MRI, except with a classic juvenile bone cyst, which is identified by its typical location, "fallen fragment sign," and ultrashort history.

Example: Ill-defined Hyperintensity

An area of increased signal intensity with ill-defined margins seen in water-sensitive MRI sequences is often described simply as "edema." This is frequently offered as a diagnosis when no other suggestive findings are seen. Edema in bone marrow or in structurally altered cortical bone is an extravascular interstitial fluid collection that may accompany, for instance, a traumatic, inflammatory, degenerative or even a neoplastic process. "Edema" is a term that runs the gamut from benign to malignant disorders. Simply put, the resulting MRI signal is based partly on an increased proton density in the imaged region, regardless of the cause, which is usually but not always edema (see below).

Based on the MR image alone, it cannot be stated with certainty whether "bone marrow edema" actually represents pure edema, meaning an extravascular interstitial fluid collection. Taking degenerative changes in the knee joint as an example, "bone marrow edema" may result from fat necrosis, fibrosis, or trabecular bone changes such as a bone bruise, as Zanetti et al[12] have shown. A pathologic process need only have enough protons to cause increased signal intensity in water-sensitive sequences. This applies to traumatic, inflammatory, degenerative, and neoplastic processes, the latter also showing an increased intracellular water content (see Case 145, Case 146, and Case 149). Even contrast administration cannot positively distinguish, for example, between tumor tissue and edema. It is clearer and more accurate, therefore, to report an edema equivalent[13,14] or an "edema-like hyperintensity," or simply to report the presence of a proton-rich area.

1.2.2 Lesion Localization

The second question raised by an abnormal finding is its location, which is considered in terms of functional anatomy. Is the finding located in a stress-exposed area (e.g., entheses), a critical area for perfusion deficits (e.g., epiphyses, toes or fingers), or a region where hematopoiesis occurs (e.g., a vertebral body)? These are key questions that aid in the classification of findings.

1.2.3 Epicenter of a Lesion

The third question relates to the epicenter of a lesion or other finding. Most neoplastic processes exhibit a concentric pattern of tumor growth. Thus, for example, if the center of a lesion is located in the cortex, it is reasonable to assume that the process originated in the cortex or periosteum (cortical osteoid osteoma, periosteal osteosarcoma, stress fracture, etc.). If there is an enthesis in the affected area, it should also be considered that stress at the insertion site may have led to cortical destruction or new bone formation (see Case 103 and Case 104).

1.2.4 Solitary, Bilateral, Multiple or Disseminated Lesions

The fourth question is whether a lesion is solitary, bilateral, multiple, or disseminated. It should also be asked whether the finding initially imaged and detected is only the "tip of an iceberg." Whole-body imaging techniques are available for answering this question. If it is believed that focal lesions (e.g., metastases) have already interacted with bone, the screening test of first choice is bone scintigraphy. Other options are whole-body MRI or, if a plasmacytoma is suspected, whole-body CT. A solitary osteolytic lesion in younger patients is more likely to be a primary bone tumor or tumorlike lesion. Multiple foci would be more consistent with fibrous dysplasia, Langerhans cell histiocytosis, sarcoidosis, angiomatosis, or a rheumatic enthesis (e.g., in a patient with psoriasis or ankylosing spondylitis). Disseminated lesions would be more consistent with, say, a generalized Langerhans cell histiocytosis, whether as single-organ or multiorgan disease. A generalized systemic process usually suggests a congenital disorder. In older patients, a solid osteolytic focus is most likely a solitary plasmacytoma or metastasis, while multiple or disseminated lesions are suspicious for a CUP syndrome (cancer from unknown primary) or systemic plasmacytoma.

These are just a few examples; the great variety of other potential causes of osteolytic, osteosclerotic, and mixed changes cannot be explored within the limited scope of this book. Imaging of the contralateral side is a tactic that may be rewarding in both children and adults who present with unusual, difficult-to-classify findings that are not located on the midline. If the same or similar findings are noted on the opposite side, this would always suggest a syndromic or dysplastic cause.

Note

When considering etiologic possibilities, always consider the prevalence of a given disease in addition to biological data and location. For practical reasons, always consider the more common entities first and the rarer ones last.

1.2.5 Assigning a Lesion to a Basic Entity

The fifth question seeks to determine to which of the seven *basic entities*, or major nosologic groups a finding should be assigned.

The seven basic entities listed below provide the basis for lesion classification:

- Normal variant (possibly symptomatic) or malformation
- Trauma (acute or chronic)
- Inflammation
- Tumor and tumorlike lesions
- Perfusion disorder with hyper- or hypoperfusion and necrosis
- Regression (degeneration)
- Systemic disease (metabolic, disease of the reticulohistiocytic system, storage disease, neoplasia)

The answer to the fifth and final question is obtained by systematically answering the first four questions and logically tying them together in a synoptic review.

In closing, we offer this useful rule to follow in making a diagnosis: be wary of Ockham's razor. This is a principle of economy in logic and problem-solving that is still employed today in scientific theory and methodology. Ockham's razor states that when faced with a choice among several possible explanations for the same phenomenon, one should always favor the explanation that requires the fewest hypotheses and thus represents the "simplest" theory. This principle encourages the scientist to recognize just one adequate explanation for any given phenomenon.

If we were to apply this principle consistently, it would mean the end of modern, rational differential diagnosis in medicine. For example, if the radiologic sign of osteosclerosis were simplified to a single cause (the "simplest" theory) such as an osteosclerotic metastasis, then the many other possible causes (e.g., a reactive process due to nonspecific osteitis, a reparative process due to bacterial osteomyelitis or trauma, a neoplastic process with an ossifying tumor matrix in osteosarcoma, or a dysplastic process in melorheostosis or osteopoikilosis) would have to be discarded. This approach would, in the author's view, yield a wrong diagnosis in at least one-third of all nontraumatic cases in skeletal radiology. It is true that if two or three rounded osteosclerotic foci of the same density were seen on one skull radiograph, it would be helpful to start by assuming one cause (e.g., metastatic lesions in a breast cancer patient). At the same time, however, one should never simplify matters by trying to place two nonidentical imaging findings in the same box (a "reverse Ockham's razor" approach; see Case 2).

Another misleading simplification is to make a diagnosis based on an uninformed image comparison between a current case and a case pictured in a textbook or other publication—that is, applying the diagnosis from a textbook image to a specific case without further deliberations. While it is true that predominantly visual disciplines in medicine (radiology, dermatology, histology) work by the principles of empirical pattern recognition, this does not mean that two cases with similar imaging features have the same etiology and classification. To stay with the example of osteosclerosis: both inflammation and a tumor can cause osteosclerosis, which may have the same imaging appearance in both entities.

It is only by linking the finding to other available imaging findings, to the history, and to clinical and laboratory data that we can arrive at a diagnosis that is correct and useful for the patient.

1.2.6 Summary

Note

The five key questions for image interpretation:

1. Pathoanatomic background (destruction, necrosis, reactive, etc.)?
2. Lesion localization from a functional anatomic standpoint (stress-exposed area, critical zone for perfusion, etc.)?
3. Epicenter of the lesion?
4. Solitary, bilateral, multiple, disseminated?
5. Assignment to one of seven basic entities:
   - Normal variant or malformation
   - Trauma (acute, chronic)
   - Inflammation
   - Tumor (including tumorlike lesions)
   - Perfusion disorder
   - Regression
   - Systemic disease (metabolic, disease of the reticulohistiocytic system, storage disease, neoplasia)

Image interpretation concludes with a clinical evaluation. At this time it is important to consider whether a finding that was assigned to one of the basic entities is symptomatic or whether it was detected incidentally. This applies particularly to imaging findings which ultimately could not be classified with complete certainty.

Note

The principle is this: an incidental finding is more likely to be innocent, and it may be safe to take a wait-and-see approach. But if an imaging finding is symptomatic, it is more likely to require histologic examination.

It should also be determined, in consultation with the referring physician, whether the clinical and laboratory data for symptomatic lesions fit with the radiologic findings. In the course of this discussion, the radiologist should communicate the data that formed the basis for his or her impression, and which the referring clinician does not yet know. The radiologist, being aware of the imaging findings, can ask the patient much more targeted questions than the clinician, who may know only the basic clinical presentation before requesting images. Typical examples of this are presented in Case 104, Case 152, Case 156, and Case 158. The prevalence of a disease for a given patient age and gender should always be considered in the synopsis, as mentioned earlier in connection with question 4.

The patient should not depart until the radiologist (not the technician) has critically reviewed the case from an imaging standpoint and discussed it with the patient. Patients expect a conversation in which they receive answers to their questions, without taking anything away from the office consultation with the treating physician. This is the only way that radiology can continue to assert its role as a clinical specialty, and the only way patients can know what the scope of radiology services should include.

In the chapters that follow, we will explore diagnostic approaches, tips, tricks, and pitfalls relating to difficult or seemingly difficult cases that are drawn from skeletal radiology and arranged by anatomic regions. The sample cases follow the approach to systematic image interpretation described above. The case discussions are selected out of the seven basic entities. For pragmatic reasons we have changed the sequence of the questions addressed during image interpretation by starting with an objective description of the finding, then proceeding to location, pathoanatomic background, and finally the assignment to a possible basic entity. Each sample case concludes with a synopsis that summarizes the essential aspects of the case.

This approach is similar to Sherlock Holmes' philosophy for investigating a criminal case: "So much is observation, the rest is deduction." We believe that a radiologist should have something of a criminologist's passion when faced with a challenging diagnosis.

► **Comment on Chapters 2 to 7** In the format that is consistently followed in the case presentations, the "prior history and clinical question" is preceded by an identification of the referring party. This is the physician, or occasionally a self-referred patient, who has asked the author for a radiology consult. The author feels that providing this information helps to make the overall problem clearer. The illustrations do not have detailed captions, as they are described fully in the text. "Unwieldy" terms are abbreviated. On the first occurrence of an abbreviation or acronym, the full term is spelled out in parentheses; each subsequent occurrence is not expanded. Some of the more common abbreviations and acronyms are explained in the List of Abbreviations.

2 Skull

2.1 Sclerotic Changes

Case 1 (▶ Fig. 2.1)

Case description

- Referring physician: radiologist.
- Prior history and clinical question: A 24-year-old woman with syndromic epilepsy underwent cranial MRI that showed generalized thickening of the cranial vault. A CT examination was then ordered for further investigation of the bony changes. The experienced radiologist made the correct interpretation (below), but she sought consultation due to the unusually pronounced changes.

Radiologic Findings

The principal finding on MRI (▶ Fig. 2.1 **a**) is a large, left-sided arachnoid cyst. The CT scout view (▶ Fig. 2.1 **b**) shows cloudy areas of increased attenuation that are most conspicuous in the frontal and high parietal areas. Axial CT scans (▶ Fig. 2.1 **c–e**) show variable, generalized thickening of the inner table. The outer table appears normal and the diploë is intact.

Location

The principal changes are confined to the inner table.

Pathoanatomic Background of the Findings

The sectional images identify the findings as primary bone changes and not as meningeal hyperostosis. Contrast-enhanced MR images (not pictured here) did not show meningeal enhancement.

Assignment to a Possible Basic Entity

▶ **Normal variant or malformation?** Yes. This case represents an incidental finding in an MRI examination for syndromic epilepsy. The patient had no complaints (e.g., bone pain) that might be referable to the bone findings. The "harmonious" thickening and increased density of the inner table are consistent with a long-standing process.

▶ **Trauma?** No. At least the patient was not known to have had any serious falls, so it would be unrealistic to suggest patchy meningeal calcifications secondary to recurrent subdural bleeds (hemorrhagic pachymeningitis; ▶ Fig. 2.2, see following section Synopsis and Discussion). This pathogenesis would also imply a

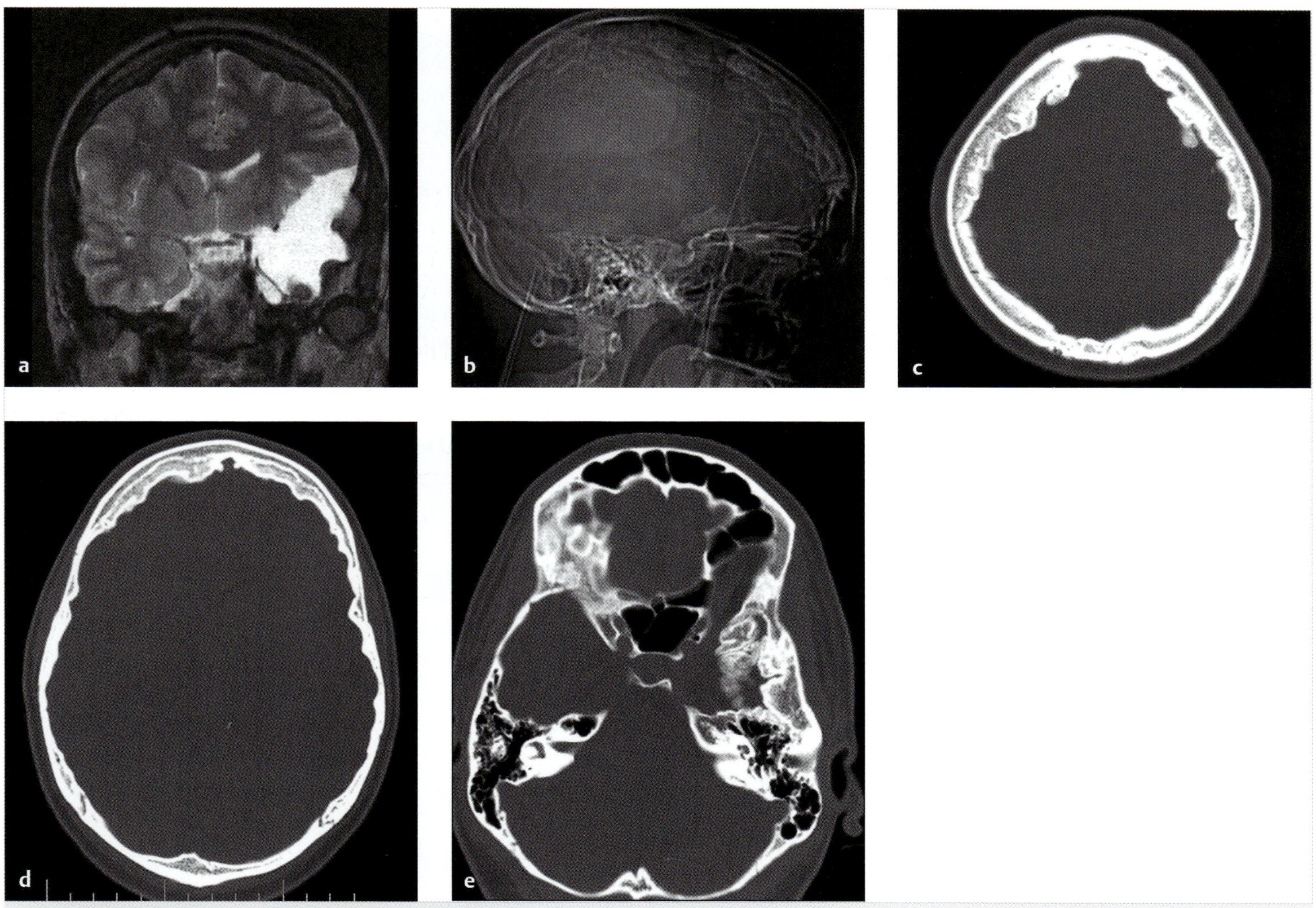

Fig. 2.1 a–e Case 1: Too much bone: normal variant or pathologic?

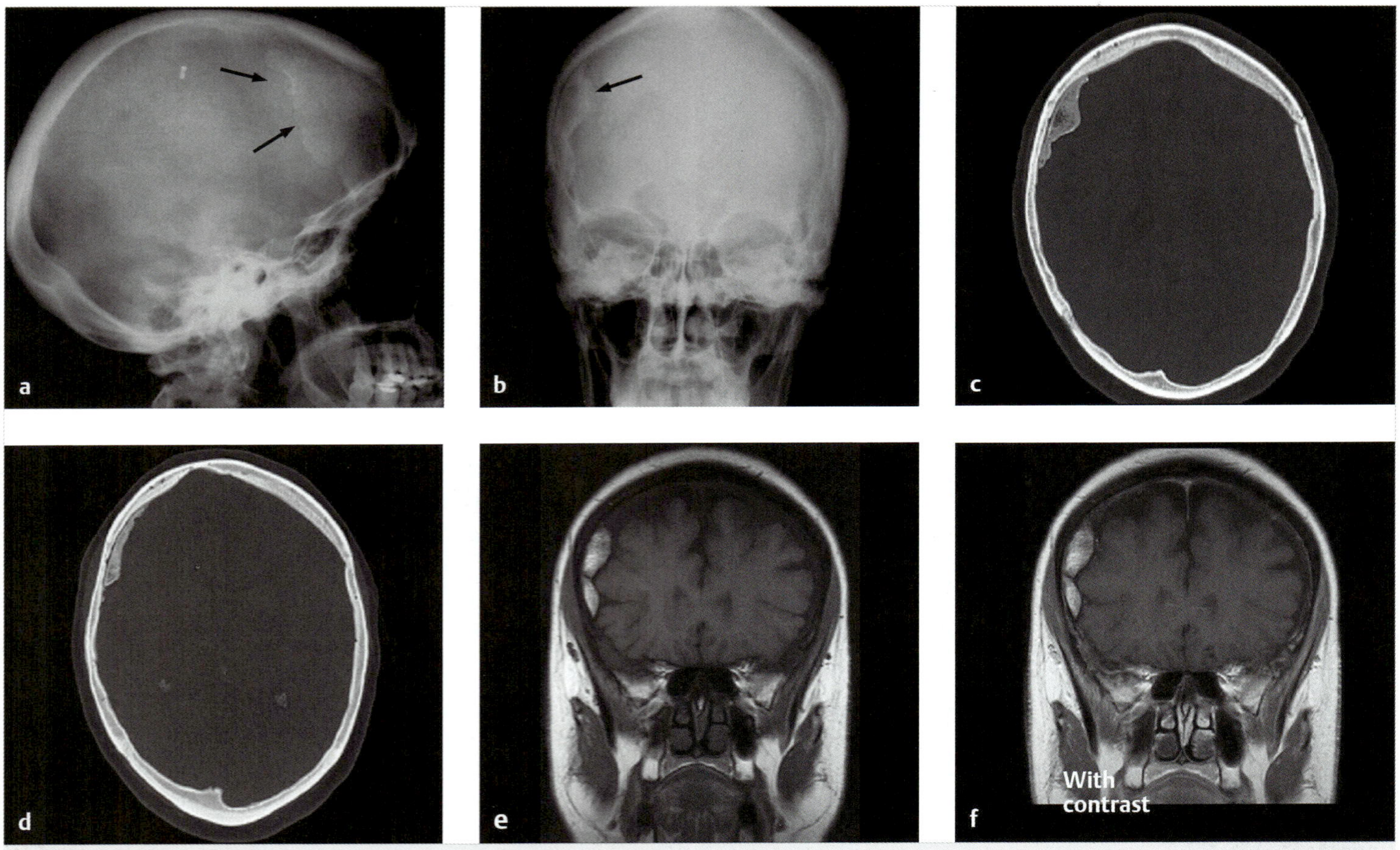

Fig. 2.2 a–f Differential diagnosis of patchy ossification.

complete "obliteration" of the subdural space, probably resulting in impaired drainage. But the MRI shows no evidence of this.

▸ **Inflammation?** The history is negative for an inflammatory process. Moreover, it is difficult to imagine a generalized osteitis confined to the inner table and not involving the diploë.

▸ **Tumor?** No. One might consider a plaque-like meningioma growing in and on the bone, but contrast-enhanced MRI shows no evidence of a meningeal process (compare with Case 2 and Case 3). Fibrous dysplasia (see also Case 4 and Case 7) is unlikely to cause hyperostosis limited to the inner table; it would almost always involve both the inner and outer tables with expansion of the intervening space.

Synopsis and Discussion

The correct diagnosis is diffuse hyperostosis cranialis interna (diffuse calvarial hyperostosis), which is not an uncommon incidental finding, especially in pre- and postmenopausal women, and can be classified as a normal variant. The hyperostotic changes are especially pronounced in both the cranial vault and the phalanges in Morgagni syndrome, which occurs in postmenopausal women and is combined with obesity and hirsutism. The 24-year-old patient had undergone premature menopause, apparently related to her complex syndromic epilepsy. The pathogenesis of the hyperostosis is not fully understood but is definitely the result of an altered hormonal status.

▸ Fig. 2.2 illustrates an old, ossified subdural hematoma for comparison. When questioned closely, this 47-year-old woman recalled that she had suffered a head injury many years ago. The plain radiographs (▸ Fig. 2.2 **a, b**) show an area of increased density in the right frontoparietal region, which appears on CT (▸ Fig. 2.2 **c, d**) as an ossified mass abutting the inner table but not fused with it. T1-weighted MRI shows no enhancement after contrast administration (▸ Fig. 2.2 **e, f**). The ossification is very mature and consists of cancellous bone that apparently contains a medullary cavity with fatty tissue. This explains the high signal intensity in T1-weighted images.

Final Diagnosis

Diffuse hyperostosis cranialis interna relating to precocious menopause.

Comments

Even pronounced skeletal changes can still be classified as a normal variant when they are asymptomatic and are encountered with some frequency.

Case 2 (▶ Fig. 2.3)

Case description

- Referring physician: oncologist.
- Prior history and clinical question: A 61-year-old woman presented with a painless swelling in the left temporo-sphenoidal region. She had been treated for right breast cancer 10 years earlier. Question: metastasis, Paget disease with sarcomatous transformation, or fibrous dysplasia?

Radiologic Findings

The CT images (▶ Fig. 2.3 **a–f**) show pronounced hyperostosis of the inner table with a normal-appearing outer table and intact diploë, similar to Case 1. In addition an unstructured, massive sclerotic lesion with marginal spiculations is visible in the left sphenoid bone and temporal bone. The spicules represent sites of new bone formation along vascular pathways. The scans also show marked swelling in the displaced masseter muscle. These findings are consistent with an active process that is quite unlike the generalized hyperostosis affecting the

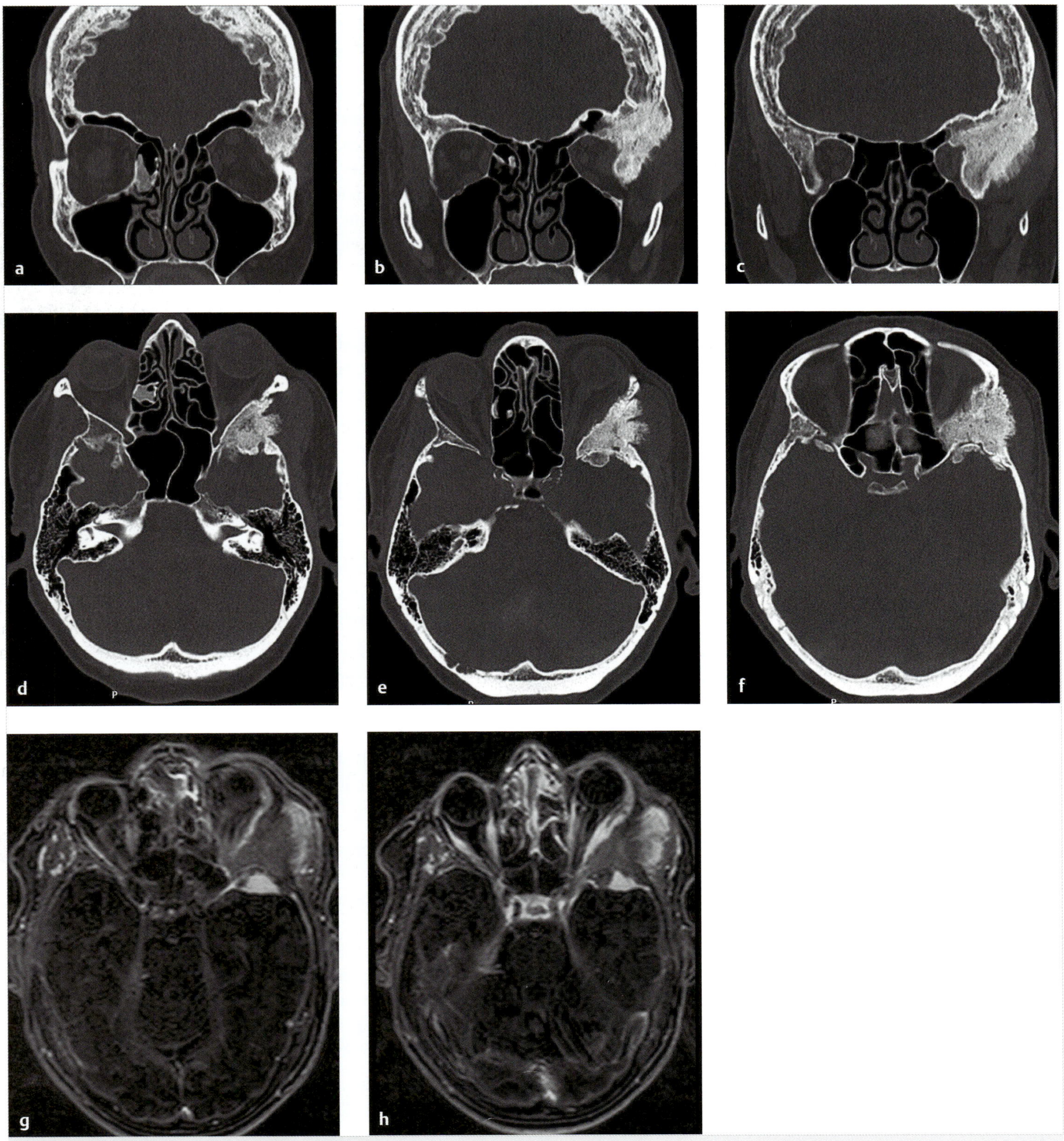

Fig. 2.3 a–h Too much bone: normal variant or pathologic?

inner table. Contrast-enhanced MRI (▶ Fig. 2.3 **g, h**) shows a very hyperintense (enhancing, therefore well-perfused) elliptical mass toward the meningeal side with concomitant enhancement of the osseous lesion, especially in its outer portion.

Location

The clinically symptomatic lesion in the left sphenoid bone and temporal bone is closely related to the adjacent mass showing meningeal enhancement.

Pathoanatomic Background of the Findings

The imaging findings show a definite relationship between the dural or meningeal mass and the osseous changes. This means that a meningeal neoplasm has apparently spread to the adjacent bone and has induced the formation of vascularized new bone along its margin. The fact that the meningeal mass has a convex boundary with the osseous lesion would not be consistent with contiguous meningeal invasion by a primary bony process (e.g., osteosclerotic metastasis or a bone-producing tumor).

Assignment to a Possible Basic Entity

▶ **Normal variant or malformation?** The diffuse hyperostosis of the inner table ranks as an incidental finding in the postmenopausal patient, but not the active hyperostotic process with associated swelling in the left sphenoid bone and temporal bone.

▶ **Trauma?** The patient has no apparent history of acute or chronic trauma involving the affected region in the left sphenoid bone and temporal bone.

▶ **Inflammation?** No. A chronic inflammation in the form of osteitis would have been painful, and imaging would probably have shown sequestra or (on MRI) abscess formation. The meningeal mass is solid and shows no signs of an inflammatory process. Serologic inflammatory markers were normal in this patient.

▶ **Tumor?** For the sclerotic process in the left temporo-sphenoidal region: yes.

Synopsis and Discussion

The left temporo-sphenoidal process is most consistent with a sphenoid meningioma that has invaded the adjacent bone. Not infrequently, the intraosseous spread of meningioma is a painless process. The sphenoid region is a site of predilection for meningiomas, and the tumor cells stimulate metaplastic new bone formation. All of these factors are present in this case. The diagnosis of sphenoid meningioma is confirmed by contrast-enhanced MRI, which shows massive enhancement of the dura bordering the osseous lesion.

The other hyperostotic changes in the inner table are interpreted as a harmless variant (see under "Normal variant or malformation" above and Case 1) and have nothing to do with the intraosseous neoplastic process. This excludes a diagnosis of

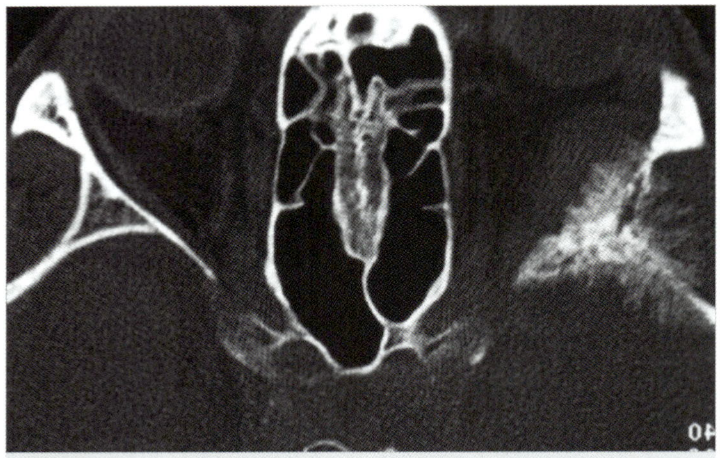

Fig. 2.4 Differential diagnosis of spiculated new bone formation.

Paget sarcoma, since the bony cranium shows no signs of Paget disease. Paget sarcoma is generally lytic and not sclerotic, and other osseous changes typically affect the full cross-section of the bone. Although the referring physician suggested that the diffuse hyperostosis of the inner table may have been due to fibrous dysplasia, we can exclude that diagnosis because fibrous dysplasia generally affects both the inner and outer tables and expands the volume of the affected cranial bone. If we were to consider the sclerosing temporo-sphenoidal process in isolation, disregarding the adjacent meningeal focus, we might entertain the possibility of an osteosclerotic (osteoblastic) metastasis (▶ Fig. 2.4) from breast cancer, for example—but that would be inconsistent with the convex interface of the meningeal neoplasm with the adjacent bone. Finally, one might consider a frequent catch-all diagnosis for sclerotic changes in the skull, namely chronic sclerosing osteomyelitis (Garré), but there appears to be little justification for the existence of this entity, which was described by Garré[16] 120 years ago!

The tumor was completely removed along with the affected dura and bone (Simpson 1). It was identified histologically as meningioma. The swelling of the masseter muscle is considered a reactive phenomenon.

Final Diagnosis

Sphenoid wing meningioma with intraosseous spread (histologically confirmed). Diffuse hyperostosis of the inner table, predominantly affecting the frontoparietal area, was noted as an incidental finding.

Comments

Two prominent radiologic findings should not necessarily be placed in the same category. The principle of "reverse Ockham's razor" does not apply in the present case. It is more accurate to interpret one of the findings as the principal diagnosis, which requires surgery, while interpreting the other finding as an incidental normal variant.

Case 3 (▶ Fig. 2.5)

Case description

- Referring physician: general surgeon.
- Prior history and clinical question: A 37-year-old woman presented with a bony-hard protuberance in the left high parietal area, which she claimed had been present since puberty but had recently enlarged. She complained of occasional paroxysmal headaches at that location. On specific questioning, she described several other anatomic anomalies: a double uvula, double gallbladder, and malpositioned teeth. CT scans were interpreted as being suspicious for a bone tumor (e.g., fibrous dysplasia, hemangioma, metastasis).

Radiologic Findings

CT scans (▶ Fig. 2.5 **b, c**) demonstrate an expansile osteosclerotic process in the high parietal region involving all three layers of the bone. Bony spicules are visible at the periphery of the raised area. The process shows very high uptake on bone scintigraphy (see ▶ Fig. 2.5 **a**). The author ordered contrast-enhanced MRI (see ▶ Fig. 2.5 **d, e**), which shows a spindle-shaped, intensely enhancing dural mass located just deep to the expanded bone area.

Location

The high parietal bony lesion directly overlies the dural mass.

Pathoanatomic Background of the Findings

The findings suggest an active, bone-producing mass that appears to have high peripheral vascularity, as evidenced by the presence of bony spicules (see under Radiologic Findings in Case 2). It is reasonable to assume that the bony lesion is related to the meningeal soft-tissue mass.

Assignment to a Possible Basic Entity

▶ **Normal variant or malformation?** No, because of the symptomatic bony change.

▶ **Trauma?** No, the patient gave no history of trauma.

▶ **Inflammation?** No. There are no clinical signs of inflammation (local warmth, etc.) about the palpable bulge. As a rule, chronic inflammatory bone changes with reparative new bone formation are not associated with the formation of bony spicules.

▶ **Tumor?** Yes. The bony lesion is expansile and produces a bony matrix. It is consistent with a meningioma that has infiltrated the bone.

Synopsis and Discussion

Based on CT and scintigraphic findings, the differential diagnosis should include *hemangioma*, since hemangiomas in flat bones tend to form bony spicules like those seen in ▶ Fig. 2.6 **b**. Also, hemangiomas commonly incite new bone formation. But we do not see the honeycomb pattern that is typical of hemangiomas (see ▶ Fig. 2.6 **a–c**). This pattern results from the juxtaposition of blood vessels and newly formed bone, appearing as bony spicules at the periphery of the mass.

The CT images of the bony lesion also raises the possibility of a very vascular osteosclerotic *metastasis* (from breast cancer in women, from prostate cancer in men). However, the absence of a

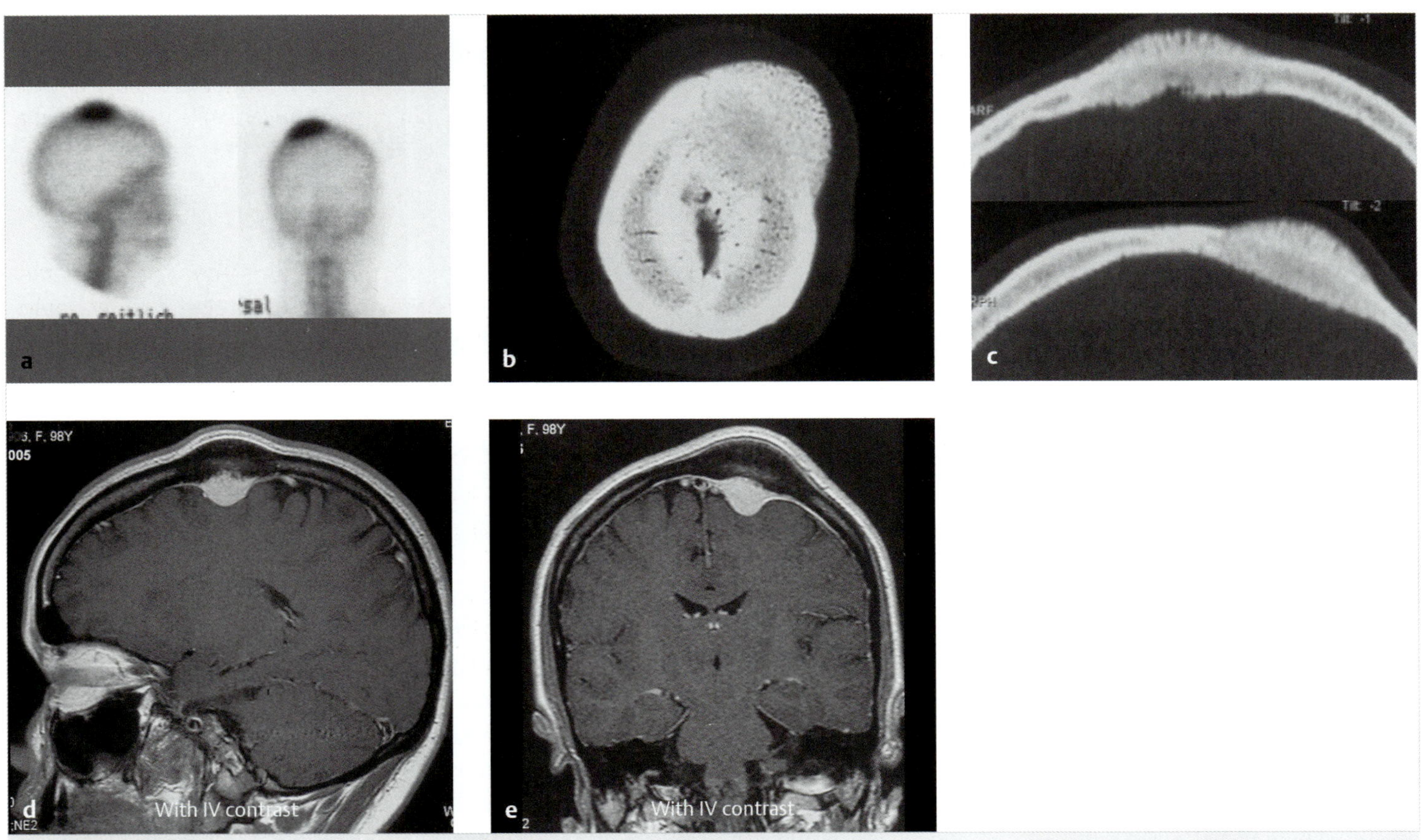

Fig. 2.5 a–e A "black and white cap" on scintigraphy and CT.

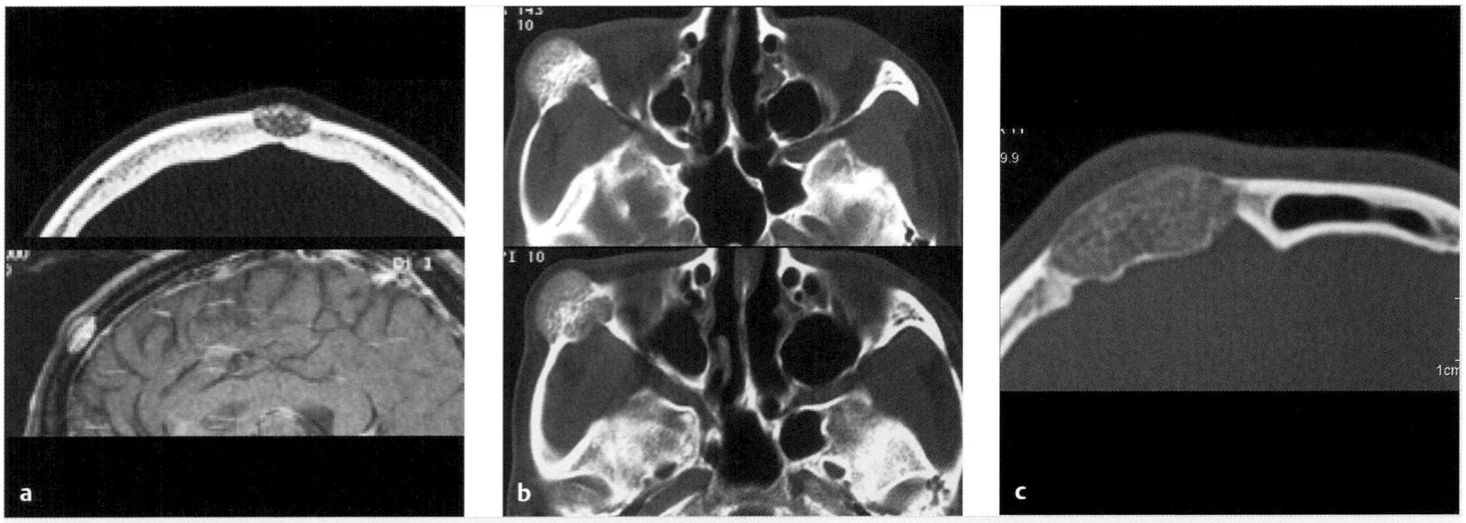

Fig. 2.6 a–c Differential diagnosis of hemangioma (three different patients).

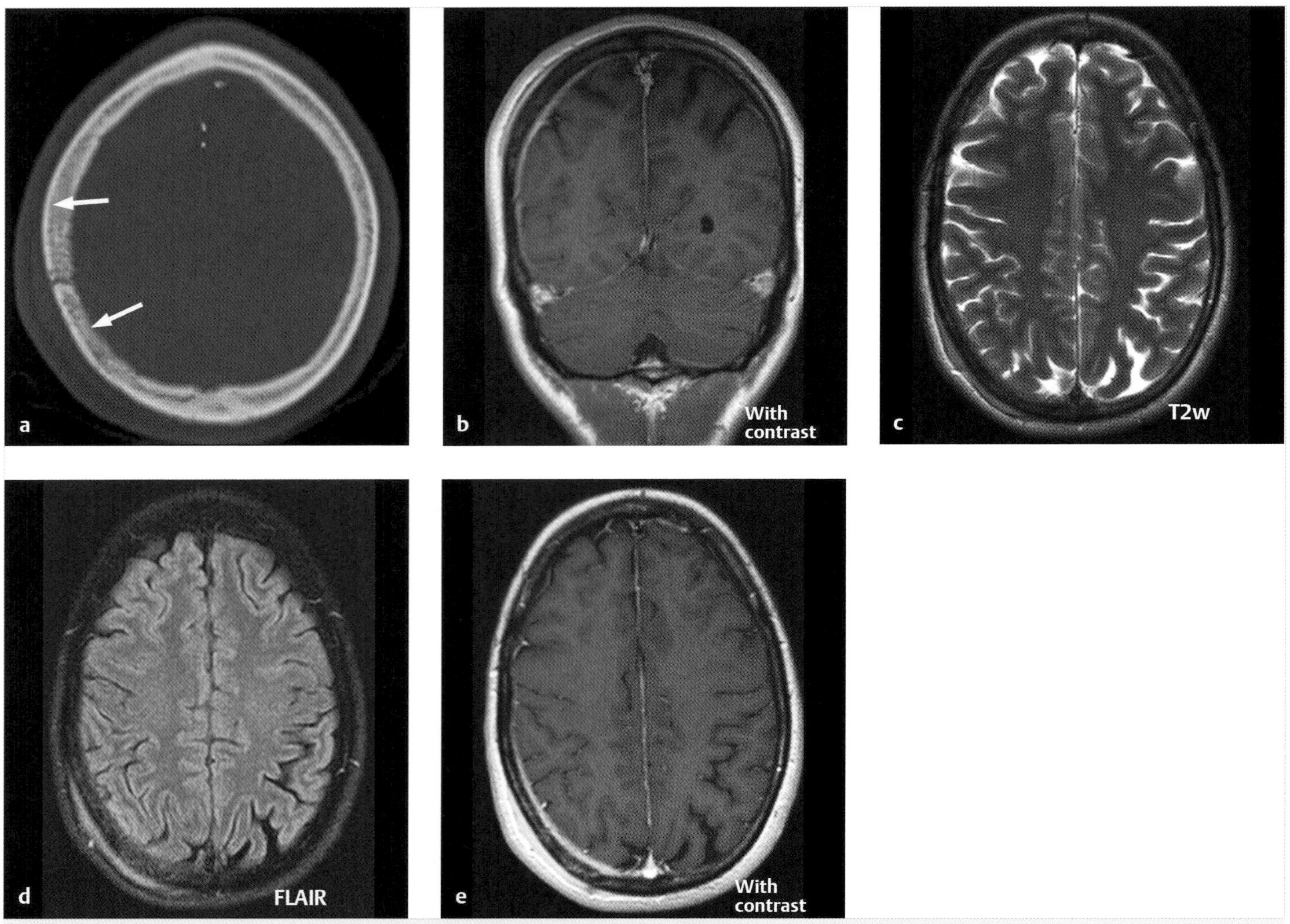

Fig. 2.7 a–e Differential diagnosis of perforating bone lesions: non-Hodgkin lymphoma (NHL) in the right parietal bone.

known primary tumor in this patient would exclude metastasis from the differential diagnosis.

Another possible diagnosis is *non-Hodgkin lymphoma* (see ▶ Fig. 2.7), which can also stimulate metaplastic new bone formation.

Because the differential diagnosis of bone-forming lesions in the calvarium would always include a *meningioma* infiltrating the bone, it was necessary to proceed with contrast-enhanced MRI in this patient. These images unequivocally showed an intensely enhancing meningioma. In the case of non-Hodgkin lymphoma, the area of dural infiltration would have been flatter and not as spindle-shaped as with meningioma (see ▶ Fig. 2.7). In the present case, a diagnosis of meningioma fits very well with the other anomalies described by the patient (see above under Prior history and clinical question). Upon questioning, she stated that she had a brother with neurofibromatosis. This fulfills the criteria for type 2 neurofibromatosis, which has an autosomal dominant mode of inheritance with many new mutations (on chromosome 22q12). These patients may develop tumors at a very early age, apparently due to a failure of genetic tumor suppression. Meningiomas are particularly common. Intraosseous meningiomas are also known to occur in young individuals.

To aid differentiation from meningioma, ▶ Fig. 2.6 shows the imaging appearance of hemangiomas in the cranial vault of three different patients. A finding common to all three cases is the presence of a honeycomb pattern on CT. None of these cases shows evidence of infiltration of adjacent bone or nearby organs. The skin and subcutaneous tissue are only displaced by the mass, resulting in a palpable bulge. Sagittal contrast-enhanced MRI (see ▶ Fig. 2.6 **a**, lower image) proves that the vascular tumor demonstrated by CT (see ▶ Fig. 2.6 **a**, upper image) is unrelated to the meninges.

▶ Fig. 2.7 illustrates a patient with non-Hodgkin lymphoma in the right parietal bone (29-year-old woman). The tumor has broken through the bone and infiltrated both the dura and the galea. On CT (see ▶ Fig. 2.7 **a**) the infiltrative growth mimics a (blurred) honeycomb pattern. This pattern, which appears moth-eaten on radiographs, is commonly seen with small-cell and round-cell tumors. Lymphoma is one of the possible diagnoses for destructive lesions in the skull and is often combined with sclerosis due to reactive and metaplastic new bone formation and necrosis. Differentiation from bony invasion by meningioma was not possible in the present case, and the final diagnosis was made histologically.

Final Diagnosis

Meningioma in the high parietal area infiltrating the adjacent bone in a patient with neurofibromatosis type 2.

Comments

Lesions in the cranial vault require contrast-enhanced imaging of adjacent brain structures, especially in adults, to confirm or exclude a meningeal process. A thorough and detailed history is helpful in making an accurate diagnosis.

Case 4 (▶ Fig. 2.8)

Case description

- *Referral:* self-referral by the patient.
- *Prior history and clinical question:* A 46-year-old man with unexplained dizziness had undergone MRI, which showed a lesion in the medial and lateral frontal region on the left side. He did not receive a definite diagnosis from various consulting physicians, which worried him. The patient stated that the lesion appeared "pitch black" on the bone scan.

Radiologic Findings

CT scans (see ▶ Fig. 2.8 **a, b**) show an expansile bone lesion of uniform "ground-glass" attenuation in the left frontomedial and frontolateral regions. On contrast-enhanced MRI (see ▶ Fig. 2.8 **c**) the lesion shows moderate inhomogeneous enhancement. Adjacent meningeal structures appear normal.

Location

The slightly expansile lesion is located within the frontal bone.

Pathoanatomic Background of the Findings

The ground-glass appearance shows that the lesion is composed of woven bone. It is purely productive and has no destructive features. It has replaced the local bone. There is no involvement of adjacent structures (meninges; see MRI). The positive bone scan confirms that the lesion is active.

Assignment to a Possible Basic Entity

▶ **Normal variant or malformation?** No. The lesion was detected incidentally, but the circumscribed replacement of normal calvarial structures (outer and inner tables and diploë) by woven bone suggests a harmless lesion rather than a normal variant. Also, the high uptake on the bone scan is not consistent with a normal variant.

▶ **Trauma?** No, the history was negative for trauma.

▶ **Inflammation?** No. An older or chronic reactive inflammatory process would be associated with pain and at least transient local warmth.

▶ **Tumor or tumorlike lesion?** Yes, the description of ground-glass attenuation in the lesion is consistent with fibrous dysplasia.

Synopsis and Discussion

Histologic examination of bone affected by fibrous dysplasia reveals fibrous tissue with a typical whorled structure and immature, nonlamellar bony trabeculae. The disease is caused by a postzygotic (somatic) mutation of the *GNAS-1* gene on chromosome 20 and, besides fibrous metaphyseal defect, is probably the most common tumorlike lesion of bone. In most cases it is solitary and clinically asymptomatic. Fibrous tissue replacement makes the bone less stable and may cause it to become bowed.

Typical radiographic and CT signs are variable expansion of the affected bone and a ground-glass pattern (compare with ▶ Fig. 2.9 **a–c**: 34-year-old woman with left-sided visual deterioration, and ▶ Fig. 2.9 **d–f**: incidental finding in a 55-year-old man) of the only moderate and disordered or nonlamellar calcifying fibrous tissue. Larger lesions (as in Case 7) tend to undergo regressive changes with circumscribed myxoid transformation, liquefaction, and eventual fatty degeneration. This may produce a variegated imaging appearance with lucent zones in bone showing ground-glass transformation (soap-bubble pattern; see Case 7). Because areas of fibrous dysplasia usually undergo constant remodeling, they typically appear as "hot spots" on bone scintigraphy. Ground-glass attenuation is also the hallmark of fibrous dysplasia on CT scans (▶ Fig. 2.8 **a, b**). MRI findings are nonspecific and depend on the momentary status of the dynamic process. The case in question meets all the criteria for a relatively small focus of fibrous dysplasia in the frontal bone (incidental finding, ground-glass attenuation on CT, positive bone scan), with the skull (especially the facial skeleton) representing the third

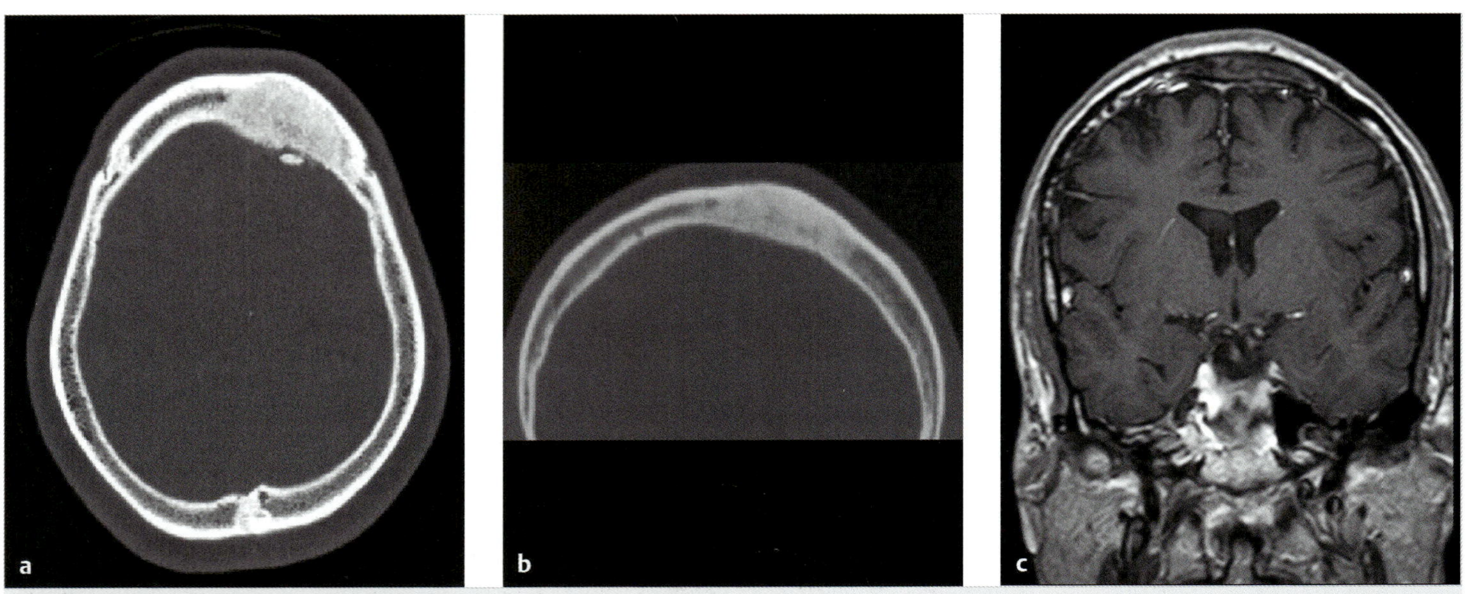

Fig. 2.8 a–c Osteoblastic metastasis?

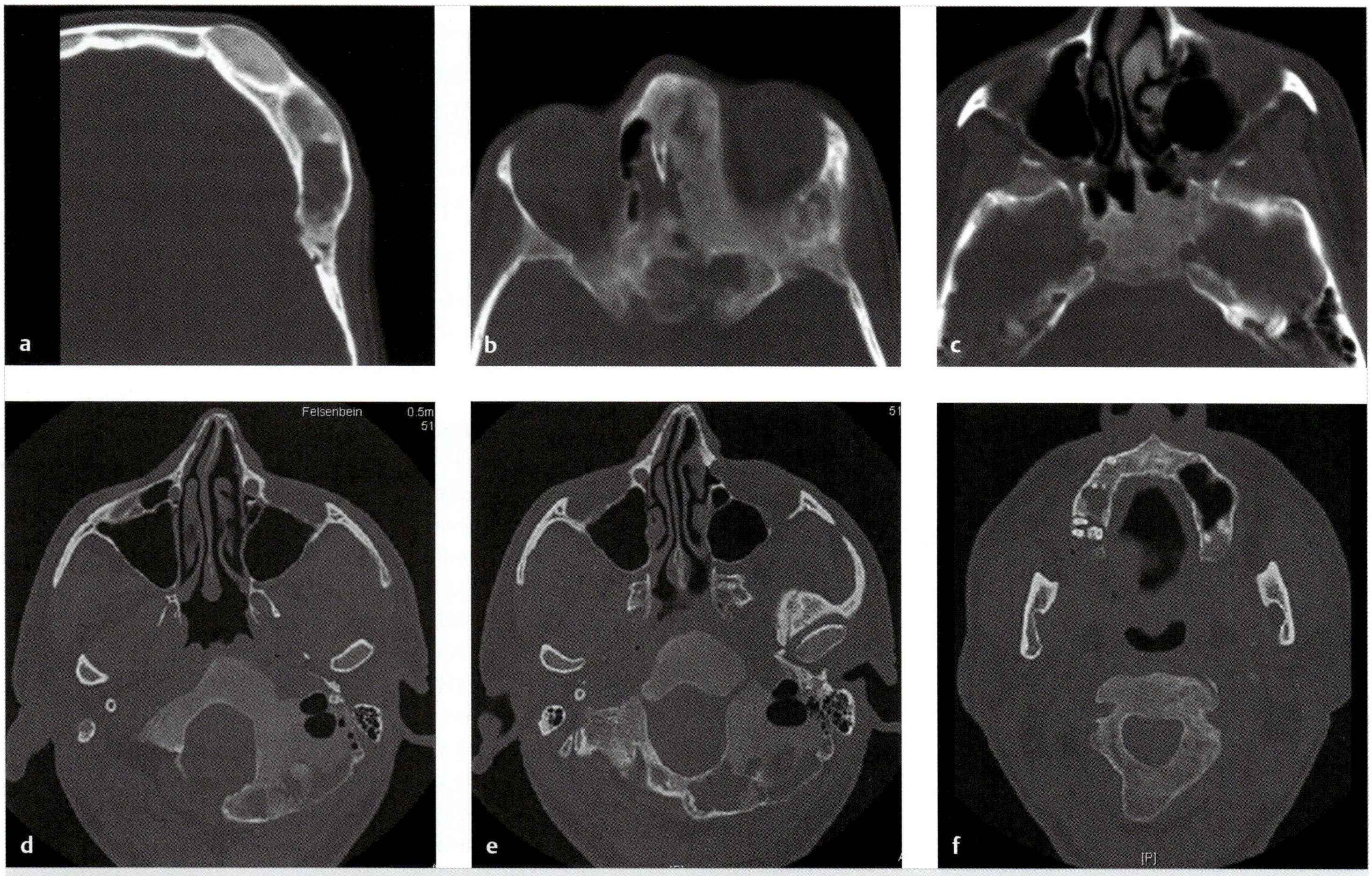

Fig. 2.9 Ground-glass pattern: **a–c** 34-year-old woman with left-sided visual deterioration; **d–f** incidental finding in a 55-year-old man.

most common site of occurrence. Actually there is no reasonable differential diagnosis for this case. The usual catch-all diagnosis of "metastasis" would be absurd because the patient—an otherwise healthy 46-year-old man—does not have a primary tumor and the lesion shows no aggressive features.

Final Diagnosis

Focus of fibrous dysplasia in the frontal bone.

Comments

CT scans, obtained as an adjunct to nonspecific incidental MRI findings, display the radiologic hallmark of ground-glass attenuation, which is diagnostic of fibrous dysplasia. There is no need for histologic confirmation.

Case 5 (▶ Fig. 2.10)

Case description

- Referring physician: surgeon.
- Prior history and clinical question: A 43-year-old woman had a long history of a painless, bony-hard protuberance in the left occipital area. The woman stated that her hairdresser had expressed concern over the bulge, and this prompted her to consult a surgeon. The surgeon ordered CT scans (see ▶ Fig. 2.10), but the radiologist was noncommittal in his report.

Radiologic Findings

CT (▶ Fig. 2.10 **a–c**) demonstrates a solid elliptical mass of osseous density expanding mostly outward from the outer table. The diploë is narrowed but still intact. In ▶ Fig. 2.10 **b** the mass has "overgrown" the bone on the lateral side, creating a narrow gap between it and the underlying bone.

Location

Outer table of the occiput.

Pathoanatomic Background of the Findings

The homogeneous mass, isoattenuating to the outer table, appears to be of an osseous nature. This is consistent with the finding of a palpable, bony-hard, nondisplaceable mass on clinical examination.

Assignment to a Possible Basic Entity

▶ **Normal variant or malformation?** No. The relevant literature (e.g., Freyschmidt[17]) shows no evidence that a mass of osseous density can occur on the outer surface of the occiput as a normal variant.

▶ **Trauma?** No, the history was negative for trauma.

▶ **Inflammation?** No. There is no evidence from the history or physical findings (e.g., pain, local warmth) that would indicate a previous or currently active, primary chronic inflammatory process.

▶ **Tumor?** Yes. The mass is solid, has displaced surrounding tissues, and is clinically benign. The differential diagnosis would include a harmless ivory osteoma or a paraosseous osteosarcoma.

Synopsis and Discussion

The unimpressive clinical findings (long history of an indolent bulge) make *osteoma* the most likely diagnosis and justify a wait-and-see approach without histologic confirmation. The mature lesion would have shown little or no uptake on bone scintigraphy. If the tumor were to enlarge and form an overlying bursa with signs of bursitis, it would be appropriate to proceed with surgical removal. Osteomas are defined as benign, slow-growing lesions composed of mature, well-differentiated bone tissue with a predominantly lamellar structure. The following types are distinguished:

- *Classic osteoma* (ivory osteoma), located almost exclusively on the skull and arising from the outer table
- *Juxtacortical (paraosseous) osteoma*, typically occurring on long bones
- *Medullary osteoma* (enostosis, bone island), often detected incidentally in cancellous bone; so common that it may be classified as a normal variant

It is still unclear whether osteomas should be classified as true bone tumors, as a reactive process with tumorlike growth, or as hamartomas. The WHO classification of bone tumors published in 2002[15] differed from the 1994 classification, in that it no longer listed osteoma as a separate entity. But in the current WHO classification (2013), osteoma can be found again under benign osteogenic tumors.

The classic *paraosseous osteosarcoma*, on the other hand, is generally associated with pain and is located almost exclusively on the metaphysis or metaphyseal–diaphyseal junction of long bones (see ▶ Fig. 7.27 in Case 144), occurring most commonly on the popliteal surface of the femur (50–70% of all cases). A cranial location would be extremely rare—another reason why this tumor is mainly of academic interest and should be excluded from the differential diagnosis for all practical purposes. A paraosseous osteosarcoma would show intense tracer uptake on bone scans.

Besides osteoma, the category of bone-forming tumors of the skull would also include the rare *osteoblastoma* (ca. 1% of all bone tumors; ca. 12% of osteoblastomas are located in the bony skull). Studies[18] indicate that *osteoid osteomas* have not yet been reported at that location, and that only 1% of *osteosarcomas* occur in the skull.

▶ Fig. 2.11 illustrates the rare case of an osteoblastoma located at the right parietotemporal junction of a 27-year-old man. Confirmed histologically by Prof. H. Ostertag of Hannover, the tumor is composed mainly of a dense soft-tissue mass (osteoid formed by the tumor). Matrix ossification is visible at the base of the lesion on CT (see ▶ Fig. 2.11) and is a fundamental property of

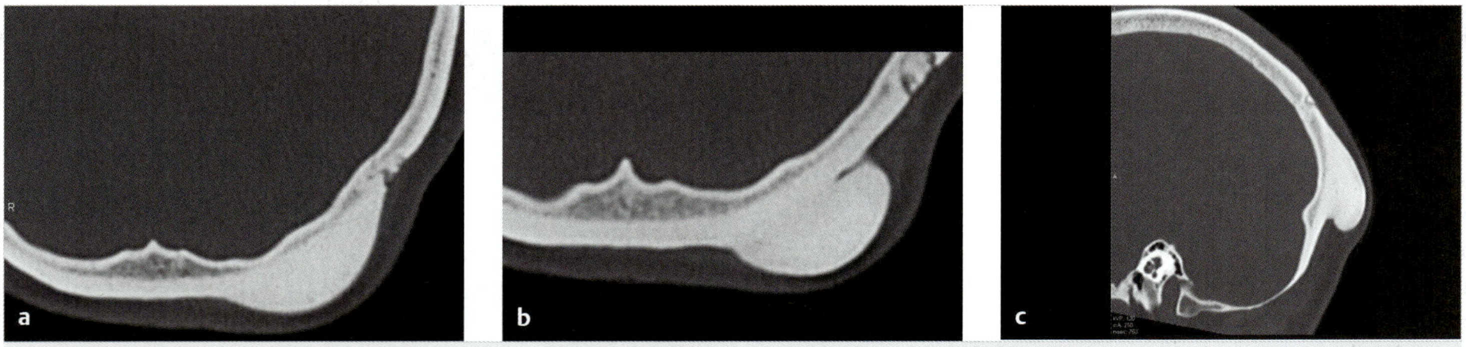

Fig. 2.10 a–c Occipital protuberance.

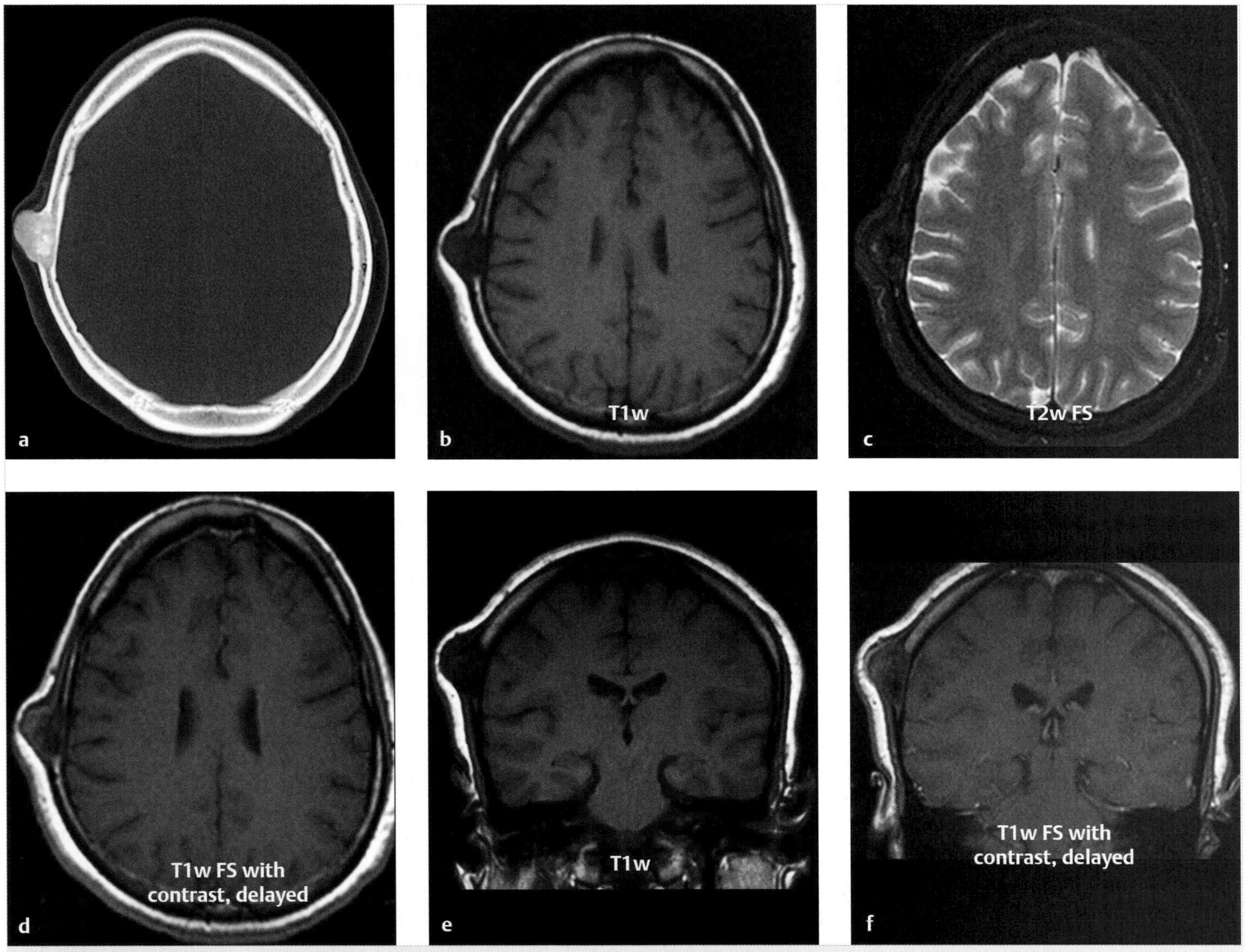

Fig. 2.11 a–f Differential diagnosis: osteoblastoma.

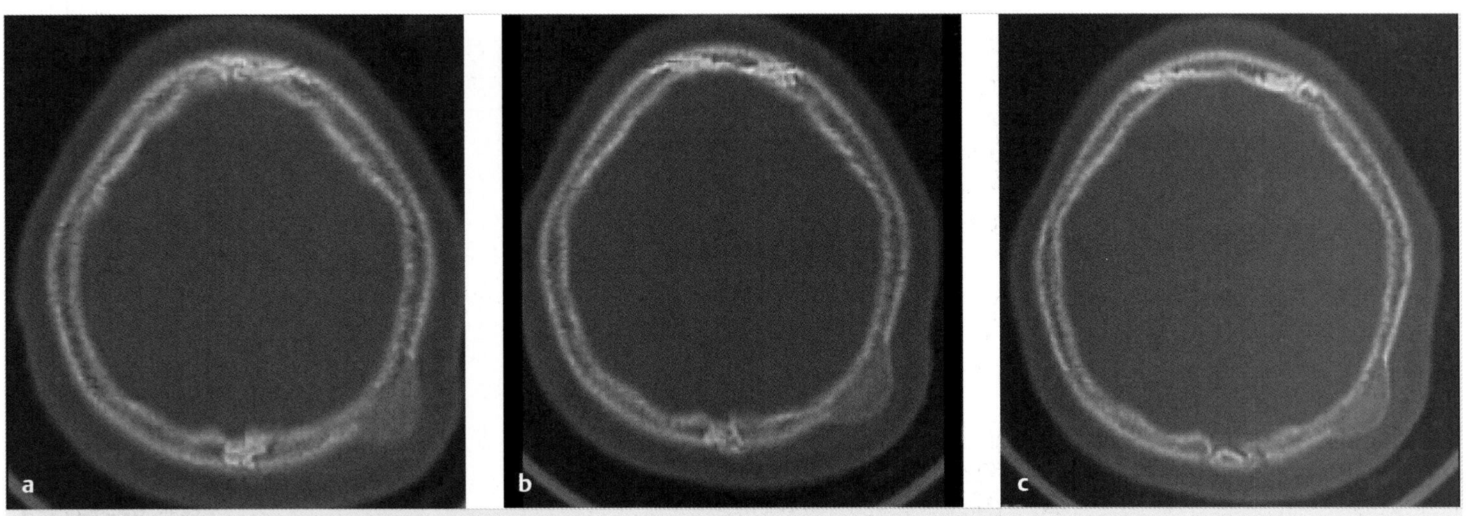

Fig. 2.12 a–c Differential diagnosis of exophytic skull lesions.

bone-forming tumors. Like the osteoma in ▶ Fig. 2.10, the lesion originates from the outer table, which it has destroyed and replaced with a thin new bony shell. The unenhanced MR images are nonspecific. Images after contrast administration show moderate enhancement—most osteoblastomas have a rich blood supply! When we run through various possible diagnoses, the obvious matrix formation leaves no reasonable alternative besides osteoblastoma or osteoblastoma-like osteosarcoma.

▶ Fig. 2.12 illustrates the case of a 17-year-old male adolescent in whom a protuberance was detected incidentally on the left side of the occiput. The young man had no complaints in that area. The site was first investigated by incisional biopsy to exclude a sebaceous cyst. When the lesion was found to be bony at operation, the patient was finally referred to an imaging center where CT scans showed "a bony protuberance on the outer table, 2 cm in diameter, with no evidence of destructive changes." Without further explanation the radiologist diagnosed it as a periosteal chondroma and recommended histology for benign/malignant differentiation. The CT lesion appears to originate from the diploë. It produces a mass effect and has gradually eroded through the outer table. Concomitant reactive-reparative periosteal new bone formation has created a protuberant bony shell. The lesion has a faint ground-glass appearance and contains very fine reticular densities that can be characterized as trabecular structures. The differential diagnosis raises three possibilities:

- Focal hematopoietic hyperplasia
- Focus of fibrous dysplasia
- Incipient osteoma arising atypically from the diploë

We favor focal hematopoietic hyperplasia, although it has previously been described only in the ribs[18] and has an unknown etiology. The purely exophytic growth pattern presumably results from the dura mater, which is adherent to the bone and does not permit reparative, protuberant new bone formation. The two other possible diagnoses are also benign; hence there is no need for histologic evaluation, and clinical follow-up is sufficient.

Final Diagnosis

Ivory osteoma of the occipital bone.

Comments

A solid, clinically indolent lesion of homogeneous bone density that arises from the outer table and remains unchanged for years can reasonably be classified as a benign process consistent with osteoma—especially since these lesions occur almost exclusively on the skull. There is no need to create a "loophole" by giving the patient a confusing differential diagnosis that includes the possibility of malignancy.

Case 6 (▶ Fig. 2.13)

Case description

- *Referring physician:* maxillofacial surgeon.
- *Prior history and clinical question:* A 54-year-old woman claimed that, after suffering a head injury 2 years before, small nodules began appearing on her forehead in increasing numbers. Clinical examination revealed innumerable small, palpable, nontender protuberances with no external signs of trauma.

Radiologic Findings

CT (▶ Fig. 2.13 **a–e**) demonstrates innumerable osteoma-like masses of bony attenuation arising from the outer table. They have left the outer table intact except for one lesion in ▶ Fig. 2.13 **c** No posttraumatic changes are found.

Location

Outer table of the frontal bone.

Pathoanatomic Background of the Findings

The small lesions are of osseous density on CT scans, enabling them to be classified as bony structures.

Assignment to a Possible Basic Entity

▶ **Normal variant or malformation?** No, the changes first appeared 2 years ago.

▶ **Trauma?** Possibly, because the patient began to notice the lesions following an unspecified trauma. Sub- or intraperiosteal trauma may lead to reactive bone changes, a mechanism that is known to occur in myositis ossificans and heterotopic ossifications. The same is true of factitious trauma.

▶ **Inflammation?** No, because the clinical manifestations show no evidence of an inflammatory cause.

▶ **Tumor?** One possibility is osteomas, whose pathogenesis is still unclear (see Case 5). Another possibility is hamartomas, which may have an adult onset.

Synopsis and Discussion

This case is still unsolved because we have no access to any further information. But previous considerations (see above, Assignment to a Possible Basic Entity) suggest the following differential diagnosis: *Multifocal periosteal or subperiosteal hemorrhages with subsequent ossification* as in myositis ossificans. This condition requires an antecedent trauma in which the forehead was struck

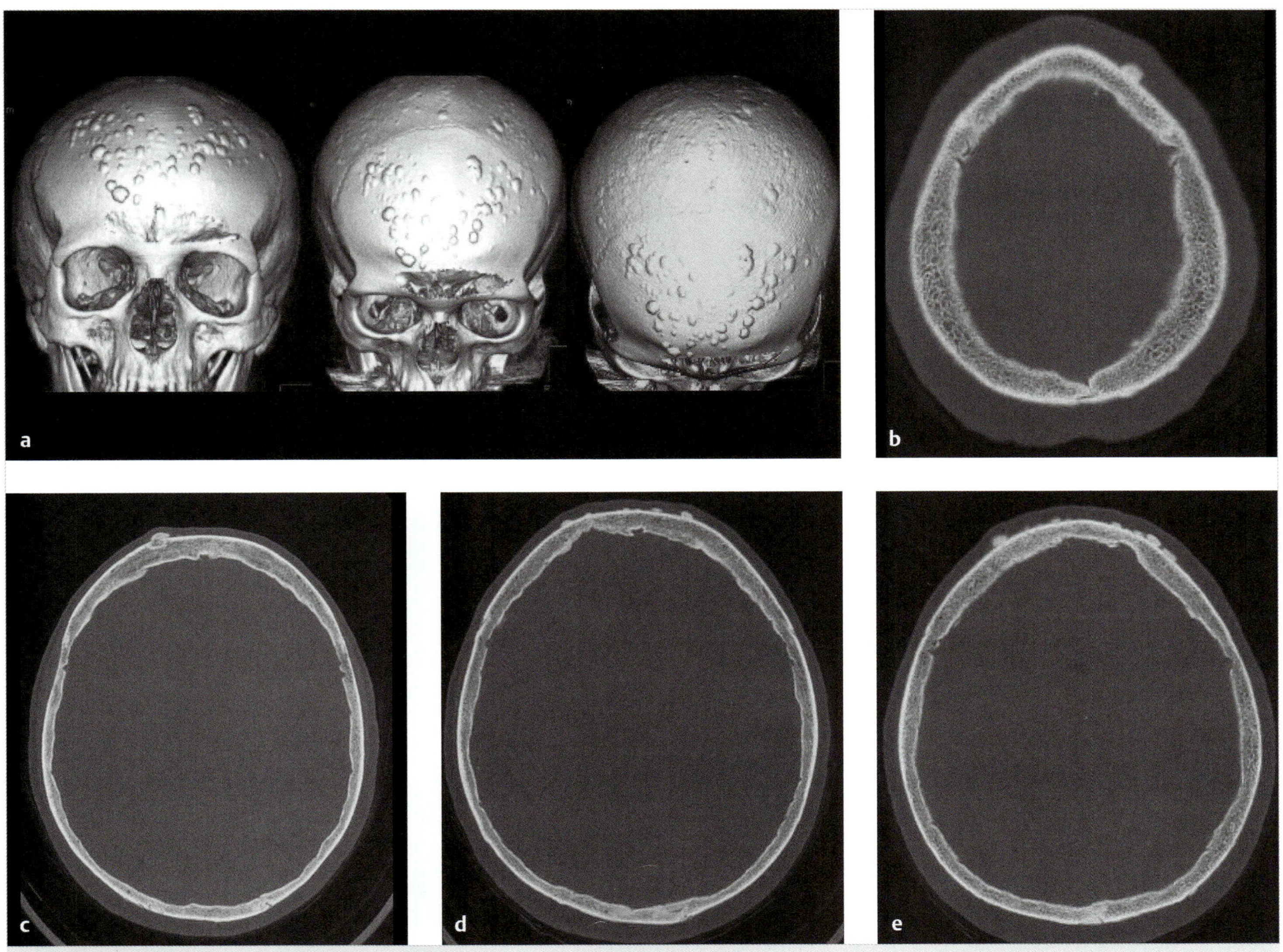

Fig. 2.13 a–e "Crumb cake" nodularity on the skull.

by a blunt, knobby object. The object would have to have been curved to produce lesions on both sides of the forehead, which is not very plausible. The injuries may have been factitious, caused by repetitive self-inflicted trauma to the forehead. We once observed a similar process in a mentally ill patient who repeatedly kicked the edge of a low kitchen table with her anterior thighs over a long period of time, resulting in periosteal and subperiosteal femoral hemorrhages with later osteoma-like ossification.

Hamartomatous osteomas, like those occurring in Gardner syndrome (familial intestinal polyposis), also arise during the course of the disease and are not necessarily congenital, see Freyschmidt.[19] We do not know whether the patient followed our recommendation for a colonoscopy to check for polyposis, nor do we know her prior family history.

Final Diagnosis

A definitive diagnosis could not be made. The two most likely diagnoses are as follows:

1. Factitious myositis ossificans–like ossifications on the outer table of the frontal bone.
2. Hamartomatous osteomas in a setting of familial colonic polyposis. The patient is actually too old for this diagnosis, however. We do not know if she already has or had colon cancer, which would be possible in a patient with colonic polyposis.

Comments

Unusual imaging findings challenge the pathogenic imagination —especially when hard facts are not available in the patient's history, as is often the case.

Case 7 (▸ Fig. 2.14)

Case description

- Referring physician: internist.
- Prior history and clinical question: A 26-year-old woman had noticed a bony-hard swelling in her right parietal area since puberty but ascribed no importance to it. She claimed to have occasional paroxysmal pain in the affected area, especially before her periods. Radiologists had already given a diagnosis of fibrous dysplasia. The internist wanted a second opinion.

Radiologic Findings

Initial examination by MRI (see ▸ Fig. 2.14 **a–h**) shows an elliptical mass in the right parietal area that originates from the bone and appears hypointense in the T1w image (▸ Fig. 2.14 **a, b**). It contains a bicentric structure isointense to brain, with postcontrast images showing an intense ring or target pattern of enhancement (see ▸ Fig. 2.14 **c–f, h**). The "lesion within a lesion" is hyperintense in water-sensitive sequences (see ▸ Fig. 2.14 **g**). CT scans (see ▸ Fig. 2.14 **i–l**) prove that the expansile process arising from the calvarium encompasses all three layers of the skull and has replaced the original bone with tissue of ground-glass attenuation. The "lesion within a lesion" pattern results from bicentric cavities that are at least devoid of bony tissue. Densitometry was not performed but we estimate an attenuation of approximately 20 HU.

Location

Right parietal bone with equal involvement of the outer and inner tables and the diploë.

Pathoanatomic Background of the Findings

The portion of the mass with ground-glass attenuation is consistent with woven bone, while the bicentric cavitation is a secondary regressive change consistent with liquefaction (see also Case 4). The adjacent dura appears normal on pre- and postcontrast MRI.

Assignment to a Possible Basic Entity

▸ **Normal variant or malformation?** No. The process apparently began in puberty and appears to be related in some way to episodes of premenstrual pain. Moreover, this type of change has not been previously described as a normal variant (see Freyschmidt[17]).

▸ **Trauma?** No, given the negative history.

▸ **Inflammation?** No, given the absence of clinical signs.

▸ **Tumor or tumorlike lesion?** Yes, but apparently benign (long history) and tumorlike. This is also suggested by the expansile growth pattern. These signs, combined with the ground-glass attenuation on CT and the cranial location, strongly support a diagnosis of fibrous dysplasia.

Synopsis and Discussion

Fibrous dysplasia is suggested by initial MRI, the prior history, lesion location, and the normal appearance of the adjacent dura (with exclusion of a meningioma penetrating the bone) and was proven by subsequent CT scans showing ground-glass attenuation. The bicentric cavitation is also consistent with fibrous dysplasia since larger lesions (as in this case) tend to undergo regressive changes with myxoid transformation of the woven bone (see also Case 4). While fibrous dysplasia is a congenital bone disease resulting from a postzygotic mutation, it is often detected in the third to fourth decade of life, either incidentally or based on relatively mild symptoms (relative to lesion size). The symptoms—usually pain, occasional swelling—are hormone-dependent in women and are explained by perfusion changes in the woven bone (hyperperfusion with edema formation, possible secondary hypoperfusion with circumscribed necrosis and/or myxoid transformation). Fibrous dysplasia belongs to the category of tumorlike bone lesions, which can be accurately diagnosed by clinical and radiologic findings and do not require biopsy (a "don't touch me" or "leave me alone" lesion).

The differential diagnosis would include *Paget disease*, but this diagnosis is unlikely for the following reasons:

- The disease history dates from puberty. Patients with Paget disease generally do not become symptomatic until the fifth or sixth decade, if at all.
- Ordinarily a uniform ground-glass appearance is not observed in Paget disease.

Final Diagnosis

Fibrous dysplasia in the right parietal bone.

Comments

Expansion and a ground-glass appearance are the radiologic hallmarks of fibrous dysplasia, but focal regressive changes are also seen.

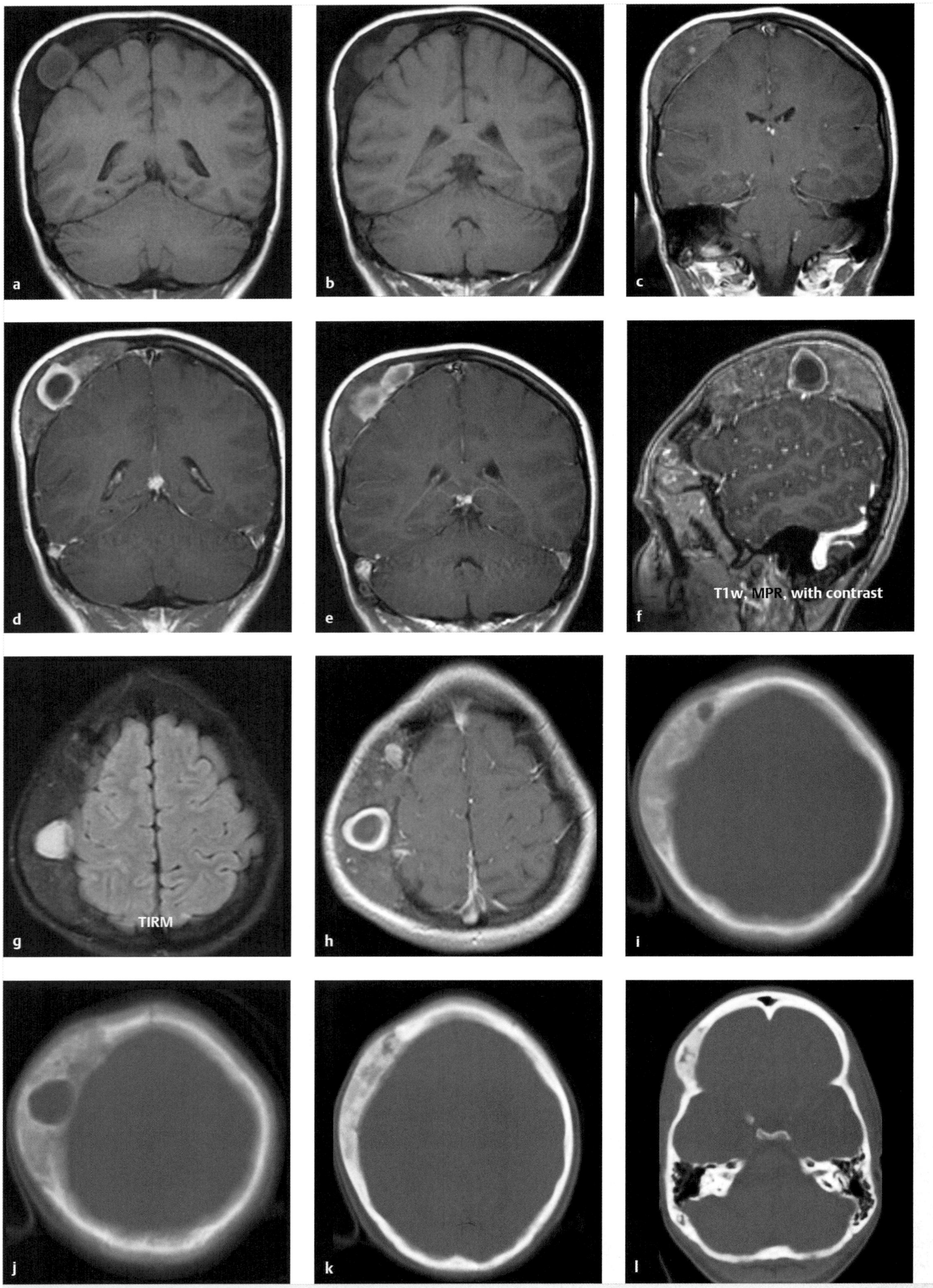

Fig. 2.14 a–l Chronic osteomyelitis?

2.2 Osteolytic Lesions and Lesions with Mixed Features

Case 8 (▶ Fig. 2.15)

Case description

- Referring physician: radiologist.
- Prior history and clinical question: A 58-year-old woman, otherwise healthy, claimed to have experienced an occasional warm sensation predominantly in her left forehead region over a long period of time. She stated that her son, who lived abroad, had noticed that her head appeared enlarged. Later she saw her family doctor, who drew blood samples. The tests showed a two-fold elevation of alkaline phosphatase levels, but her doctor was unsure how to proceed. Finally her son insisted that she have her head imaged. The radiologist recommended that we should narrow the differential diagnosis between Paget disease and fibrous dysplasia. His practice is in southern Germany, where doctors have had relatively little experience with Paget disease. (This is absolutely correct, because Paget disease is rare in southern Germany but almost endemic in northern Germany, occurring mainly in older individuals.)

Radiologic Findings

The lateral skull radiograph (▶ Fig. 2.15 **a**) shows cloudy structural changes consisting of a mixture of lucencies and opacities. The radiologist correctly followed the radiographs with CT scans (▶ Fig. 2.15 **b**), which show generalized thickening of the calvarium that is most pronounced in the left frontoparietal region. The normal three-layered structure of the calvarium has been almost completely lost. While irregular ossification is found in the diploë on the right side, the left frontoparietal region is hypodense and contains islands of ossification. Other hyperdense islands and lytic areas are noted farther posteriorly on the left side.

Location

The skull radiograph and CT show involvement of all three wall layers throughout the calvarium.

Pathoanatomic Background of the Findings

The imaging findings show that normal bony structures in the skull have been replaced by irregular ossifications that expand the skull volume. The images show an alternation of bone resorption and irregular new bone formation, suggesting that the process is still active.

Assignment to a Possible Basic Entity

▶ **Normal variant or malformation?** No. The remodeling process had its clinical onset in adulthood (note the history!). The elevated serum alkaline phosphatase level is also inconsistent with a normal variant.

▶ **Trauma?** No, the patient gave no history of trauma.

▶ **Inflammation?** Yes. Bone destruction and reparative new bone formation are typical features of bone inflammation. Common osteomyelitis is definitely excluded by the absence of clinical signs (local heat, pain, fistulation, etc.) and larger areas of bone destruction. Thus, we must be dealing with an inflammation-like disorder, and the only possibility is Paget disease (osteitis deformans).

▶ **Tumor?** No. The process is much too extensive and diffuse for a neoplasm.

▶ **Systemic disease (metabolic, reticulohistiocytosis, storage disease)?** No. Except for elevated serum alkaline phosphatase, there is no clinical or laboratory evidence for these conditions. A bone scan (not pictured here) showed intense uptake only in the skull, similar to Case 14. This would also exclude hyperparathyroidism (see Case 15).

Synopsis and Discussion

The coexisting signs of bone resorption and irregular reparative new bone formation (woven bone) with an expansion of cranial volume are hallmarks of the intermediate stage of Paget disease (see below under Intermediate or mixed stage). This diagnosis is also consistent with patient age, lesion location (the skull is the fourth most common site of occurrence after the pelvis, femur, and tibia), and elevated alkaline phosphatase. Note that if the volume of the changes were small, the osteoblast burden would be insufficient to raise the serum alkaline phosphatase level.

Paget disease is an inflammationlike disease of bone that progresses through three characteristic pathologic, clinical and radiologic stages and may involve one or multiple bones:

- *Lytic stage:* The classic model starts with a lytic stage initiated by a viral infection stimulating osteoclastic activity. The osteoclasts cause a very rapid breakdown of bone, resulting in osteolysis (see Case 9 and Case 12).
- *Intermediate or mixed stage:* Bone remodeling at this stage is marked by a reaction of osteoblasts and activated fibroblasts with the exuberant formation of new, nonlamellar, primitive woven bone.

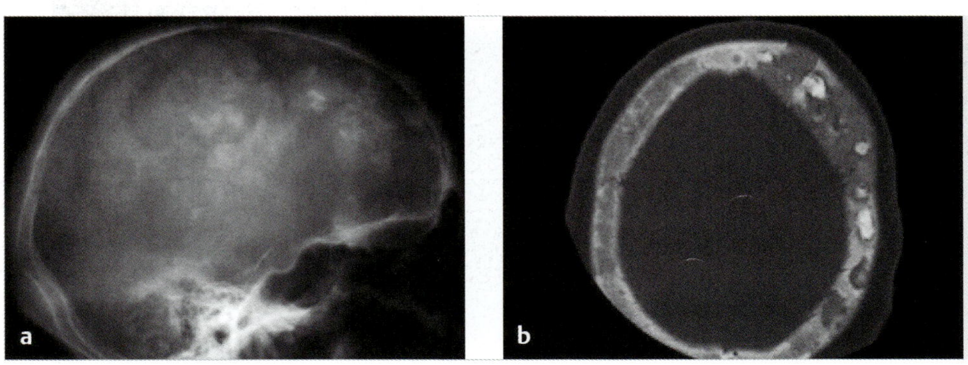

Fig. 2.15 a, b Cloudy appearance of the skull.

- *Sclerotic stage:* A predominance of bone formation over bone resorption leads over time to a dense network of calcified woven bone with a high fiber content, which creates irregular coarsened structures that are particularly characteristic of Paget disease in the pelvis and long bones.

Bone scintigraphy generally shows intense uptake in the early and intermediate stages. This is seen even on early images since the remodeling bone area has a rich blood supply and the mineralizing woven bone is very avid in its uptake of radiotracer. The onset of Paget disease may occur as early as the fourth decade. Since it usually runs an asymptomatic course, it often goes undiagnosed until the sixth to eighth decade when it is often detected incidentally, sometimes from an elevated serum alkaline phosphatase level.

Paget disease of the skull mainly requires differentiation from *fibrous dysplasia*. The main differentiating criterion is the ground-glass appearance on imaging, described fully in Case 4 and Case 7. Moreover, patients with fibrous dysplasia are younger when the change is first detected. The changes in Paget disease are generally symmetrical. Fibrous dysplasia tends to spare the cranial sutures. Sites of predilection for fibrous dysplasia are the sphenoid bone and paranasal sinuses, while Paget disease most commonly affects the calvarium. The outer and inner tables are typically thickened in Paget disease; this finding is less pronounced in fibrous dysplasia.

When the radiologic changes in the skull are considered in isolation, the differential diagnosis would also have to include hyperparathyroidism (see Case 15), but this disease is excluded because in the latter abnormal tracer uptake is not limited to the skull, as it is in Paget disease. It is sometimes difficult histologically to distinguish between Paget disease and hyperparathyroidism.

Final Diagnosis

Mixed (intermediate) stage of Paget disease.

Comments

Lytic lesions in the calvarium coexisting with irregular new bone formation and volume expansion are strongly suggestive of Paget disease when found in an older, otherwise healthy patient. An elevated serum alkaline phosphatase level can further aid the diagnosis, although this value will not be elevated if the structural changes have affected only a small bone volume.

Case 9 (▶ Fig. 2.16)

Case description

- Referring physician: radiologist.
- Prior history and clinical question: A routine checkup in a 76-year-old man revealed an elevated serum alkaline phosphatase level. Subsequent whole-body bone scintigraphy (not shown) demonstrated focal areas of intense uptake in the calvarium. Because the radiograph showed large osteolytic areas, a metastatic tumor was suspected. This prompted comprehensive inpatient screening for a primary tumor, which was unsuccessful. Afterward we were asked to perform a percutaneous biopsy. Based on the geographic pattern of the osteolytic areas and absence of clinical abnormalities (e.g., palpable soft-tissue masses over the lytic areas), we doubted the previous diagnosis of metastases and suspected osteoporosis circumscripta. A subsequent cranial CT examination confirmed our suspicion.

Radiologic Findings

The lateral skull radiograph (▶ Fig. 2.16 **a**) demonstrates large geographic lucencies in the parietal region, consistent with scintigraphic findings (not shown). Axial CT (▶ Fig. 2.16 **b**) shows a long demineralized area in the parietal bone with an intact basic architecture of the bone.

Location

Parietal region, involving all layers of the calvarium.

Pathoanatomic Background of the Findings

The process in this case is associated with a loss of bone substance without signs of osteolytic destruction. The elevated alkaline phosphatase level also indicates concomitant bone formation. Overall, however, the process is predominantly catabolic.

Assignment to a Possible Basic Entity

▶ **Normal variant or malformation?** No. Circumscribed "atrophic" processes that are associated with decreased bone density and a normal bone shape are not known to occur as normal variants in the calvarium (compare with Case 10 and Case 13).

▶ **Trauma?** Negative history.

▶ **Inflammation?** Certainly not in the traditional sense, given the absence of true destructive and reparative elements and the absence of sequestra on CT. On the other hand, a very early stage of Paget disease presents as an inflammationlike condition marked by osteoclastic resorption, known also as *osteoporosis circumscripta* (see below under Synopsis and Discussion). This early "osteolytic" stage starts with multiple small foci in the skull and may last for years. Osteoblastic and fibroblastic areas with fiber bone formation are detectable microscopically at this stage but not radiologically (see Case 8 for further pathoanatomic details).

▶ **Tumor?** No. It would be most unusual for a destructive neoplastic process to leave the shape and basic architecture of the bone intact while tumor cells simply "demineralized" the affected bone area.

▶ **Perfusion disorder?** Hyperperfusion due to a trophic disturbance with subsequent demineralization (transient edema followed by transient osteoporosis) has not yet been observed at this location. Sites of predilection for transient osteoporosis are juxta-articular bone areas about the hip, knee, ankle, and subtalar joints.

Synopsis and Discussion

The descriptive term *osteoporosis circumscripta* (see Inflammation? above) is reserved exclusively for the early osteolytic stage of Paget disease. If the radiologist notes circumscribed demineralization of the cranial vault without destructive changes on radiographs, and then proceeds with CT to confirm the nondestructive character of the lesion(s), this process in itself will supply the correct diagnosis—*without* histologic confirmation. The determination of serum alkaline phosphatase may also be helpful.

In this case it would be unrealistic to include *metastasis* in the differential diagnosis.

Eosinophilic granuloma (focal Langerhans cell histiocytosis, ▶ Fig. 2.17) is also highly unlikely because it is a disease of preschool and school-age children. To date we have observed a few isolated cases in the sixth and seventh decades and have seen none in the eighth decade. The child in ▶ Fig. 2.17 was asymptomatic. The temporal bone lesion enlarged noticeably over a 1-year period and was joined by a second lesion in the occipital bone. In this case there is no reasonable alternative to a diagnosis of eosinophilic granuloma.

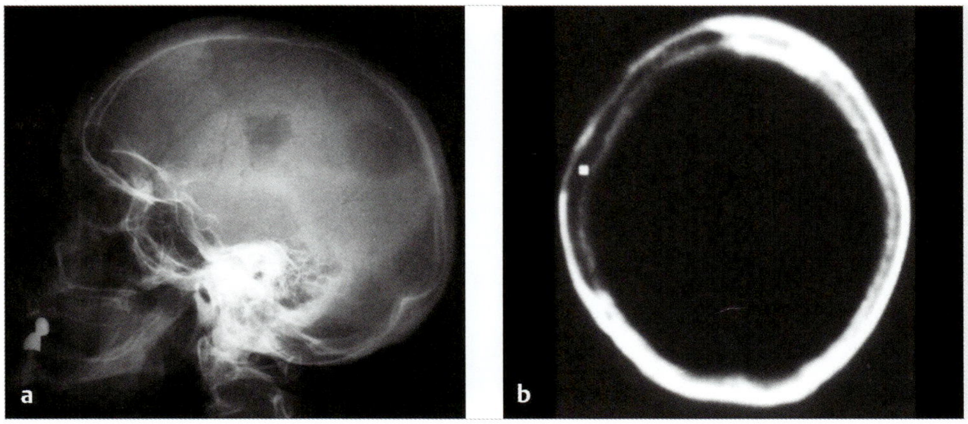

Fig. 2.16 a, b Metastases?

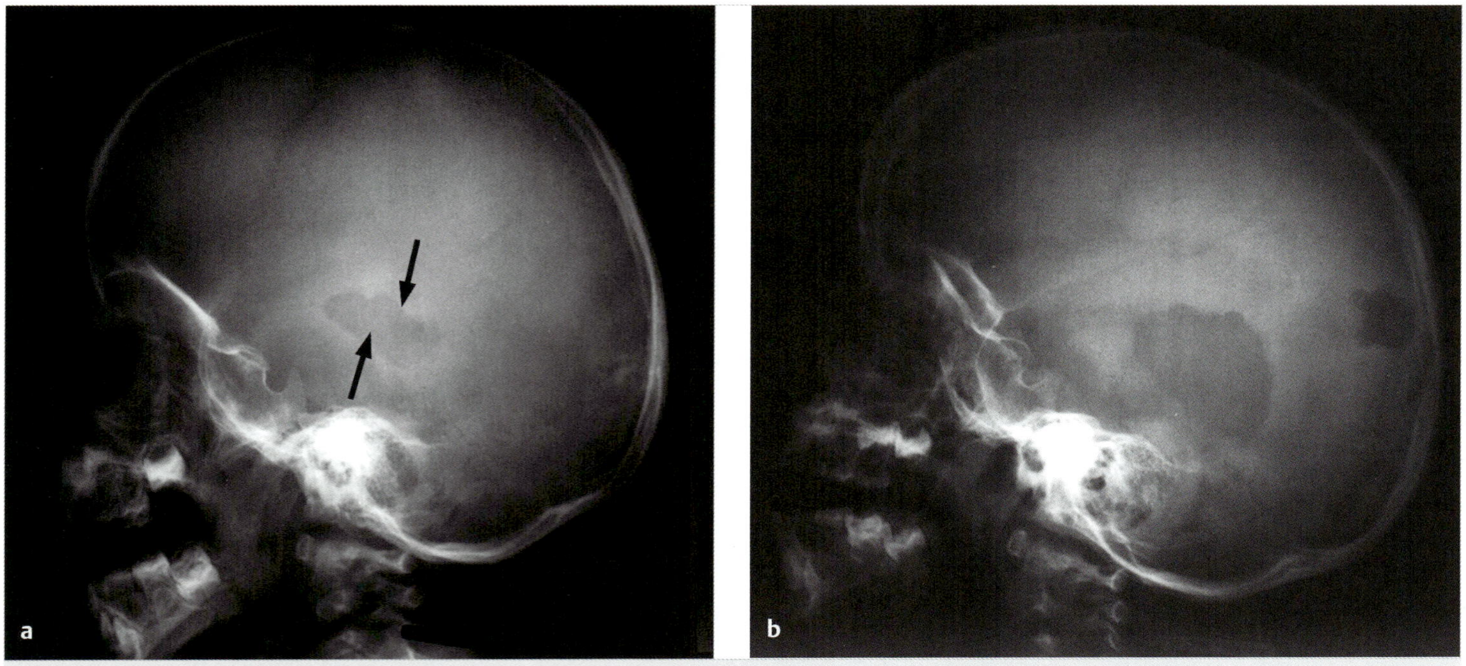

Fig. 2.17 a, b Differential diagnosis of osteolytic changes.

Final Diagnosis

Early lytic stage of Paget disease.

Comments

Remember: not every osteolytic lesion on radiographs or CT scans is a metastasis. There are other diseases! Metastasis should be diagnosed sparingly, as it can be very distressful for an otherwise healthy patient.

Case 10 (▶ Fig. 2.18)

Case description

- Referring physician: oncologist.
- Prior history and clinical question: A 68-year-old woman presented with recurrent episodes of occipital pain and swelling. A previous imaging examination was interpreted as showing areas of occipital bone destruction suspicious for bone metastasis. A primary tumor is not known.

Radiologic Findings (Primary)

The projection radiograph (▶ Fig. 2.18 **a**) demonstrates three well-circumscribed osteolytic areas that are "cold" on scintigraphy (▶ Fig. 2.18 **c**). CT displays the areas as smoothly marginated defects with paper-thin outer and inner tables (▶ Fig. 2.18 **b**). No paraosseous component is seen.

Location

The epicenter of the lesions is in the diploë.

Pathoanatomic Background of the Findings

It is important to ask what is occupying the defects in place of bone tissue and diploë (fluid, fat, connective tissue?). MRI is the best modality for distinguishing between connective tissue and fluid. T2-weighted (T2w) image slices through the defects (▶ Fig. 2.18 **d**) show a structure that is isointense to cerebrospinal fluid (CSF). To determine whether this is actually CSF, a FLAIR (fluid-attenuated inversion recovery) sequence is acquired which suppresses the signal from CSF. This sequence (▶ Fig. 2.18 **e**) shows an absence of signal from the CSF spaces and the defects, confirming that the defects are occupied by CSF-filled arachnoid diverticula.

Assignment to a Possible Basic Entity

▶ **Normal variant or malformation?** Yes. Arachnoid diverticula are among the most familiar normal variants in the cranial vault. They are also called Pacchionian granulations or arachnoid villi. CSF is reabsorbed by intradural arachnoid villi or Pacchionian granulations and drains into the dural sinuses. These arachnoid villi can form pitlike recesses of variable size (10 mm to several centimeters) in the inner table and diploë, which may cause extreme thinning of the outer table with an associated watch-glass bulge. The most common sites of occurrence are the frontal bone and parietal bone. The granulations are distributed along major venous sinuses, so it is helpful to check the proximity of the diverticula to vascular channels on the images.

▶ **Trauma?** No history.

▶ **Inflammation?** No clinical manifestations.

▶ **Tumor?** This is the main entity requiring differentiation from large arachnoid diverticula on plain radiographs. The most likely possibilities are eosinophilic granuloma, multiple myeloma, and metastases. The negative bone scan virtually excludes metastases but does not exclude multiple myeloma. It would be unusual for metastasis or multiple myeloma to affect only one area of the cranial vault—in this case the occipital bone. This also applies to eosinophilic granuloma (focal Langerhans cell histiocytosis, see ▶ Fig. 2.17 in Case 9). The latter diagnosis is also inconsistent with the advanced age of the patient. In any case, the information supplied by the FLAIR sequence is sufficient to exclude these tumors.

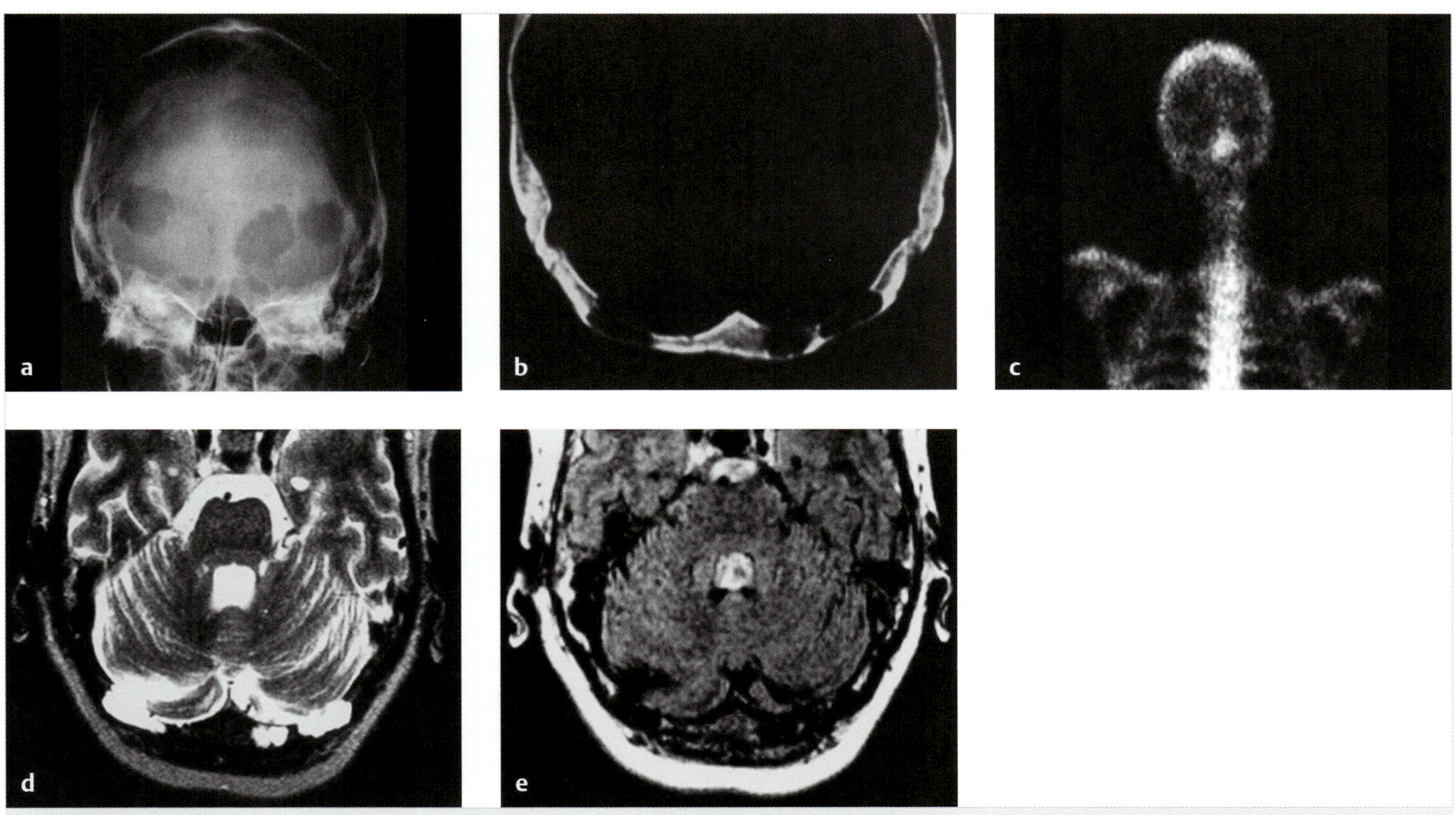

Fig. 2.18 a–e Metastases?

Synopsis and Discussion

Normal variants, especially Pacchionian granulations, should be considered whenever osteolytic areas are detected radiographically in the cranial vault. This is particularly true when the changes are confined, atypically, to one cranial bone. If subsequent CT scans demonstrate smooth-bordered masses with no paraosseous spread or adjacent reactive sclerosis, a normal variant is even more likely. Because the patient in this case had complaints which prompted diagnostic imaging, it is reasonable to proceed with further imaging studies; the first-line option is MRI with a FLAIR sequence. If this modality is not available, bone scintigraphy is a second-line option which, when negative, will at least make metastasis a very unlikely diagnosis.

We cannot explain the clinical symptoms (recurrent occipital pain and swelling) that this patient manifested in connection with Pacchionian granulations or arachnoid diverticula.[20] Cases published to date in the literature have described similar symptoms, for which no plausible explanation has been found.

To aid the diagnostician in differentiation from Pacchionian granulations, ▶ Fig. 2.19 illustrates the case of a 46-year-old woman with an intraosseous epidermoid (synonyms: epithelial cyst, epidermoid cyst in bone) in the left occipital area. Whole-body bone scans in this patient demonstrated slight uptake in the left occipital area. Because the patient had breast cancer, further imaging studies were performed. The CT scans in ▶ Fig. 2.19 **a–f** show a large, central osteolytic lesion in the calvarium with smooth margins and slight internal expansion. The lesion is covered partly by a very thin remnant of the inner and outer tables, producing a watch-glass bulge, and partly by periosteum alone. There is no apparent infiltration of adjacent structures. The attenuation values in the lesion range from 10 to 50 HU. These images are almost identical to the one in ▶ Fig. 2.18 **b**. On T1w MRI (▶ Fig. 2.19 **g**) the lesion is slightly hyperintense to cerebellum and shows only faint enhancement after contrast administration (▶ Fig. 2.19 **h**). In the T2w image (▶ Fig. 2.19 **i**) the lesion exhibits an outer proton-rich zone and an inner or central hypointense zone. The CSF-suppressed FLAIR sequence in ▶ Fig. 2.19 **j** identifies the outer hyperintense zone in image ▶ Fig. 2.19 **h** as fluid. Further crucial information is supplied by the diffusion-weighted EPI (echo planar imaging) sequence (▶ Fig. 2.19 **k, l**) and the ADC (apparent diffusion coefficient) image (▶ Fig. 2.19 **m**). The lesion appears hyperintense in the EPI sequence. The ADC image shows that the high signal intensity in ▶ Fig. 2.19 **k, l** is caused by a diffusion abnormality and not by T2w shine-through effects. Taken with the clinical presentation (incidental discovery), these findings are strongly suggestive of an intraosseous epidermoid. This case is very similar to one published by Dammert et al. (2003),[21] who stated that the diffusion abnormality documented by diffusion-weighted imaging and the ADC image is highly specific for an epidermoid. An intraosseous epidermoid develops when epidermis becomes displaced beneath the periosteum or into the bone. The active germinal matrix produces hyperkeratosis as well as para- and dyskeratosis. This creates an osteoclastic stimulus leading to local bone resorption. The epidermal tissue may become misplaced as a result of trauma, but a dysontogenetic origin is thought to be more likely in the skull. Histologically, the cyst wall is formed by a uniform layer of squamous epithelium that develops a granular cell layer on the luminal side as it matures. It is covered externally by a thin fibrotic layer. The cyst lumen is lined by desquamated and compressed keratin lamellae.

Another epidermoid case, illustrated in ▶ Fig. 2.20, confirms the claim of Dammert et al. This 18-year-old patient had struck the right side of her head on a bar while playing sports at school. Afterward she noticed an indentation in the right posterior parietal area, which subsequently enlarged, so she and her parents claimed. She was diagnosed clinically with a minor head injury, which was not thought to be related to the indentation. CT, which was not performed until 3 months later, showed a full-thickness bone defect in the right posterior parietal area (▶ Fig. 2.20 **a–c**). The differential diagnosis consisted of eosinophilic granuloma and epidermoid cyst. On T1w MRI (▶ Fig. 2.20 **d**) the lesion appears hypointense to brain and slightly hyperintense to bone. It shows only a slight degree of peripheral enhancement (▶ Fig. 2.20 **e**). In the T2w image (▶ Fig. 2.20 **f**) the lesion is isointense to CSF, and in the FLAIR sequence (▶ Fig. 2.20 **g**) it is isointense to brain. Finally, the lesion is isointense to brain structures in the ADC images (▶ Fig. 2.20 **h**). All of the findings are consistent with an intraosseous epidermoid. Because the patient was asymptomatic—and it is ultimately unknown whether eosinophilic granulomas may pass through stages in which they resemble an intraosseous epidermoid on MRI—we recommended surgical excision. Histology at 7 months after the traumatic event identified the lesion as an *epidermoid cyst with a focal granulating and fibrotic inflammatory reaction*, interpreted partly as a foreign-body reaction.

This last case naturally raises the question of whether the head trauma induced the epidermoid cyst, as the clinical presentation suggests. But epidermoid cysts or intraosseous epidermoids in the calvarium are generally asymptomatic. The young woman first noticed a depression in the right calvarium after the impact trauma and claimed that the palpable depression had enlarged over time. But this would have been possible only if the skin over the lesion area had been disrupted, allowing epithelium to become displaced beneath the periosteum or directly into the bone through a fractured outer table. This would most likely have caused a hematoma with an associated bulge, not an indentation. We believe, rather, that the head impact ruptured a pre-existing cyst, thereby reducing its volume and forming a palpable depression in the skull. The histologic finding of an inflammatory foreign-body reaction suggests that the rupture had been present for some time. This case is quite interesting from a forensic standpoint as well.

Final Diagnosis

Pacchionian granulations (arachnoid diverticula).

Comments

"Holes" in the calvarium should not automatically be interpreted as metastases. An unusual normal variant such as Pacchionian granulations should also be considered following a thorough and systematic analysis. One or more "holes" in the skull of younger patients often represents eosinophilic granuloma and, in rare cases, an epidermoid cyst—which MRI can confirm with some certainty by diffusion-weighted and ADC imaging.

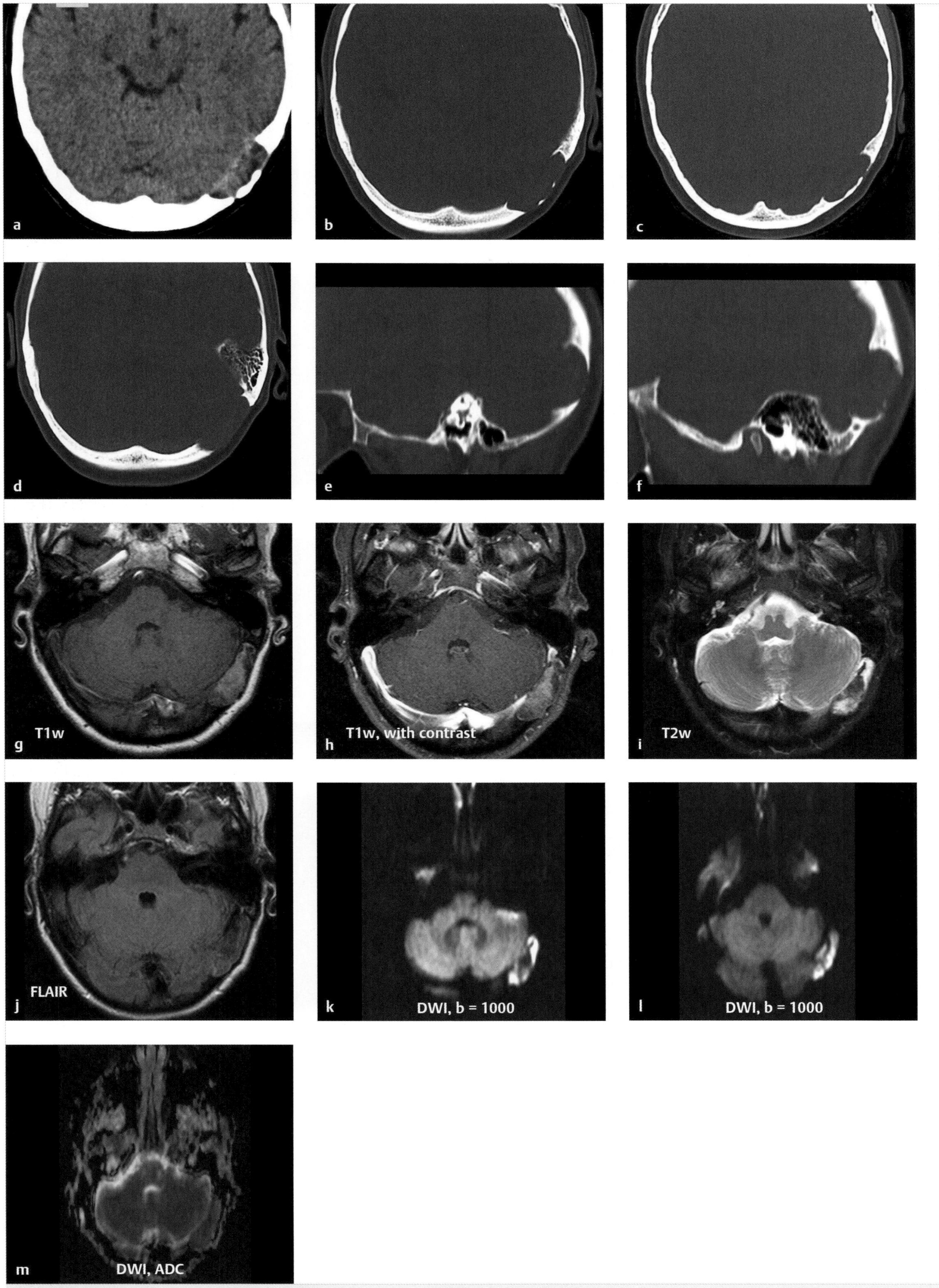

Fig. 2.19 a–m Differential diagnosis: epidermoid?

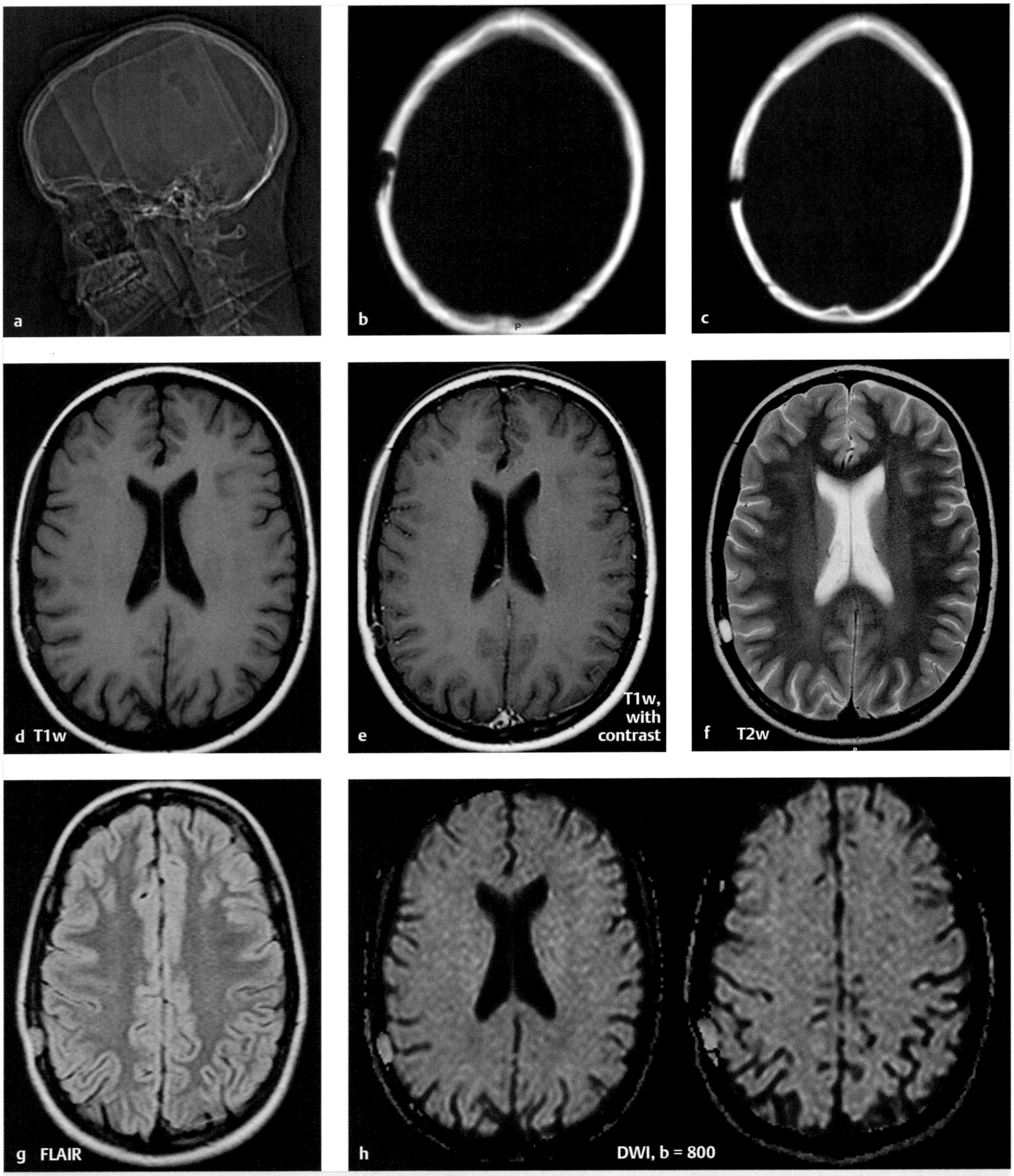

Fig. 2.20 a–h Could this also be an epidermoid (18-year-old female)?

Case 11 (▶ Fig. 2.21)

Case description

- Referring physician: radiologist.
- Prior history and clinical question: A 26-year-old woman had been aware of a depression in her left forehead for some time.

Radiologic Findings

Imaging revealed thinning of the anterior and central portions of the left frontal calvarium with no associated sclerosis or periosteal reaction. The affected area was bounded deeply by a paper-thin segment of inner table. The thinning of the calvarium was less pronounced on a prior image taken 4 years earlier (not shown).

Pathoanatomic Background of the Findings

The absence of any reaction in adjacent structures (sclerosis, periosteal reaction) indicates a gradual osteoclastic resorption of the bone. The remaining bone is little more than a "war memorial," that is, there are no macroscopic traces of the actual cause. This process of nonreactive bone resorption has been fittingly referred to as "vanishing bone disease."

Assignment to a Possible Basic Entity

▶ **Normal variant or malformation?** No, because the process is only a few years old.

▶ **Trauma?** No, there is no corresponding history.

▶ **Inflammation?** No, at least not in the traditional sense of osteitis or osteomyelitis, which in their florid stage are generally marked by pain and local warmth. The inflammatory process also incites local reactions such as periosteal calcification, sclerosis, etc. A burned-out inflammation would have been reflected in the prior history.

▶ **Tumor?** Possibly. There are angiomatoses (especially the lymphatic kind) that stimulate osteoclastic bone resorption. In most cases, however, angiomatosis is no longer detectable at the time of radiologic and pathologic examination; this is possible only in isolated cases (see Case 32 and Case 33). In the case of a burned-out angiomatosis, the bone is replaced by connective tissue.

▶ **Perfusion disorder?** Possibly. Besides angiomatosis, a trophic process has been discussed as a potential cause of vanishing bone disease. This would involve a disturbance of vascular innervation leading to intense local hyperperfusion including neovascularization (due to stimulation of vascular growth factor), which stimulates the osteoclasts and creates an imbalance in bone remodeling with predominant bone resorption. It may be that angiomatosis is histologically indistinguishable from the features of extremely hyperperfused bone with neovascularization, at least using conventional histologic methods. The stimulation of osteoclasts by hyperperfusion due to neurovascular dysfunction bears a strong resemblance to the pathogenesis of neurogenic osteoarthropathy.

Synopsis and Discussion

Based on the above considerations, the only reasonable clinical and radiologic diagnosis is vanishing bone disease, known also as phantom bone disease, Gorham–Stout disease, or massive osteolysis syndrome. This condition is marked by a gradual and inexorable resorption of the affected bone (for pathogenesis, see under Tumor? above). Sites of predilection are the bones of the shoulder girdle (clavicle, proximal humerus, scapula) and pelvis (ilium [see Case 54], ischium), sacrum, and proximal femur. Not infrequently, the disease process is self-limiting; a fatal outcome is somewhat rare. The case described has certain special features: A known dermatologic disease is *circumscribed scleroderma*, which leads to shrinkage and atrophy of the skin and subcutaneous tissue and may also affect the underlying bone. If this process occurs in the frontoparietal area and creates a palpable depression, it is often called *scleroderma en coup de sabre* in the flowery and Francophile language of dermatologists. Its etiology and pathogenesis are not fully understood but may relate to an angiomatosis or angiomatosislike mechanism. In our case, focal scleroderma was confirmed clinically and the patient was placed on methotrexate therapy following an initial course of high-dose penicillin.

▶ Fig. 2.22 illustrates another case with nonreactive destruction of an initially circumscribed bone area in the posterior parie-

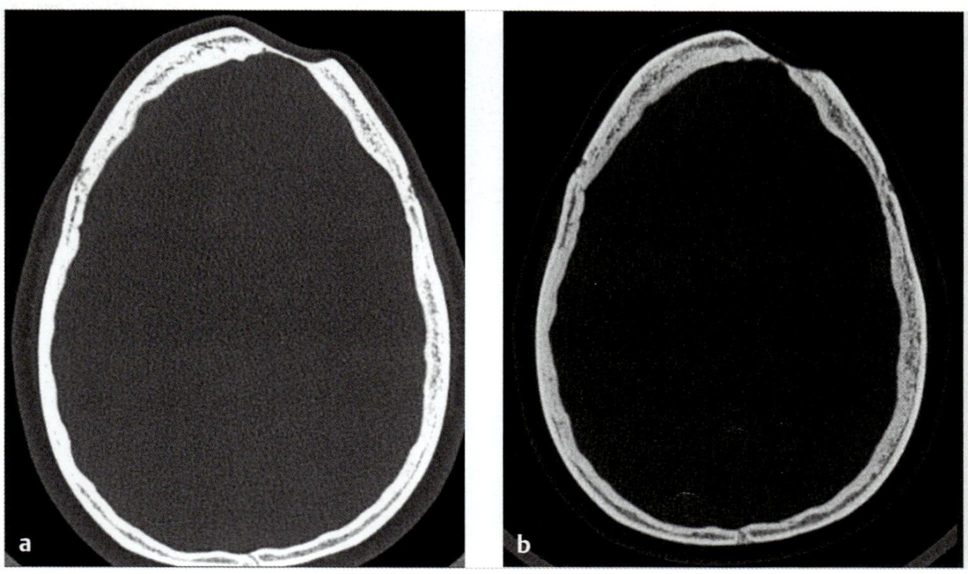

Fig. 2.21 a, b A depression in the skull.

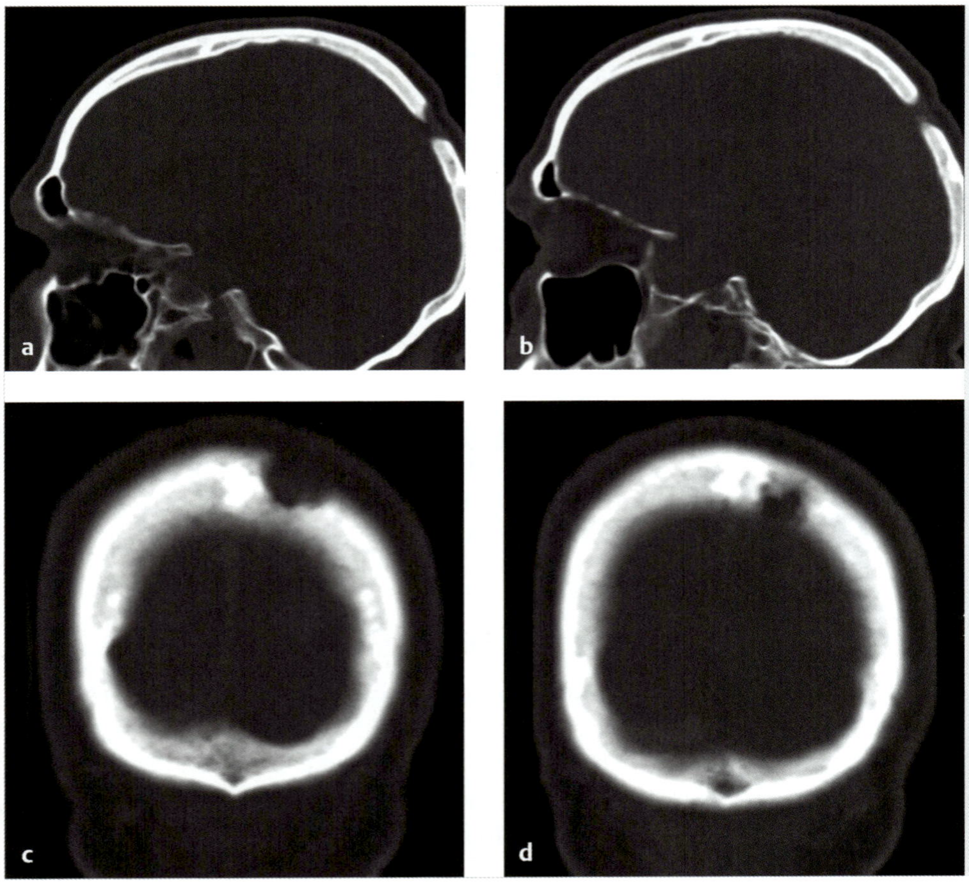

Fig. 2.22 a–d Circumscribed nonreactive bone destruction in the posterior parietal region of a 60-year-old man.

tal region of a 60-year-old man. Another case of vanishing bone disease is presented in Case 54.

Final Diagnosis

Vanishing bone disease (phantom bone disease, massive osteolysis, Gorham–Stout disease).

Comments

When the term “vanishing bone” or “phantom bone” is applied to the nonreactive, circumscribed resorption of bone, this already has the status of a diagnosis—quite unlike the eponymic term “Gorham–Stout disease.”

Dermatologic examination by a specialist may provide a broader perspective on a complex disease process: Is there a primary skin disease, or are cutaneous manifestations just the visible tip of an iceberg below the skin, that is, in the bone?

Case 12 (▶ Fig. 2.23)

Case description

- Referring physician: radiologist.
- Prior history and clinical question: A 59-year-old man suffered a fall and a skull radiograph was taken to exclude a fracture. The radiograph revealed a large area of decreased density in the calvarium. The change was investigated further by CT and scintigraphy.

Radiologic Findings

The lateral skull radiograph (▶ Fig. 2.23 **a**) demonstrates a large area of decreased density. Only the posterosuperior region of the calvarium still shows normal radiographic density. Arrows indicate the boundary between normal and pathologic bone. CT (▶ Fig. 2.23 **b**) shows irregular, bilateral hypodensities in the parietal and frontal regions of the skull; only the posterior parietal and high occipital regions still show normal density. Scintigraphy (▶ Fig. 2.23 **c**) shows large areas of high uptake in the affected regions with minimal uptake in the normal posterior calvarium.

Location

The structural changes involve the entire frontal and parietal regions of the calvarium, crossing the sutures and sparing only a posterior parietal and high occipital area.

Pathoanatomic Background of the Findings

As in Case 8, this bone-remodeling process is active (denoted by tracer uptake) and is characterized by demineralization, reparative calcifying woven bone formation, and an absence of destructive changes with preservation of the basic "matrix" (architecture) of the affected calvarium. In contrast to Case 8, there is not yet an appreciable increase in bone volume.

Assignment to a Possible Basic Entity

See Case 8.

Synopsis and Discussion

When the large demineralized area in the radiograph is described as osteoporosis circumscripta, it is not difficult to identify the condition as Paget disease. This case lies between the purely osteolytic (demineralizing) early stage of Paget disease as illustrated

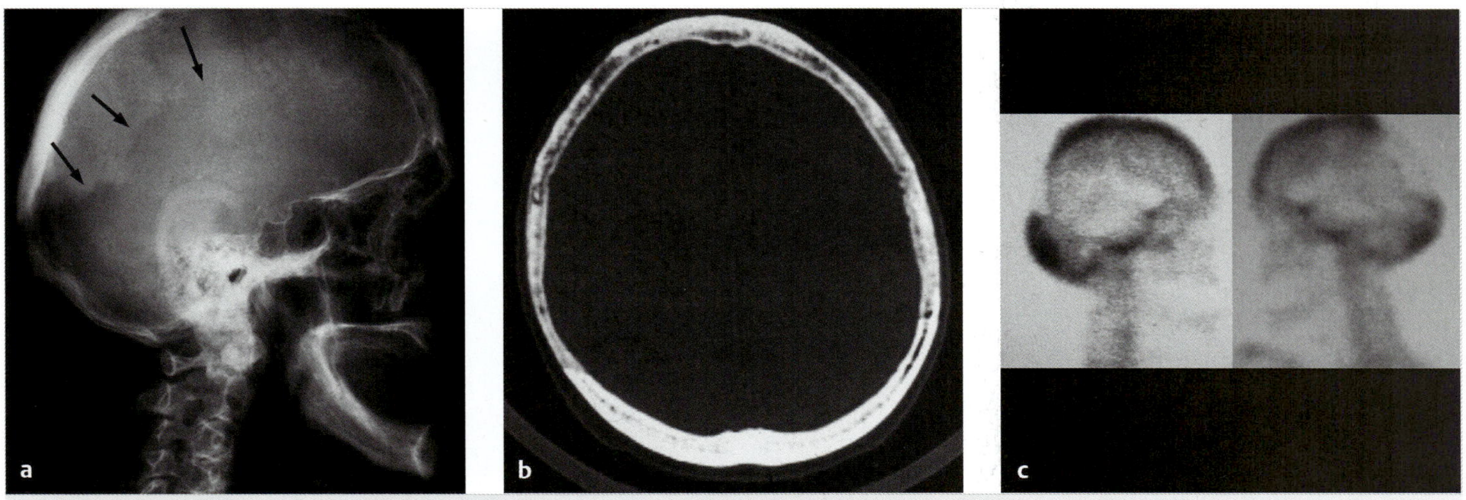

Fig. 2.23 a–c Large metastasis or lymphoma?

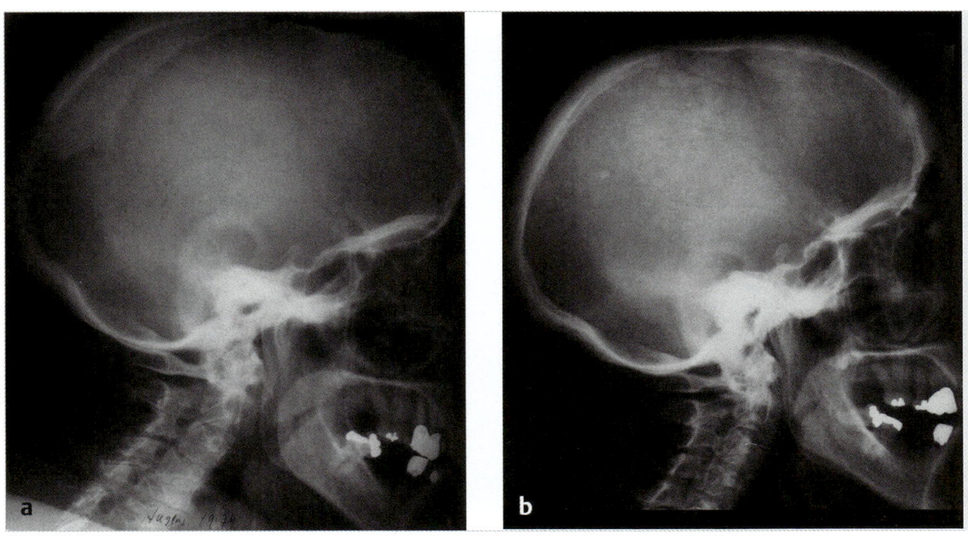

Fig. 2.24 a, b Extensive cranial involvement by Paget disease in a 58-year-old woman before and after treatment.

in Case 9 and the mixed (intermediate) stage shown in Case 8. The bone scan is instructive: it accurately reflects the extensive remodeling process and helps to classify the radiographic finding. *The large areas of increased uptake form the typical scintigraphic pattern of Paget disease.* This pattern may also occur with bone-infiltrating processes such as malignant lymphoma, but we have not previously seen it to this extent in the skull. Another advantage of bone scintigraphy is that it displays or excludes possible additional lesions on a single whole-body scan (see Case 14 and Case 140 versus Case 107). If a typical bone scan (with a large area of increased tracer uptake) is combined with a typical radiograph, no further work-up is needed. A biopsy is unnecessary.

▸ Fig. 2.24 illustrates another case of extensive cranial involvement by Paget disease in a 58-year-old woman, initially (▸ Fig. 2.24 **a**) and 6 years later after treatment with calcitonin and bisphosphonates (▸ Fig. 2.24 **b**). The posttreatment film documents significant remineralization.

Final Diagnosis

Early intermediate stage of Paget disease.

Comments

A large area of increased radiotracer uptake in the skull of an older, asymptomatic patient is strongly suggestive of Paget disease. Bone scintigraphy is a rapid, cost-effective adjunct that can noninvasively classify osteolysis as osteoporosis circumscripta. Even when a bone scan is obtained primarily to screen for metastases, a large area of increased uptake in the skull and perhaps in other skeletal regions should always raise initial suspicion of Paget disease (see also the Synopsis in Case 9).

Case 13 (▶ Fig. 2.25)

Case description

- Referring physician: oncologist.
- Prior history and clinical question: An 80-year-old woman was initially treated for headaches by a neurologist. She was treated with corticosteroids for suspected temporal arteritis. The inflammatory markers improved while pains persisted. When "osteolytic areas" were found on the skull radiograph and CT, she was transferred to internal medicine and underwent a very thorough examination that did not reveal a tumor. Finally, the treating oncologist looked at prior CT scans from 9 years earlier, which showed identical findings. The oncologist correctly excluded neoplasia as the cause of the skull changes but would like to know the actual cause.

Radiologic Findings

The calvarium is of normal shape and shows irregular structural lucencies that are partially confluent in the parietal and frontal regions (▶ Fig. 2.25 **a**). The diploë appears slightly expanded. On closer scrutiny a radiologist, who is experienced in conventional imaging, notes very prominent vascular markings from the venous sinuses and the vascular channels and lacunae in the diploë. The CT images (▶ Fig. 2.25 **b, c**) would prove to a less experienced reader that the tortuous and serpiginous lucencies represent vascular grooves or vascular prints. Considering the different level of the scans, there is essentially no difference in the findings between ▶ Fig. 2.25 **b** and ▶ Fig. 2.25 **c**.

Location

Entire calvarium, encompassing all three elements (inner table, diploë, outer table).

Pathoanatomic Background of the Findings

The described lucencies may be collectively classified as vascular grooves or channels, and a few may be identified as small Pacchionian granulations. The slight expansion of the diploic spaces seen in the lateral radiograph, with associated thinning of the inner and outer tables, can be interpreted as atrophy.

Assignment to a Possible Basic Entity

▸ **Normal variant or malformation?** We need not consider whether this condition should be classified either as severe age-related atrophy due to osteoporosis or as a normal variant of age-related atrophy. After a thorough image analysis showed that the lucencies were vascular grooves or channels in a skull with age-related atrophy and had remained unchanged for 9 years, there is no need to consider any other possible diagnoses.

Final Diagnosis

Age-related atrophy of the skull.

Comments

Atypical or unusual skull radiographs in older patients may very well represent ordinary age-related atrophy.

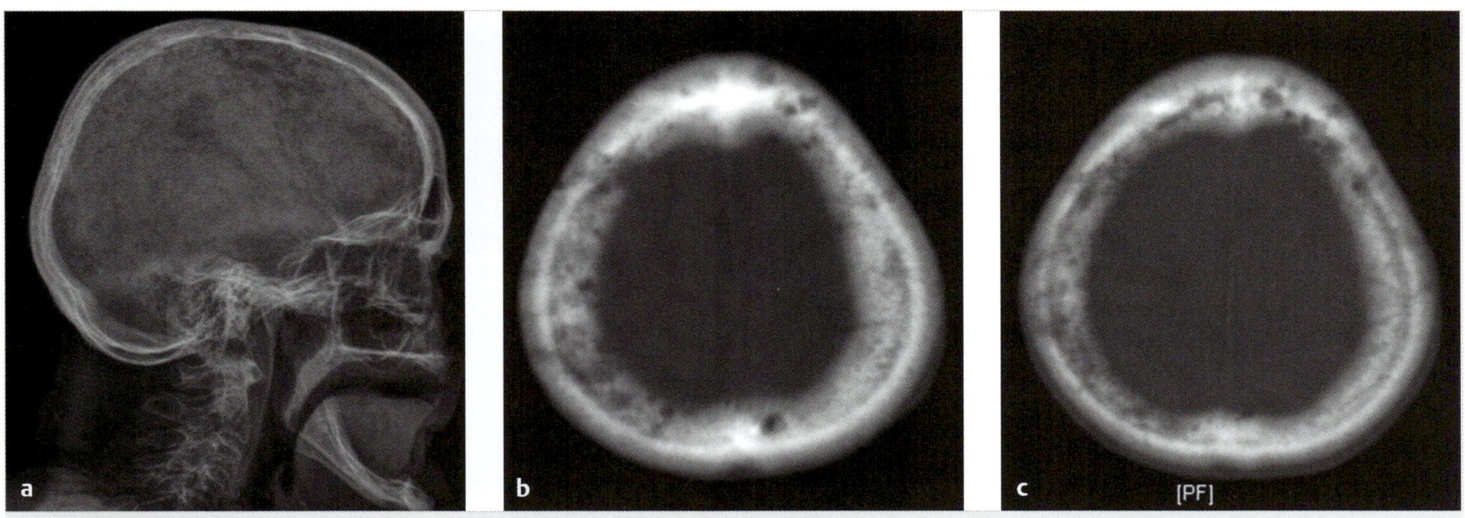

Fig. 2.25 Cranial metastases? The image in b is from 2002; the images in a and c are from 2011.

Case 14 (▸ Fig. 2.26)

Case description

- Referring physician: radiologist.
- Prior history and clinical question: A 76-year-old woman was hospitalized with a highly febrile infection and cephalgia, nausea and vomiting. The patient suffers from type 2 diabetes mellitus and mild hypertension. She gave no musculoskeletal complaints. Laboratory tests showed a two-fold elevation of serum alkaline phosphatase. Subsequent whole-body bone scintigraphy showed greatly increased radiotracer uptake in the skull with no other abnormalities. Subsequent radiographs and CT scans yielded findings that cannot be classified.

Radiologic Findings

Except for intense uptake in the skull, whole-body scintigraphy (▸ Fig. 2.26 **a**) shows no abnormalities other than slight uptake in the right manubrioclavicular joint, patellae and ankles, which can be interpreted as age-related phenomena without clinical relevance. The skull radiographs (▸ Fig. 2.26 **b, c**) show diffuse patchy opacities. It is unclear whether the intervening lucencies are real or apparent. This is also unclear on the CT scans (▸ Fig. 2.26 **d**) because the irregular hyperdensities are too close together. Two other findings are crucial, however: the marked thickening of the calvarium with expansion of the diploë and the ill-defined markings on the inner and outer tables. The changes extend into the skull base (▸ Fig. 2.26 **e**). The coarse, bilateral focal densities in the frontal areas closely resemble ▸ Fig. 2.15 **b** in Case 8.

Location

The skull radiograph and CT scans document complete involvement of all three components of the calvarium.

Pathoanatomic Background of the Findings

Same as in Case 8.

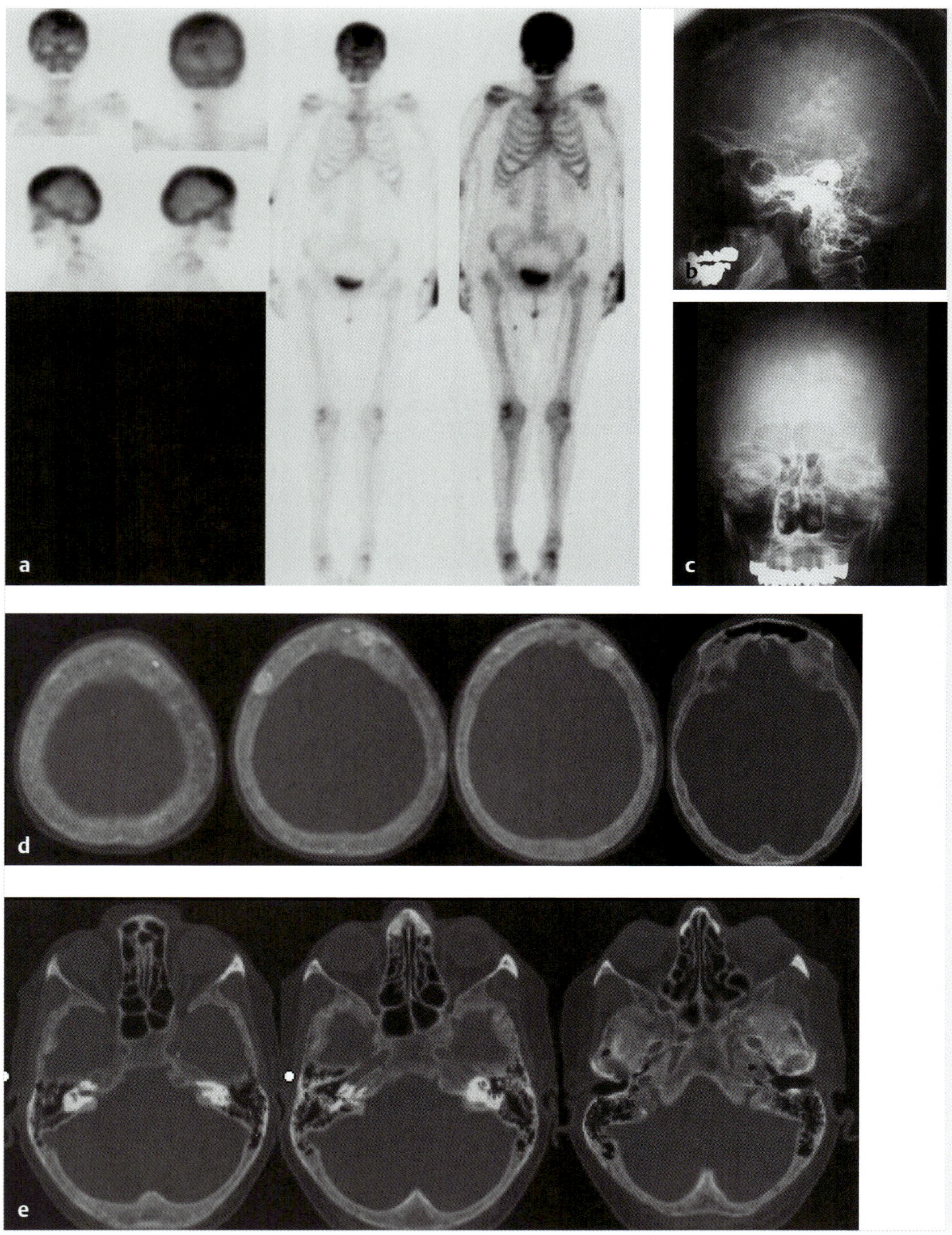

Fig. 2.26 a–e Black skull.

Assignment to a Possible Basic Entity

See under Case 8.

Synopsis and Discussion

The patient has an intermediate stage of Paget disease. The imaging findings are highly specific for this disease, as described in Case 8. There is practically no reasonable differential diagnosis. Even hyperparathyroidism, which produces the same phenomena on radiographs and CT (see Case 15), is excluded by the absence of other abnormalities in the whole-body bone scan. According to generally accepted guidelines for the management of Paget disease, the case requires treatment (with bisphosphonates) to prevent compression effects on cranial nerves (e.g., the acoustic nerve).

▶ Fig. 2.27 illustrates the findings in a late sclerotic stage of Paget disease, marked by an extreme "cloudy skull" and significant volume expansion. This pattern of findings is unmistakable and should be familiar to all younger radiologists, so that they can diagnose similar findings at a glance. There is no realistic differential diagnosis. Scintigraphy may be negative in the late stage (late inactive phase), and even the alkaline phosphatase level may be normal. Biopsy is unnecessary.

Final Diagnosis

Mixed (intermediate) stage of Paget disease.

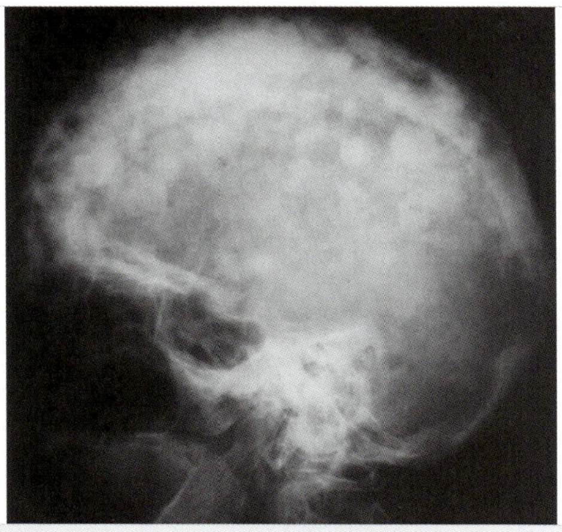

Fig. 2.27 Cloudy skull.

Comments

The most frequent cause of extensive radiotracer uptake in the skull in older patients is Paget disease (see also Case 12). The "cloudy skull" is also pathognomonic for this disease.

Case 15 (▶ Fig. 2.28)

Case description

- Referring physician: internist.
- Prior history and clinical question: A 34-year-old woman visited her internist complaining of cardiac arrhythmia, lethargy, and depression. Laboratory tests showed an elevated serum calcium level and elevated alkaline phosphatase. The internist ordered a bone scan, which showed very high uptake in the skull (▶ Fig. 2.28 **c**). A supplemental skull radiograph showed "curious" structural changes that could not be classified. Paget disease was considered, however.

Radiologic Findings

The radiographic appearance of the skull (▶ Fig. 2.28 **a**) can be described as a pepper-pot or "salt-and-pepper" pattern, meaning a mixture of countless small osteolytic foci and fine focal densities. We ordered CT scans (▶ Fig. 2.28 **b**), which explain this finding: the calvarium is permeated by innumerable tiny lytic zones and densities with no alteration of cranial shape. The diploë is no longer delineated.

Location

The structural changes involve all portions of the calvarium, that is, the inner and outer tables and the diploë.

Pathoanatomic Background of the Findings

The extreme structural transformation of the calvarium with a positive bone scan and normal skull shape suggest a systemic alteration of bone metabolism. This is also supported by the clinical presentation and laboratory data. When we reevaluated the patient's bone scan, we noticed that tracer uptake was absent in the soft tissues, kidneys, and bladder but was relatively high in the bone, particularly the skull. This pattern, called a "superscan," is found only in processes that cause generalized bone remodeling with an extremely high bone turnover (e.g., disseminated metastasis, hyperparathyroidism, mastocytosis, osteomyelosclerosis syndrome, etc.). The combination of a salt-and-pepper skull with a superscan then provided the engrammatic link to hyperparathyroidism.

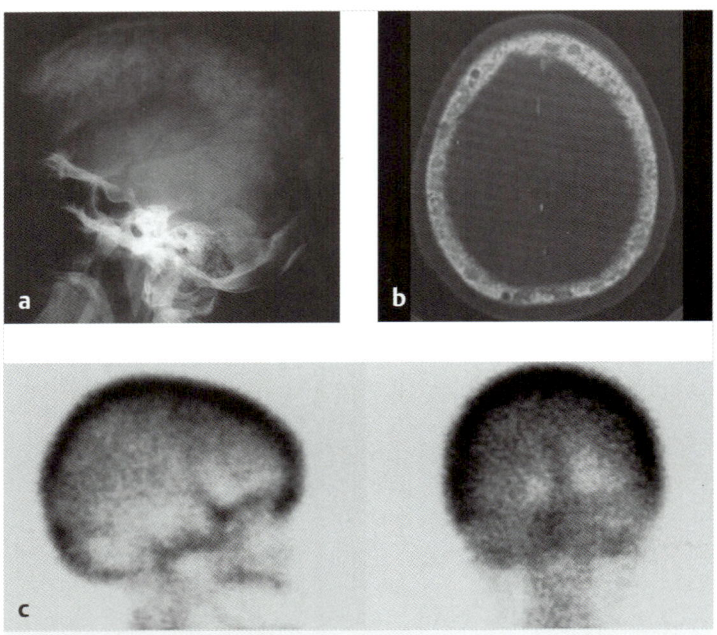

Fig. 2.28 a–c Age-related atrophy?

Assignment to a Possible Basic Entity

Our considerations on the pathoanatomic background of the skull changes raised a strong index of suspicion for hyperparathyroidism. From a radiologic standpoint, only one more piece was needed to establish the diagnosis: a radiograph of the hand skeleton (▶ Fig. 2.29). The hand radiograph in hyperparathyroidism shows highly specific changes such as phalangeal tuft resorption (acro-osteolysis), subperiosteal resorption mainly affecting the phalanges, intracortical striation, and a coarsened bony trabecular pattern.

Synopsis and Discussion

The present case of primary hyperparathyroidism could ultimately be solved based on pathognomonic imaging findings alone. The keys were choosing the proper supplemental imaging study and conducting a detailed review of the findings: The initial study was a bone scan that had been only partially interpreted as showing high uptake in the skull. A subsequent skull radiograph demonstrated structural changes best characterized as the pepper-pot or salt-and-pepper pattern of hyperparathyroidism. But the differential diagnosis for this finding also includes Paget disease, which may closely resemble hyperparathyroidism on plain radiographs (compare with Case 14). But a careful review of the bone scans showed definite signs of a generalized change in bone

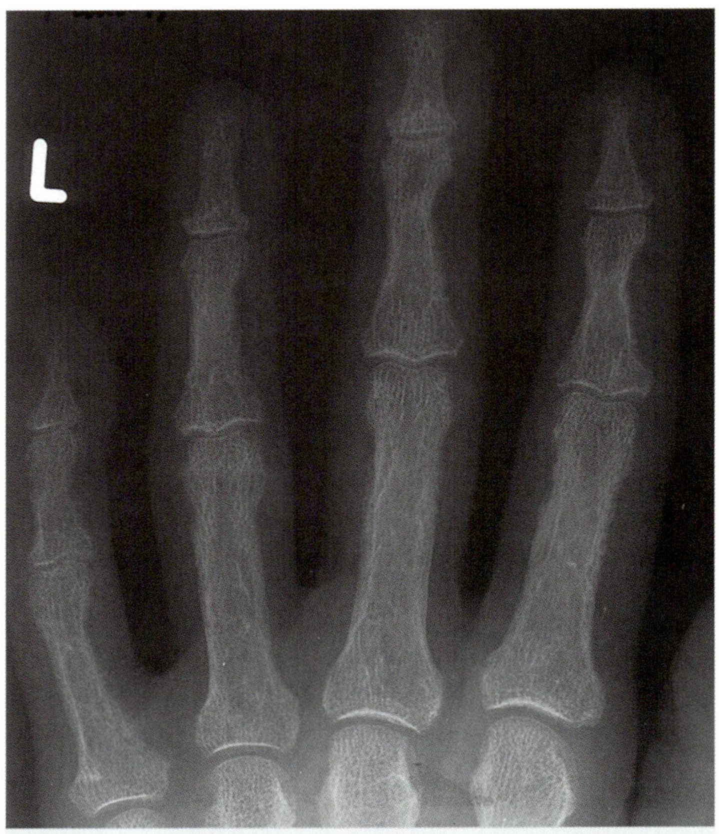

Fig. 2.29 Radiograph of the hand in the 34-year-old female patient with suspected age-related atrophy (see ▶ Fig. 2.28).

metabolism that ruled out Paget disease. When the radiograph also excluded the other systemic skeletal diseases noted above, we needed only a hand radiograph to provide the crowning proof of hyperparathyroidism.

Further information on hyperparathyroidism is presented in Case 137.

Final Diagnosis

Primary hyperparathyroidism.

Comments

The appropriate combination of imaging studies in the proper sequence leads to the correct diagnosis of hyperparathyroidism. The most specific changes are found in the phalangeal bones of the hand.

Case 16 (▶ Fig. 2.30)

Case description

- Referring physician: nephrologist.
- Prior history and clinical question: A 45-year-old man with malignant hypertension and chronic renal failure had been on dialysis for 3 years. His parathormone level was found to be elevated to 160 pmol/L (normal: 6 pmol/L), which prompted a referral for whole-body bone scintigraphy. The bone scan showed massive tracer uptake in the occiput (a "black occiput"), which raised the following differential diagnosis:
  - Brown tumor of hyperparathyroidism
  - Paget disease
  - Vanishing bone disease (Gorham–Stout disease)
  - Metastasis from an unknown primary tumor
  - Angiomatosis

Radiologic Findings

The bone scan shows extreme, very conspicuous uptake in the occiput but is otherwise normal (▶ Fig. 2.30 **a**). A lateral radiograph of the skull (▶ Fig. 2.30 **b**) shows coarse osteolysis of the occipital bone that precisely fits the area of the scintigraphic finding—a vanishing occiput! The remaining portions of the calvarium show a pepper-pot or salt-and-pepper pattern as evidence of secondary hyperparathyroidism (see also Case 15). We then performed a CT examination to gain more information on the condition of the calvarium (▶ Fig. 2.30 **c**). The occiput shows a completely normal basic architecture on CT but it is extremely demineralized.

Location

The finding is limited entirely to the occiput—that is, to one anatomic unit.

Pathoanatomic Background of the Findings

The occiput has undergone extreme demineralization while maintaining a normal shape. The demineralizing process is very active metabolically.

Assignment to a Possible Basic Entity

▶ **Normal variant or malformation?** No, this pattern is not known to occur as a normal variant or malformation.

▶ **Trauma?** The patient gave no history of mechanical trauma (see below Synopsis and Discussion for further details).

▶ **Inflammation?** There are no clinical manifestations of a bacterial inflammation. The absence of volume expansion is inconsistent with Paget disease (osteitis *deformans*). Thus, bone resorption has occurred without bone deformation.

▶ **Tumor?** No, the bone is demineralized but not destroyed. This excludes a brown tumor from the differential diagnosis. This is also an argument against angiomatosis or vanishing bone disease (see Case 11 and Case 54), as the bone is still present.

▶ **Perfusion disorder, etc.?** See Synopsis and Discussion below.

Synopsis and Discussion

After the differential diagnosis raised by the abnormal bone scan was narrowed on the basis of radiographic and CT findings, the only plausible remaining cause was an unexplained perfusion disorder which, when combined with secondary hyperparathyroidism, led to extreme occipital demineralization. The easiest way to determine this was by *asking the patient*. We discovered that, prior to his illness, he had worked in a coal-fired power plant for 5 years. His job was to measure the filling level of the coal by using a radioactive telecobalt source. In the course of his work, he was supposed to change his position relative to the telecobalt source at frequent intervals, alternating between the right and left sides. For convenience, and contrary to safety regulations, he did this by turning his head quickly to one side while in front of the source rather than changing sides behind the source. This maneuver resulted in greater relative exposure of the occiput to the cobalt gamma radiation. We estimate that he received a cumulative dose of approximately 0.2–2 Gy to the occiput. This dose is sufficient to increase regional vascularization and perfusion of the occipital bone (as an anatomic unit). In the setting of hyperparathyroidism, this greater blood flow led to excessive oc-

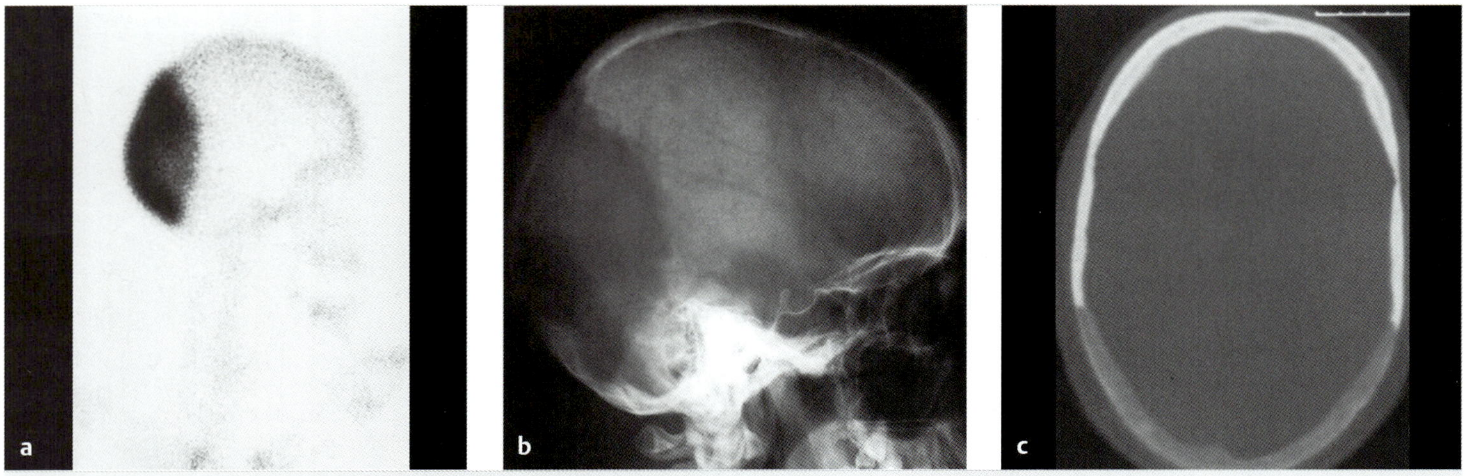

Fig. 2.30 a–c "Vanishing occiput."

cipital bone resorption accompanied by limited parathormone-induced resorption in the rest of the skull creating the typical pepper-pot or salt-and-pepper skull in hyperparathyroidism (see Case 15).

A follow-up radiograph of the skull after parathyroidectomy (▶ Fig. 2.31) showed complete remineralization of the occiput, proving that our pathogenetic hypothesis was correct.[22]

Final Diagnosis

The "black" occiput on the bone scan and the "vanished" occiput on the skull film resulted from the patient being a victim of radiation-induced excessive bone resorption in a setting of secondary hyperparathyroidism.

Comments

Often the simplest and most intelligent way to solve an unusual case is to ask the patient.

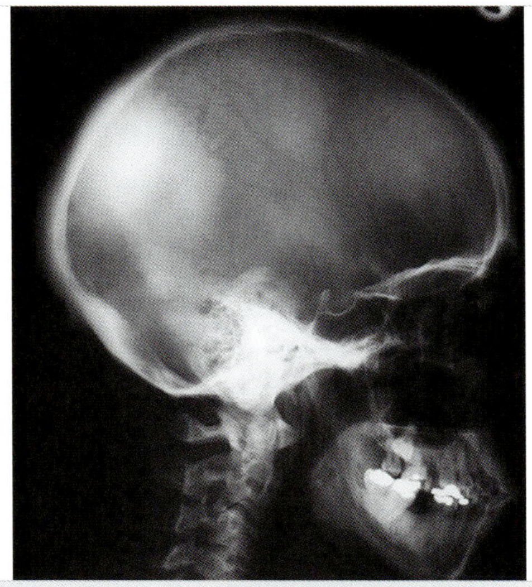

Fig. 2.31 Follow-up skull radiograph after parathyroidectomy in the patient with secondary hyperparathyroidism and a vanished occiput (see ▶ Fig. 2.30).

3 Spine

3.1 Mono- and Bisegmental Changes

Case 17 (▶ Fig. 3.1)

Case description

- Referring physician: radiologist.
- Prior history and clinical question: A 28-year-old man presented with posterior neck pain on yawning and occasional dysphagia with no other complaints. His personal and family history was otherwise normal. The referring radiologist submitted the MR images and requested identification of changes noted in the C1 and C2 vertebrae.

Radiologic Findings

The MR images after intravenous (IV) contrast administration (▶ Fig. 3.1 **a, b**) show lobulated masses with very low signal intensity located in and around the craniovertebral joints.

Location

Multicentric processes located in and around the bones of the craniovertebral joints.

Pathoanatomic Background of the Findings

The pathoanatomic background cannot reasonably be interpreted based on the MR images alone. Very likely, however, the findings represent an ossifying process.

Assignment to a Possible Basic Entity

Accurate interpretation of the MRI findings requires projection radiographs and CT scans using methods that directly visualize the bone (▶ Fig. 3.1 **c–e**).

▶ **Normal variant or malformation?** Yes. The lobulated masses are located in the right half of the atlas, the dens, and the right arch of the atlas. They are solid, smoothly marginated, and have no discernible soft-tissue component. They resemble a multicentric extra- and intraosseous osteoma that appears to *flow down* uniformly in and on the bone. This in itself suggests a diagnosis of melorheostosis.

▶ **Trauma?** No, the history is negative for trauma. Otherwise we might consider old myositis ossificans, but CT in that case would show spongy bone rather than compact bone (see Case 30). Moreover, myositis ossificans does not involve the interior of a bone.

▶ **Inflammation?** No, the history is negative and the process has no destructive features.

▶ **Tumor?** Solid ossifications do occur in paraosseous osteosarcoma, but this tumor is a more coherent mass that does not resemble flowing candle wax on the cortex. A classic paraosseous osteosarcoma is typically painful and occurs almost exclusively on the metaphyses and metadiaphyses of the long bones (see ▶ Fig. 7.27 in Case 144) with a predilection for the popliteal surface of the femur (50–70% of all cases). The involvement of two bones (in our case, C1 and C2) is extremely unusual. Also, the unilateral involvement does not suggest a tumor.

Synopsis and Discussion

The correct diagnosis is melorheostosis at a somewhat unusual location. Biopsy is unnecessary. The disease, associated with typical epi- and endosteal ossification, occurs sporadically and most likely results from a postzygotic mutation that interferes with embryonic metameric differentiation. This accounts for the typical *radial and segmental pattern of unilateral involvement*. The term "melorheostosis" is derived from the Greek *melos* (limb) and *rheos* (flow) and fittingly describes the characteristic finding of ossifications that appear to flow down the outer and inner sides of the involved bone. In over 60% of cases the disease is associated with variable skin lesions, subcutaneous fibrosis, muscle contractures, and vascular malformations. We described five different basic radiologic patterns in 23 cases,[23] and since then we have confirmed these results in more than 40 cases:

- Osteoma-like form
- Classic "flowing candle wax" form
- Myositis ossificans–like ossifications, especially near joints
- Osteopathia striata–like form
- Mixed forms

Two additional cases with an unusual spinal location are presented in ▶ Fig. 3.2 (47-year-old woman, incidental finding) and in ▶ Fig. 3.3 (30-year-old woman, incidental finding). Note again the *segmental unilateral distribution of the ossifications*.

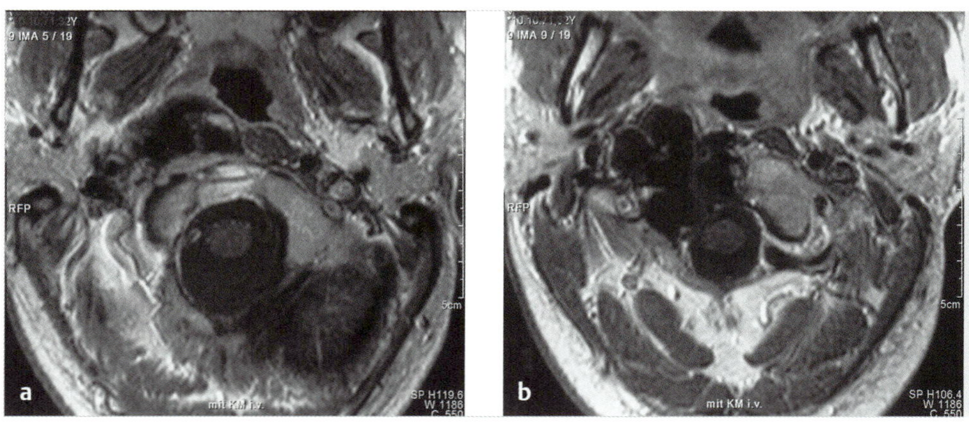

Fig. 3.1 a–e Unexplained findings on MRI in a 65-year-old woman.

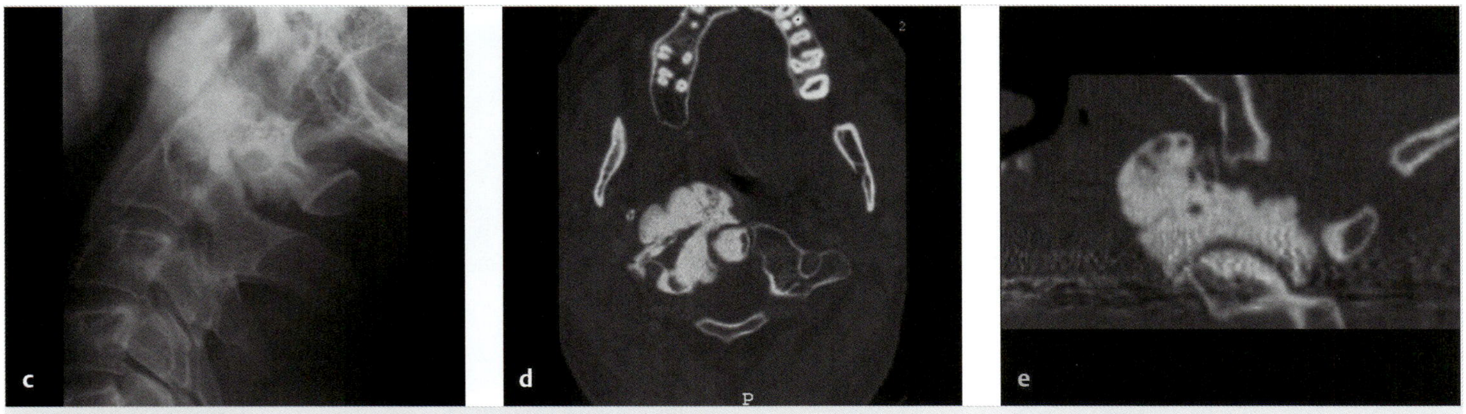

Fig. 3.1 (continued) Unexplained findings on MRI in a 65-year-old woman.

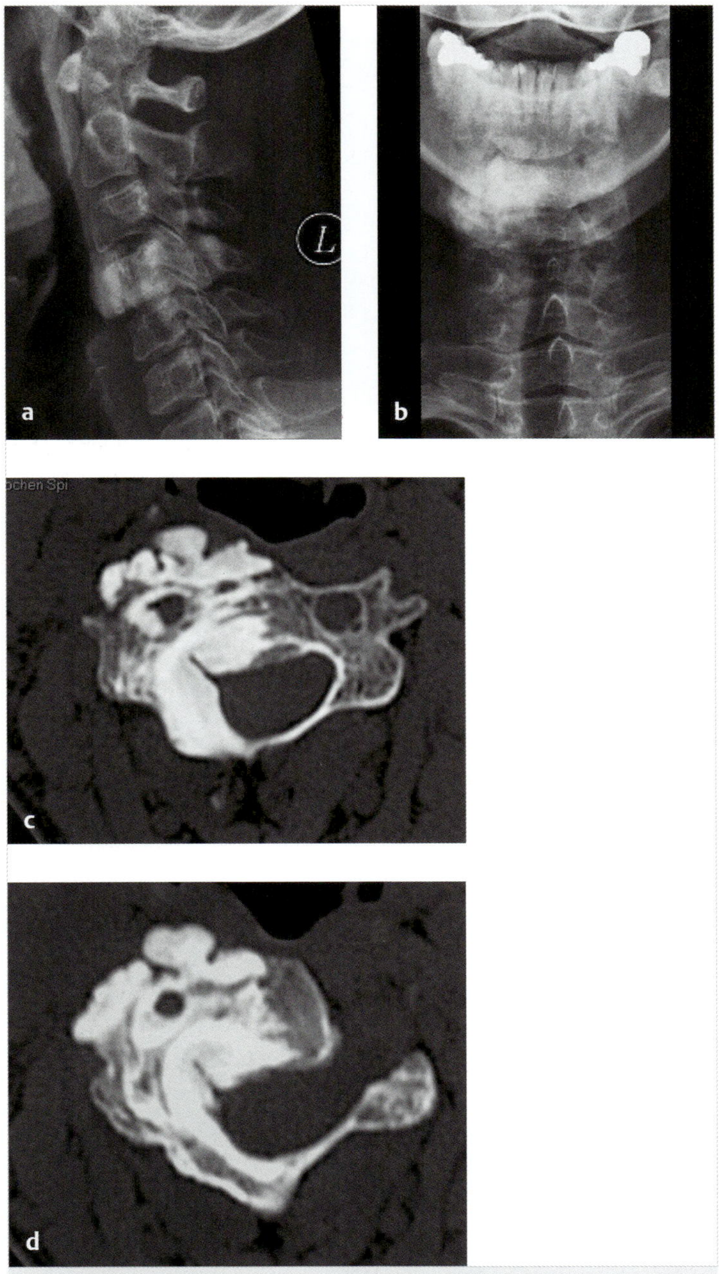

Fig. 3.2 a–d Melorheostosis in a 47-year-old woman.

Final Diagnosis

Melorheostosis in C1 and C2.

Comments

Lesions that correspond ontogenetically to specific anatomic structures (in this case a segmental, unilateral distribution of ossifications) are very suspicious for a developmental anomaly and make an inflammatory or neoplastic process unlikely. Because melorheostosis has a nonspecific histology, a correct radiologic diagnosis is of crucial importance!

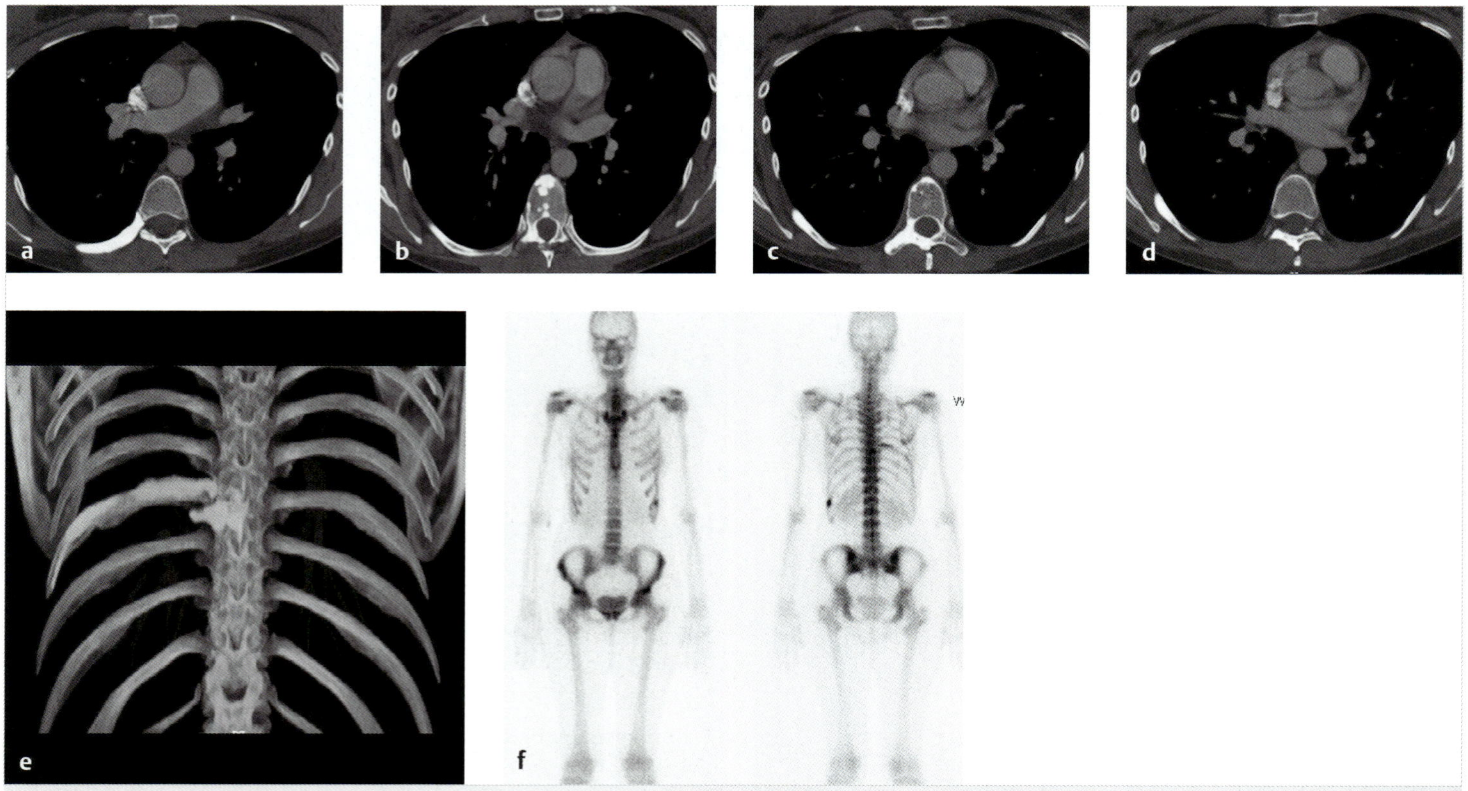

Fig. 3.3 a–f Melorheostosis in a 30-year-old woman

Case 18 (▶ Fig. 3.4)

Case description

- Referring physician: radiologist.
- Prior history and clinical question: A 57-year-old man underwent a routine checkup in which ultrasound detected a hepatic lesion (incidentaloma). Subsequent CT scans revealed (again incidentally) an intraosseous lesion in the T11 vertebral body. Further investigation of this lesion by CT, MRI, and scintigraphy raised suspicion of an atypical osteoma. The radiologist requested a consult to confirm this diagnosis.

Radiologic Findings

Whole-body bone scans (▶ Fig. 3.4 **a**) show moderately increased uptake in the T11 vertebra. Axial CT scans (▶ Fig. 3.4 **b, c**) show an extremely dense mass in T11 with small spicules radiating into the surrounding cancellous bone (▶ Fig. 3.4 **c**). As the sagittal (▶ Fig. 3.4 **d, e**) and coronal reformatted CT images (▶ Fig. 3.4 **f**) demonstrate, the "white" mass contains a bicentric lucent area, the upper portion of which has a sclerotic margin. The lucent area on CT shows increased signal intensity in the STIR (short-tau inversion recovery) sequence (▶ Fig. 3.4 **g**) and after IV contrast administration (▶ Fig. 3.4 **i**), while in T1-weighted (T1w) images (▶ Fig. 3.4 **h**) it is isointense to spinal cord. The signal intensity surrounding the mass is very slightly increased (▶ Fig. 3.4 **g**).

Location

The bony mass is located predominantly in the posterior half of T11. The lower portion of the lesion is located at the center of the vertebral body while its upper portion is more posterosuperior. The lower portion of the mass is very closely related to the nutrient canal (Hahn cleft) through which blood vessels enter and exit the vertebra.

Pathoanatomic Background of the Findings

The "white" mass on CT represents solid (compact) bone with very little bone turnover, as indicated by only moderately increased uptake on the bone scan. The lucencies in the mass may correspond to vascular structures.

Assignment to a Possible Basic Entity

▶ **Normal variant or malformation?** No, this type of entity is not known to occur as a normal variant. A smaller version of the lesion could be a bone island (enostosis), which is one of the most common incidental findings in skeletal radiology (see also Case 5).

▶ **Trauma?** No, the history is negative for spinal trauma.

▶ **Inflammation?** No, the lesion was detected incidentally and the history is negative.

▶ **Tumor or tumorlike lesion?** Yes, if we include osteoma and giant osteoma among the benign bone-forming tumors.

Synopsis and Discussion

The following findings are suggestive of a *giant osteoma:*

- Location in cancellous bone
- Very high lesion density consistent with compact bone in the trabecular meshwork (hence the term "bone island")
- Fine spicules that "anchor" the lesion in the cancellous bone
- Relatively low uptake on bone scintigraphy (small osteomas show no uptake at all, while larger lesions show low to moder-

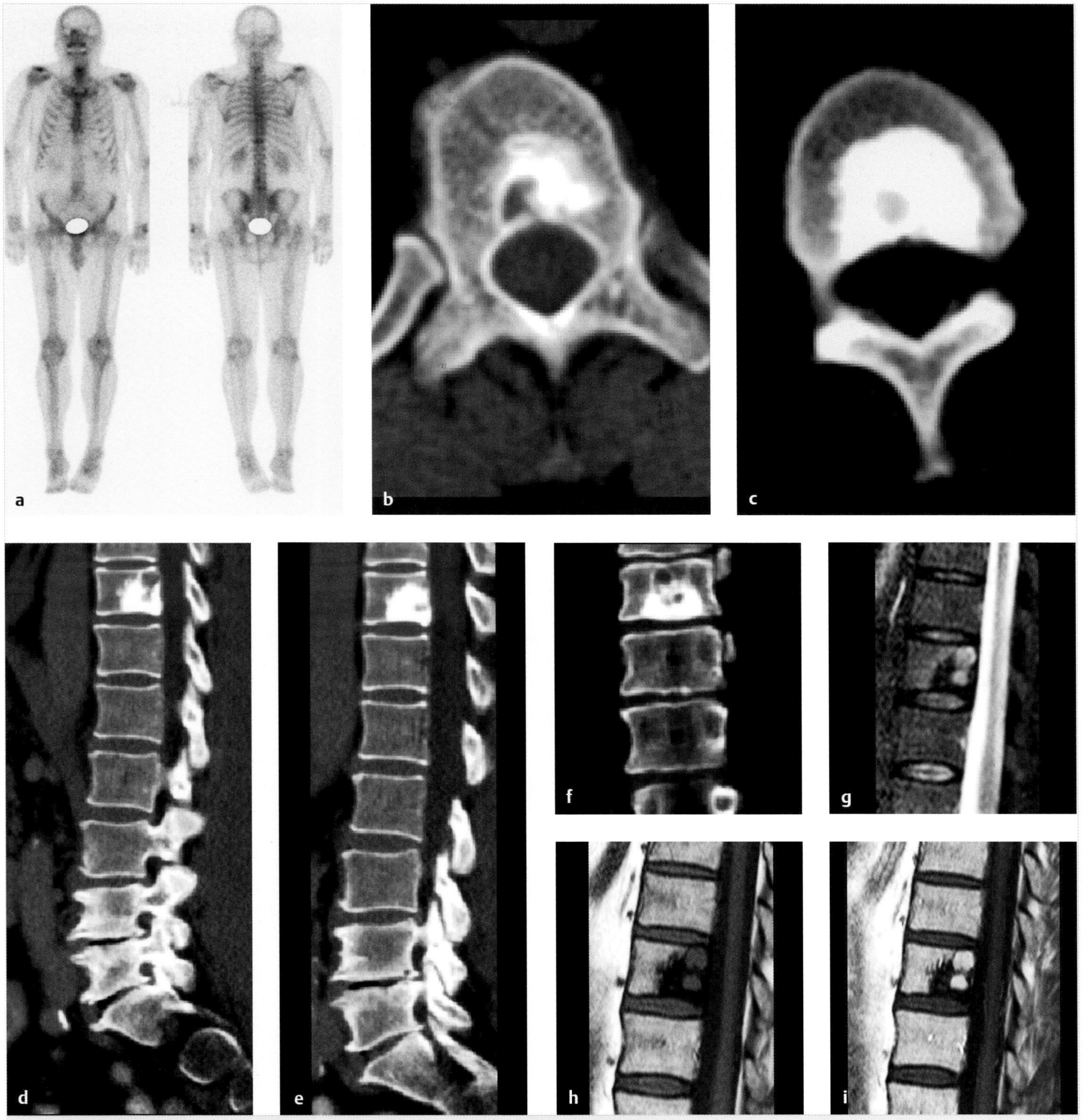

Fig. 3.4 a–i Metastasis?

ate uptake—even though the lesions participate in normal, continuous bone remodeling, but apparently at a low level)

- Incidental finding

The bicentric or dumbbell-shaped lucency in the lesion most likely represents vascular channels. It is not unusual to detect relatively large vessels in giant osteomas. In the present case they may be collateral vessels if we assume that the slow-growing osteoma occluded the central vascular system in the Hahn cleft. This could also account for the slightly increased signal intensity surrounding the osteoma, which may be interpreted as mild congestive edema.

We can exclude a *malignant bone-forming tumor* because the lesion is asymptomatic and shows only slight local bone metabolism. This means that the lesion does have a physiologic basic metabolism necessary for its nutrition but does not produce new tumorous bone—which would be a criterion for osteosarcoma, for example.

We might also consider *melorheostosis*, but this is not consistent with the central location of the lesion relative to the coronal plane. Melorheostosis also tends to be unilateral (see Case 17).

The lesion is too dense for a *giant notochordal hamartoma* (see Case 19).

A biopsy is unnecessary, especially since biopsies from lesions of such high density are generally nondiagnostic.

Final Diagnosis

Giant osteoma in T11, detected as an incidental finding.

Comments

A relatively large mass of compact bone density located within trabecular bone is generally a large osteoma, especially if it is detected incidentally and shows little tracer uptake on bone scans. Giant osteomas may contain vascular channels.

Case 19 (▶ Fig. 3.5)

Case description

- Referring physician: radiologist.
- Prior history and clinical question: A 55-year-old woman underwent a "routine MRI" of the cervical spine, which showed a signal abnormality in C2. Further investigation by CT and ^{18}F-FDG PET showed changes that were suspicious for, among other things, a giant notochordal hamartoma.

Radiologic Findings

C2 has no signal in the T1w image (▶ Fig. 3.5 **a**). It is minimally hyperintense to adjacent vertebral bodies in the T2w image (▶ Fig. 3.5 **b**) but shows uniformly high signal intensity in the coronal STIR image (▶ Fig. 3.5 **c**). C2 appears sclerotic on sagittal CT (▶ Fig. 3.5 **d**). It appears as a cold lesion on ^{18}F-FDG PET (arrow in ▶ Fig. 3.5 **e**, which is a magnified view from ▶ Fig. 3.5 **f**).

Location

Lesion is confined to C2.

Pathoanatomic Background of the Findings

C2 has become involved by a process associated with new bone formation (reactive, reparative, tumor matrix?). The fact that the process is negative on ^{18}F-FDG PET suggests that it is now inactive and that the sclerotic changes are old (no regional increase in blood flow, no measurable regional bone turnover). The sclerosis must still have an active soft-tissue component, however, otherwise we could not explain the relative proton abundance on MRI.

Assignment to a Possible Basic Entity

▶ **Normal variant or malformation?** This type of finding has not been previously described as a normal variant or malformation.

▶ **Trauma?** No, the patient gave no trauma history.

▶ **Inflammation?** Yes, in principle. The findings may result from an old, nonspecific, nondestructive inflammatory process that healed with sclerosis. But this does not necessarily explain the relative abundance of protons in C2, which is also at odds with the negative bone scan.

▶ **Tumor?** Yes, and apparently an inactive one. It could be a nonaggressive tumor that has caused reactive sclerosis. The negative bone scan indicates that the sclerosis is old or is smoldering "at a low flame." Tumor tissue must still be present, however, due to the relative abundance of protons in water-sensitive MRI sequences. Thus, the findings basically point to a benign tumor. The location within a vertebral body suggests a tumor of notochordal origin. While a "white" vertebral body is always suspicious for malignant lymphoma, the negative bone scan and absence of clinical complaints essentially rule out this diagnosis.

▶ **Perfusion disorder?** Old, nonfragmented foci of osteonecrosis may present with osteosclerosis with no shape distortion of the affected bone. This does not explain the relative proton abundance of the lesion in C2, however.

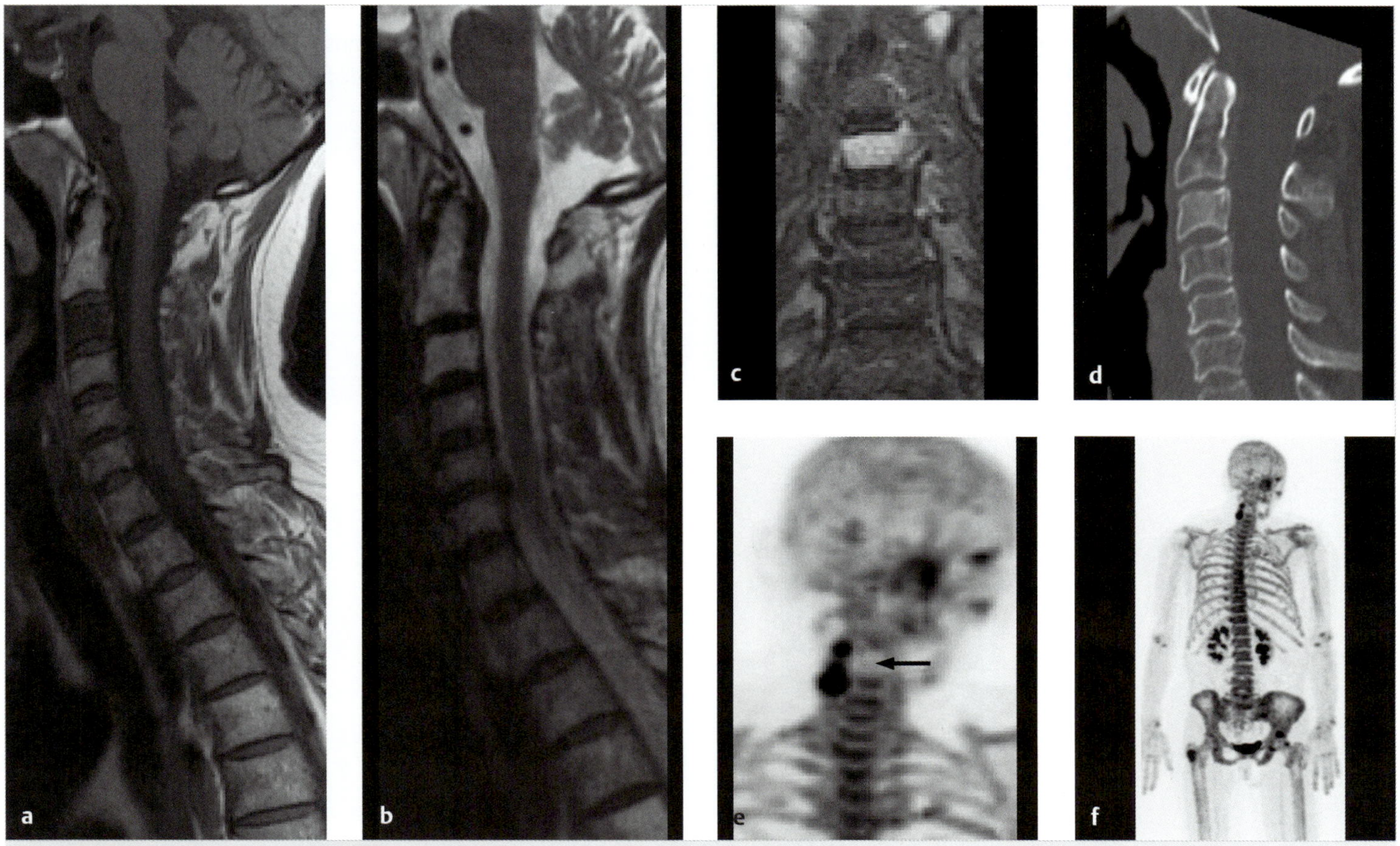

Fig. 3.5 a–f More than just a metastasis?

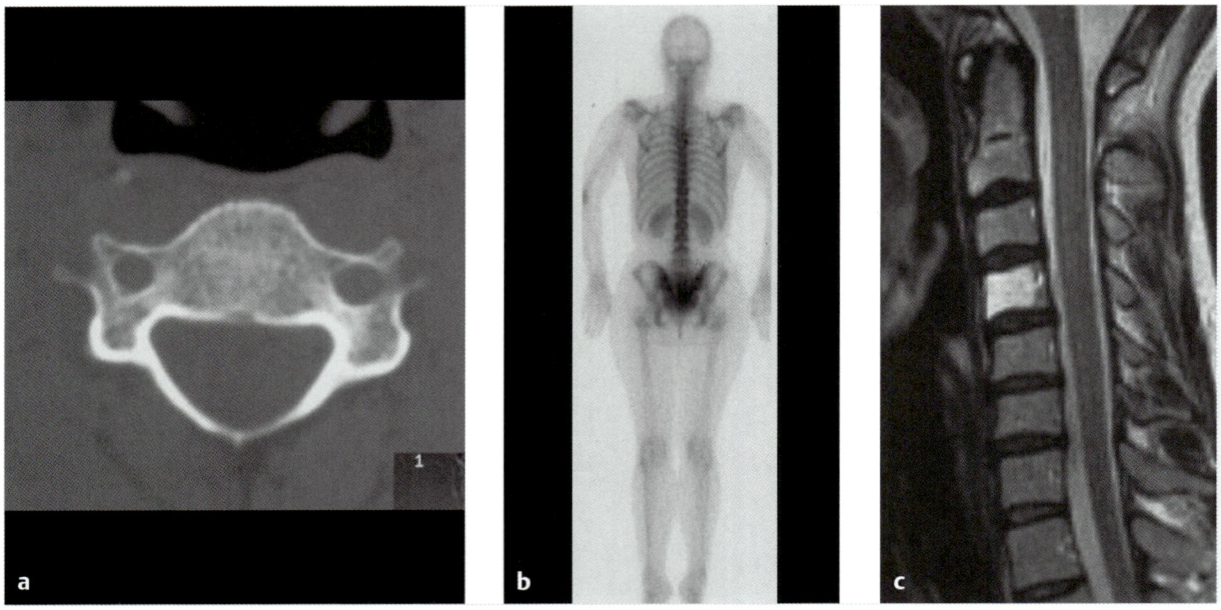

Fig. 3.6 a–c Giant notochordal hamartoma in C4.

Synopsis and Discussion

The following triad is very specific for a *giant notochordal hamartoma* as described by Mirra and Brien[24]:

1. Negative ^{18}F-FDG PET-CT or negative ^{99m}Tc-MDP bone scan
2. Osteosclerosis in a vertebral body
3. Absence of T1w signal intensity plus high T2w signal intensity (in the case of moderate sclerosis)

The authors interpret these tumors as notochordal lesions which, unlike the harmless notochordal rests that occur as normal variants, tend to grow until puberty, may occupy an entire vertebral body by their end stage, but then stop growing and do not cause destructive changes like a true chordoma. The two cases observed by the authors were very similar histologically to chordomas but did not meet all the criteria for true chordoma. Thus they were merely followed for a long period of time without showing any radiologic change. Yamaguchi et al.[25] refer to this lesion as a *benign intraosseous notochordal cell tumor* to express its neoplastic nature. This means that these lesions should be closely followed to allow for prompt detection of possible malignant transformation, making them similar in behavior to large enchondromas in large bones. Kyriakos (2011)[26] has published a review of benign notochordal lesions. To date we have seen five patients with these lesions and have advised long-term observation (yearly MRI follow-ups), without histologic confirmation. The differential diagnosis should include nonfragmented osteonecrosis, which we have seen with identical radiologic findings—also in a cervical vertebral body—and had histologically confirmed in a patient with a history of pancreatitis. This case explains our wait-and-see approach for a lesion that exhibits the above triad in a vertebral body.

► Fig. 3.6 illustrates another case of giant notochordal hamartoma drawn from our files. This lesion was located in the C4 vertebra and was also detected incidentally.

Final Diagnosis

High index of suspicion for a giant notochordal hamartoma in C2. Long-term clinical and radiologic follow-up is recommended.

Comments

When faced with unusual incidental findings, one should be well-prepared enough to consider even an unusual diagnosis.

Case 20 (▶ Fig. 3.7)

Case description

- Referring physician: oncologist.
- Prior history and clinical question: A 47-year-old woman with breast cancer had undergone mastectomy, postoperative radiation to the chest wall, and tamoxifen therapy. Her bone scan showed circumscribed uptake in the C5 spinous process, which was considered suspicious for metastasis. Subsequent MRI upheld this suspicion, and a percutaneous biopsy under CT guidance was recommended. The biopsy was terminated due to severe pain, but CT scans acquired during the procedure cast doubt on the diagnosis of metastasis. A repeat biopsy was still recommended, but the patient refused. The treating oncologist then requested our radiologic consultation.

Radiologic Findings

The T2w MR image in ▶ Fig. 3.7 **a** shows a nonspecific expansion of the C5 spinous process. The other sequences added no information except for the finding of moderate contrast enhancement. The CT scans (▶ Fig. 3.7 **b–d**), which directly visualize bone, show harmonious expansion of the fifth spinous process and adjacent portions of the vertebral arch with intact contours. The normal cancellous bone as in the vertebral body has been replaced by an ossified material with a ground-glass pattern. The small white dots within the material in ▶ Fig. 3.7 **c** may represent a cartilaginous calcification pattern. The bone scan (not pictured here) showed circumscribed tracer uptake in the C5 spinous process.

Pathoanatomic Background of the Findings

The circumscribed uptake on the bone scan signifies an active process. The only notable MRI finding is expansion of the C5 spinous process. CT shows that the spinous process is structurally altered but not destroyed. The ground-glass pattern suggests that normal bone has been replaced by woven bone and that this change has been present for some time (harmonious expansion).

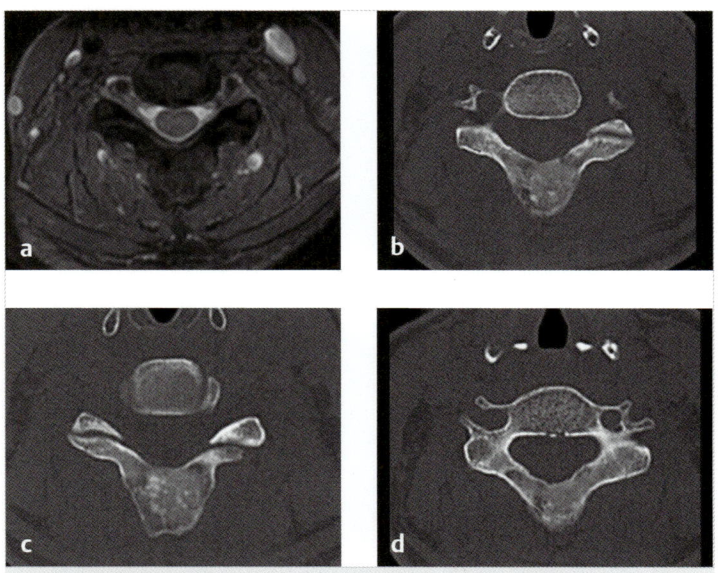

Fig. 3.7 a–d Metastasis from breast cancer?

Location

The lesion is solitary by bone scintigraphy. It is not located in a region rich in bone marrow, where metastases principally tend to occur.

Assignment to a Possible Basic Entity

▶ **Normal variant or malformation?** No. The positive bone scan indicates an active process. Most normal variants are negative on bone scans unless, for example, they interfere with activities in a way that incites reactive new bone formation. But then they would probably be symptomatic. We are unaware of a comparable malformation.

▶ **Trauma?** No, there is no trauma history. The lesion is an incidental finding!

▶ **Tumor?** The patient is at increased risk for metastasis, but this location is not typical (see Location above). The absence of apparent destructive changes is not consistent with a malignant process. The harmonious expansion of the affected bone and the ground-glass appearance are proof of a harmless connective-tissue lesion.

Synopsis and Discussion

The above findings and their interpretation immediately suggest fibrous dysplasia in the posterior elements of C5. This is supported by the following:

- Incidental finding.
- Lesion morphology: The expansion is harmonious and is accompanied by ground-glass pattern and cartilaginous deposits.
- Solitary occurrence: Foci of fibrous dysplasia are usually solitary.

Several factors do not support a diagnosis of metastasis:

- Incidental finding.
- Solitary occurrence at a highly atypical site. Metastatic involvement of a spinous process (which contains little bone marrow) would ordinarily occur only in a patient with disseminated disease.
- Lesion morphology: A metastasis should present as an osteosclerotic (osteoblastic) lesion, which would be more irregular or sclerotic and would not cause harmonious bone expansion. Only a previously osteolytic and irradiated metastasis could develop a fibrous dysplasia–like morphology, but that is not the case here.

To aid differentiation, ▶ Fig. 3.8 shows the case of a 79-year-old man with another incidentally detected lesion, this time in L3. The volume expansion and ground-glass pattern are virtually pathognomonic for fibrous dysplasia. The honeycomb component is caused by vascular channels and may represent residua from an earlier hyperperfusion phase or a vascular process within fibrous dysplasia. We can definitely exclude an active vascular process, since that would have produced symptoms, especially given the very pronounced encroachment on the spinal canal.

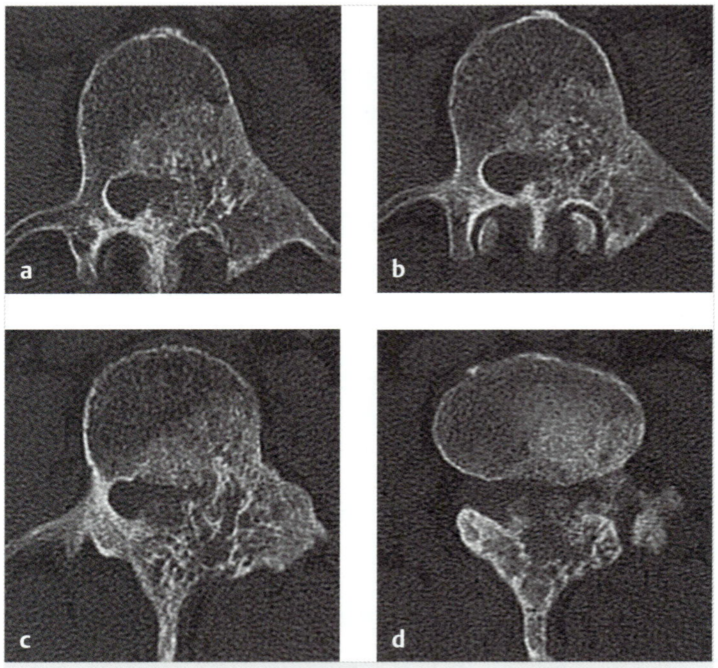

Fig. 3.8 a–d Fibrous dysplasia in L3.

Comments

When a solitary focus of moderately increased uptake in a cervical spinous process is noted incidentally on a whole-body bone scan in a breast cancer patient, it is highly unlikely that the lesion is metastatic. MRI is not a useful adjunct to the bone scan in this case because the bone information supplied by MRI is not very specific (see Chapter 1). CT is better for this purpose as it gives direct visualization of bone details and evokes the "engram" that calls fibrous dysplasia to mind: harmonious expansion of a bone or bone segment with a ground-glass pattern. Biopsy confirmation is unnecessary, nor is there a need for radiologic follow-up as long as the patient remains asymptomatic.

Final Diagnosis

Fibrous dysplasia with cartilaginous components in the posterior elements (arch and spinous process) of C5, detected incidentally.

Case 21 (▶ Fig. 3.9)

Case description

- *Referral:* The patient herself wanted a second opinion.
- *Prior history and clinical question:* A 32-year-old woman had a 2-year history of increasing posterior neck pain ("at lower right") that was resistant to medication. Projection radiographs were unrewarding. MR images (not shown here) were interpreted as showing "edema" in C5. Further investigation by scintigraphy and CT led to a presumptive diagnosis of osteochondroma.

Radiologic Findings

The bone scan (▶ Fig. 3.9 **a**, posteroanterior) shows a focus of intense uptake in C6 just to the right of the midline. Intense uptake was already noted on early images (not pictured here). Axial CT scans (▶ Fig. 3.9 **b, c**) show a round defect on the right posterolateral side of C5 that contains an irregularly ossified structure. The lesion is also clearly displayed in coronal (▶ Fig. 3.9 **d**) and sagittal (▶ Fig. 3.9 **e**) reformatted sections.

Location

The defect has an eccentric location in a vertebral body.

Pathoanatomic Background of the Findings

The most likely pathoanatomic interpretation is neoplastic destruction with an ossified matrix filling the defect. A sequestrum associated with sypondylitis or eosinophilic granuloma, for example, would have an amorphous structure quite unlike the relatively ordered structure of the ossifications seen in this case (see also Case 24 and Case 35).

Assignment to a Possible Basic Entity

▶ **Normal variant or malformation?** No, they are not known to occur in this form. The clinical presentation is also inconsistent with a normal variant or malformation.

▶ **Trauma?** No history.

▶ **Inflammation?** No, this does not fit the clinical presentation. Spondylitis with a sequestrum of this size would produce much more severe symptoms with a shorter history. Also, imaging would show pronounced marginal sclerosis around the defect.

▶ **Tumor?** Yes, specifically a bone-forming tumor.

Synopsis and Discussion

The most likely diagnosis is osteoblastoma for the following reasons:

- The history is relatively long; this would not be characteristic of osteoid osteoma or osteosarcoma.
- The lesion is approximately 1.5 cm in diameter, which is the cut-off between osteoid osteoma and osteoblastoma (the larger variant of osteoid osteoma), especially if the tumor is located in the spine.
- The ossification pattern indicates a bony matrix.
- The multiphase bone scan indicates a very well-perfused tumor. This is typical of osteoblastoma.

The following factors do not support a diagnosis of osteochondroma:

- CT does not demonstrate a stalk.
- The ossification pattern does not fit. The main body of an osteochondroma generally consists of well-differentiated cancellous bone, with ingrowth into adjacent bone creating a sclerotic

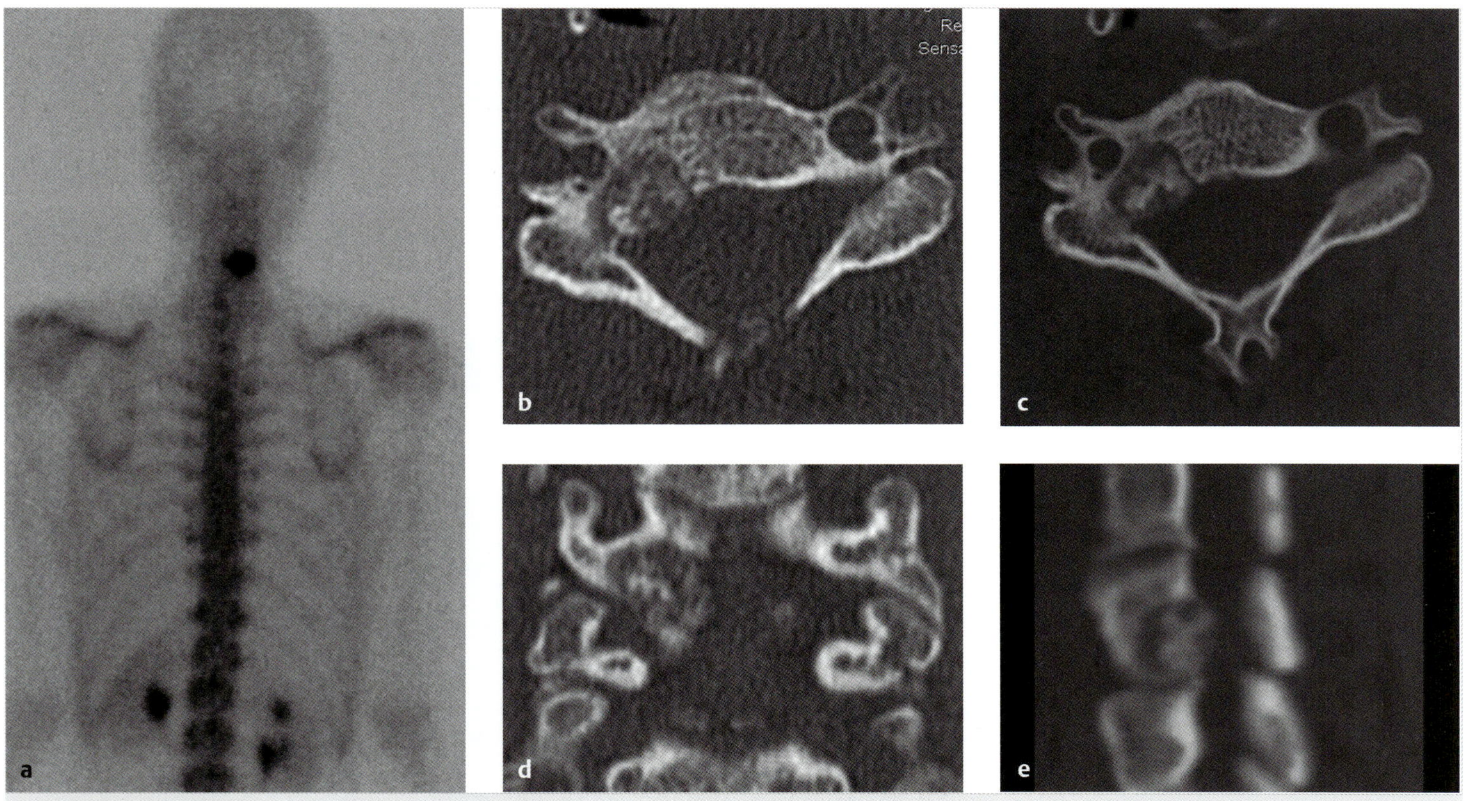

Fig. 3.9 a–e A simple case?

margin. Imaging (CT) shows a translucent gap between the sclerotic margin and the outer contour of the osteochondroma, which represents a cartilaginous cap.

The diagnosis was established preoperatively by CT-guided percutaneous biopsy, followed by an en bloc resection of the tumor (Prof. Harms, Langensteinbach).

Final Diagnosis

Osteoblastoma in C5.

Comments

A well-perfused tumor that is located in a vertebral body or its appendages and forms an ossifying matrix is most likely an osteoblastoma when detected in a younger patient. Approximately one-third of all osteoblastomas occur in the spine.

Case 22 (▶ Fig. 3.10)

Case description

- *Referring physician:* pediatric oncologist.
- *Prior history and clinical question:* A 14-year-old girl in puberty complained of unpleasant "sensations" in the back of her neck. MRI was ordered "as a precaution." Physical examination showed no abnormalities. MRI incidentally revealed a lesion in T1 that was not further specified. The worried parents sought advice from a very experienced pediatric oncologist, who in turn consulted us.

Radiologic Findings

The T1w images (▶ Fig. 3.10 **a, d**) show a slightly hyperintense area in the anterior portion of T1. It is very hyperintense in the T2w image (▶ Fig. 3.10 **b**) and enhances after contrast administration (▶ Fig. 3.10 **c, e**). ▶ Fig. 3.10 **e** shows linear structures that may be interpreted as vessels. This description of findings is strongly suggestive of an active hemangioma. Several low-dose CT scans through C7 and T1 (▶ Fig. 3.10 **f–i**) were additionally obtained in order to calm the parents and because "something needed to be done" (*ut aliquid fiat*). In any case, the familiar engram of a "honeycomb pattern with the presence of intralesional fat" suggests the diagnosis of hemangioma and increases diagnostic confidence. Indeed, CT revealed a honeycomb pattern in the suspected finding on T1w images (arrows in ▶ Fig. 3.10 **f**). The interspaces contain fine fatty structures that explain the T1w imaging appearance.

Location

The lesion occupies an eccentric location in a vertebral body.

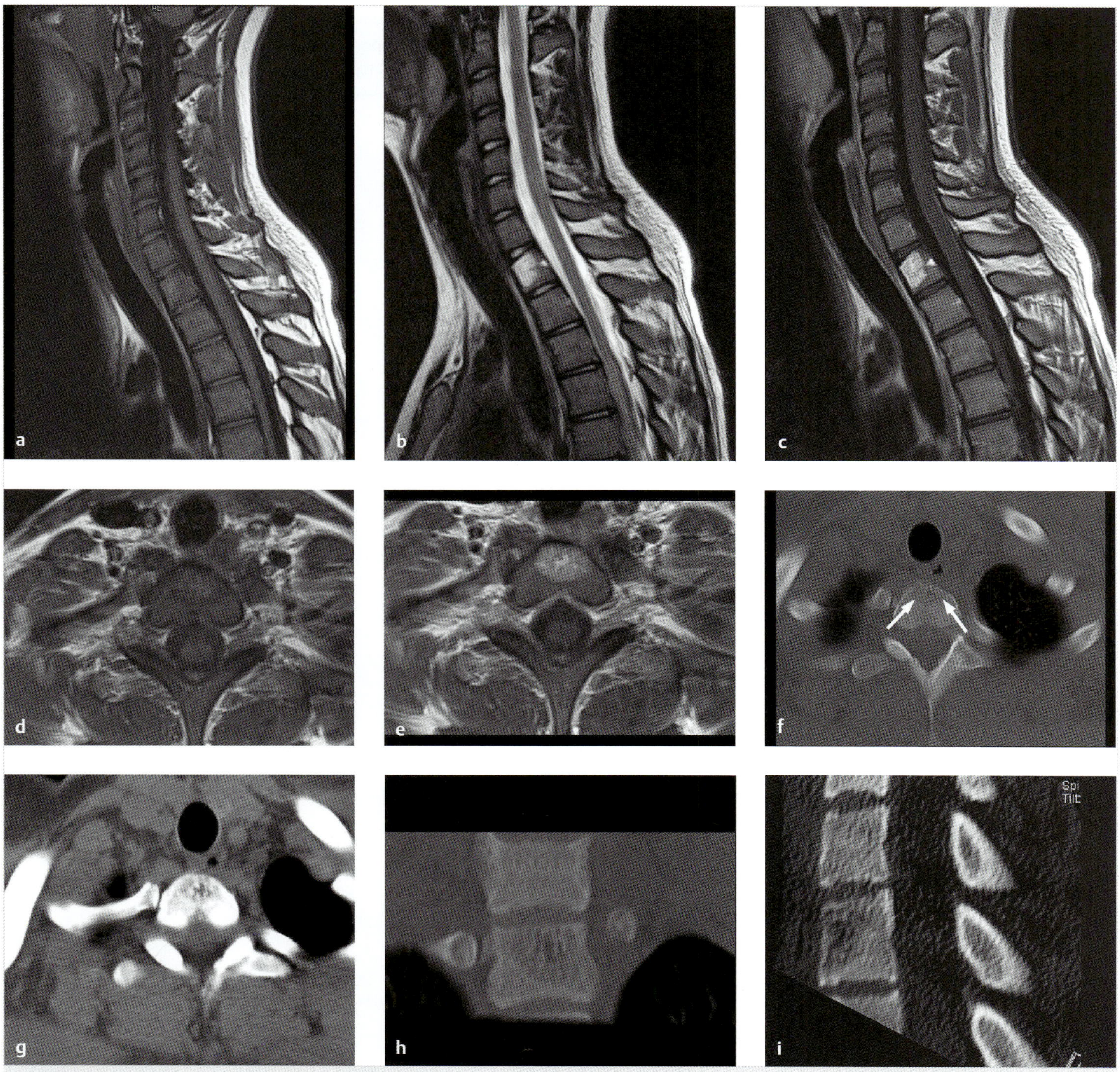

Fig. 3.10 a–i Unexplained findings on MRI.

Pathoanatomic Background of the Findings

Well-perfused intracancellous lesion that contains fat—probably hemangioma.

Assignment to a Possible Basic Entity

▸ **Normal variant or malformation?** Probably, since hemangiomas in the spine or their outcome, a hemangiomatous vertebra ("war memorial"), are very often noted as incidental findings (in approximately one-third of all MRI examinations of the spine).

Synopsis and Discussion

All findings are consistent with a still-active hemangioma in T1:

- Incidental finding
- Intralesional fat on T1w images and CT
- Circumscribed honeycomb pattern on CT
- Subtle vascular structures and marked enhancement on post-contrast MRI

We assume that most congenital hemangiomas in the bone, especially in the spine, spontaneously regress by puberty, like hemangiomas in the skin. What remains is rarefied cancellous bone with residual trabeculae that may show compensatory thickening with interspersed fatty proliferation (vacuum fat), resulting in the "war memorial" of a hemangiomatous vertebra. Regression of the vascular structures follows a variable timetable from one case to the next. In our case we assume that the regression is not yet complete; the hemangioma is still active, therefore. Active angiomatous lesions that do not appear until adulthood and are usually symptomatic would consist of either vascular malformations or one of the multiple lesions of hemangiomatosis (see also Case 154). There is no need to proceed with histologic evaluation in the present case.

Final Diagnosis

Still-active hemangioma in the T1 vertebra.

Comments

MRI examinations that are defensively motivated and do not have a strict medical indication may "uncover" incidental findings that initiate a chain of additional tests. When the imaging findings are interpreted, it is important to consider that we are dealing with incidental findings in an asymptomatic individual (not a patient!).

Case 23 (▶ Fig. 3.11)

Case description

- Referring physician: neurosurgeon.
- Prior history and clinical question: A 17-year-old male presented with low back pain of acute onset. Based on imaging findings, the neurosurgeon formulated a differential diagnosis consisting of "intravertebral disk herniation, chordoma, or spondylodiskitis." The young man was otherwise in good health and showed no inflammatory markers.

Radiologic Findings

On MRI the L4–L5 intervertebral disk (▶ Fig. 3.11 **a, b**) shows significant morphologic change and is decreased in height. Hyperintense material has tracked upward from the L4–L5 disk space through a defect in the lower endplate in the cancellous bone of L4, where it has formed a globular mass of high signal intensity, isointense to the healthy disks. There is a marked posterior protrusion of nucleus pulposus at L4–L5, also significant edema-like signal throughout L4 and a thin area of edema-like signal beneath the anterior upper endplate of L5. Axial CT (▶ Fig. 3.11 **c**) shows a gross defect located close to the L4 lower endplate surrounded by a somewhat diffuse area of sclerosis.

Location

The principal lesions visible in the L4–L5 intervertebral disk space and in the lower portion of L4 are in close topographic relation to one another.

Pathoanatomic Background of the Findings

Given the close topographic relation of the disk lesion to the intraosseous defect, it is not difficult to interpret the findings as an intravertebral disk herniation.

Assignment to a Possible Basic Entity

▶ **Normal variant or malformation?** No, the clinical presentation alone would refute this interpretation.

▶ **Trauma?** No prior history.

▶ **Inflammation?** No. The young patient has no signs of spondylodiskitis such as a long pain history, serum inflammatory markers, etc. Moreover, there are no signs of diskitis.

▶ **Tumor?** Yes, if it is assumed that a subchondral lesion broke through the lower endplate and caused secondary intralesional disk herniation. But what kind of tumor would do this?

▶ **Degeneration?** Very likely, since the imaging findings strongly suggest an intravertebral disk herniation.

Synopsis and Discussion

Overall, the following findings are consistent with an unusually large, two-stage internal *disk herniation:*

- Low back pain of sudden onset
- Gross degeneration of the L4–L5 intervertebral disk
- Direct relationship between the hyperintense track in the disk space and the globular isointense mass in the defect in the

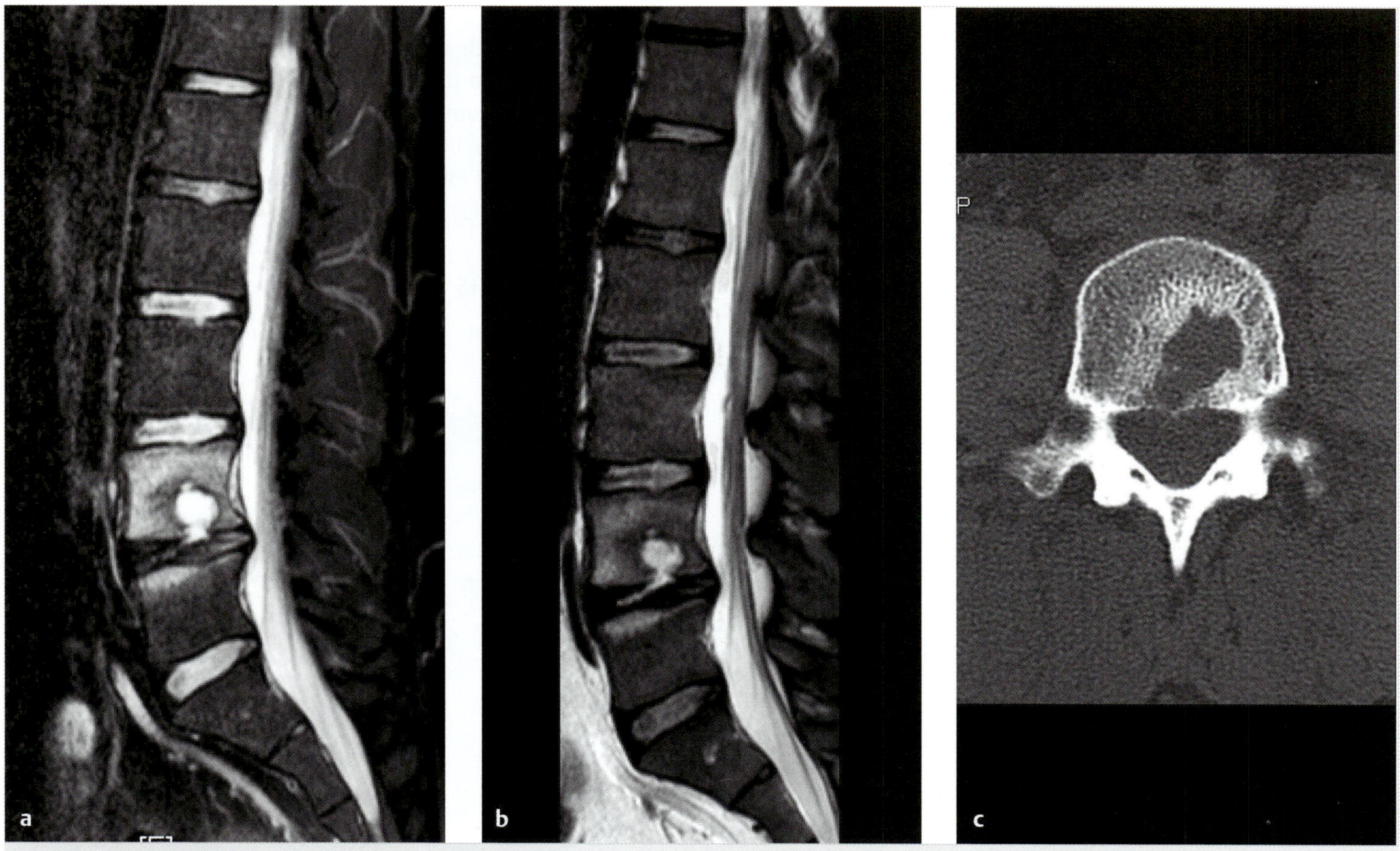

Fig. 3.11 a–c Metastatic destruction?

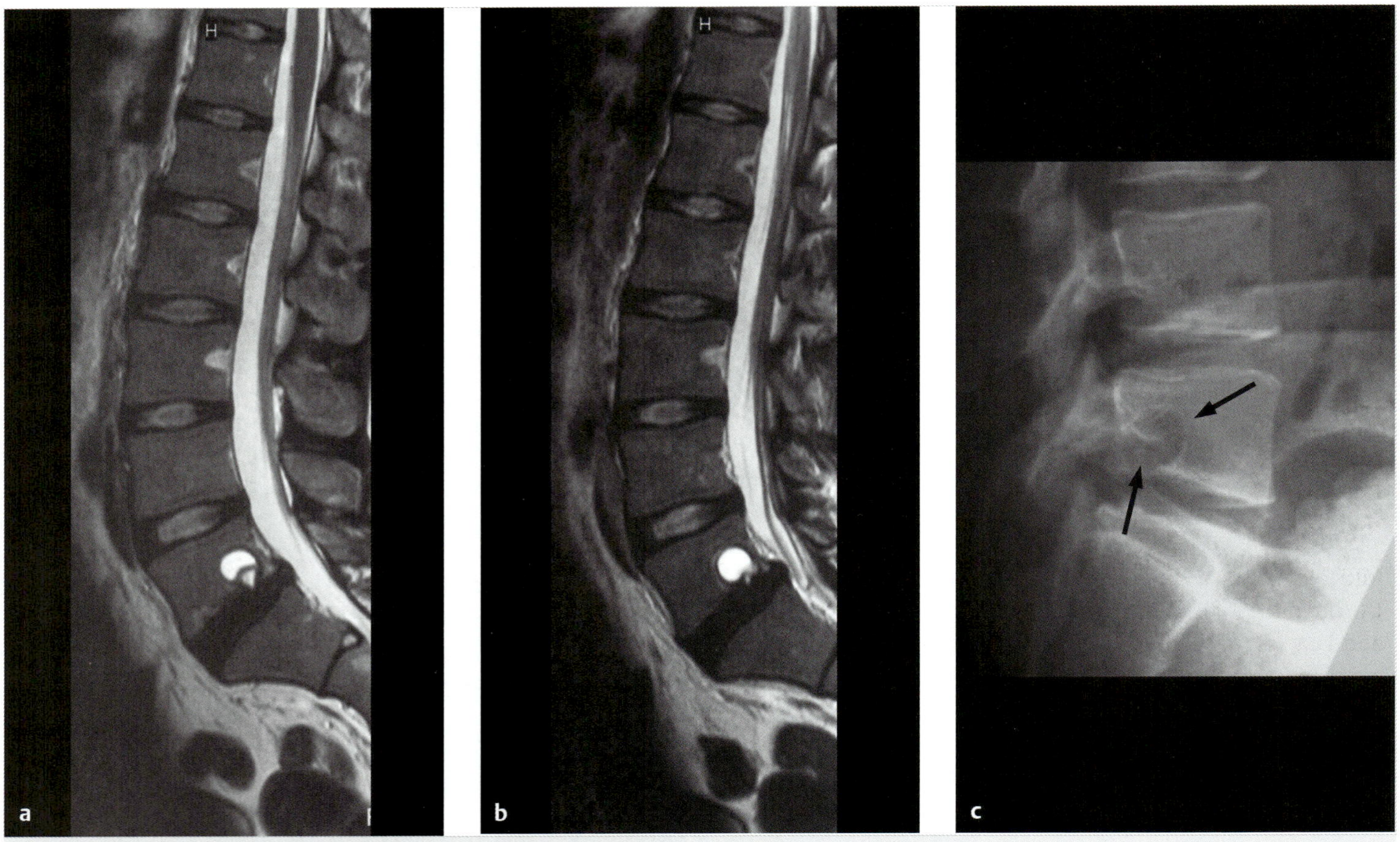

Fig. 3.12 a–c Intraosseous ganglion in a 24-year-old man.

lower portion of L4, apparently representing freshly herniated disk material (the high MRI signal is isointense to the other healthy disk spaces)
- Gross associated edema-like signal in L4
- Posterior protrusion of nucleus pulposus at L4–L5 suggesting a propensity for degenerative disk disease

Degeneration of the L4–L5 intervertebral disk must have been present for some time. This would explain the sclerosis under the perforated lower endplate of L4. At the same time, however, a degenerative defect must have formed in the lower endplate allowing a kind of ganglion (see also ▶ Fig. 3.12) to form in the adjacent cancellous bone. The nucleus pulposus then herniated "in two stages" through the pre-existing defect.

Chordoma is unlikely because this tumor generally respects the adjacent intervertebral disk and tends to break through the side of the affected vertebral body, spread by upward or downward paravertebral extension, and then invades an adjacent vertebra. Chordoma originates from ectopic chordal tissue in a vertebral body, never from the nucleus pulposus. The peak age incidence of chordomas is in the fifth and sixth decades, although the tumor may occur at any age.

The last diagnosis to be considered is a *neoplastic process* that has spread from L4 to the adjacent disk space, but this is inconsistent with the tracklike spread of the presumed tumor tissue in the L4–L5 disk space (see also Case 24).

The case was treated surgically and the diagnosis was confirmed histologically.

For comparison, ▶ Fig. 3.12 shows an intraosseous ganglion, a tumorlike lesion with a fibrous wall and gelatinous contents. This lesion develops from the coalescence of smaller "cysts," which in turn arise from myxomatous degeneration of the subchondral tissue or in adjacent structures. In the case shown, the 24-year-old man had occasional low back pain, which may or may not have been caused by the ganglion.

Final Diagnosis

Gross, two-stage intravertebral disk herniation (deep Schmorl node) in L4.

Comments

An intravertebral disk herniation should always be considered in the differential diagnosis of destructive changes in a vertebral body located near the intervertebral disk.

Case 24 (▶ Fig. 3.13)

Case description

- Referring physician: neurosurgeon.
- Prior history and clinical question: A 46-year-old man had a 5-month history of back pain that did not radiate in a radicular pattern. MRI of the lumbar spine showed an abnormality in L4 that was interpreted as "suspicious for metastatic lung cancer," as the patient was a heavy smoker. Subsequent thoracic CT revealed "pulmonary nodules." Open biopsy of the L4 lesion was performed at a different institution specializing in tumor surgery but was inconclusive. The current attending neurosurgeon wants a diagnosis.

Radiologic Findings

MRI demonstrates a mass below the collapsed upper endplate of L4. The mass is isointense to the adjacent disk tissue in both T1w and T2w images (▶ Fig. 3.13 **a, b**), and the disk shows severe degenerative changes. ▶ Fig. 3.13 **b** shows a connection between the intracancellous mass and the nucleus pulposus. This connection is clearly documented in the coronal STIR image (▶ Fig. 3.13 **c**), showing high signal intensity in the water-sensitive sequence. Axial CT scans (▶ Fig. 3.13 **d–f**) demonstrate a gross subchondral defect, with panel "d" showing a "sequestrum" inside the defect. CT scans through the upper lung zones (▶ Fig. 3.13 **g**) show multiple very fine nodules, especially in the right lung, which on closer scrutiny are found to contain small central lucencies.

Location

Much as in Case 23, the principal lesions in the L3–L4 disk space and the upper portion of L4 are in close topographic relation to one another.

Pathoanatomic Background of the Findings

As in Case 23, there is the strong impression of a primary internal disk herniation, but the imaging findings may also reflect a primarily neoplastic or other destructive process in L4 which destroyed the L4 upper endplate prior to causing an intravertebral disk herniation. The pulmonary foci may represent Langerhans-cell histiocytosis and are actually typical of that disease.

Assignment to a Possible Basic Entity

▶ **Normal variant or malformation?** No, a normal variant or malformation is not known to occur in this form.

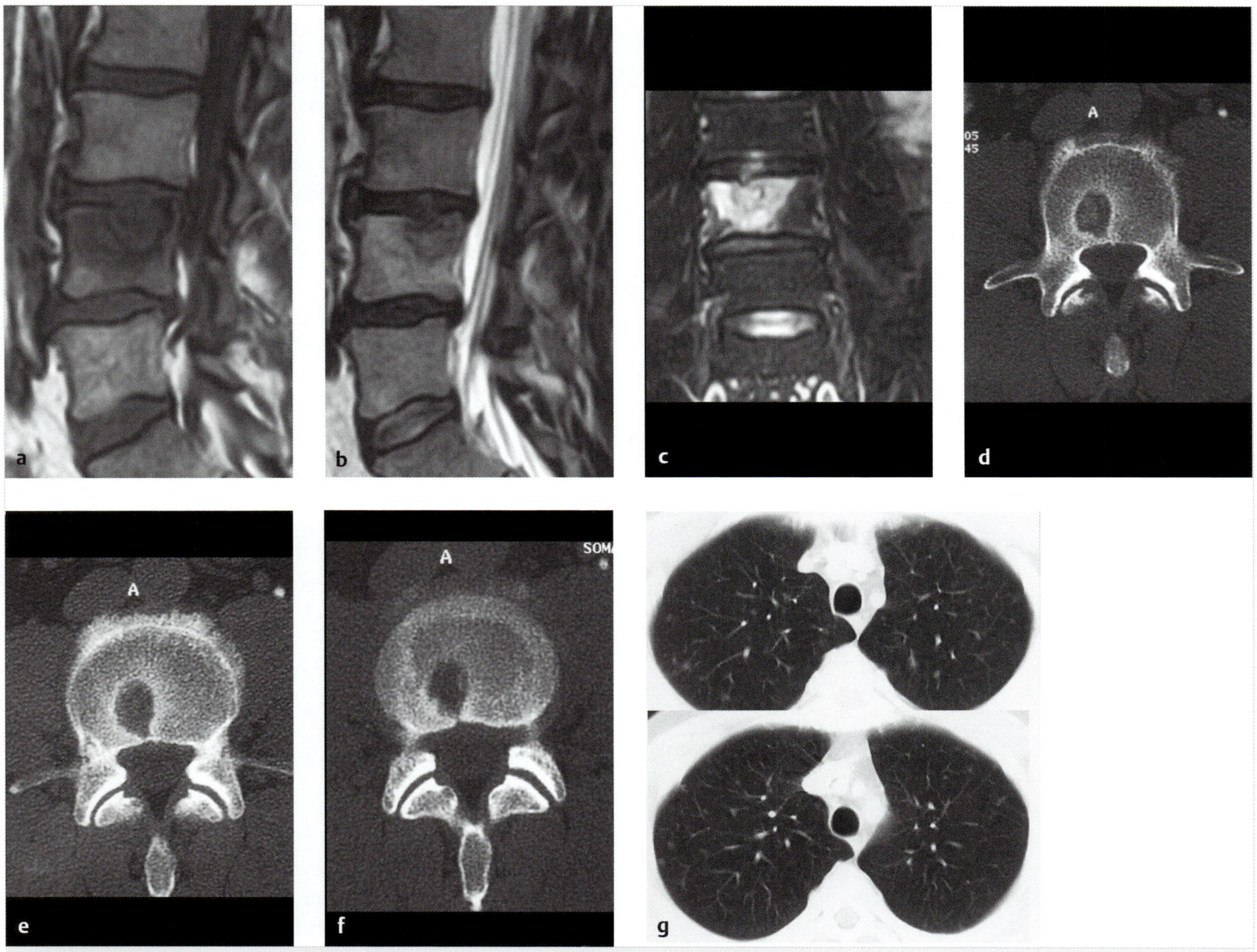

Fig. 3.13 a–g Spondylitis with a sequestrum?

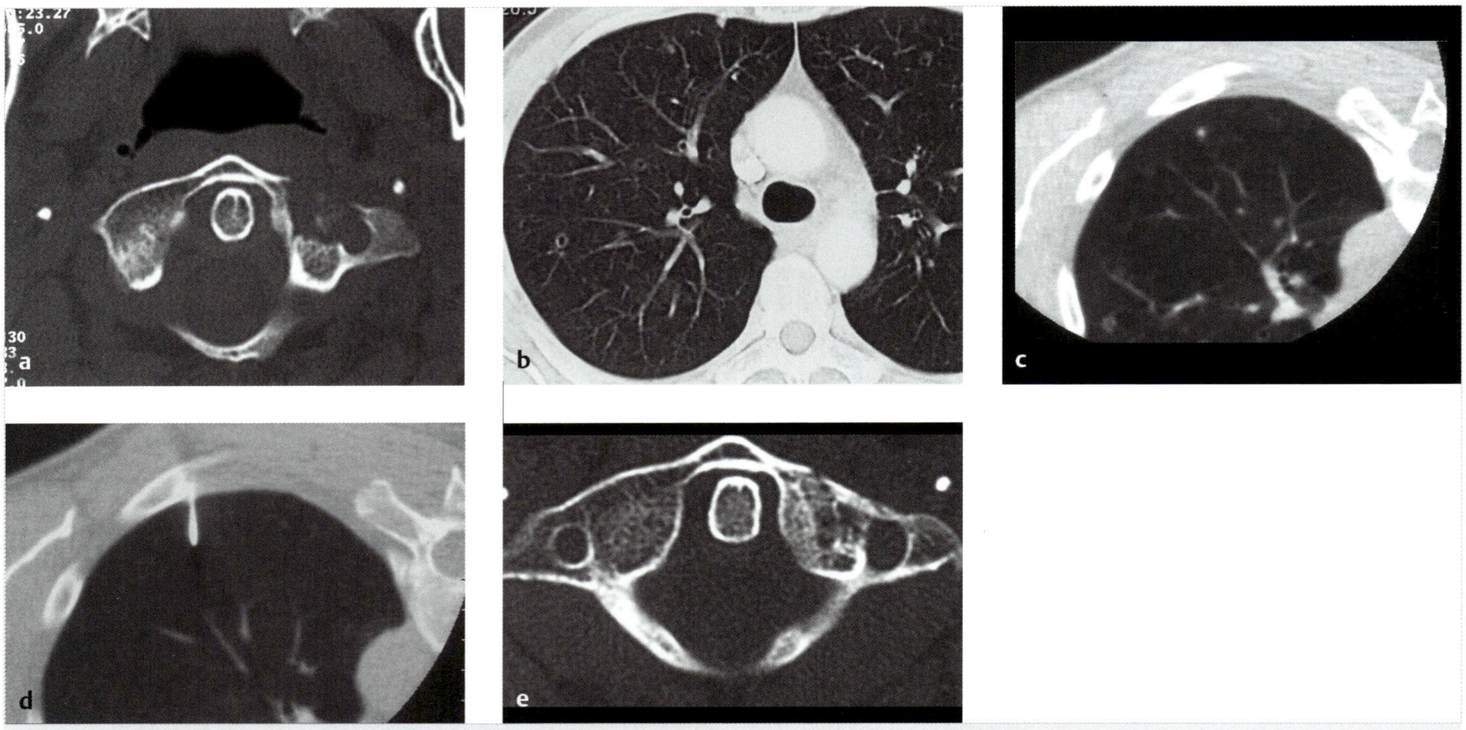

Fig. 3.14 a–e Systemic Langerhans-cell histiocytosis with osseous involvement in a 44-year-old man.

▸ **Trauma?** No, the history is negative for spinal trauma.

▸ **Inflammation?** No. Water-sensitive sequences in spondylodiskitis would show more extensive involvement of the affected disk space. Contrast-enhanced images (not shown here) did not reveal an abscess. Bone sequestra are discussed below.

▸ **Tumor?** Possibly. See under Pathoanatomic Background above.

▸ **Systemic process?** When the bony involvement is considered in relation to the pulmonary lesions, it is not difficult to relate all the findings to systemic Langerhans-cell histiocytosis.

Synopsis and Discussion

The present case could be interpreted as a primary intravertebral disk herniation as in Case 23, were it not for the pulmonary lesions and the history of heavy smoking. These are features of Langerhans-cell histiocytosis, which frequently shows osseous involvement. It is very likely, therefore, that a focus of Langerhans-cell histiocytosis (eosinophilic granuloma) developed in the subchondral bone of L4 and led to secondary collapse of the upper endplate. It is unclear whether the "sequestrum" is the collapsed endplate, residual bone tissue, or necrotic material (see also Case 35). In any case the "sequestrum" suggests either bacterial spondylitis or an eosinophilic granuloma (see ▸ Fig. 3.14 **a–e**). But why was the open biopsy of the bone lesion negative? Experience with biopsies in Langerhans-cell histiocytosis has shown that they often yield a specific result only after repeated biopsy attempts. In some cases, however, the diagnosis must be based entirely on clinical and radiologic data. This is because Langerhans-cell histiocytosis may run a very dynamic course. Some sites in a lesion may show regressive changes with fibrillation and cyst formation, while other sites may show viable or revitalized histiocytic tissue. These dynamics also explain the frequently long course of the disease. In the present case, the patient appears to have multisystem Langerhans-cell histiocytosis with pulmonary involvement (5–15% of cases), which has an uncertain prognosis without systemic therapy (corticosteroids, methotrexate). The link between smoking and the development of Langerhans-cell histiocytosis of the lung is well established. It should be added that in Langerhans-cell histiocytosis, osteolytic lesions in the spine and skull are especially likely to show sequestra.

▸ Fig. 3.14 illustrates another case of systemic Langerhans-cell histiocytosis with osseous involvement in a 44-year-old man with a history of smoking. He complained of posterior neck pain, rapid fatigability, and a sudden decline in activity level. MRI of the craniovertebral joints (not pictured here) showed an indeterminate process in the left lateral mass of the atlas. We ordered CT scans, which showed a large defect in the left lateral mass (▸ Fig. 3.14 **a**) that contained a small sequestrum. This finding (destruction with a sequestrum) was strongly suspicious for eosinophilic granuloma or Langerhans-cell histiocytosis. We then proceeded with pulmonary CT scans, which showed multiple small nodules with central intranodular cavitation in the upper lung zones (▸ Fig. 3.14 **b, c**). These lesions are highly specific for Langerhans-cell histiocytosis of the lungs. CT did not yet show evidence of fibrosis. The oncologist requested histologic confirmation, which we obtained by CT-guided biopsy of the right lung due to the unfavorable location of the bony lesion in the atlas (▸ Fig. 3.14 **d**). Histology confirmed Langerhans-cell histiocytosis. The patient quit smoking, was placed on steroid therapy for 3 weeks, and 6 months later he was free of complaints. By 1 year the lesion in the atlas was fully consolidated (▸ Fig. 3.14 **e**).

Final Diagnosis

Systemic Langerhans-cell histiocytosis with a focus (eosinophilic granuloma) in L4, upper endplate collapse, and secondary intravertebral disk herniation. Another case of systemic Langerhans-cell histiocytosis is illustrated in ▸ Fig. 5.32.

Comments

If a negative biopsy from a destructive bone lesion does not yield a clinically useful diagnosis, the radiologist should delve more deeply into the patient's history and clinical presentation. A look at nearby organs such as the lungs may be very rewarding.

Case 25 (▸ Fig. 3.15)

Case description

- Referring physician: orthopedist.
- Prior history and clinical question: A 26-year-old man had been experiencing low back pain for several weeks. He was found to have an indeterminate lesion in L3.

Radiologic Findings

The MR images (▸ Fig. 3.15 **a–c**) show extensive destruction of the L2–L3 intervertebral disk. A hyperintense "track" extends downward from the residual structures, running through the middle of L3 to the opposing lower endplate. Edema-like signal is noted around the track in L3 and below the L2 lower endplate. The axial CT series in ▸ Fig. 3.15 **d** demonstrates a cancellous bone defect in the posterior third of L3, which shows a targetlike pattern as well as a multicentric arrangement. The defect extends through the entire vertebral body from the disrupted upper endplate (upper left image in ▸ Fig. 3.15) to the still-intact lower endplate (lower right image).

Location

The epicenter of the changes below the L2 lower endplate and in L3 is located in the intervertebral disk or its nucleus pulposus.

Pathoanatomic Background of the Findings

The close topographic relationship between the destroyed intervertebral disk and the tunnel-like structure in L3 suggests a deep internal disk herniation. The nuclear tissue missing between L2 and L3 has entered the tunnel in L3. This suggests an immediate assignment to a possible basic entity: a degenerative process affecting the intervertebral disk and adjacent bony structures.

Synopsis and Discussion

Deep Schmorl nodes are especially likely to occur in patients with developmental disorders of the spine. In the present case this is evidenced by the narrowed disk spaces in the lower thoracic spine and by the unusual bulging of the upper and lower endplates of T11, T12, L1, and L2, apparently as a result of previous Scheuermann disease. These deep Schmorl nodes or intravertebral disk herniations may extend from one disrupted intervertebral

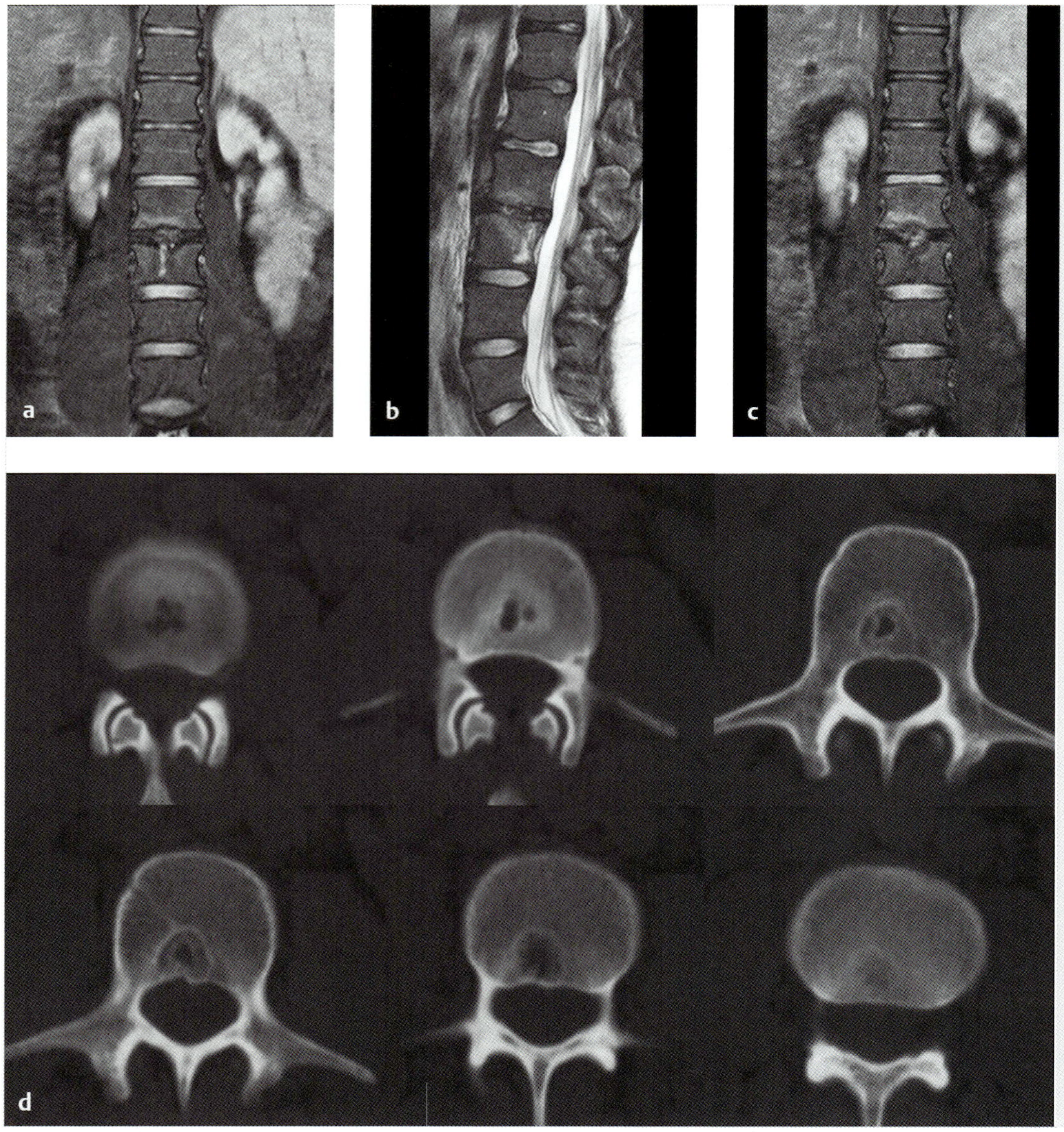

Fig. 3.15 a–d Spondylodiscitis?

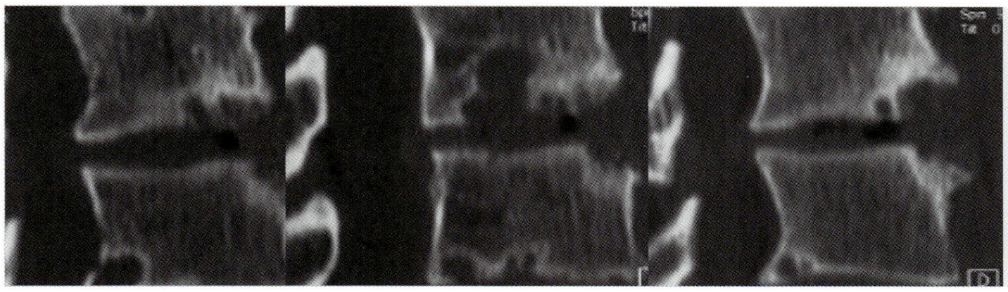

Fig. 3.16 Neoplastic destruction?

disk to another and can mimic a burst fracture on cursory examination. There is no reasonable differential diagnosis in the present case.

The CT images in ▶ Fig. 3.16 demonstrate *multiple intravertebral disk herniations* and an anterior retromarginal disk herniation in the lumbar segment of a 40-year-old woman who had childhood Scheuermann disease and osteopenia. The degenerative nature of the findings is indicated by a vacuum phenomenon between the affected vertebral bodies ("air and fat are the radiologist's friend!").

Final Diagnosis

Deep, chronic intravertebral disk herniation, known also as a deep Schmorl node.

Comments

Deep Schmorl nodes, though rare, should not be confused with neoplastic or inflammatory changes owing to their unmistakable pathoanatomic features in sectional images.

Case 26 (▶ Fig. 3.17)

Case description

- Referring physician: radiologist.
- Prior history and clinical question: A 42-year-old man complained of severe posterior chest pain. He had no prior history of cancer. The differential diagnosis consisted of spondylitis, tumor, and necrosis.

Radiologic Findings

CT images of T11 (▶ Fig. 3.17 **a–c**) look as if the bone has disintegrated into small fragments. A large, geographic osteolytic area is noted at the junction of the right vertebral arch and transverse process. The imaged structures are sclerotic. The paraosseous soft tissues are thickened.

Location

The changes are located primarily in the cancellous bone of the vertebra and show initial spread to paravertebral soft tissues.

Pathoanatomic Background of the Findings

There are two ways of interpreting the pathoanatomic changes of the radiologic findings:

1. The vertebral body has disintegrated into many sclerotic fragments. This may occur in osteonecrosis.
2. Some pathologic process (inflammation, tumor?) caused moth-eaten destruction of the cancellous bone, and this was followed by reactive/reparative sclerosis. This mechanism is supported by the relatively large osteolytic area at the junction of the right vertebral arch and transverse process.

Assignment to a Possible Basic Entity

▶ **Inflammation?** Probably not, since spondylitis more commonly originates from the well-perfused areas of the vertebral body near the upper and lower endplates and causes early destruction of the adjacent endplates. They appear to be intact, however (▶ Fig. 3.17 **c**).

▶ **Tumor?** Very likely. Moth-eaten destructive changes and sclerosis are typical radiologic features of osseous involvement by small-cell and blue-cell tumors such as non-Hodgkin lymphoma and Ewing sarcoma.

▶ **Necrosis?** Probably not, as indicated by the relatively large, coherent osteolytic area in the right posterior elements.

A definite radiologic diagnosis cannot be made, so CT-guided percutaneous biopsy was performed. Histology revealed involvement by non-Hodgkin lymphoma. A thorough examination of the patient showed no additional manifestations, so we are dealing with primary non-Hodgkin lymphoma of bone.

Synopsis and Discussion

When we interpret the innumerable fragments in T11 as residual sclerotic bony trabeculae and the gaps between them as destructive tumor tissue, it is not difficult to recognize a moth-eaten pattern of tumor destruction. It is known that bone lymphoma, whether primary or secondary, may incite reactive/reparative connective-tissue formation with primitive woven bone. Of course, the differential diagnosis would also include an osteosclerotic metastasis from an aggressive unknown primary tumor (CUP syndrome), but that is less common than bone lymphoma.

Final Diagnosis

Primary non-Hodgkin lymphoma of bone.

Comments

A combination of destructive and sclerotic changes in a vertebra rich in red marrow or in the metaphysis of a major long bone is always suspicion for non-Hodgkin lymphoma in a patient of any age who does not have a known primary tumor.

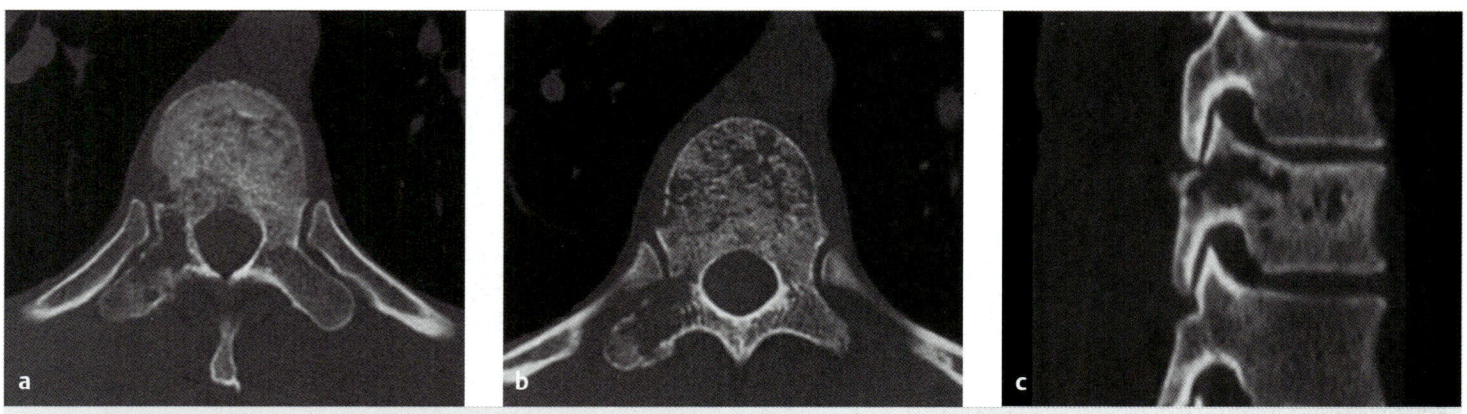

Fig. 3.17 a–c Necrosis?

3.2 Oligo- and Multisegmental Changes

Case 27 (▶ Fig. 3.18)

Case description

- Referring physician: orthopedist.
- Prior history and clinical question: A 12-year-old girl presented with nonspecific posterior neck pain. A radiograph of her cervical spine showed calcifications in the C4–C5 and C5–C6 disk spaces and wedging of the C5 vertebra, which were considered suspicious for a tumor. The case was investigated further by MRI, but without a conclusive diagnosis.

Radiologic Findings

The lateral radiograph of the cervical spine (▶ Fig. 3.18 **a**) shows disk-shaped calcifications in the C4–C5 and C5–C6 disk spaces with anterior wedging of the C5 vertebral body. The sagittal T2w image (▶ Fig. 3.18 **b**) shows that the nucleus above C5 is shortened and tilted anteriorly. Its anterior tip points toward a defect devoid of MR signal. Other projections and sequences added no information, so it was decided to obtain low-dose CT scans of C4 through C6. The reformatted images in ▶ Fig. 3.18 **c, d** show a defect in the upper endplate of the wedged C5 vertebra, and below the defect is a space devoid of cancellous bone. ▶ Fig. 3.18 **c** also shows a small defect in the lower endplate of C5. Clumped calcifications are present in the C4–C5 and C5–C6 disk spaces. The larger calcification at C5–C6 is shaped like a synthetic intervertebral disk. Small flecks of calcification are visible within the defect in C5. The vertebral body height of C5 is significantly reduced.

Pathoanatomic Background of the Findings

The intervertebral disk calcifications, endplate defects, and the defect in C5 are obviously interrelated. Dense clumps of calcification generally result from a previous (old) necrotic process, here involving the nuclei pulposi. Partial necrosis of the anterior apophysis of C5 could account for its diminished height, and an intervertebral disk herniation could explain the defect in C5.

Assignment to a Possible Basic Entity

▶ **Normal variant or malformation?** Not known to occur in this form.

▶ **Trauma?** No history.

▶ **Inflammation?** Possibly; it would have to be an aseptic inflammation culminating in necrosis.

▶ **Tumor?** No, because where would the tumor be located? In the defect in C5? And how could the other findings be explained?

▶ **Perfusion defect with necrosis?** As noted under Pathoanatomic Background, necrosis could explain all the findings (see Synopsis and Discussion below), though it would have to represent the end stage of an ultimately unidentified disease process (inflammation, primary perforation disorder, trauma?).

Synopsis and Discussion

All the findings are consistent with a condition known in the literature as “calcifying discitis.” This entity is observed in children and adolescents but its etiology is poorly understood. Approximately 75% of affected children present clinically with pain, limited motion, and torticollis. Fever and leukocytosis have also been reported and suggest an inflammatory etiology.[27] Some children also have a history of trauma. The cervical spine is a site of predilection. The calcifications may be transient, lasting for a period of weeks or months, or they may persist. Perforation of the calcium collections into the vertebral bodies, intervertebral foramina, spinal canal, or surrounding soft tissues has been described.

In the present case we can reconstruct the pathogenesis as follows: nonspecific, nonbacterial inflammation of the disk space structures at C4–C5 and C5–C6, followed by destruction of the intervertebral anatomic structures with necrosis and secondary calcification (necrotic tissue is a “calcium sink”), leading to pres-

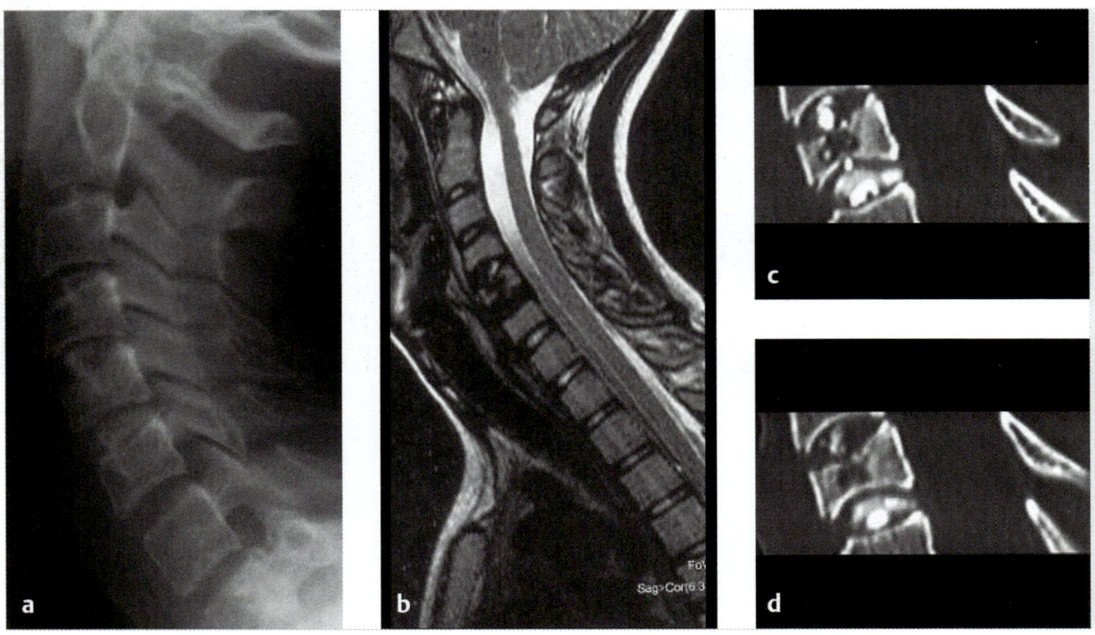

Fig. 3.18 a–d Calcium pyrophosphate deposition disease (CPPD)? Chondrocalcinosis?

sure on the adjacent endplates causing rupture and intravertebral disk herniation.

Final Diagnosis

Calcifying discitis in the C4–C5 and C5–C6 disk spaces.

Comments

Structures in the intervertebral disk spaces that resemble synthetic disks may signify calcifying discitis.

Case 28 (▶ Fig. 3.19)

Case description

- Referring physician: orthopedist.
- Prior history and clinical question: A 64-year-old colleague noticed increasing stiffness of the spine with an inability to bend his neck backward. He has gout and type 2 diabetes mellitus. He was concerned that he may have ankylosing spondylitis. He submitted a prior radiograph of the cervical spine taken 6 years previously, stating that the large spondylophyte visible on C5 was interpreted as a degenerative osteophyte in a setting of osteochondrosis.

Radiologic Findings

The cervical spine radiograph from 1986 (▶ Fig. 3.19 **a**) shows a large spondylophyte projecting downward from the lower anterior half of C5. The corresponding disk space is of normal height. Another, more band-shaped ossification arises from the lower anterior half of C2. A radiograph taken in 1992 (▶ Fig. 3.19 **b**) shows more pronounced, ankylosing (flowing, "sugar-coated") ossifications from C2 to C7. All the disk spaces are of normal height, and the endplates show no abnormalities. A posteroanterior radiograph of T12–L3 taken in 1992 (▶ Fig. 3.19 **c**) shows conspicuous, ankylosing ossifications along the sides of the vertebrae.

Location

The ossifications do not originate from the vertebral margins (diskovertebral junctions) but from the anterior and lateral ligamentous structures.

Pathoanatomic Background of the Findings

The ossifications are solid and apparently developed in the absence of previous or associated spinal disease. They originate from ligamentous structures.

Assignment to a Possible Basic Entity

▶ **Normal variant or malformation?** Both are excluded by the progression of the changes over time.

▶ **Trauma?** No history.

▶ **Inflammation?** No corresponding signs (e.g., destruction of vertebral structures, clinical findings).

▶ **Tumor?** No, there is no evidence of a "space-occupying" process.

▶ **Regressive process?** Very likely. This interpretation is supported by the age of the patient and the absence of any inflammatory signs.

Synopsis and Discussion

The hyperostotic changes on the outer surfaces of the affected vertebral bodies are characteristic of diffuse idiopathic skeletal hyperostosis (DISH), known also as hyperostotic spondylosis deformans or Forestier disease. The criteria for this diagnosis are as follows:

- Flowing, ankylosing spondylophyte formation along the front and sides of at least four contiguous vertebrae
- No signs of osteochondrosis

Additional criteria:

- Ligament ossifications (e.g., posterior longitudinal ligament, pelvic ligaments)
- Productive fibro-ostosis (proliferative enthesophathy)

Exclusion criteria:

- Degenerative changes in intervertebral disks
- Sacroiliitis

The etiology is unknown. There is a definite association with diabetes mellitus and gout, both of which have a certain "osteoplastic disposition." The patient in this case had diabetes mellitus and gout. The hyperostosis is manifested chiefly in structures with dense connective tissue, especially ligaments. This distinguishes DISH from ordinary spondylosis deformans.

In any type of spondyloarthritis (ankylosing spondylitis, psoriatic spondyloarthritis, etc.), the ossifications (syndesmophytes, parasyndesmophytes) arise from the vertebral margins or diskoligamentous junctions, which represent entheses. Other enthesitic changes occur in the vertebral endplates, which are also entheses.

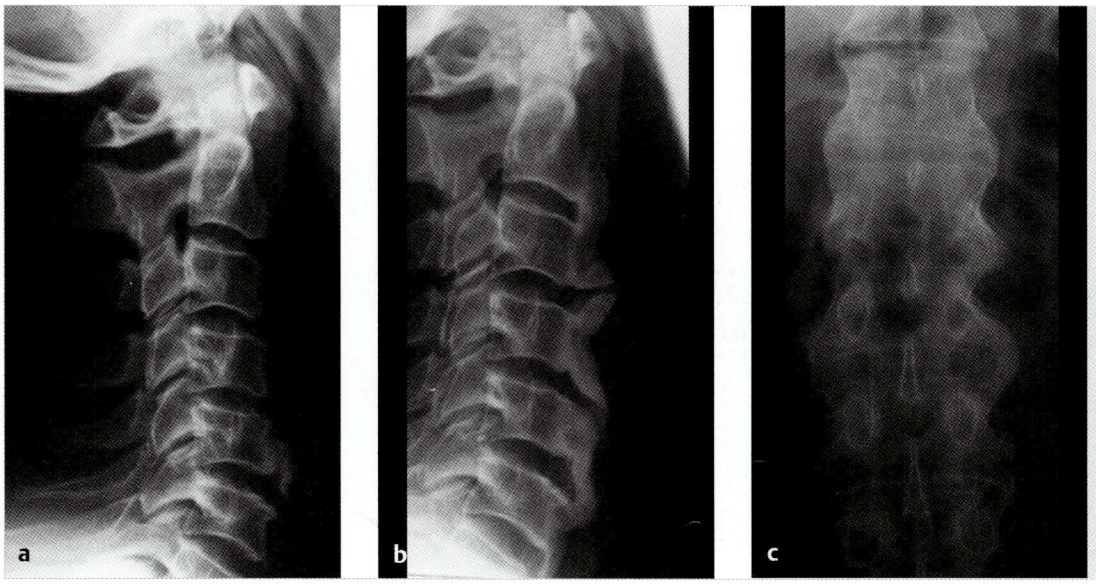

Fig. 3.19 Ankylosing spondylitis? The earlier radiograph was taken in 1986 (a); the later ones were taken in 1992 (b, c).

In the florid stage the inflammatory changes are characterized by simultaneous bone destruction and proliferation. The sacroiliac synchondroses ("joints") and/or manubriosternal synchondrosis are commonly affected, as are the capsular and ligamentous insertions (see also Case 39, Case 40, Case 48, Case 49, Case 84, Case 97, and Case 145).

Comments

DISH mainly requires differentiation from spondyloarthritis and ordinary osteochondrosis with spondylophyte formation. Noting the diagnostic criteria for DISH permits an accurate classification of the hyperostotic changes in the spine.

Final Diagnosis

DISH.

Case 29 (▶ Fig. 3.20)

Case description

- Referring physician: radiologist.
- Prior history and clinical question: A 51-year-old woman had pain and increasing stiffness in her cervical spine, 1 year after sustaining a basal skull fracture. MRI of the cervical spine showed unusual paravertebral soft-tissue changes on the left side at the C3–C7 level in addition to vertebral changes (hypointense in T1w images, hyperintense in T2w and TIRM images) that could not be definitely classified. The next logical study, CT examination of the neck, yielded a surprising result.

Radiologic Findings

On MRI the C3–C5 vertebrae have low signal intensity in the T1w sequence (▶ Fig. 3.20 **a**) and appear eroded anteriorly. An anteriorly convex mass, isointense to muscle, is visible along the anterior aspect of the vertebrae, extending inferiorly to the C7 level. The changes have high signal intensity in water-sensitive sequences (▶ Fig. 3.20 **b, c**). The CT scans in ▶ Fig. 3.20 **d–r** show sclerosis in C3 and C4 and partial sclerosis in C5, which appears slightly eroded anteriorly. The vertebrae are bordered by an irregularly ossified mass that shows anterior and anterolateral extension on the left side. The mass is bordered in turn by a still-unossified soft-tissue mass that has displaced the left retropharyngeal structures anteriorly. Bone scintigraphy (▶ Fig. 3.20 **s**) shows intense uptake in the left anterolateral portion of the cervical spine.

Location

The epicenter of the ossifications is located in the space between the anterior vertebral margins and anterior longitudinal ligament.

Pathoanatomic Background of the Findings

The findings indicate an ossifying or bone-forming process, still in a florid stage (positive bone scan), with associated erosion of the affected anterior vertebral contours and sclerosis of the underlying cancellous bone. Anterior to the ossifying process is a purely soft-tissue mass at a left anterolateral location.

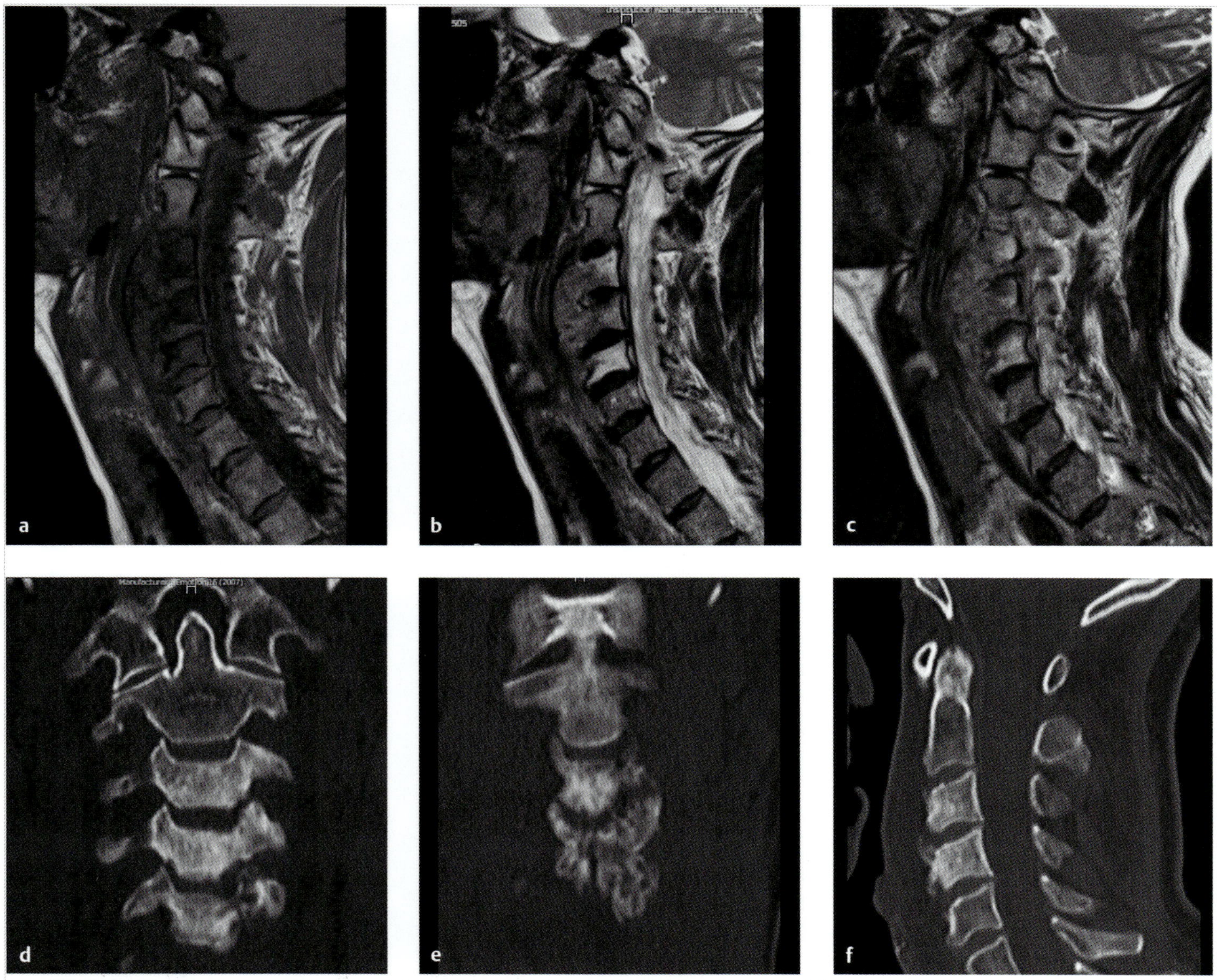

Fig. 3.20 a–s An incredible case with contradictory features: myositis ossificans?

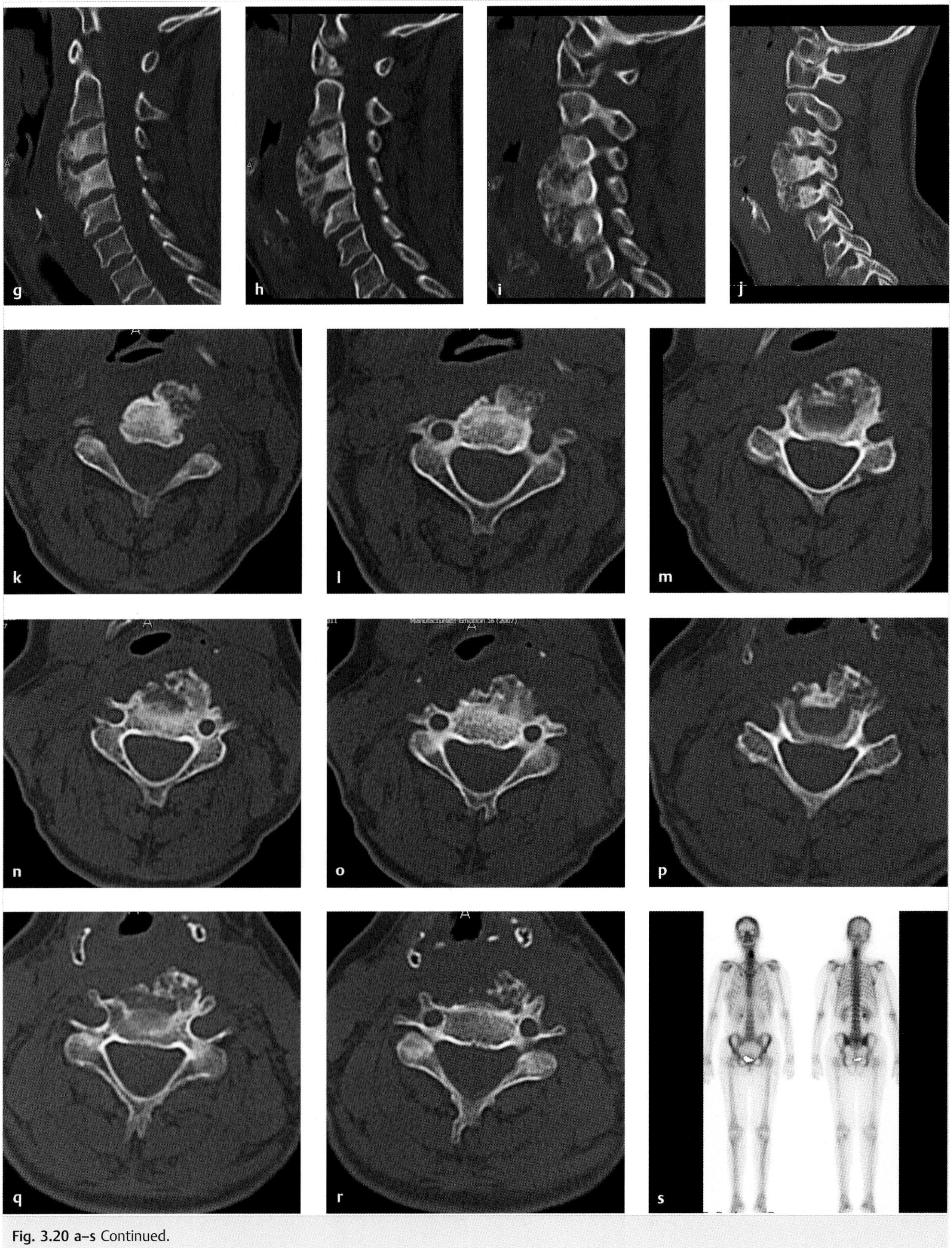

Fig. 3.20 a–s Continued.

Assignment to a Possible Basic Entity

► **Inflammation?** Possibly. Nonbacterial inflammatory changes in tendons often have significant fibroblastic potential. Trauma has been suggested as a precipitating cause for most cases. The histologic detection of inflammatory cells does not necessarily mean that a process has a primary inflammatory cause. Inflammatory cells are also found as an epiphenomenon following trauma, as in myositis ossificans.

► **Trauma?** The patient has a positive trauma history, having suffered a basal skull fracture a year earlier. There may have been trauma to pre- and paravertebral soft tissues inciting the development of myositis ossificans. Florid myositis ossificans presents a characteristic trizonal pattern (peripheral ossification followed by an intermediate zone, then an immature zone), which reflects the maturation of the process and is clearly apparent on the CT scans (► Fig. 3.20 **g–j**). But this alone does not explain the unossified mass, unless we assume that myositis ossificans occurred as a two-stage process.

► **Tumor?** Periosteal osteosarcoma may invade the bone, but the portion near the bone ossifies first while the peripheral portion ossifies last ("reverse trizonal pattern").

Synopsis and Discussion

There are three realistic differential diagnoses for the partly contradictory findings:

1. Myositis ossificans (heterotopic ossification) progressing in two stages
2. Periosteal (juxtacortical) or high-grade surface osteosarcoma
3. Prevertebral tendinitis

► **On differential diagnosis 1** The most frequent cause of *myositis ossificans* is trauma (traumatic myositis ossificans; see also Case 156). The patient was seen 1 year after sustaining a basal skull fracture, with the complaint of neck pain and increasing neck stiffness. It is likely that the trauma caused bleeding beneath the tough anterior longitudinal ligament, which precipitated the development of myositis ossificans. This could also explain the anterior convexity of the prevertebral ossifications. The density of the ossifications is consistent with a 1-year history of myositis ossificans. The pressure from the firm anterior longitudinal ligament led to erosions in the affected anterior vertebral margins and intracancellous sclerosis. It is also conceivable that a primary bony injury may have caused the anterior vertebral erosions and intraosseous sclerosis. It is not unusual for myositis ossificans to progress in two stages; we have repeatedly observed this in the pelvis and appendicular skeleton (see Case 156). This process is marked by a solid ossification with cancellous bone formation coexisting with a soft-tissue mass that has not yet ossified. The soft-tissue mass might also be caused by tendinitis of the prevertebral muscles developing as a result of anatomic changes from the myositis ossificans (see On differential diagnosis 3 below).

► **On differential diagnosis 2** Periosteal osteosarcomas grow on the bone surface. They develop predominantly in the adjacent soft tissues; infiltration of the medullary cavity is somewhat rare. Cases of this kind always raise the possibility of a high-grade surface osteosarcoma. The above-mentioned "reverse trizonal pattern" of ossifications in periosteal osteosarcoma is not found in the present case. The most common sites of occurrence of periosteal osteosarcoma are the femur and tibia. Uncommon sites are the ribs, maxilla, and pelvis. We know of no instances of vertebral involvement. Periosteal osteosarcoma accounts for only 1% of all osteosarcomas. When we consider probabilities in the diagnosis of borderline cases like this one, we must acknowledge that myositis ossificans after a basal skull fracture is a far more likely diagnosis than a rare periosteal osteosarcoma occurring at a previously unknown site. The same considerations apply to high-grade surface osteosarcoma, which is even rarer than periosteal osteosarcoma and most commonly involves the femur and tibia.

► **On differential diagnosis 3** Prevertebral tendinitis (also called retropharyngeal tendinitis) is an acute self-limiting disease of the longus colli muscle.[28,29] Its etiology is unknown but may relate to crystal deposits with a secondary inflammatory response, trauma, hemorrhage, a primary idiopathic inflammation, or necrotic processes. The site of predilection is the upper cervical spine. Most patients with this very rare disease are in the fifth or sixth decade of life. Our case involves very pronounced ossifications and adjacent osseous changes that do not fit the usual presentation or location of prevertebral tendinitis. At most, we might refer the unossified mass to prevertebral tendinitis, considering it a result of chronic trauma to the prevertebral muscles due to anatomic changes (see above On differential diagnosis 1).

It is questionable whether a histologic examination would yield a definitive result. These processes are difficult to distinguish from one another by their histology. The lesion may very well contain areas with cellular atypias, increased mitosis, etc. that would be interpreted as malignant. Conversely, there are cases in which ossifications recurring over a period of years are classified histologically as myositis ossificans until a juxtacortical osteosarcoma is eventually identified. Due in part to difficult access, this case is still being followed while symptoms are managed with NSAIDs.

Working Diagnosis

Traumatic myositis ossificans for further observation.

Comments

Rare disease entities that are manifested at even rarer sites can often be identified only by long-term follow-up.

Case 30 (▶ Fig. 3.21)

Case description

Prior history and clinical question: This case, fully elucidated, was kindly furnished to the author for teaching purposes by Dr. M. Venator, a radiologist practicing in Cologne. A 23-year-old woman had been experiencing severe right paravertebral pain in the lower thoracic spine for approximately 4 weeks. She could not recall acute antecedent trauma. The patient works as a geriatric nurse. This requires considerable lifting, and occasionally she must catch a falling patient without warning. Her family doctor found elevated serum inflammatory markers. Initial MRI demonstrated a conspicuous but initially indeterminate mass in the right T9–T10 region, which was correctly investigated further by CT on the same day. Finally a CT-guided percutaneous biopsy was performed (▶ Fig. 3.21 **j**) for a presumptive diagnosis of myositis ossificans. The pathologist confirmed myositis ossificans of the thoracic spine.

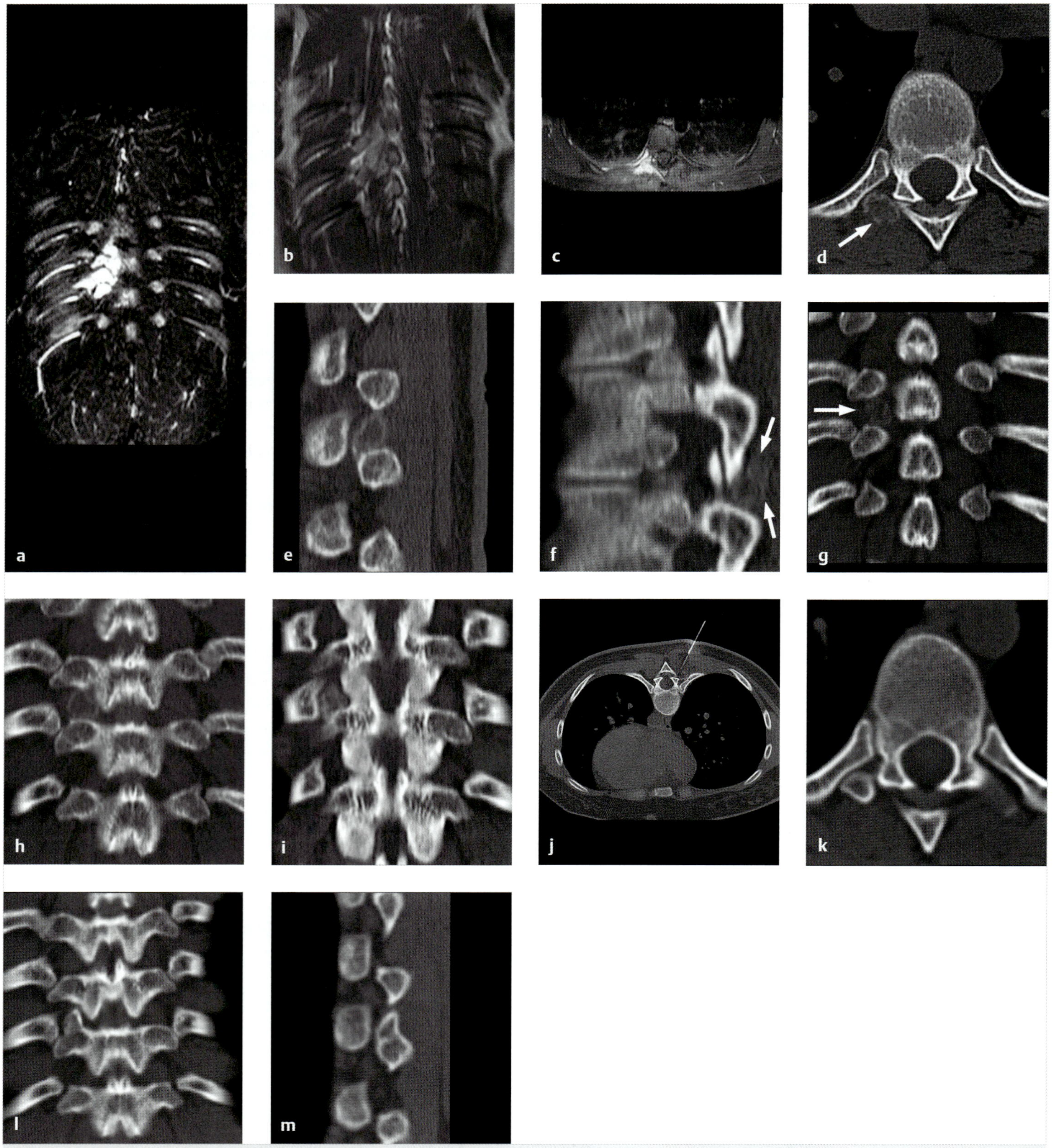

Fig. 3.21 a–m Intercostal soft-tissue mass on MRI.

Radiologic Findings

The initial MR images (▶ Fig. 3.21 **a–c**) show a hyperintense right inter- and paravertebral process at the T9–T10 level that extends into the corresponding intercostal space and enhances markedly after contrast administration. The T1w images show possible evidence of an underlying osseous process, but this is not definite. The CT images in ▶ Fig. 3.21 **d–i** demonstrate a mass with a calcified rim (see arrows in ▶ Fig. 3.21 **d, f**) located in the angle between the pedicle and transverse process of T9 and T10 on the right side. No ossification is visible at the center of the lesion. CT images 1 year later (▶ Fig. 3.21 **k–m**) show the now-solid ossified mass with a well-defined cortex and central medullary cavity. It has fused to the upper border of the right pedicle of T10, like an exostosis.

Location

The epicenter of the mass with the calcified or ossified rim is located in the soft tissues between two vertebral pedicles.

Pathoanatomic Background of the Findings

The MRI and CT findings can be interpreted as showing a proliferating and ossifying connective-tissue mass, but a bone-forming tumor with perifocal edema should also be considered.

Assignment to a Possible Basic Entity

▶ **Inflammation?** The good perfusion of the mass on contrast-enhanced MRI could be interpreted as inflammation-related, but not the ringlike ossification. If the term “myositis ossificans” is taken literally, since the process does appear inflammatory by its clinical and MRI features, then we are justified in classifying the mass as inflammatory.

▶ **Tumor?** Bone-forming tumors of soft tissues are extremely rare. Possibilities in the present case might include an osteoblastoma or osteosarcoma of the soft tissues.

Synopsis and Discussion

The classification of the process between the T9 and T10 pedicles on the right side as “myositis ossificans” is justifiable on radiologic grounds: an ossification develops at the center of a traumatized soft-tissue area with reactive connective-tissue proliferation. Although the patient could not recall a specific injury, her occupation as a geriatric nurse is consistent with a sudden straining movement leading to hemorrhage. On the other hand, gross trauma need not always be present as a precipitating cause of myositis ossificans; it is sufficient to have several muscular and collagen fiber tears occurring in response to minor trauma.

It is beyond our scope to explore the complex histomorphologic background of myositis ossificans, but we can briefly review its pathogenesis[18] (see also Case 156):

- The proliferation of spindle cells with *mitotic* activity occurs during the first week after soft-tissue trauma.
- At 7 to 10 days, primitive osteoid is formed by fibroblasts, starting at the periphery of the traumatized area.
- The second week is marked by the formation of primitive cartilage and woven bone, which differentiates to trabecular bone within 2 to 5 weeks.
- By approximately 6 weeks, a cellular center with large mesenchymal cells can be seen that is surrounded by osteoid and a rim of lamellar bone. This trizonal pattern is demonstrable on radiographs and CT scans by 4 to 6 weeks at the latest.

The present case fits with the above timetable of myositis ossificans. One year after the initial visualization of ringlike ossification in a pseudoinflammatory setting, the lesion has fully differentiated and matured and has fused to the upper cortex of the T10 pedicle, like an exostosis. If these images were interpreted without knowing the prior history, the initial interpretation would probably be a hyperostotic normal variant or even a mature cartilaginous exostosis (which would then be included in the sixth edition of Freyschmidt's “Koehler/Zimmer: Borderlands of Normal and Early Pathological Findings in Skeletal Radiography”).

Final Diagnosis

Myositis ossificans (heterotopic ossification) between the T9 and T10 pedicles (histologically confirmed, see ▶ Fig. 3.21 **j**).

Comments

The detection of ossification in a trizonal pattern in a soft-tissue mass 4 weeks after the onset of pain should suggest a diagnosis of myositis ossificans, even at an unusual location.

Case 31 (▶ Fig. 3.22)

Case description

- Referring physician: urologist.
- Prior history and clinical question: A 52-year-old woman with left hydronephrosis was found to have fine "spots" in the bone on urologic imaging. Metastases?

Radiologic Findings

Plain radiographs (not pictured here) showed sclerotic foci in all the lumbar vertebral bodies and in the pelvis. For better visualization of details, several representative CT scans (▶ Fig. 3.22 **a–h**) are presented here which show solid bone islands of variable size in the medullary cavities. These osteoma-like foci are partially confluent. To determine whether the foci were active, a bone scan (▶ Fig. 3.22 **i**) was obtained and was negative.

Pathoanatomic Background of the Findings

The foci most likely consist of solid lamellar bone.

Assignment to a Possible Basic Entity

▶ **Normal variant or malformation?** Because the patient has no current or prior history of skeletal complaints, it is reasonable to assume that the inactive bone foci (negative bone scan) have

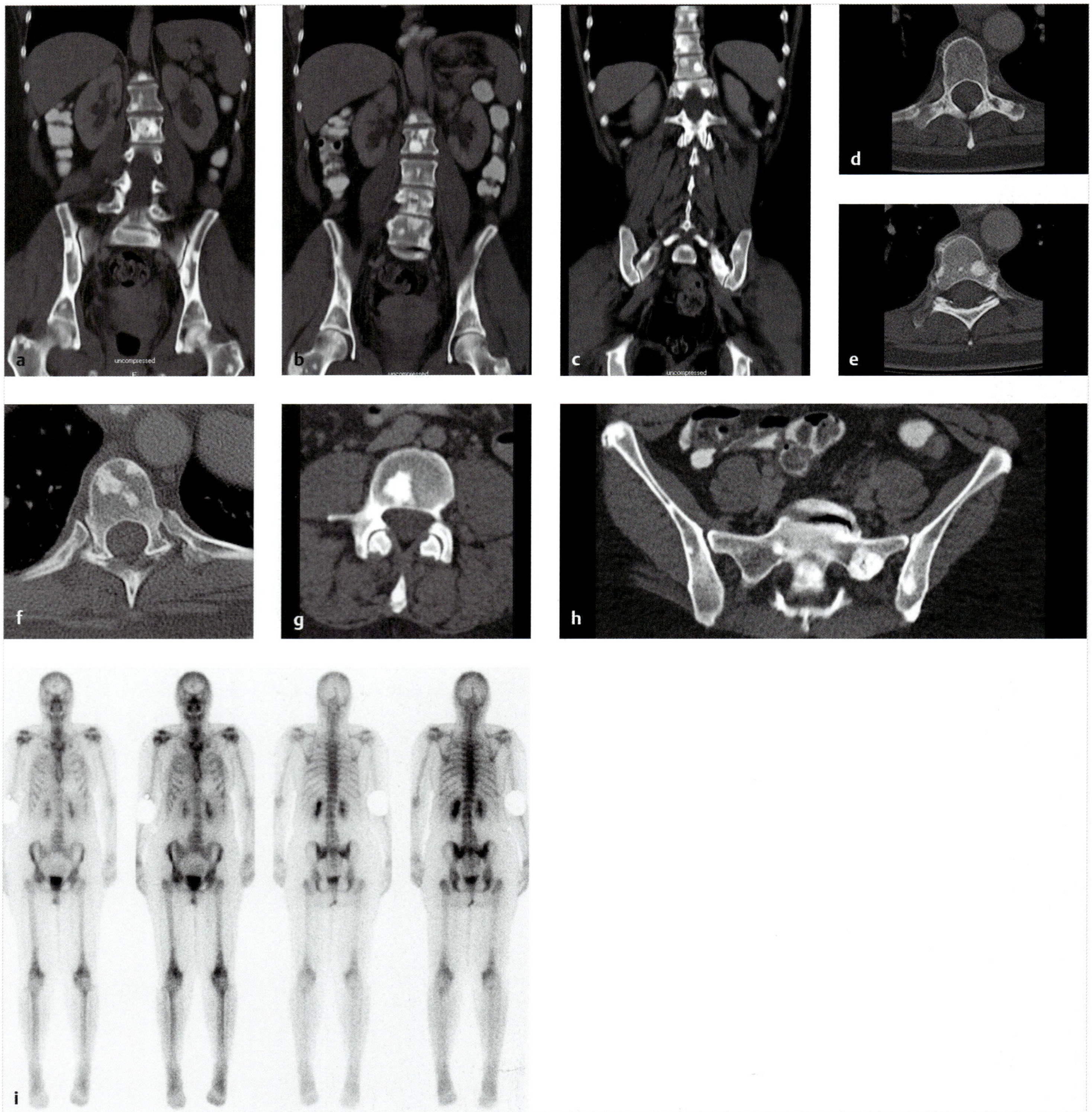

Fig. 3.22 a–i Osteosclerotic metastases?

been present for a long time and are most likely congenital. Spotted bones or osteopoikilosis is almost the only underlying entity that could produce disseminated osteoma-like foci.

► **Tumor?** No, the negative bone scan practically rules out metastasis and multicentric osteosarcoma.

Synopsis and Discussion

Osteopoikilosis, or spotted bone disease, is a rare (prevalence 12: 100,000 population) autosomal dominant bone disease characterized by sharply circumscribed densities 2 to 5 mm in diameter in the cancellous bone, most commonly involving the epimetaphyses of the appendicular skeleton. The pelvis and spine may also be involved in extreme cases. The densities correspond histologically to densely packed bony trabeculae with a lamellar structure. The changes do not have pathologic significance, and the diagnosis is based entirely on radiologic findings (radiographs, bone scan if required). Cutaneous manifestations are occasionally present: dermatofibrosis lenticularis disseminata, keratoma hereditarium dissipatum palmare et plantare, and a propensity for keloid formation. A speckled or lenticular form is distinguished from a striate form and mixed form. Associations with melorheostosis (see Case 99) have been described. Because some of the spots in the present case do not fit with one of the classic forms of osteopoikilosis, we assume a mixed form. Mixed forms of congenital multifocal sclerosis are also referred to as "mixed sclerosing bone dysplasia."

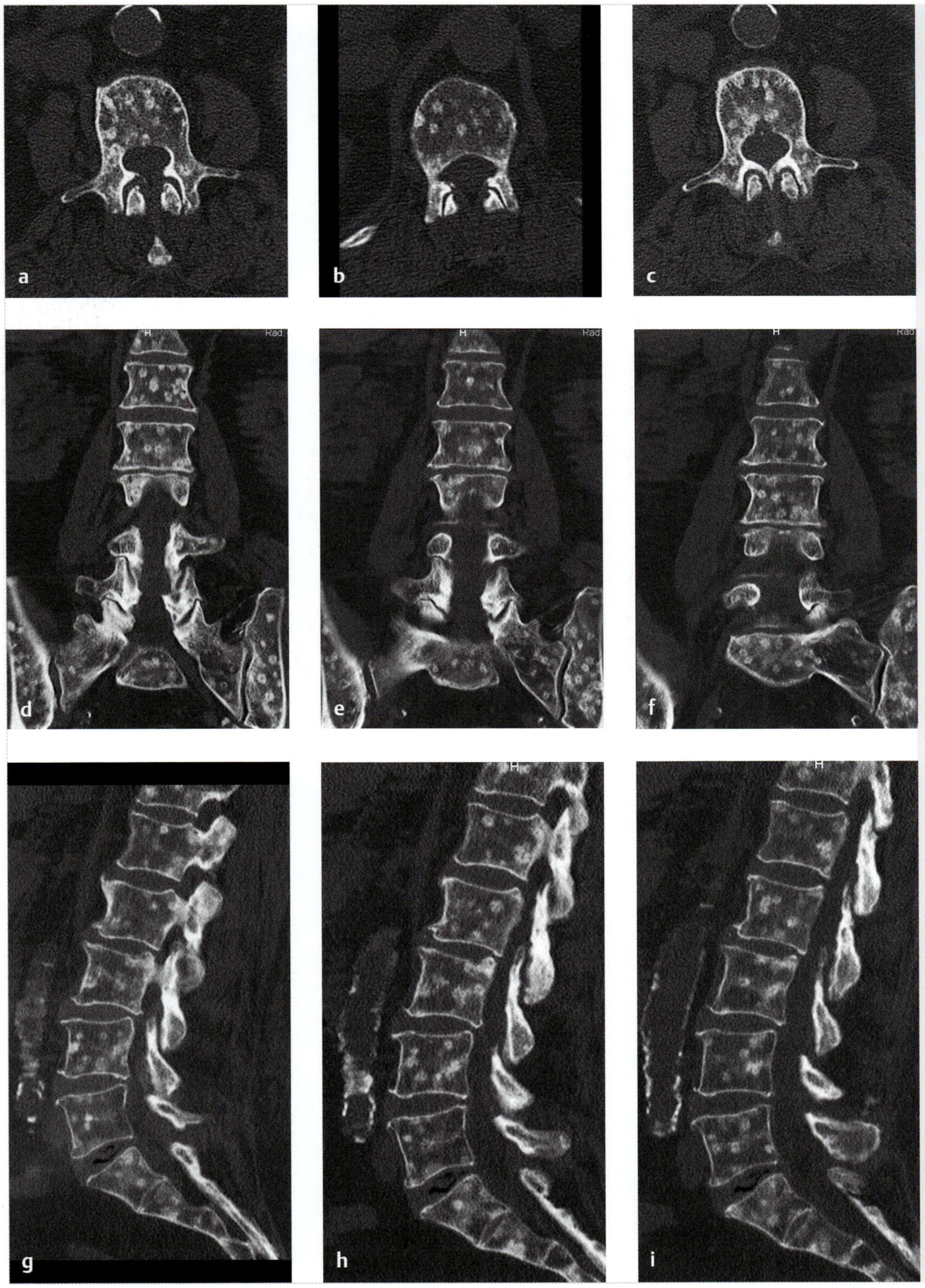

Fig. 3.23 a–j Osteopoikilosis (spotted bones) in the axial skeleton and hands.

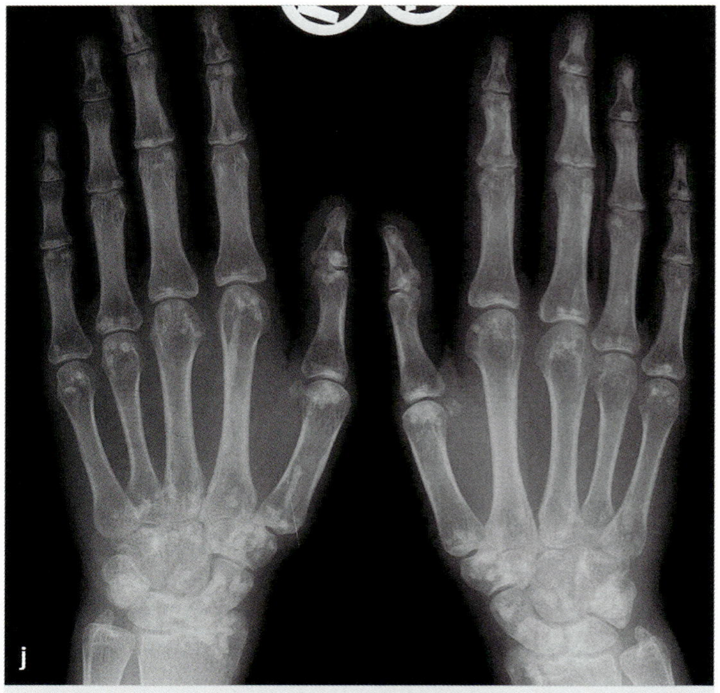

Fig. 3.23 a–j Continued.

▶ Fig. 3.23 illustrates the classic appearance of osteopoikilosis in the axial skeleton and hand (a test region for osteopoikilosis) in a different patient. We believe that the small central lucencies in some of the densities represent central vessels or tiny medullary cavities. We have observed this phenomenon more frequently in the last two decades because increasingly we visualize the spots with CT or MRI.

Final Diagnosis

Unusual presentation of spotted bones (osteopoikilosis).

Comments

The differential diagnosis of disseminated, unusually dense foci in the cancellous bone should always include osteopoikilosis or other forms of congenital sclerosis, even in patients with a tumor history. Bone scintigraphy is extremely helpful in narrowing the diagnosis.

Case 32 (▶ Fig. 3.24)

Case description

- Referring physician: oncologist.
- Prior history and clinical question: A 60-year-old woman presented with disseminated skeletal pain, 5 years after undergoing a splenectomy for angiosarcoma. At that time no metastases were detectable in the abdomen, lungs, or bone. No further treatment was performed, and the patient was clinically and radiologically free of disease (by ultrasound and abdominal CT) for 4 years after her initial treatment. Then she developed pain in the right groin area, with MRI showing edema-like signal in the head and neck of the right femur. Further investigations showed a disseminated process with mostly sclerotic foci, but osteolytic lesions were also noted in approximately one-third of all the lesions. The process was not confined to the right hip but involved the entire pelvis and spine. Given the previous clear R0 resection of splenic angiosarcoma and 4 years without recurrence or metastasis, it was reasonable to ask whether the skeletal lesions were metastatic angiosarcoma or whether an aggressive angiomatosis might be responsible for this unusual course. It was noteworthy that imaging studies (MRI, PET-CT) showed no evidence of malignancy other than the skeletal changes.

Radiologic Findings

Reformatted CT images of the spine and pelvis (▶ Fig. 3.24 **a–c**) show disseminated osteosclerotic and osteolytic lesions of variable size (e.g., T12 and S1, see arrows in ▶ Fig. 3.24 **c**). But other images (not pictured here) showed additional involvement of the shoulder girdle and proximal long bones. A whole-body bone scan (not pictured) revealed disseminated foci of increased uptake in the spine, shoulder girdle, proximal long bones, and pelvis.

Location

The disseminated lesions are confined to skeletal areas rich in cancellous bone while sparing the cortex and paraosseous soft tissues.

Pathoanatomic Background of the Findings

The patient's prior history raises a suspicion that the lesions may be disseminated osteosclerotic and osteolytic metastases. But the unusually long disease-free interval of 4 years also suggests an aggressive form of angiomatosis that was not properly identified on initial histology.

Assignment to a Possible Basic Entity

See under Pathoanatomic Background of the Findings. Osteopoikilosis (see Case 31) is excluded by the positive bone scan, coexisting lytic lesions, and clinical presentation.

Synopsis and Discussion

The differential diagnosis in this case consisted of aggressive angiomatosis on the one hand and a disseminated vascular tumor such as hemangioenthelioma or angiosarcoma on the other. This distinction had therapeutic implications, making it necessary to obtain histology for one of the lesions and compare it critically with the primary histology of the splenic tumor, taking into account the progression of findings. A CT-guided percutaneous biopsy was taken from the neck of the right femur. Based on morphologic analysis and immunohistology, three experienced bone pathologists identified the lesion as a malignant vascular process consistent with *angiosarcoma* and noted a similarity to the histology of the splenic tumor. The difficulty in distinguishing the lesion from an aggressive form of angiomatosis was also noted. We nevertheless recommended treatment with a vascular proliferation inhibitor (tha-

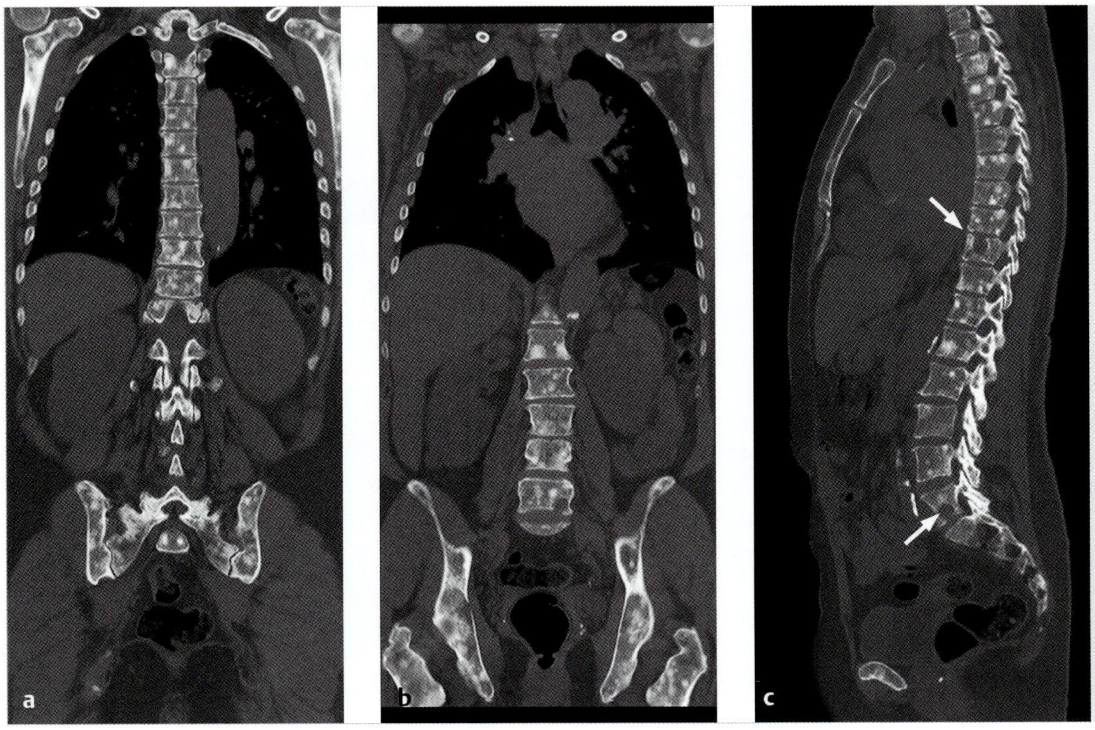

Fig. 3.24 a–c Osteopoikilosis?

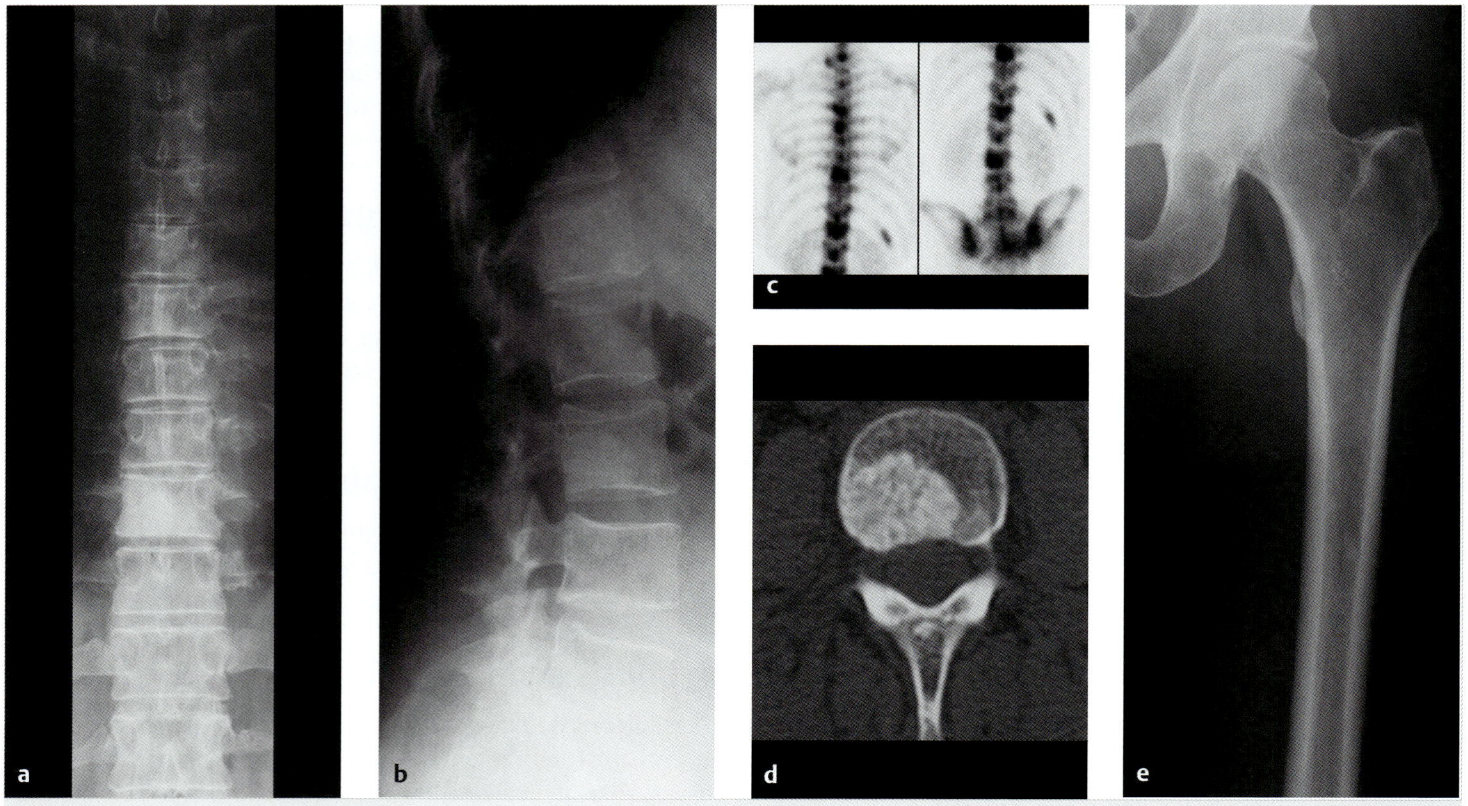

Fig. 3.25 a–e Sclerosing form of skeletal angiomatosis.

lidomide), but it did not positively affect the further course. The patient then declined further treatment and eventually died from consumption coagulopathy in the form of Kasabach–Merritt syndrome.

Angiomatosis (hemangiomatosis) is characterized by the development of multiple or disseminated hemangiomas that have the same histology as an ordinary angioma. See Case 59 for critical comments on this issue. The angiomas may be venous, lymphatic, or of a mixed type. If the angiomas cause osteolytic bone lesions, the disease is described as "cystic skeletal angiomatosis." When skeletal angiomatosis is combined with angiomatous changes in the soft tissues (liver, spleen, pleura, etc.), the prognosis tends to be unfavorable. Histology also shows more aggressive features. Pure skeletal angiomatosis will generally resolve over a period of many years, either by reparative osteosclerosis or fatty infiltration, see Case 34. Most forms of skeletal angiomatosis have a primary osteolytic presentation (see Case 33). Primary sclerosing forms are less common (▶ Fig. 3.25) and there is controversy as to whether they represent a resolution stage of previously asymptomatic osteolytic angiomatosis.

In the case presented here, we felt that the clinical course was more consistent with an aggressive form of angiomatosis that began with a splenic focus accompanied by skeletal foci that were still clinically and radiologically occult. This impression was strengthened when the pathologists noted the difficulty of positively distinguishing between pure angiosarcoma and aggressive angiomatosis.

▶ Fig. 3.25 illustrates the case of an asymptomatic patient with the sclerosing form of pure skeletal angiomatosis, which was referred to us for biopsy investigation of a "suspected osteosclerotic metastasis from an unknown primary tumor." We were able to follow this biopsy-confirmed case for 15 years. Over time the foci decreased in size and intensity on both radiographs and bone scans.

Final Diagnosis

Angiosarcoma of the spleen with multicentric growth or late skeletal metastasis. Presumably not an aggressive form of angiomatosis.

Comments

The differential diagnosis of disseminated focal lesions in cancellous bone includes osteosclerotic metastases, osteopoikilosis (spotted bone) or other congenital skeletal diseases, and even rare instances of angiomatosis.

Case 33 (▶ Fig. 3.26)

Case description

- Referring physician: orthopedist.
- Prior history and clinical question: A 48-year-old woman presented with nonspecific abdominal complaints. Abdominal CT demonstrated a splenic focus plus numerous osteolytic lesions in the lumbar spine. A metastatic process was suspected, and a comprehensive tumor search was initiated. This work-up included thoracic CT, which showed additional foci in the thoracic spine; the lungs and pleura appeared normal. Laboratory findings were also normal. A bone biopsy performed at another institution (we could not ascertain the exact biopsy site) was negative. The patient was then referred to an orthopedist, who correctly questioned the initial suspicion of metastasis and consulted us about the possibility of a different cause.

Radiologic Findings

The reformatted CT images (▶ Fig. 3.26 **a–c**) show multiple punched-out lesions in the cancellous bone. The lesions in L2 and L4 contain faint sequestrum-like structures. Postcontrast CT (▶ Fig. 3.26 **d**) shows one larger and one very small hypodense lesion in the spleen. Unfortunately, delayed views of the spleen at 10 to 15 minutes were not obtained.

Pathoanatomic Background of the Findings

It is reasonable to suspect a single cause for the defects in the vertebral cancellous bone and in the spleen. The tissue replacing the normal structures would probably have a neoplastic or tumorlike origin (e.g., granuloma). The small sequestrum-like densities may represent residual bone or reactive ossification.

Assignment to a Possible Basic Entity

▶ **Normal variant or malformation?** No. Multiple defects in vertebral bodies and in the spleen are not known to occur as a normal variant or malformation.

▶ **Trauma?** No history. Moreover, acute or chronic trauma would not cause cancellous bone defects or “holes” in the spleen.

▶ **Inflammation?** No, given the absence of clinical and laboratory abnormalities.

▶ **Tumor?** Very likely, though not in the form of metastasis since the relatively young patient had no known primary tumor and no clinical or laboratory signs of metastasis. We know from experience that multicentric tumors of the bone and a parenchymal organ (like the spleen) most commonly result from angiomatosis.

▶ **Systemic process?** Possibly. Granulomatous diseases such as systemic Langerhans-cell histiocytosis or sarcoidosis may produce lesions in both the spleen and the bone, as in the present case.

Synopsis and Discussion

Cystic angiomatosis (see Case 32) is supported by the following findings:

- No specific clinical symptoms, normal laboratory findings.

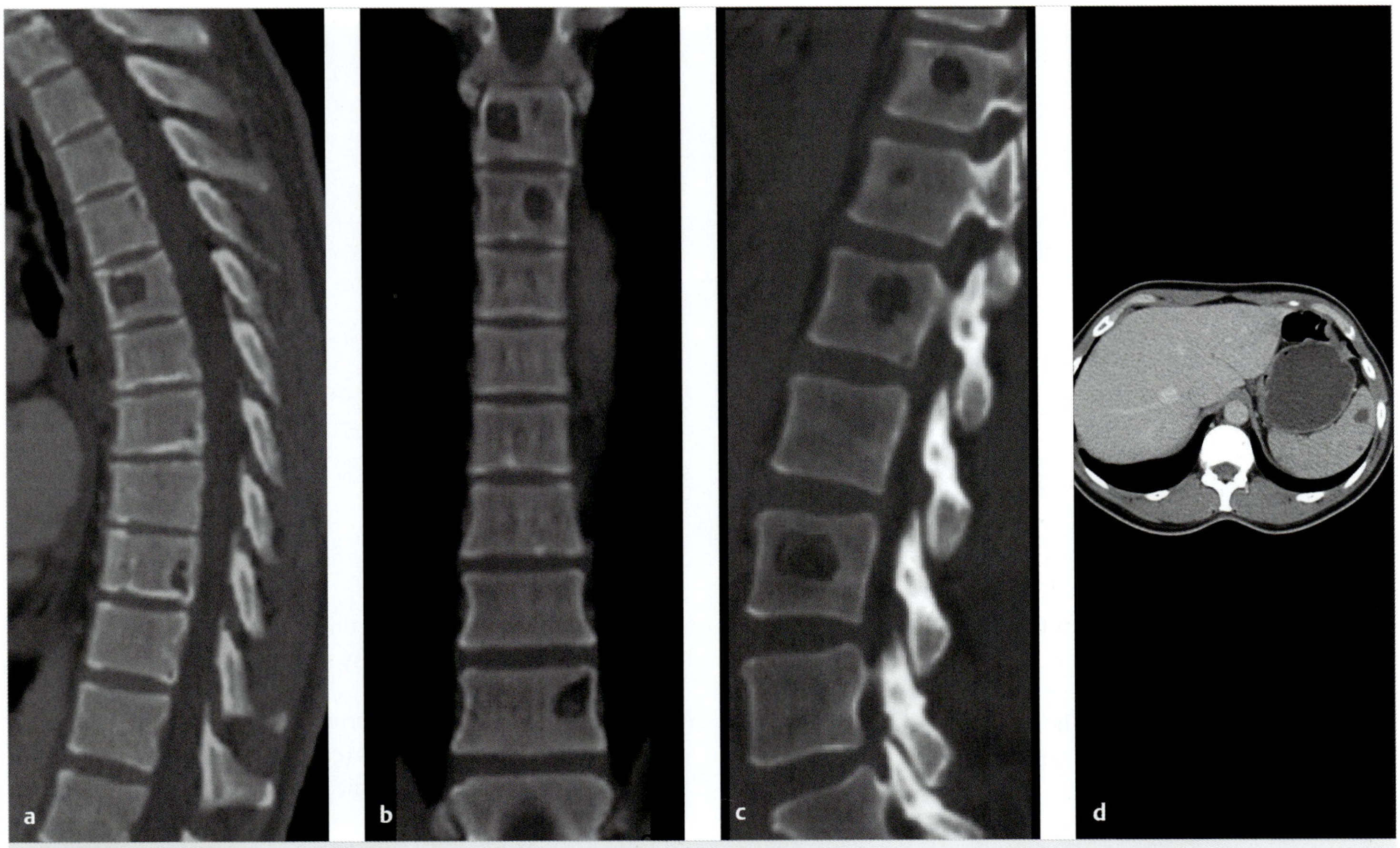

Fig. 3.26 a–d Metastases?

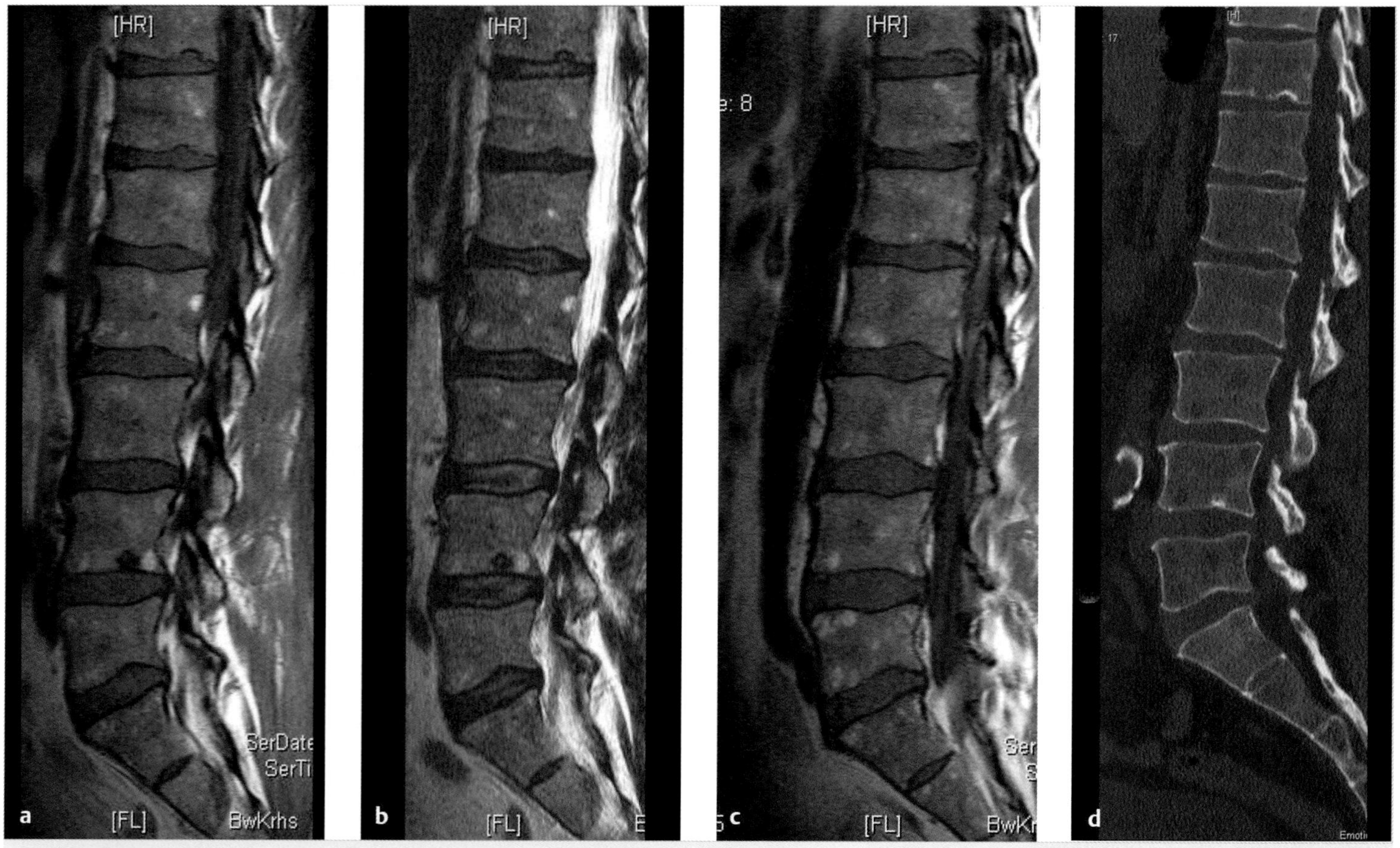

Fig. 3.27 a–d Minimal form of angiomatosis in a 58-year-old man (incidental finding).

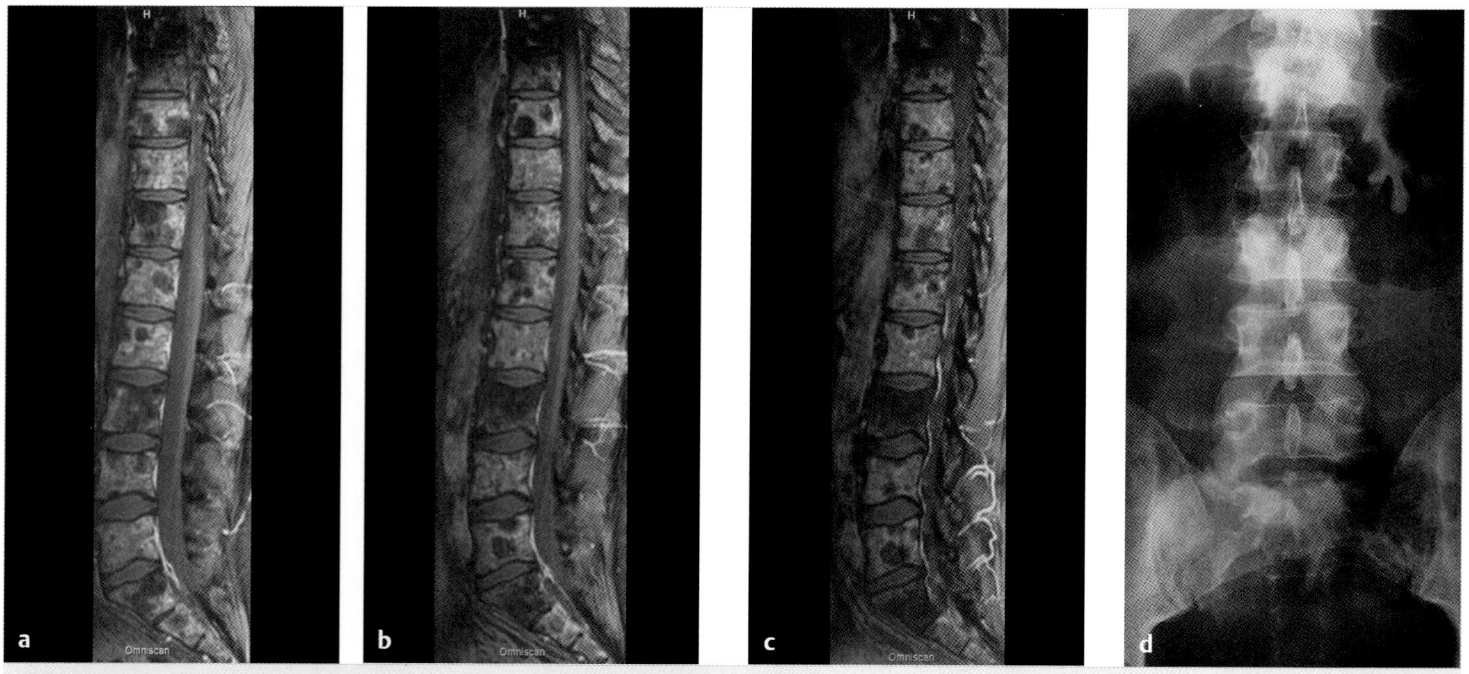

Fig. 3.28 a–d Excessive disseminated angiomatosis in a 48-year-old man.

- Age of the patient: We have over 40 cases of angiomatosis in our files, with most occurring in women in the fourth and fifth decades of life.
- Simultaneous involvement of bone and spleen: Besides the pleura, the spleen is the parenchymal organ most commonly affected by angiomatosis.
- Initial negative histology: In our experience it is not unusual to have a negative or nonspecific histology for angiomatosis if the pathologist is unprepared for this diagnosis and does not perform special tests on the biopsy material.

Metastases from an unknown primary tumor are unlikely, owing to the lack of clinical symptoms (e.g., B symptoms) and the highly improbable association of splenic metastases with skeletal metastases.

A diagnosis of *Langerhans-cell histiocytosis* is not supported by the age of the patient (most cases occur in school-age children) or the absence of pulmonary lesions on CT. *Sarcoidosis* is not consistent with negative pulmonary and mediastinal CT, because florid sarcoidosis of the bone is almost always associated with thoracic imaging abnormalities.

At the request of the oncologist, percutaneous biopsy was performed on one of the spinal lesions, which provided histologic confirmation of angiomatosis.

▶ Fig. 3.27 illustrates a minimal form of angiomatosis detected incidentally in a 58-year-old man. The tiny, disseminated angiomatous lesions have high signal intensity in both T1w and T2w MR images (very specific for hemangiomas) but produce only very small, subtle hypodensities on CT scans. In contrast to Case 32 and ▶ Fig. 3.28, this case does not require histologic confirmation because the patient is asymptomatic and a biopsy would not have therapeutic implications.

▶ Fig. 3.28 illustrates a case of widely disseminated angiomatosis in a 48-year-old man who died from the disease. The T1w MR images of the lumbar spine after contrast administration (▶ Fig. 3.28 **a–c**) show a variegated pattern of diffuse irregular and spotty hyperintensities interspersed with focal hypointense areas, confluent in L3, which represent areas of reactive or reparative sclerosis (▶ Fig. 3.28 **d**). The diagnosis was confirmed histologically.

Final Diagnosis

Cystic angiomatosis with involvement of the spleen.

Comments

The combination of lytic skeletal foci with splenic lesions in a 48-year-old woman without a known primary tumor is more suggestive of cystic angiomatosis than metastatic cancer from an unknown primary (CUP) or Langerhans-cell histiocytosis.

Case 34 (► Fig. 3.29)

Case description

- Referring physician: radiologist.
- Prior history and clinical question: A 60-year-old man had pain at the thoracolumbar junction after a bicycle fall with no other trauma history. His nutritional status and general health were good. Radiographs of the lumbar spine and pelvis (► Fig. 3.29 **a, b**) showed a mixed pattern of spotty and streaky demineralization that is typical of multiple myeloma (diffuse plasmocytoma). The upper endplate of L1 is collapsed. These findings warranted further investigation by whole-body bone scintigraphy, CT, and MRI.

Radiologic Findings

The whole-body bone scan (► Fig. 3.29 **q**) shows focal increased uptake in L1 with no other abnormalities. Radiographic findings in the lumbar spine and pelvis are described above. Radiographs of test regions for multiple myeloma, like the skull and proximal long bones, were obtained to confirm or exclude this disease. Additional osteolytic lesions are visible in the proximal femurs (► Fig. 3.29 **n**). The skull (► Fig. 3.29 **p**) and humeri (► Fig. 3.29 **o**) show no osteolytic changes. CT images of the lumbar spine (► Fig. 3.29 **c–i**) show a predominantly honeycomb pattern of cancellous bone destruction, which is also seen in the posterior vertebral elements. The remaining trabeculae appear accentuated. Overall, the images call to mind the structural changes in hemangiomatous vertebrae. On imaging with a soft-tissue window (not shown here), mostly fatty tissue was found occupying the spaces between the residual trabeculae. The collapsed upper endplate of L1 is depicted very clearly in the CT images (► Fig. 3.29 **e, f**). The MR images (► Fig. 3.29 **j–m**) also demonstrate copious fat, which is clearly documented in the fat-suppressed image (► Fig. 3.29 **m**). As expected, the postcontrast images (not pictured here) did not show significant enhancement in areas devoid of cancellous bone. Edema-like signal is noted below the collapsed upper endplate of L1.

Location

Abnormal findings are limited to the medullary cavities of the spine including the posterior elements, to the pelvis, and to the proximal femur.

Pathoanatomic Background of the Findings

The multiple foci of gross cancellous bone destruction in the spine, pelvis, and proximal femurs with fatty replacement may be the end stage (the "war memorial") of an abnormal, probably neoplastic process. The tissue that destroyed the bone and/or stimulated its destruction has disappeared and has been replaced by fat (vacuum fat).

Assignment to a Possible Basic Entity

► **Normal variant or malformation?** No.

► **Trauma?** Only relating to the compression fracture of L1.

► **Inflammation?** There is no prior history of a conventional inflammatory process. Paget disease (osteitis deformans) is not consistent with the honeycomb pattern of bone destruction, the absence of bone expansion, and the negative bone scan.

► **Tumor?** Yes, because tumor can destroy bone both directly and indirectly (by osteoclast stimulation). Multicentric honeycomb bone destruction is known to occur with angiomatosis. The predilection for certain skeletal regions (see below, Synopsis and Discussion) is another typical feature. In the present case, the angiomatous tissue that destroyed the bone was replaced by fat.

► **Perfusion disorder?** Perfusion disorders can lead to regional bone loss (e.g., in transient osteoporosis), but this mechanism could not reasonably apply to the entire spine, pelvis, and proximal femur, each of which has its own blood supply. Perfusion disorders were once cited as possible triggers for ordinary menopausal and senile osteoporosis, in which fine cancellous trabeculae are resorbed and replaced by fat. But the process in the present case involves a honeycomb pattern of bone destruction that does not fit with ordinary osteoporosis.

Synopsis and Discussion

The description of multicentric bone destruction as "honeycomb" should evoke the engrammatic memory link "honeycomb → hemangioma." Multiple and disseminated osteolytic hemangiomas and lymphangiomas, which may also occur in a clustered pattern, are referred to as *cystic angiomatosis* (see also Case 33). They may occur regionally (e.g., in the bones of one foot) or may involve entire skeletal segments (spine and/or pelvis and/or femur). In the absence of visceral involvement, there is a relatively good prognosis for spontaneous recovery in which the hemangiomatous defects resolve by osseous repair or fatty replacement. A somewhat unusual aspect of this case is the fact that the patient had no previous complaints and his disease was discovered only after a bicycle accident resulting in a painful compression fracture of the L1 vertebra.

A review of the radiographs and CT scans might also suggest multiple myeloma (diffuse plasmocytoma), but this diagnosis is not supported by the presence of fat in the osteolytic lesions. Nor is it compatible with the sparing of the skull, which is a region of predilection for diffuse plasmacytoma (multiple myeloma).

The radiologic diagnosis is clear-cut. There is no need for excisional biopsy, which would at most reveal fatty tissue, residual bone, and possible residual hemangiomatous and connective tissue—since the "party" ended long ago. What we see now may also be described as a "war memorial." If treatment with an angioneogenesis inhibitor (thalidomide) is considered in order to expedite the healing of any residual angiomatous tissue, despite the absence of complaints, then it might be reasonable to proceed with an excisional biopsy.

To aid differentiation, ► Fig. 3.30 presents the case of a woman with metastatic breast cancer. We do not see a honeycomb pattern of bone destruction like that occurring with angiomatosis that resolves by fat replacement. Instead the bone is permeated by irregular, ill-defined defects of variable size that are much more dense than the "fatty defects" in angiomatosis. In this case one would be justified in making a snap diagnosis of "osteolytic metastases" or "diffuse plasmacytoma."

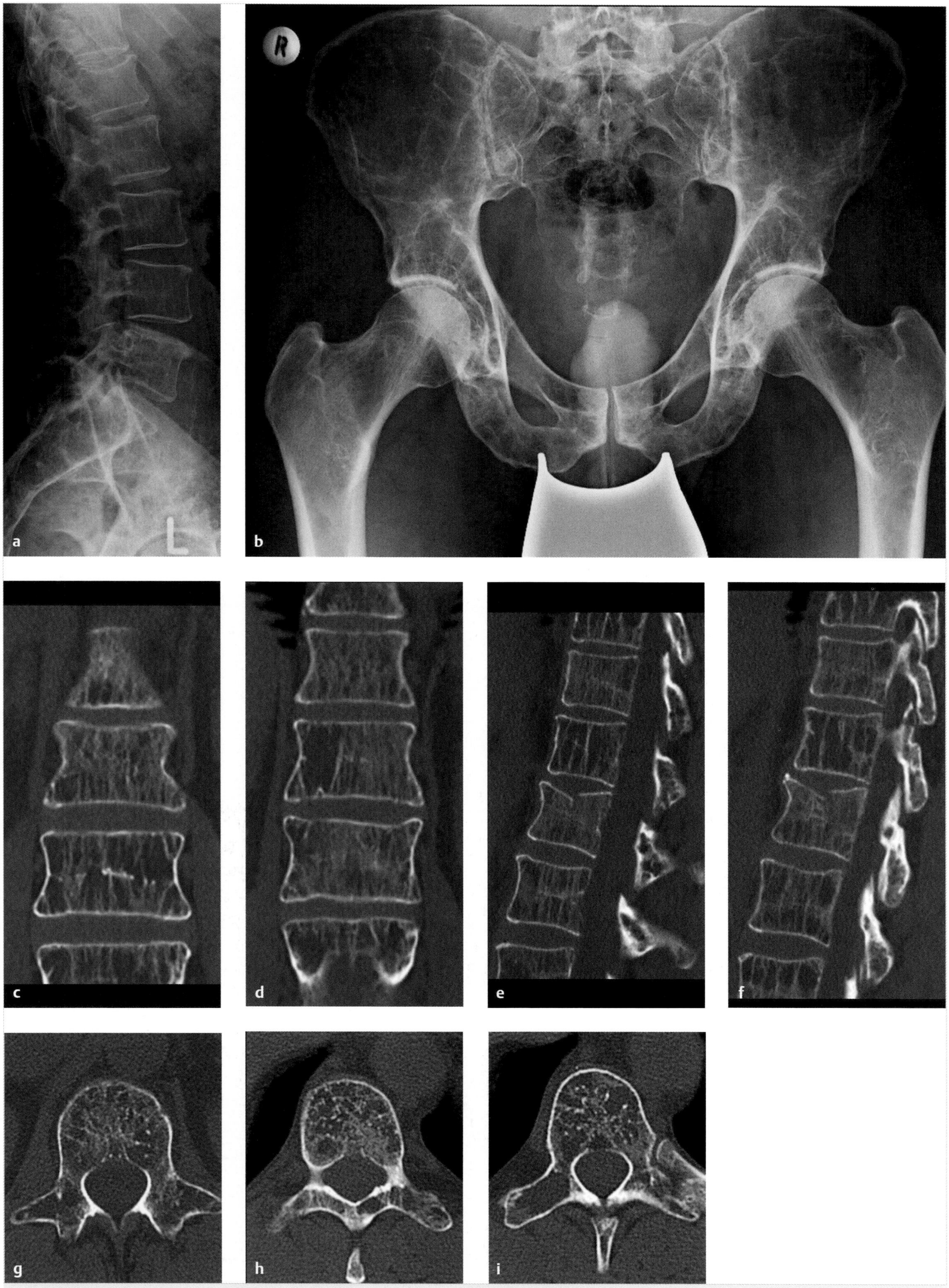

Fig. 3.29 a–q Multiple myeloma (diffuse plasmocytoma)?

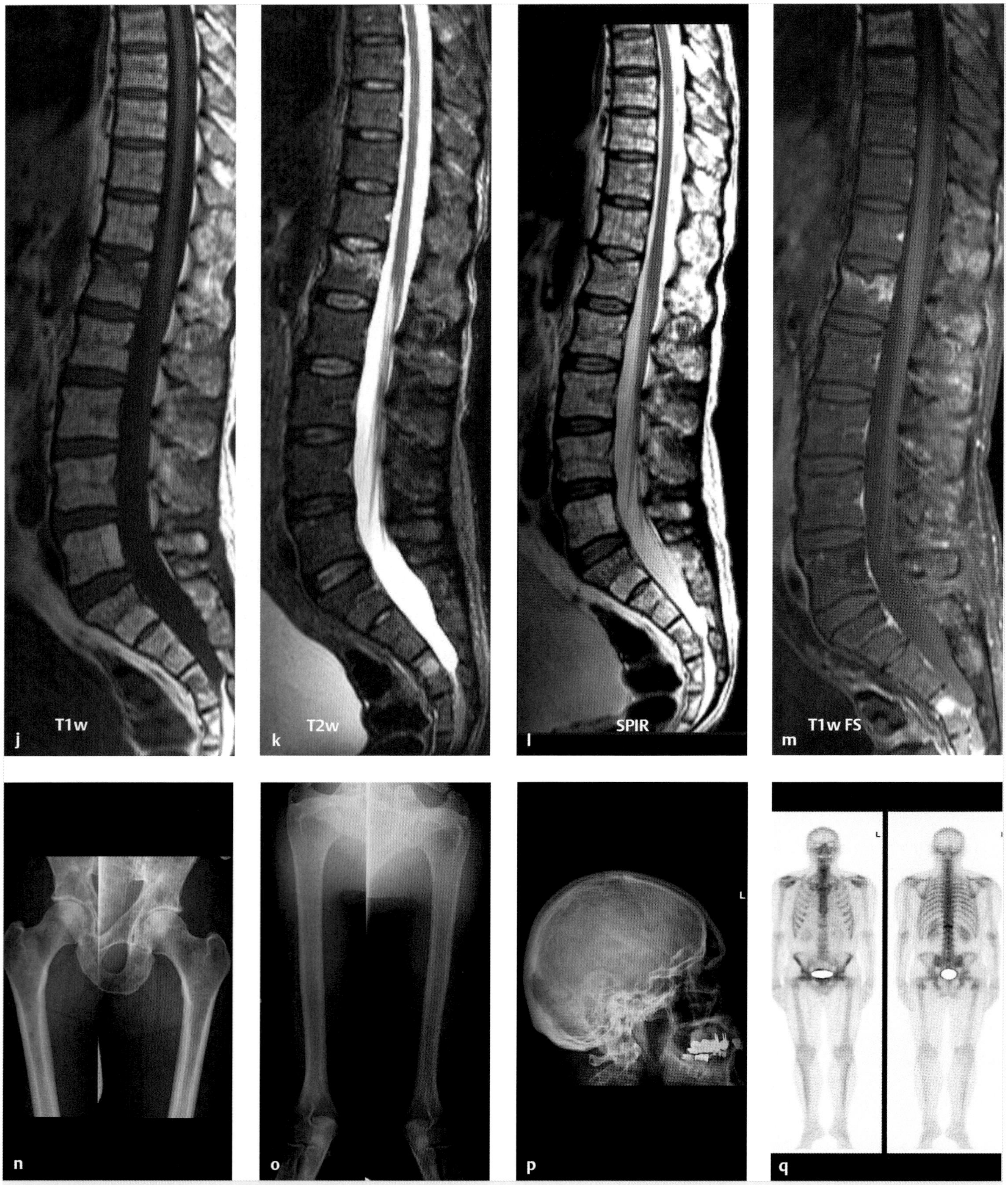

Fig. 3.29 a–q Continued.

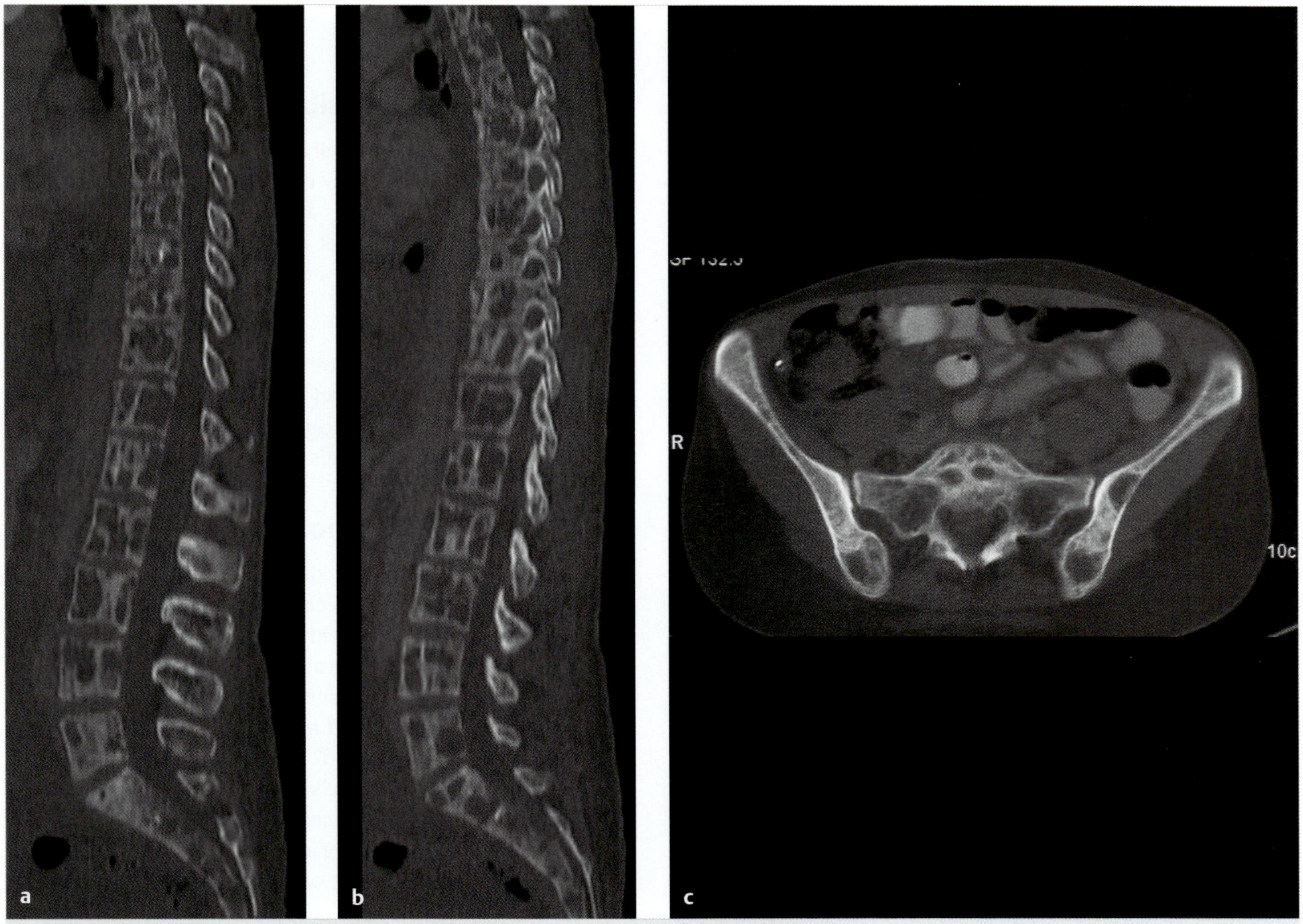

Fig. 3.30 a–c For comparison: metastatic breast cancer.

Final Diagnosis

Cystic angiomatosis of the spine, pelvis, and femur, healed with fatty replacement and accompanied by a (spontaneous) fracture of L1 following a bicycle accident.

Comments

Even in rare diseases like cystic angiomatosis, the use of memory links such as "honeycomb bone destruction → hemangioma" may provide the key to an accurate clinical and radiologic diagnosis.

Case 35 (▶ Fig. 3.31)

Case description

- Referring physician: internist.
- Prior history and clinical question: A 26-year-old woman, HIV-positive, presented with diffuse skeletal pain. A consult was sought to determine the cause of the innumerable lesions in the spine. She was known to have pulmonary tuberculosis. There were no skin abnormalities.

Radiologic Findings

The CT-sections of the lumbar spine (▶ Fig. 3.31 **a–e**) show relatively well-circumscribed osteolytic defects that contain bone sequestra. Identical lesions were present in the thoracic spine (not shown here).

Pathoanatomic Background of the Findings

Bone sequestra generally signify a necrotizing process. Inflammatory exudation with associated edema in the nondistensible and confined medullary cavity leads to a rise of intraosseous pressure that compresses the blood vessels, especially the veins. This perfusion disorder inevitably leads to toxic edema with cytokine release, oxygen radical formation, release of proteases, and eventual necrosis. Neutrophils (pus) and inflammatory pannus wall off the necrotic area, and a sequestrum (sloughed dead bone fragment) is formed. Sequestra make an ideal culture medium for pathogenic organisms. Sequestra are also found occasionally in various noninfectious, granulomatous diseases such as eosinophilic granuloma (Langerhans-cell histiocytosis) and, rarely, in areas destroyed by tumor.[30]

Assignment to a Possible Basic Entity

▶ **Inflammation?** Yes, very likely given the prior history of tuberculosis. A rare inflammatory entity in AIDS patients is bacillary angiomatosis (see Synopsis and Discussion below). If an inflammatory reactive component is not excluded in Langerhans-cell histiocytosis, we could also include this entity in the differential diagnosis.

▶ **Tumor?** Aside from a large-cell non-Hodgkin lymphoma with bone necrosis, ordinary metastatic bone destruction with sequestrum formation would be conceivable in theory but would be highly unlikely given the patient's prior history.

Synopsis and Discussion

The above considerations provide a definite indication for CT-guided percutaneous biopsy to obtain material for histology and microbiology. Histology indicated a "severe purulent necrotizing and caseating osteomyelitis, already chronic, most likely tuberculosis," and that diagnosis was confirmed by microbiologic testing.

This excludes *Langerhans-cell histiocytosis* as well as *bacillary angiomatosis* (see Inflammation? above), a multisystem disease involving the reticulohistiocytic system, skin, and mucous membranes. It is caused by *Rochalimaea quintana* and *R. henselae*, bacteria similar to the causative organism of cat-scratch disease. Cutaneous manifestations consist of multiple friable angiomatous papules that resemble pyogenic granulomas or the lesions of Ka-

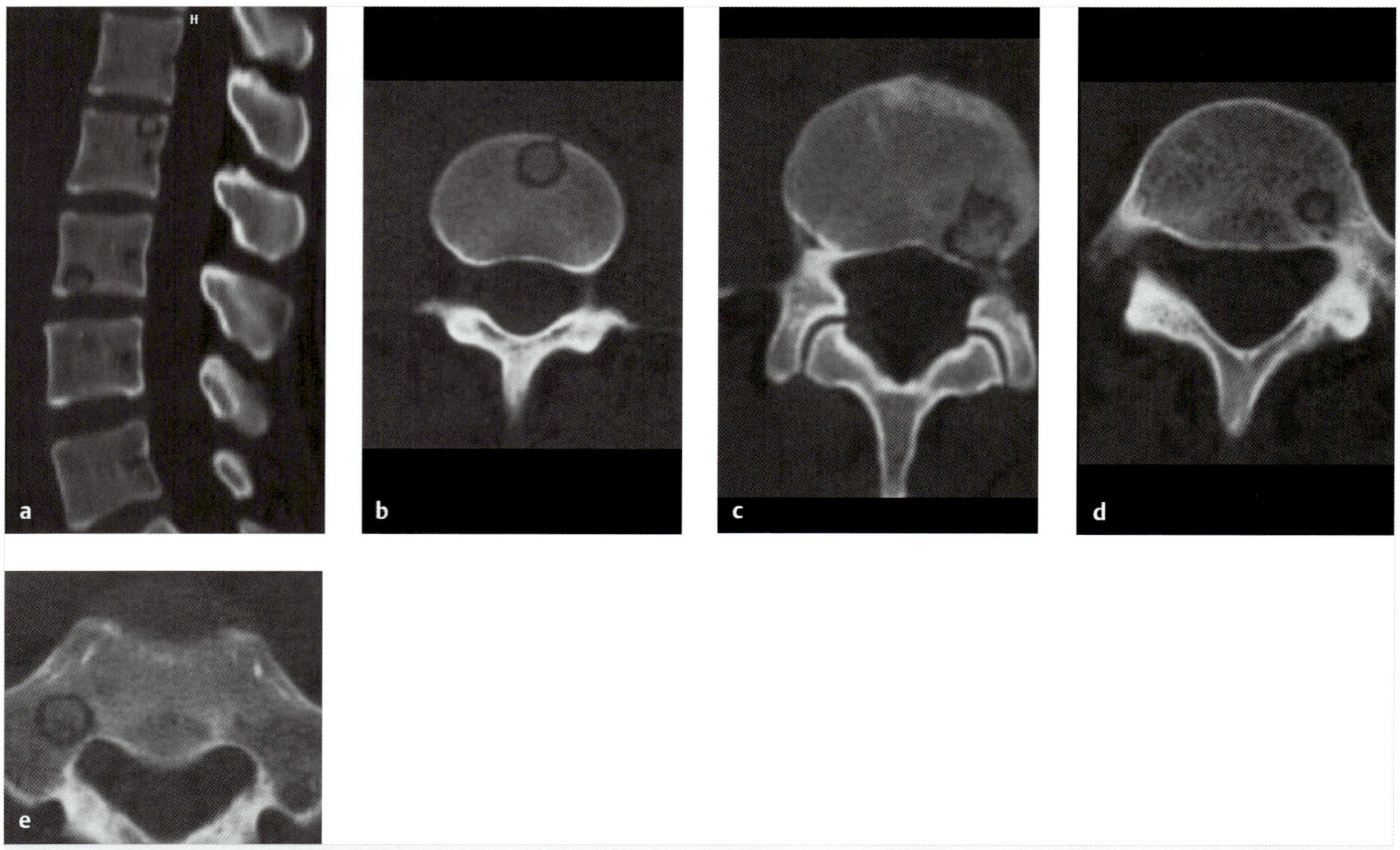

Fig. 3.31 a–e Sequestrum?

posi sarcoma. The bone changes consist of destructive lesions, which have a moth-eaten appearance and a somewhat ragged periosteal reaction. Sequestra also occur.

A final possibility would be *syphilitic (gummous) osteomyelitis*, which may also be associated with sequestra, if it is assumed that the patient has syphilis.

Final Diagnosis

Tuberculous spondylitis in AIDS.

Comments

Multiple osteolytic lesions with sequestra, when found in an HIV-positive patient with pre-existing pulmonary tuberculosis, are suggestive of bone tuberculous.

Case 36 (▶ Fig. 3.32)

Case description

- Referring physician: pathologist.
- Prior history and clinical question: A 57-year-old man complained of nonspecific ("ordinary") low back pain. On MRI of the lumbar spine, water-sensitive sequences and contrast-enhanced images revealed lesions in L2, L4, L5, and S1. An example is shown in ▶ Fig. 3.32 **i**, which demonstrates a lesion in L2.

The usual suspicion of metastasis from an unknown primary was voiced, and one of the lesions was investigated by percutaneous CT-guided biopsy. The pathologist found no tumor tissue suspicious for a metastasis but did find evidence of fibrous dysplasia. He sent the images to our institution to determine whether his presumptive diagnosis of fibrous dysplasia was compatible with the radiology. The possibility of angiomatosis was also raised at a different institution.

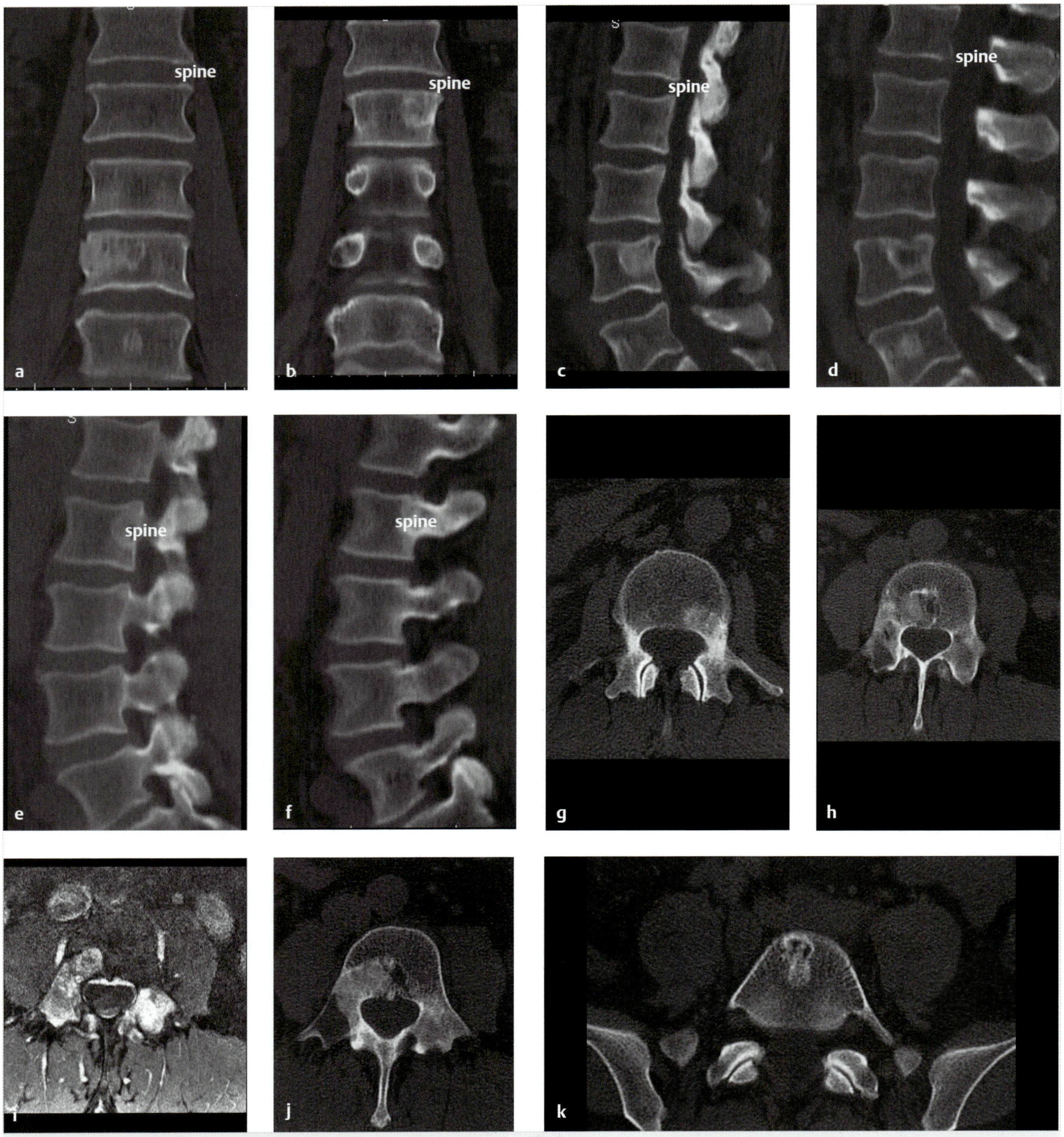

Fig. 3.32 a–k Sclerosing angiomatosis?

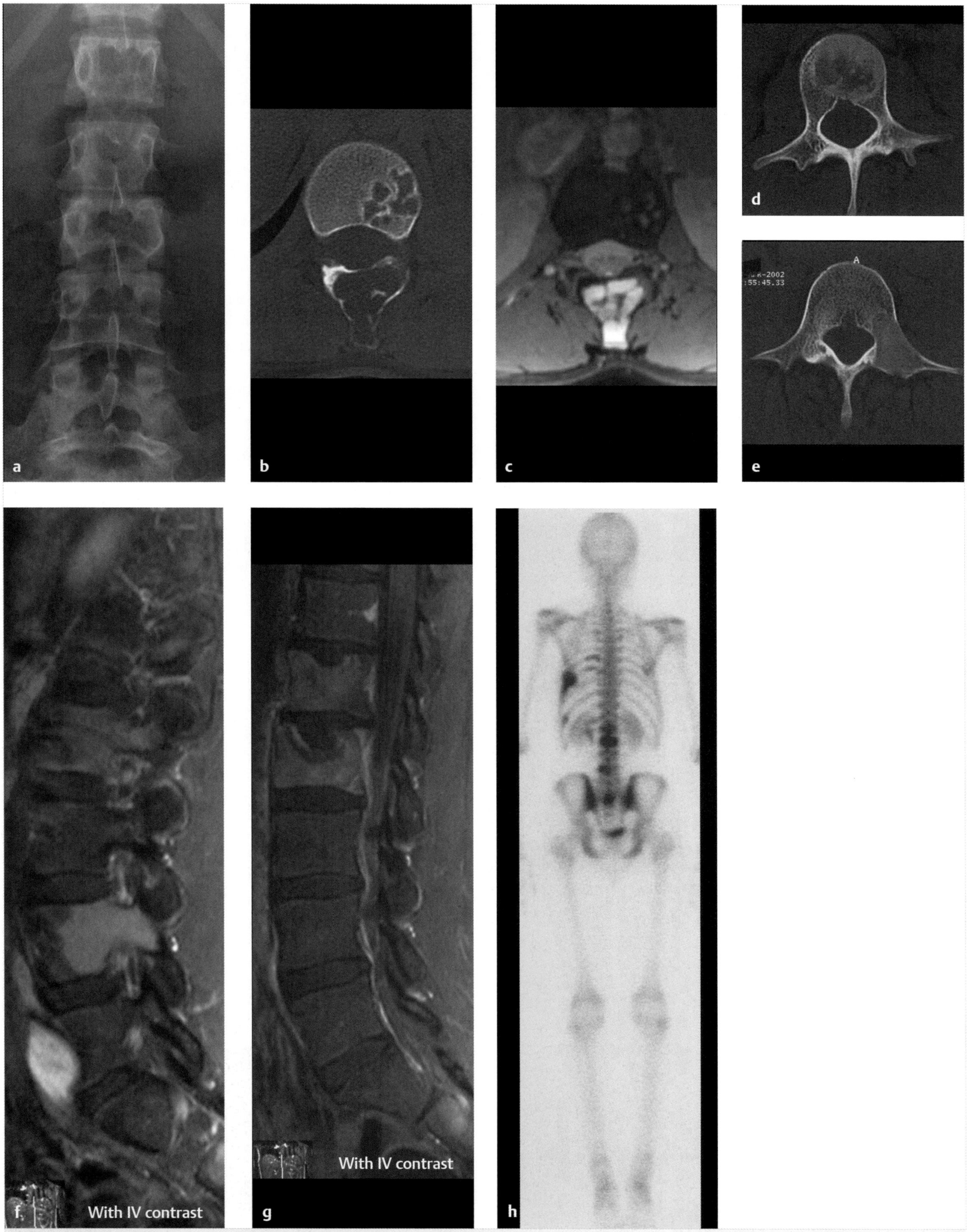

Fig. 3.33 a–h Another case of fibrous dysplasia of the lumbar spine?

Radiologic Findings

The CT images (▶ Fig. 3.32 **a–h, j, k**) demonstrate lesions of varying size in L2, L4, and L5 with predominantly ground-glass sclerosis in addition to smaller lytic elements. The lesions in L2 extend to both pedicles, and the right pedicle appears slightly expanded (▶ Fig. 3.32 **g, h**). The lesions also extend to the pedicles in L4, where both pedicles appear slightly broadened (▶ Fig. 3.32 **j**). Two panels (▶ Fig. 3.32 **c, j**) show almost homogeneous ground-glass attenuation in L4. In the MR image in ▶ Fig. 3.32 **i** (at a slightly higher level than the CT scan in ▶ Fig. 3.32 **h**), the lesions show intense enhancement after contrast administration.

Location

Some of the lesions occupy an eccentric location in the cancellous bone and are in contact with the cortex (▶ Fig. 3.32 **a, h, j**). They have spread to the vertebral appendages. ▶ Fig. 3.32 **d** shows a compression fracture in the upper endplate of L4.

Pathoanatomic Background of the Findings

A ground-glass pattern is the hallmark of nonlamellar woven bone in fibrous dysplasia and is not seen in any other type of new bone formation, be it reactive, reparative (due to metastatic destruction), or neoplastic (fibrosarcoma). Volume expansion is also a typical feature of fibrous dysplasia, as is the eccentric location with cortical bone involvement (see also ▶ Fig. 3.8 in Case 20). The good perfusion of the lesions (contrast-enhanced MRI) indicates that they are still active.

Assignment to a Possible Basic Entity

▶ **Normal variant or malformation?** Since fibrous dysplasia is considered a somatic mutation of the gene that codes for G protein, leading to the mono- or multifocal replacement of normal bone by fibrous connective tissue and immature nonlamellar bone, the findings may be loosely interpreted as a malformation.

▶ **Trauma?** No, although the collapsed upper endplate over the lesion in L4 may have occurred as a pathologic fracture in response to a fall or heavy lifting.

▶ **Inflammation?** No history or clinical signs. Reparative or inflammatory reactive bone does not have a ground-glass appearance but tends to show irregular streaks or very high density.

▶ **Tumor?** From a radiologic standpoint, angiomatosis could be considered for at least some of the lesions, but the ground-glass attenuation does not support this diagnosis. Reparative bone in angiomatosis would be more dense.

Synopsis and Discussion

The following arguments support a diagnosis of fibrous dysplasia in L2, L4, and L5:

- Nonspecific symptomatology with lesions detected fortuitously —true in most cases with small foci of fibrous dysplasia
- Eccentric lesion location with involvement of the cortex *and* vertebral appendages
- Ground-glass pattern, which always means "woven bone" and is typical of fibrous dysplasia

To establish a definitive diagnosis, the *GNAS-1* gene was identified as proof of fibrous dysplasia. This also eliminated angiomatosis from consideration.

▶ Fig. 3.33 **a–h** illustrates another case of fibrous dysplasia of the lumbar spine with lytic and ground-glass lesions. Again, note the volume expansion shown in ▶ Fig. 3.33 **e**. The MRI features (▶ Fig. 3.33 **c, f, g**) are nonspecific and do not add useful information.

Final Diagnosis

Foci of fibrous dysplasia in the lumbar spine.

Comments

If doubt exists, identification of the *GNAS-1* gene in the tissue helps to confirm a diagnosis of fibrous dysplasia.

Case 37 (▶ Fig. 3.34)

Case description

- Referring physician: radiologist.
- Prior history and clinical question: A 58-year-old man underwent a comprehensive preoperative work-up for prostate cancer that had recently been confirmed by biopsy. Intense tracer uptake was noted in the skull base and in C2. Further investigation by MRI was inconclusive. This prompted a CT examination of the skull base and upper cervical spine, which yielded two findings that could not be reconciled with each other. It should be added that the patient had sustained a traumatic impact to the skull several weeks before the radiologic examination. Since then he experienced moderate posterior neck pain during head movements.

Radiologic Findings

The right sphenoid bone appears expanded, and normal cancellous bone has been replaced by a ground-glass texture (▶ Fig. 3.34 **a**). C2 has lost its normal trabecular structure, due either to moth-eaten destruction or irregular spotty demineralization. Its volume is not significantly increased in either plane (▶ Fig. 3.34 **b, c**). Step-offs are visible at the base of the dens, and demineralization is most pronounced in that area.

Location

Bone changes are noted at two different sites, raising the question of whether there is an etiologic link between them.

Pathoanatomic Background of the Findings

The ground-glass pattern and volume expansion in the right sphenoid bone suggest fibrous dysplasia, while the moth-eaten cancellous bone destruction in the body of C2 suggests neoplasia. But do the structural changes in C2 really represent moth-eaten cancellous bone destruction, or does the irregular spotty demineralization result from a severe trophic disturbance in the form of a regional acceleratory phenomenon (RAP; see Synopsis and Discussion below) initiated by a dens fracture?

Assignment to a Possible Basic Entity

▶ **Normal variant or malformation?** If the change in the sphenoid bone is interpreted as fibrous dysplasia, then that lesion at least could be classified as a malformation (see also Case 36). But this definitely does not apply to the findings in C2 with its fractured dens.

▶ **Trauma?** The basal dens fracture is related to the impact trauma, since afterward the patient experienced posterior neck pain during head movements.

▶ **Inflammation?** No clinical manifestations.

▶ **Tumor?** The changes in C2 may represent tumor destruction with a spontaneous fracture; thus it is reasonable to classify them as metastatic to the confirmed prostate cancer.

▶ **Perfusion disorder?** The spotty demineralization in C2 may result from the dens fracture with an exaggerated activation of the RAP (see Synopsis and Discussion below). But since the skull trauma was not violent enough to cause a fracture in healthy bone, we must ask whether the bone in C2 was already structurally weakened before the trauma, so that the impact was sufficient to cause a pathologic fracture. It is still unclear whether fibrous dysplasia or a metastasis lay behind the presumed pathologic fracture, with or without an associated RAP.

These considerations provide a compelling indication for biopsy. The question of whether the prostate cancer metastasized to C2 will ultimately determine all further actions in this patient (radical prostatectomy, palliative therapy, radiation to C2?).

Synopsis and Discussion

A CT-guided percutaneous biopsy of C2 was finally performed and confirmed a metastasis from the histologically confirmed prostate cancer.

Was this case overdiagnosed? Radiology was by no means conclusive either for a metastasis or for a basal dens fracture and RAP related to pre-existing fibrous dysplasia. Meanwhile a confident diagnosis was essential in determining the scope of further management.

As its name implies, RAP (see also Pathoanatomic Background and Perfusion disorder) is an accelerating process that triggers the individual stages of fracture healing, increasing the rate of these activities by a factor of 2 to 10.[13,31] It is always conspicuous by its absence, in which case imaging will not show an often speckled pattern of postoperative demineralization, and fracture healing will be absent or delayed. The RAP is related to blood flow at the fracture site and its surroundings; it is an active process. That is why "inactivity atrophy" is an unfortunate term for demineralization at a fracture site and its surroundings. Not infrequently, the RAP is so pronounced that the bone looks demineralized as it would due to inflammation, a tumor, or the lytic (hypervascular) stage of Paget disease. In the present case, this phenomenon had to be considered in the interpretation of the CT

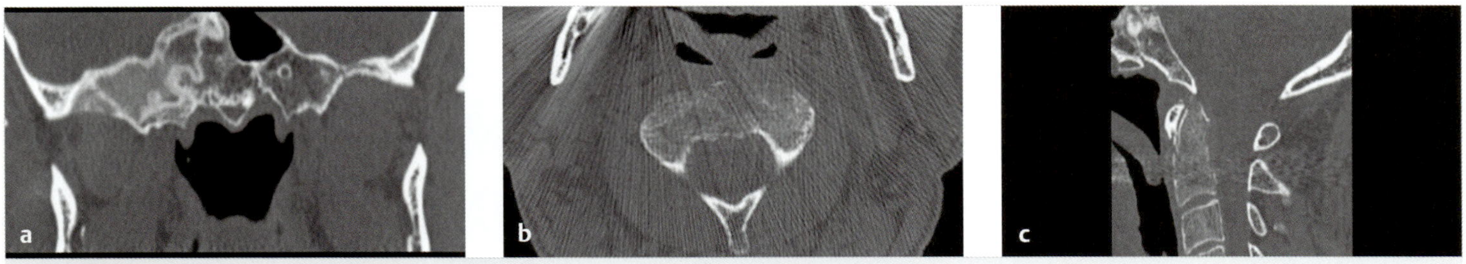

Fig. 3.34 a–c One disease or two?

images of C2, but definitive evidence required percutaneous biopsy.

In this context we refer the reader to Case 112, in which fibrous dysplasia was so demineralized after trauma that it mimicked the appearance of an aggressive tumor.

Final Diagnosis

Fibrous dysplasia in the right sphenoid bone, and bone metastasis from prostate cancer in C2 with a spontaneous fracture.

Comments

When a lesion with classic imaging features is located in proximity to an atypical second lesion, it is tempting to classify the second lesion like the first if one assumes that the atypical features of the second lesion are the result of an RAP. The differentiation of a strong RAP with spotty demineralization from moth-eaten metastatic destruction may be problematic and in some cases can be established only by biopsy.

Case 38 (▶ Fig. 3.35)

Case description

- Referring physician: radiologist.
- Prior history and clinical question: An 89-year-old woman complained of severe back pain 4 weeks after sustaining a backward fall. When she was examined on admission, pain to pressure and percussion were noted at the thoracolumbar junction. Subsequent radiographs, CT, and MRI showed unusual findings in T11 and T12, which were initially suspicious for a tumor. When questioned specifically in the light of imaging findings, the patient acknowledged that she had suffered for years from spondyloarthritis (initially undifferentiated).

Radiologic Findings

The CT images (▶ Fig. 3.35 **a–h**) show an almost complete loss of trabecular structure in the vertebral bodies. Moreover, ankylosing syndesmophytes have formed on various vertebral margins and corners, and ankylosis is noted in the intervertebral facet joints. T11 shows anterior wedging due to upward displacement of its lower endplate, and its posterior margin bulges toward the spinal canal. The upper endplate of T12 has followed the upward shift of the T11 lower endplate, causing an anterior fish-mouth splaying of T12. Its posterior margin appears compressed and, like T11, is protruding into the spinal canal. No trabecular markings are visible in T12. The lower endplate of T10 is infractured. Water-sensitive MRI sequences (▶ Fig. 3.35 **i, j**) show fluid-equivalent signal intensities throughout T12 with increased signal intensity in the compressed T11. Increased signal intensity is also noted in the paravertebral soft tissues (▶ Fig. 3.35 **k**).

Pathoanatomic Background of the Findings

Very severe cancellous bone loss is present, based on the criterion of lost structures in the vertebral bodies. This signifies advanced osteoporosis. T12 is splayed open anteriorly and appears to contain mostly fluid. T11 is severely compressed. The pronounced ankylosing processes are a result of the inflammatory destructive process and proliferative underlying disease (spondyloarthritis).

Assignment to a Possible Basic Entity

▶ **Trauma?** Yes, a fall definitely initiated the severe fracture-related deformities of T11 and T12.

▶ **Tumor?** It is appropriate to ask whether the gross loss of trabecular structure in all the vertebral bodies results from a generalized neoplastic process that destroys bone, such as diffuse plasmacytoma.

▶ **Systemic disease?** Yes, there is severe osteoporosis which is apparently a result of the radiologically documented spondyloarthritis.

Synopsis and Discussion

The further course and clinical presentation made it unlikely that the severe osteoporosis resulted from a generalized plasmacytoma (multiple myeloma). It is more likely a result of the inflammatory systemic enthesitis (spondyloarthritis), since chronic inflammatory rheumatic diseases with a long and severe course are generally associated with osteoporosis. The advanced age of the patient is definitely a factor as well. Now it is a question of determining the pathogenesis of the unusual fracture configuration of T11 and T12, which can be aptly described as a "wedged vertebra turned backwards."[32]

The unusual configuration of the T12 fracture was most likely caused by the gross osteoporotic compression fracture of T11. Because the T11–T12 diskovertebral junction was apparently more stable (due in part to ankylosing processes) than the practically hollow T12, the disk and upper endplate of T12 followed the collapse of the T11 lower endplate, causing T12 to splay open anteriorly. Bleeding from ruptured vessels then filled the space previously occupied by T12.

Final Diagnosis

Unusual osteoporotic fractures at the thoracolumbar junction in a setting of spondyloarthritis.

Comments

In interpreting the mechanics of unusual spinal fractures, it is helpful to consider easily recognized underlying diseases of the spine.

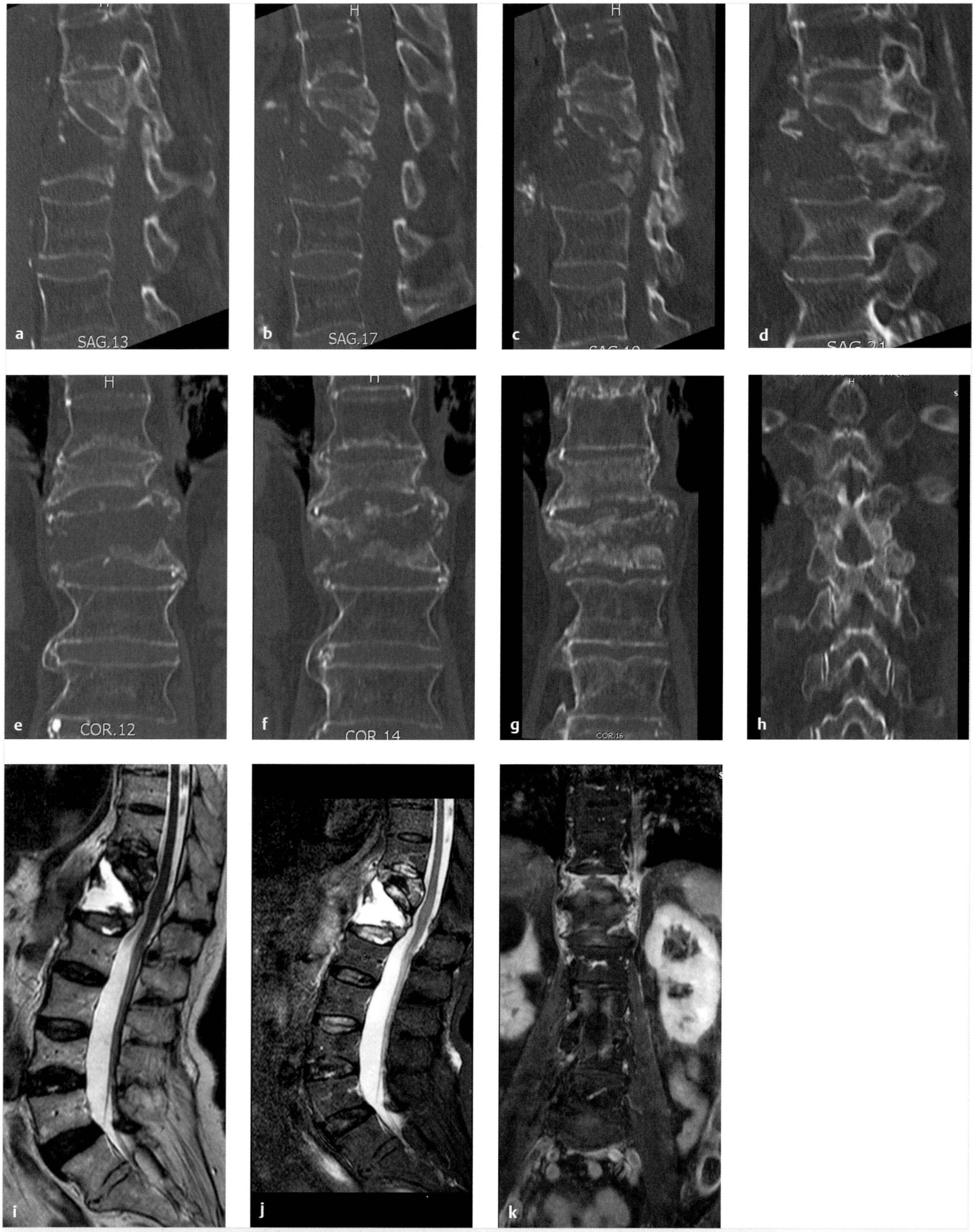

Fig. 3.35 a–k Pathologic fractures due to multiple myeloma?

3.3 Diseases of Spinal Entheses and Joints

Case 39 (▶ Fig. 3.36)

Case description

- *Referring physicians:* orthopedist and rheumatologist.
- *Prior history and clinical question:* A 52-year-old man complained of chest pain radiating to the neck and the left arm, most noticeable in the morning. He did not have typical signs of inflammatory back pain. HLA-B27 was negative and C-reactive protein (CRP) was within normal limits. The thoracic spine was examined by MRI. The radiologist presumed spondyloarthritis and added CT scans, which confirmed his working diagnosis. The patient was referred to a dermatologist to confirm or exclude psoriasis. The dermatologist wrote: "Approximately 2 weeks ago the patient had two coin-sized inflammatory lesions on the lower limbs. The lesions responded to local treatment with betamethasone, and currently the sites show postinflammatory hyperpigmentation. One possible diagnosis is nummular eczema." The treating orthopedist, like the radiologist, is convinced of a rheumatic systemic disease and requests a definitive diagnosis.

Radiologic Findings

The T2w MR images of the thoracic spine (▶ Fig. 3.36 **a, b**) show almost homogeneous high signal intensity throughout T7, in the anterosuperior corner of T9, in the upper anterior portions of T10, and under the lower endplate of T11. The T7 vertebra appears sclerotic on CT images (▶ Fig. 3.36 **c–e**), its lower endplate is destroyed, and its upper endplate shows irregular sclerosis. Parasyndesmophytes are visible in ▶ Fig. 3.36 **d, e**. The anterior portion of the upper endplate of T10 is destroyed and sclerotic (▶ Fig. 3.36 **c**). CT scans of the thoracic spine also reveal a combined destructive and proliferative process in the left anterosuperior chest wall (▶ Fig. 3.36 **f–i**).

Location

The changes are reflected in the upper and lower endplates, the vertebral margins and corners, and the anterior chest wall—areas in which numerous entheses occur. Multiple vertebral bodies are involved.

Pathoanatomic Background of the Findings

The essential features on CT are a combination of destructive changes and new bone formation or proliferation (sclerosis, parasyndesmophytes). The changes with edema-like signal intensity can be interpreted as an accompanying phenomenon of osteitis, and the whole may be interpreted as a nonbacterial inflammatory process. The similar pathoanatomy of the changes in the anterior chest wall suggests a systemic disease.

Assignment to a Possible Basic Entity

▶ **Normal variant or malformation?** No.

▶ **Trauma?** No history, not even for chronic trauma.

▶ **Inflammation?** Yes. This is consistent with the pathoanatomic background. Parasyndesmophytes plus simultaneous destructive/proliferative changes in the diskovertebral junctions, and the destructive-proliferative changes in the anterior chest wall, all suggest a psoriatic spondyloarthritis or Reiter syndrome. A bacterial inflammation is not supported by the simultaneous destructive and reparative changes, which are usually metachronous in a bacterial inflammation.

▶ **Tumor or metastasis (e.g., from prostate cancer)?** No. The history is negative in this regard and the patient has no known risk factors. In any case the eccentric distribution of the changes in the affected vertebral bodies are not consistent with a neoplastic process. Nor could a tumor explain the parasyndesmophytes.

▶ **Regressive (degenerative) process?** No. Sclerosis under the upper and lower endplates would predominate in osteochondrosis, and there would be spondylophytes rather than parasyndesmophytes.

Synopsis and Discussion

The radiologic findings strongly suggest the presence of a psoriasis-associated spondyloarthritis or Reiter syndrome. The latter diagnosis is not supported by the history and clinical data, however (e.g., urethritis, keratoconjunctivitis, etc.). But is psoriasis-associated spondyloarthritis possible if the dermatologist finds no typical signs of psoriasis in the patient (▶ Fig. 3.37, different patient)? Certainly, because the dermatologic examination in this case took place at a time when "coin-sized inflammatory lesions" on the lower leg had already subsided. This is not sufficient to exclude psoriasis, which requires a histologic examination. We ordered a biopsy which confirmed psoriasis vulgaris. Apparently the dermatologist lacked the necessary awareness of the problem at the time of initial presentation; otherwise he would have done an immediate biopsy.

When he presented at our institution, the patient stated in response to specific questioning that some time ago he had pain in the anterior chest wall radiating to the left arm. This fits with the findings in the left manubriocostal region (▶ Fig. 3.36 **f–i**), which represent asymmetric sternocostoclavicular hyperostosis (SCCH; see also Case 97) and are a common feature of psoriatic spondyloarthritis.

Finally, it should be noted that psoriatic spondyloarthritis belongs to the group of seronegative spondyloarthropathies.

Final Diagnosis

Psoriatic spondyloarthritis with involvement of the anterior chest wall (SCCH).

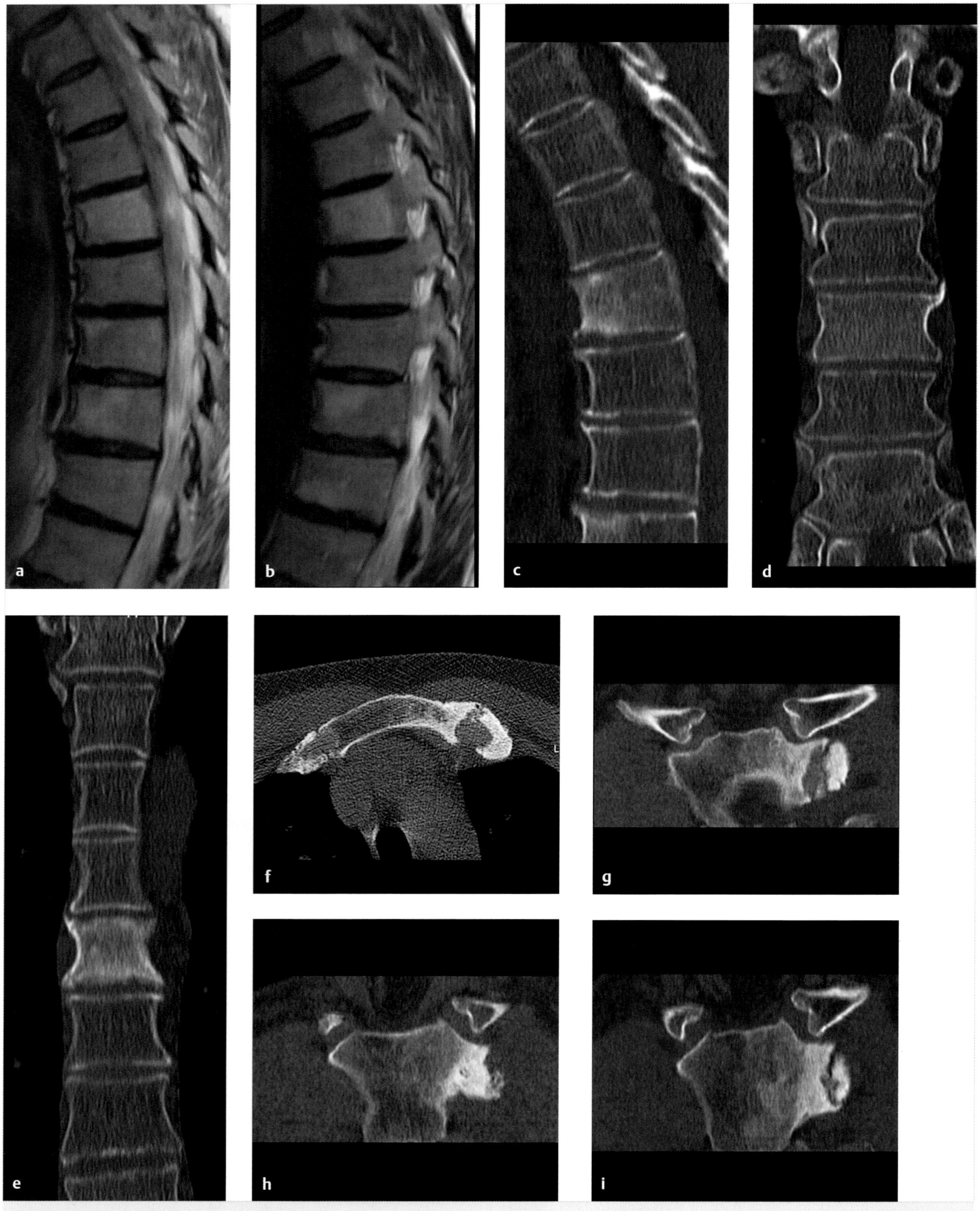

Fig. 3.36 a–i Spondylitis or metastases?

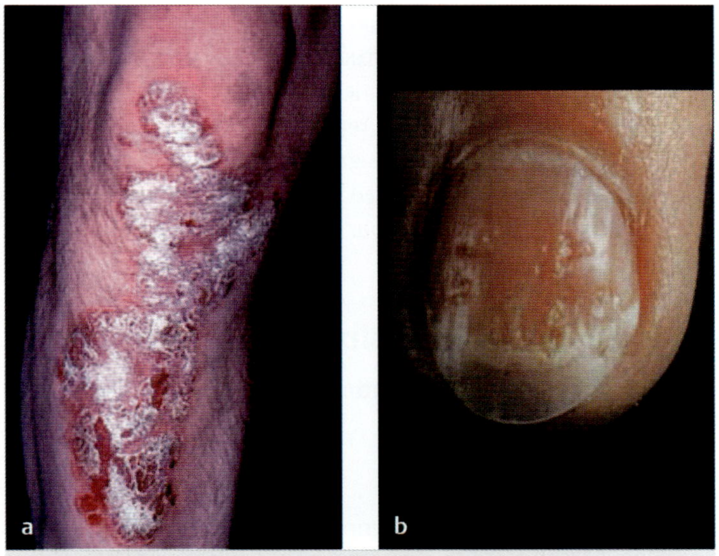

Fig. 3.37 a, b Classic signs of psoriasis in a different patient.

Comments

The orthopedist, rheumatologist, and radiologist were on the right track clinically and radiologically (following MRI with CT to investigate simultaneous destruction and reactive-reparative proliferation and parasyndesmophytes) but were misled by the inconclusive dermatology report. Insistence upon a histologic evaluation finally yielded a definitive diagnosis, without having to biopsy the spinal lesions or undertake a pointless and invasive search for a primary tumor.

Case 40 (▶ Fig. 3.38)

Case description

- *Referring physician:* general practitioner.
- *Prior history and clinical question:* A 65-year-old woman presented with a long history of nonspecific lumbar pain. Imaging revealed marked sclerotic changes in the lumbar spine, which were interpreted initially as osteosclerotic metastases from an unknown primary tumor. Tuberculous spondylitis was also considered in the differential diagnosis. The family doctor did not believe these diagnoses because the patient appeared clinically well. Before ordering a comprehensive tumor search and biopsy of the sclerotic lesions, the doctor wanted to know if there was a plausible alternative diagnosis for the radiologic changes.

Radiologic Findings

The initial MR images (▶ Fig. 3.38 **a**, T2w) show areas of markedly increased signal intensity in L3 and L5, which correlate with pronounced sclerotic changes on CT scans (▶ Fig. 3.38 **b**). The anterosuperior corners of both vertebral bodies are destroyed. Bone spurs project from the inferior edge of the erosions, and both can be characterized as syndesmophytes. These findings were the original basis for the radiology consult. We ordered additional imaging studies as described below.

Location

Based on the CT images in particular, we can definitely relate the destructive (erosive) and proliferative changes to the diskovertebral junctions (at the anterosuperior vertebral margins and upper endplates), which are entheses.

Pathoanatomic Background of the Findings

Bone destruction and new bone formation (syndesmophytes, sclerosis) are apparently taking place simultaneously. The detection of edema-like signal on MRI proves that the process is still florid. This combination of destruction and repair is a typical feature of inflammatory rheumatic enthesitis and is unlike the metachronous destruction and repair that occurs in bacterial inflammations. The edema-like signal in the bone is referable to associated osteitis. Now we need only obtain further clinical information in order to advance our interpretation and move closer to a clinical diagnosis.

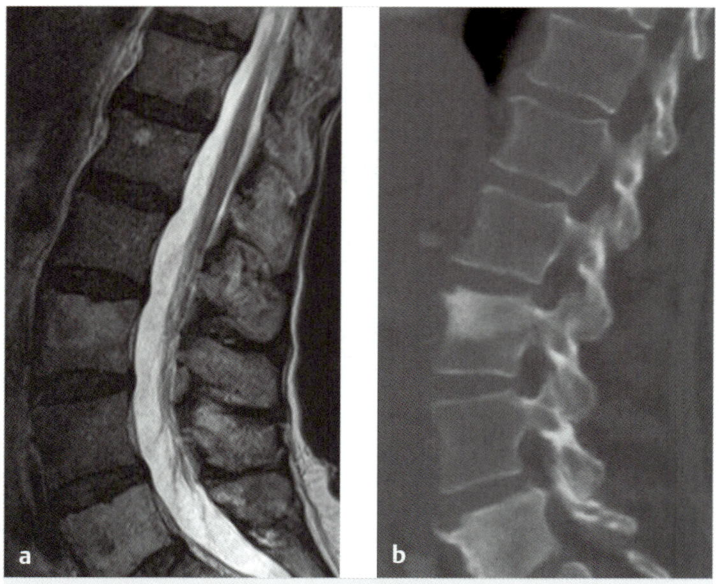

Fig. 3.38 a, b Tuberculous spondylitis or metastases?

Assignment to a Possible Basic Entity

▶ **Normal variant or malformation?** No.

▶ **Trauma?** No history.

▶ **Inflammation?** Yes. The arguments are the same as in Case 39. Further clinical information is now needed (see Synopsis and Discussion below).

▶ **Tumor?** No. What kind of tumor would we consider? Two factors are inconsistent with an osteoplastic (osteosclerotic) metastasis: the healthy-looking patient does not have a known primary tumor, and the changes are localized mainly to the vertebral margins and corners. How could an osteoplastic metastasis account for the simultaneous destruction and proliferation at the diskovertebral junctions?

▶ **Necrosis?** No. We could indeed assume a nonfragmenting necrosis with reparative new bone formation in L3 and L5, but then how would we explain the other notable findings (syndesmophytes, eroded corners)?

▶ **Synopsis and Discussion** The imaging findings discussed above clearly point in the direction of a systemic inflammatory-rheumatic enthesitis and thus to a form of spondyloarthritis. We needed only clinical information to determine what type of spondyloarthritis is present. When the author of this book contacted the patient, we learned that she had a long history of a “special kind of psoriasis,” namely pustulosis palmoplantaris (▶ Fig. 3.39 **d**). She has been receiving successful psoriasis-specific dermatologic treatment for that condition, and formerly severe pains in the spine and anterior chest wall have improved significantly.

This information allows us to make a diagnosis of *pustular arthro-osteitis or enthesio-osteitis*, which is the same as the more vaguely defined *SAPHO syndrome* (synovitis, acne, pustulosis, hyperostosis, osteitis). Pustulosis palmoplantaris (▶ Fig. 3.39 **b**) is a special form of psoriasis that may sometimes be associated with classic psoriasis (pustular psoriasis). Several features distinguish it from psoriasis as far as skeletal involvement is concerned: Instead of the sacroiliac joints, the anterior chest wall, which is rich in entheses, is more commonly affected by simultaneous destructive and proliferative changes with plaquelike ankylosis in later stages (SCCH) (see also Case 97).

Finally, we ordered a bone scan (▶ Fig. 3.39 **a**) to look for additional manifestations and found sites of abnormal uptake in the sternocostoclavicular region and thoracic spine. CT images (▶ Fig. 3.39 **c–f**) displayed the typical appearance of SCCH with additional involvement of the manubriosternal synchondrosis

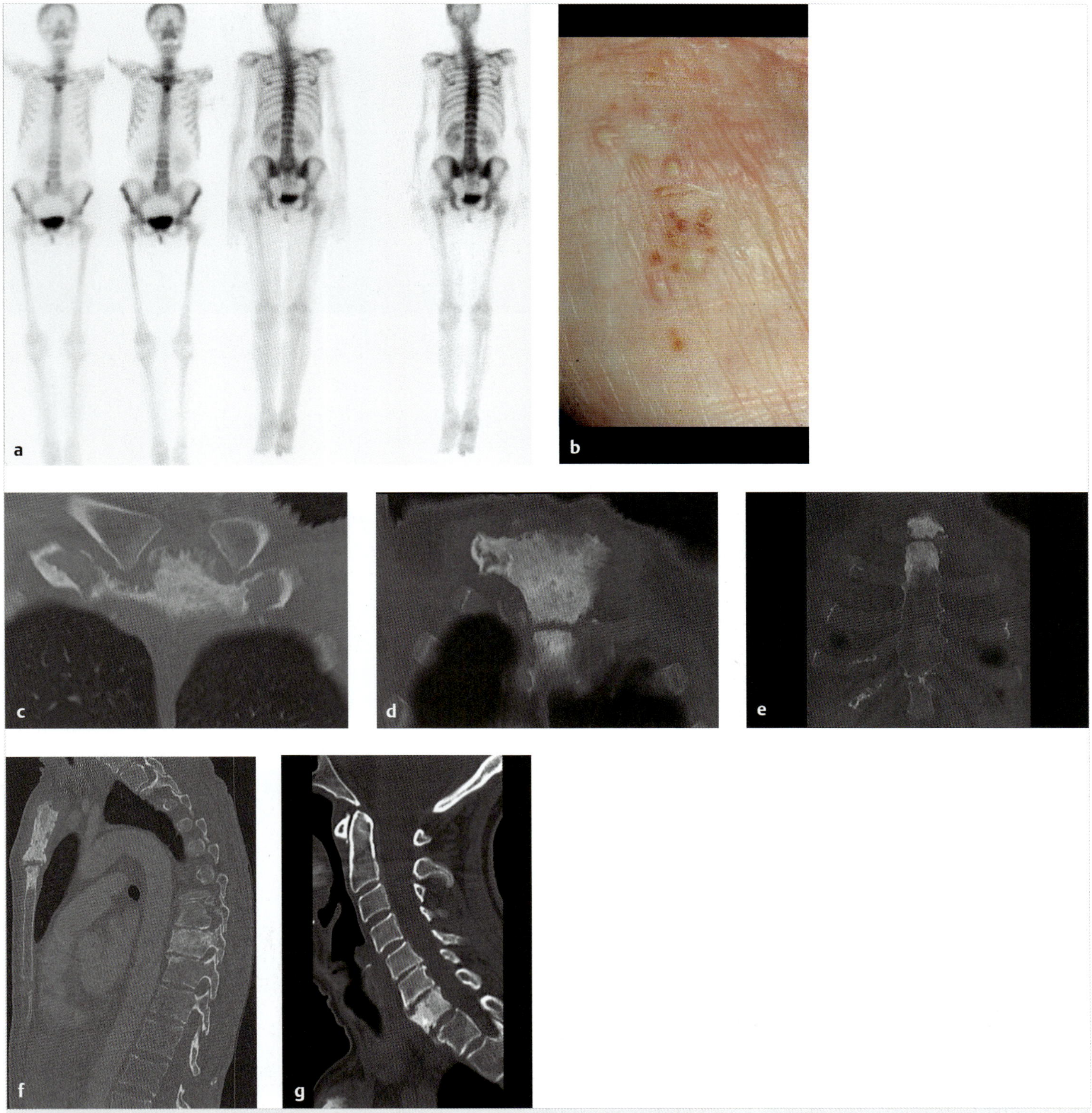

Fig. 3.39 a–g Bone scans and CT images of the patient in ▶ Fig. 3.38.

(which is also an enthesis!). The changes visible in C7 (▶ Fig. 3.39 **g**) were identical to those in L3, and both T8–T9 and T9–T10 showed the features of advanced spondylodiskitis, known also by the eponym "inflammatory Andersson lesion." The sagittal reformatted thoracic CT image (▶ Fig. 3.39 **f**) defines the true extent of the destructive-proliferative (enthesitic-osteitic) changes in the manubrium and body of the sternum.

▶ Fig. 3.40 illustrates the case of a 52-year-old woman with back pain who underwent two open biopsies to investigate radiologic changes in the thoracic spine. The biopsies were useless and showed only nonspecific osteitis, as might be expected. Clinically, however, the woman had a pronounced pustular form of psoriasis!

Final Diagnosis

Pustulotic arthro-osteitis or enthesio-osteitis (SAPHO syndrome) with involvement of the spine and anterior chest wall.

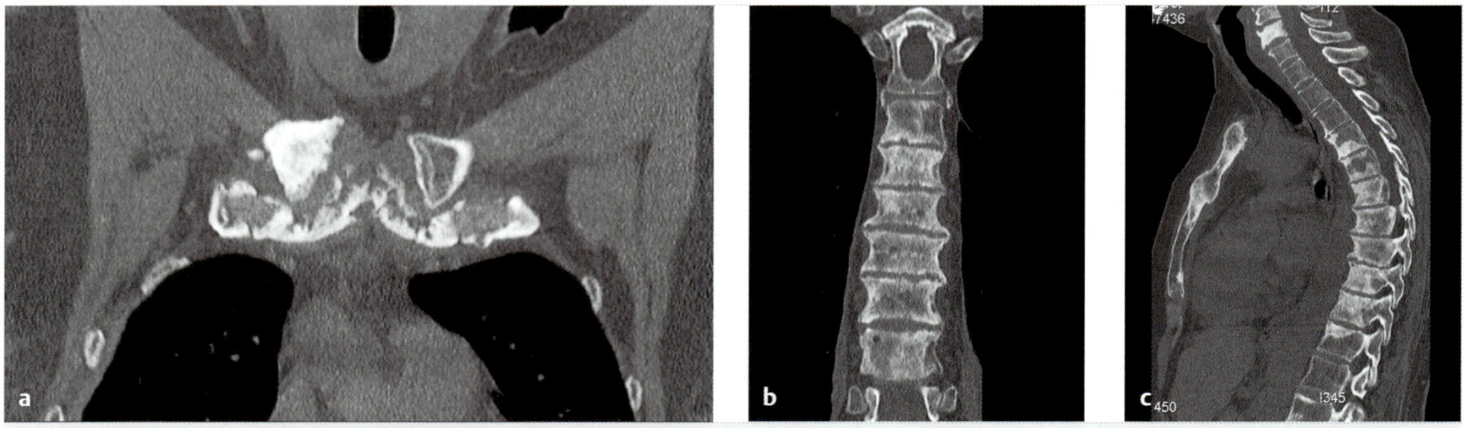

Fig. 3.40 a–c CT findings in a patient with pustular psoriasis.

Comments

Not everything that looks "white" in bone is a metastasis. Only clinical information and a whole-body bone scan can furnish a correct diagnosis and define the true extent of skeletal involvement in complex disorders such as pustulotic arthro-osteitis or SAPHO syndrome.

Case 41 (▶ Fig. 3.41)

Case description

- Referring physician: internist.
- Prior history and clinical question: A 61-year-old man presented with significant neck pain, overweight, metabolic syndrome with hyperuricemia, and a prior history of knee replacement. Question: tumor of the dens?

Radiologic Findings

CT images (▶ Fig. 3.41 **a–g**) show gross destructive changes in the odontoid process (dens). The transverse ligament of the atlas shows curvilinear calcifications (▶ Fig. 3.41 **c, d**). Crown-shaped calcium deposits surrounding the odontoid process are also visualized by the CT images. In addition there is gross destruction of the left C2–C3 facet joint (▶ Fig. 3.41 **c, d, h**). The mass around the odontoid process narrows the anterior subarachnoid canal and impresses on the medulla oblongata (▶ Fig. 3.41 **f, g, i–k**). The C2–C3 intervertebral space is greatly narrowed; almost all the disks are calcified (▶ Fig. 3.41 **f, g**). All the facet joints except the destroyed joint at C2–C3 are narrowed on the left side, and the subchondral plates are sclerotic (▶ Fig. 3.41 **c, d, h**).

Location

The destructive changes in the dens and C2–C3 facet joint are definitely related to the anatomic articular structures (cartilage, synovial membrane, capsule, ligaments). This also applies to the changes in the other facet joints.

Pathoanatomic Background of the Findings

The extensive destructive changes in articular structures (atlantoaxial joint, left C2–C3 facet joint) are definitely inflammatory in nature and originate from the synovial membrane. The calcifications in the mass located behind the dens and replacing the partially destroyed dens are either necrotic bone tissue or tophus, hydroxyapatite or calcium pyrophosphate dehydrate material. The disk calcifications may be regressive changes or may reflect a disease with calcium deposition. Thus, we are probably dealing with a complex articular process involving a combination of synovial arthropathy and chondroarthropathy.

Assignment to a Possible Basic Entity

▶ **Inflammation?** Yes, see under Pathoanatomic Background of the Findings above.

▶ **Tumor?** This question relates to the mass and the residual dens. No. It is logical to link the additional findings described above to this pseudotumor.

▶ **Necrosis?** It is certain that histology will show partial necrosis of the dens, and that necrotic material will be found in the destroyed C2–C3 facet joint.

Synopsis and Discussion

The above findings and discussions limit the differential diagnosis to two possible conditions:

1. Gout
2. Chondrocalcinosis (calcium pyrophosphate deposition disease)

▶ **On differential diagnosis 1 (see also Case 136)** Uric acid deposits in the joint incite a crystal synovitis and cartilage damage with tophus formation in the subchondral bone. The following findings are suggestive of gout in the present case:

- The patient has hyperuricemia.
- The destructive changes in the atlantoaxial joint and left C2–C3 facet joint are a result of synovitis.
- The pseudotumor around the damaged dens can be classified as tophus; this interpretation is also supported by the calcifications.
- The degenerative changes in the other facet joints are a manifestation of chronic gout.
- The disk calcifications are signs of secondary chondrocalcinosis.
- The patient has a history of knee replacement. Often the tissue is not examined for uric acid crystals, especially if the pathologist is not instructed to do so.

▶ **On differential diagnosis 2 (see also Case 155)** Primary chondrocalcinosis (pseudogout, crystal synovitis, pyrophosphate arthropathy also known as CPPD (calcium pyrophosphate dehydrate deposition disease) is a usually chronic systemic joint disease in which calcium pyrophosphate crystals are deposited in hyaline cartilage and fibrocartilage and in the periarticular soft tissues, which may produce the clinical and radiologic features of osteoarthritis and/or arthritis (pseudogout). As a rule, the deposits in the articular cartilage are visible on images. All pathologic changes in the present case, including the pseudotumor, may occur in chondrocalcinosis. Secondary chondrocalcinosis may occur in the setting of gout. A site of predilection in the spine is the fibrocartilage of the intervertebral disks. Involvement of the hyaline cartilage of the facet joints incites a synovitis with destructive changes in bony, cartilaginous, and capsuloligamentous structures. A feared complication of chondrocalcinosis in the spine is involvement of the craniovertebral joints, which may lead to cord compression and to dens destruction and fractures with a pseudotumor. The "crowned dens" sign (▶ Fig. 3.41 **a–d**), with calcifications around the dens, is very specific for primary chondrocalcinosis of the craniovertebral joints. According to Masami et Satoshi,[66] a "crowned dens" syndrome is characterized by recurrent neck pain related to radiodense deposits of hydroxyapatite or calcium pyrophosphate dehydrate in ligaments around the odontoid process, which create the appearance of a crown or halo surrounding the odontoid process on radiographic imaging.

The present case probably involves a combination of gout and chondrocalcinosis. Unfortunately, we know nothing about the extremity joints, where typical manifestations of each disease may be found (gout: big toe; chondrocalcinosis: metacarpophalangeal joints, carpal destruction with scapholunate dissociation, etc.; see Case 121, Case 127, and Case 155).

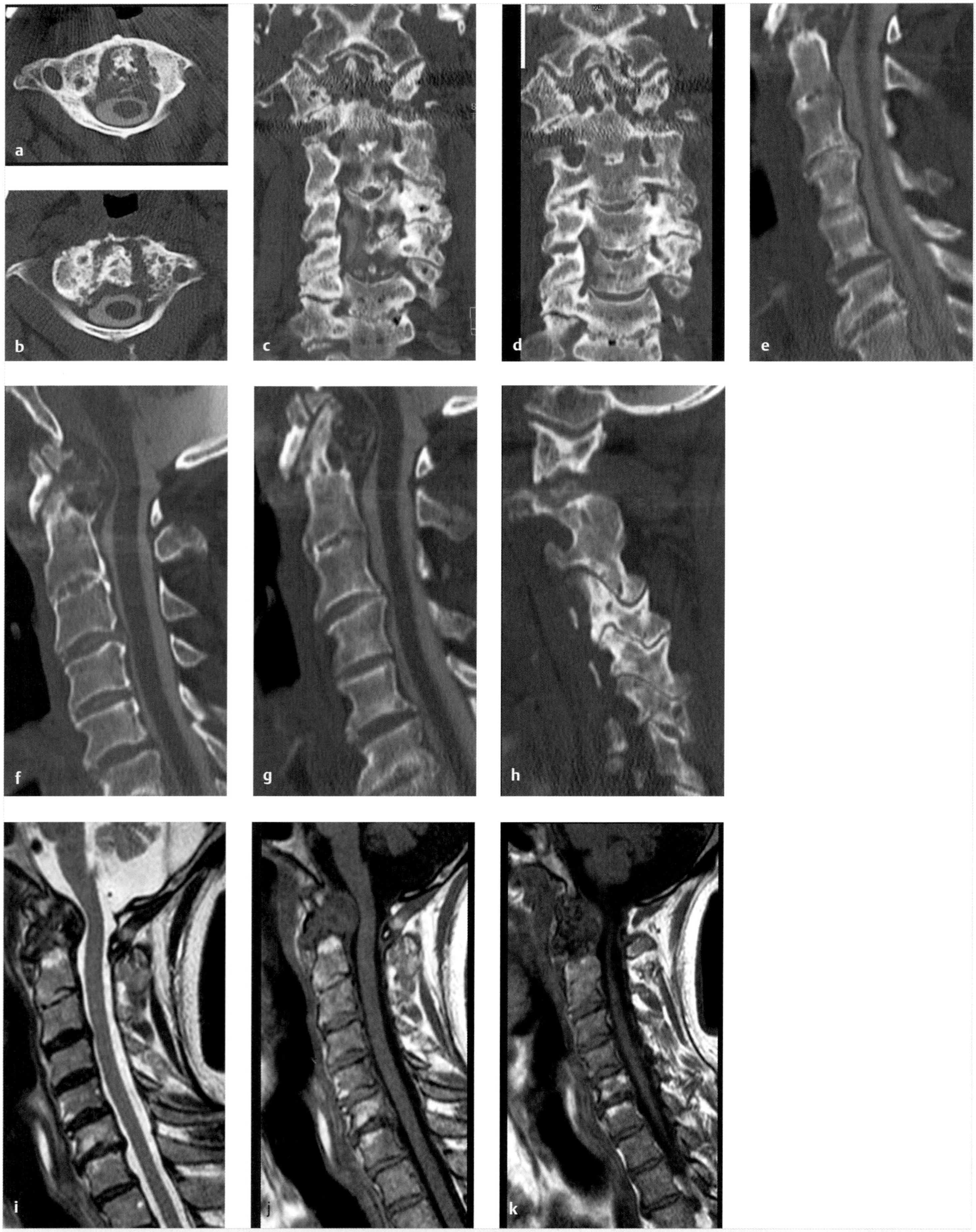

Fig. 3.41 a–k Destruction of the dens by a tumor?

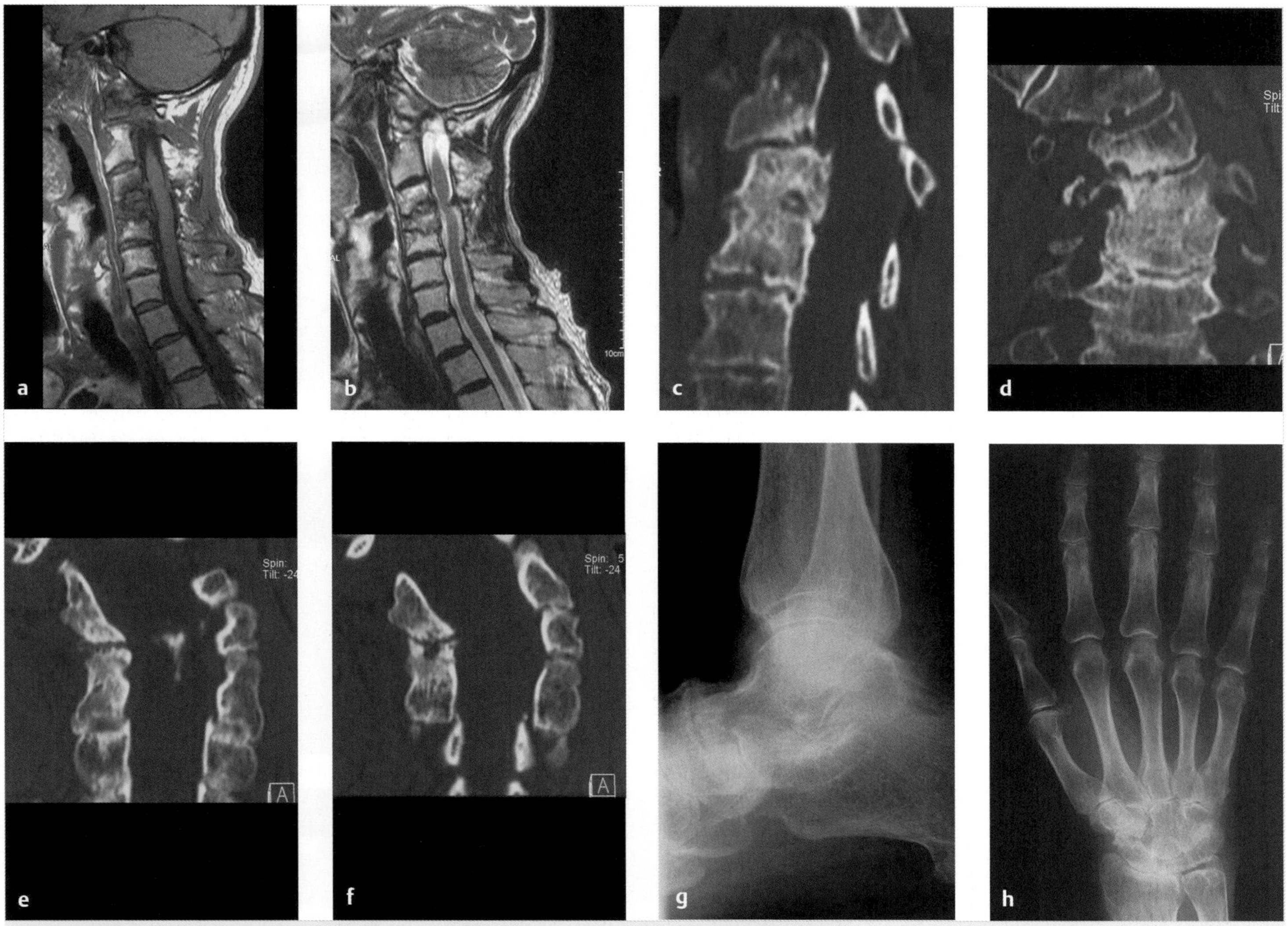

Fig. 3.42 a–h Severe chondrocalcinosis (CPPD) of the cervical spine with fixed torticollis.

▶ Fig. 3.42 illustrates another case of severe chondrocalcinosis of the cervical spine with fixed torticollis in an elderly man. The radiologic test joints for chondrocalcinosis in the hands and feet were examined in this patient. Severe bilateral degenerative changes were found in the carpal joints, ankle joints, and talonavicular joints, where ordinary primary degenerative arthritis is normally not found in the absence of pre-existing disease.

▶ Fig. 3.43 presents the case of an 85-year-old man in whom PET-CT (a–c) for melanoma staging showed increased uptake in the L4–L5 and L5–S1 facet joints and in the left foot. The CT scans (▶ Fig. 3.43 **d, e**) show marked expansion and destruction of the affected bone and joint structures. Scattered small calcified areas are also visible in the soft-tissue structures. The epicenters of the destructive changes were located in the joints, and it was logical to interpret the changes as gross tumorlike gouty arthritis with associated bone and joint destruction. Because the involvement of intervertebral facet joints with pseudotumor formation is very rare in gout, a biopsy was taken from the L5–S1 facet joint on the right side (▶ Fig. 3.43 **e**) and confirmed a gouty tophus with uric acid crystals (▶ Fig. 3.43 **f**). This case was furnished to us by Prof. Dr. Hierholzer of Potsdam.

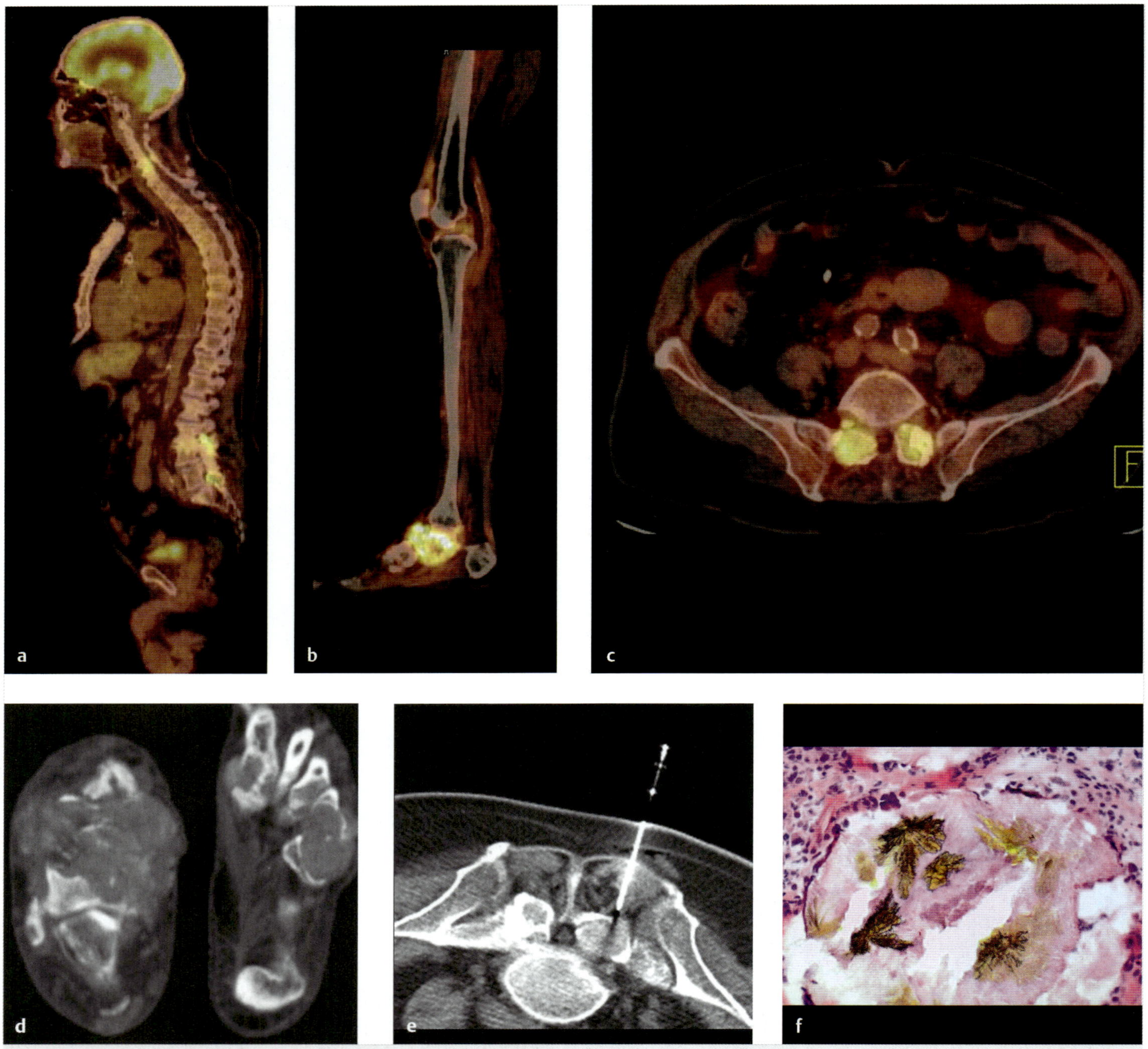

Fig. 3.43 a–f Gouty arthritis in an 85-year-old man.

Final Diagnosis

Gouty arthritis and/or chondrocalcinosis (CPPD).

Comments

Gout and/or chondrocalcinosis should be considered in the differential diagnosis of unusually pronounced erosive and destructive changes in the joints of the cervical spine.

Case 42 (▶ Fig. 3.44)

Case description

- Referring physician: internist.
- Prior history and clinical question: A 33-year-old man with back pain had been on chronic hemodialysis for 8 years. He was referred for investigation of possible bacterial spondylitis at the L1–L2 level. The patient brought along radiographs of the thoracic and lumbar spine (▶ Fig. 3.44 **a–d**).

Radiologic Findings

The patient has thoracic kyphosis with a maximum at T5–T6 in addition to S-shaped scoliosis. Slight kyphotic angulation is noted between L1 and L2. Gross erosive changes in the upper and lower endplates are seen particularly well on the anteroposterior radiograph of the thoracic spine. Intervertebral disk structures are completely destroyed at the T5–T6 and L1–L2 levels. The adjacent bony portions of T5–T6 are destroyed, as are the distal portions of L1. Overall, the cancellous trabeculae appear blurry and ill-defined (India-rubber sign).

Location

The radiologic changes are confined to the intervertebral spaces and adjacent structures and to the altered, ill-defined bone trabeculae.

Pathoanatomic Background of the Findings

Blurring of the trabeculae is an expression of osteomalacia in the setting of renal osteopathy. Given the fact that the patient is on chronic hemodialysis, the changes in the structures of the intervertebral spaces and adjacent subchondral bone, especially at T5–T6 and L1–L2, can be interpreted as erosive and destructive osteochondrosis. The absence of paravertebral soft-tissue swelling makes infectious spondylitis unlikely, especially at the T5–T6 and L1–L2 levels.

Assignment to a Possible Basic Entity

► **Inflammation?** The gross destructive changes in the upper and lower endplates and adjacent bone areas naturally raise the question of infectious spondylitis, especially since patients on chronic hemodialysis are often immunocompromised. However, the absence of soft-tissue swelling around T5–T6 and L1–L2 due to paravertebral abscess formation does not support a diagnosis of spondylitis. The presence of erosive changes in the upper and lower endplates of the other thoracic vertebral bodies also points to erosive osteochondrosis (spondylopathy).

► **Regressive process?** No, the processes in the upper and lower endplates could not be interpreted as "ordinary" osteochondrotic changes. The erosive changes are too ill-defined and are not dense enough for this interpretation.

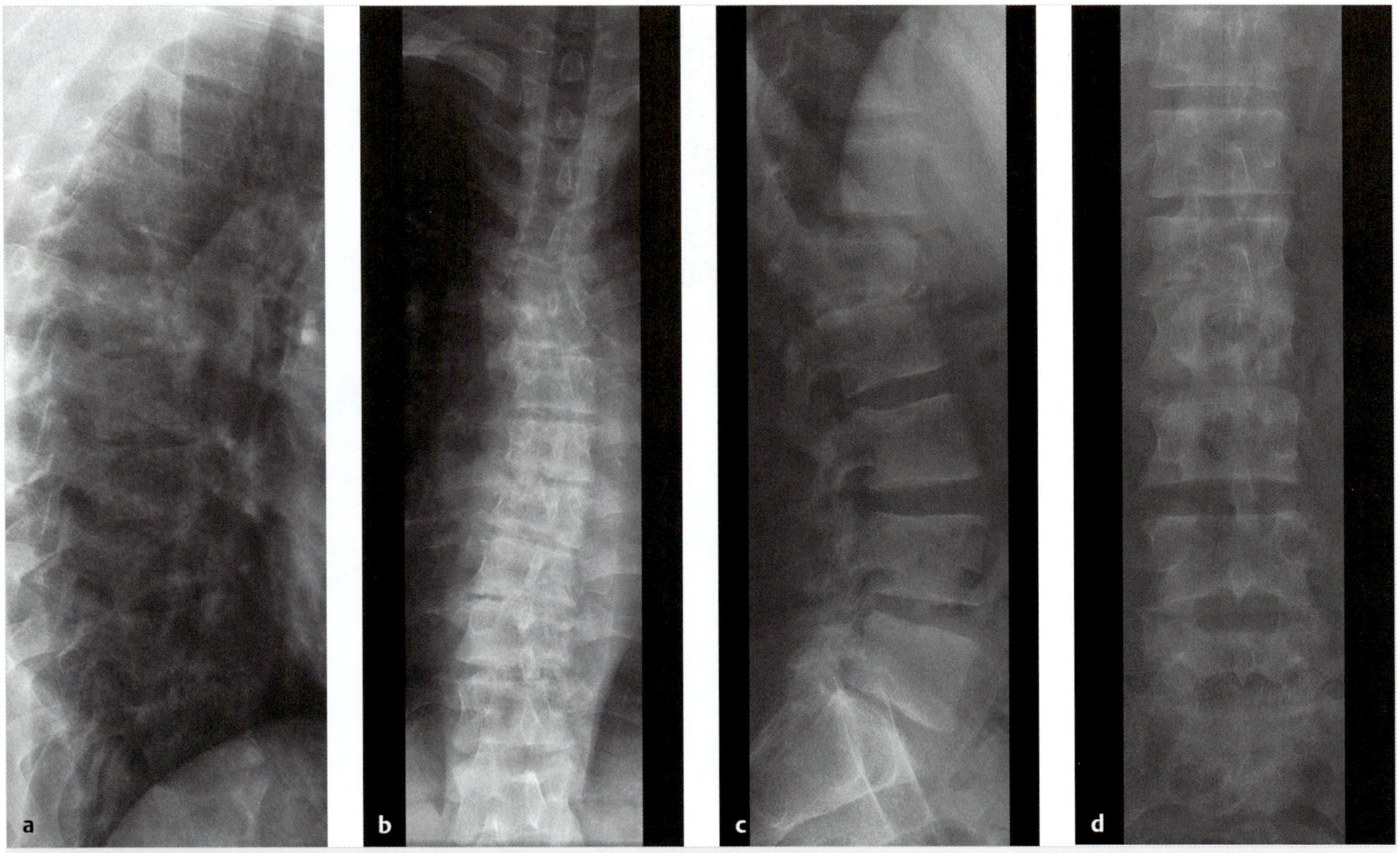

Fig. 3.44 a–d Bacterial spondylitis?

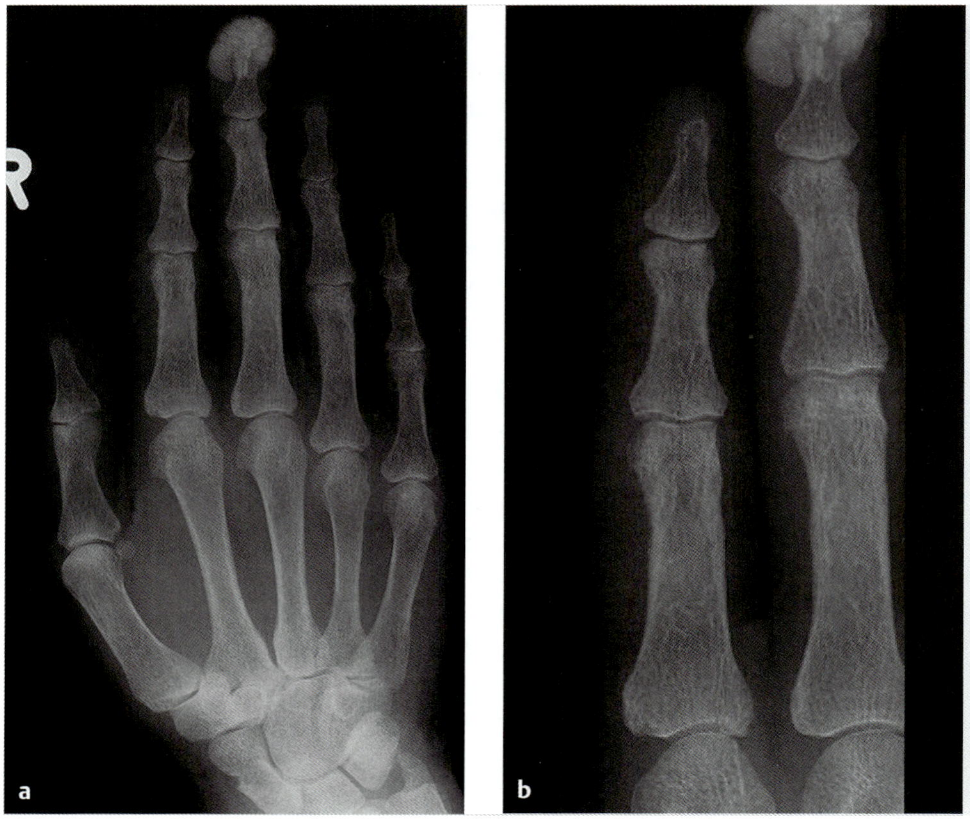

Fig. 3.45 a, b Hand radiographs of the patient in ▶ Fig. 3.44.

▶ **Systemic disease?** Yes, the blurring of the trabeculae suggests a systemic disease and is consistent with osteomalacia in a setting of renal osteodystrophy.

Synopsis and Discussion

The above findings and considerations basically allow for only one diagnosis: renal osteodystrophy with erosive spondylopathy (osteochondrosis). This is supported by the following arguments:

- Renal osteodystrophy is relatively common after 8 years of dialysis and several years of preterminal renal failure.
- A common associated finding in renal osteopathy is erosive spondylopathy or osteochondrosis, whose pathogenesis is very complex (crystal deposition, amyloid deposition, weakening of ligaments due to incorporation of foreign material, etc.). Erosive spondylopathy may also lead to bone destruction near the upper and lower vertebral endplates, sites already damaged due to renal osteodystrophy. The result of all these processes is kyphoscoliosis.
- Blurring of the trabeculae proves the presence of renal osteodystrophy, which results from a combination of secondary or tertiary hyperparathyroidism and osteomalacia.
- The final imaging proof of renal osteodystrophy with erosive spondylopathy is furnished by a simple radiograph of the hand (▶ Fig. 3.45 **a, b**), which yields highly specific findings:
  - Decreased bone density, ill-defined coarsened trabecular pattern (India-rubber sign)
  - Thinning of the cortex with subperiosteal resorption and intracortical striations (see magnified view in ▶ Fig. 3.45 **b**)
  - Loss of cortical bone over the phalangeal tufts (acro-osteolysis)
  - Soft-tissue calcification (tumorlike calcinosis) in the tip of the third finger, probably a result of vitamin D intoxication or poorly managed hyperphosphatemia
- Laboratory tests showing no significant inflammatory activity, even on follow-ups.

Final Diagnosis

Renal osteodystrophy with erosive spondylopathy.

Comments

Erosive and destructive spinal changes in patients on chronic hemodialysis with no clinical signs of increased inflammatory activity should be interpreted as erosive spondylopathy. If paravertebral soft-tissue swelling is present (by CT or MRI), the process should be investigated by CT-guided percutaneous biopsy.

3.4 Sacrum

Case 43 (▶ Fig. 3.46)

Case description

- Referring physician: radiologist.
- Prior history and clinical question: A 12-year-old girl had a 2-week history of nonspecific pain in the right hip, predominantly on the lateral side, which first occurred after a 2½-hour automobile ride followed by a walk around town. Her parents claimed that the girl did not have a visibly strained posture while riding in the car. Regarding sports activities, the girl has participated in school sports, horse riding, and is an avid trampoline jumper. Her history was otherwise unremarkable, and lab tests showed no increase in inflammatory markers. She had no clinical signs of sacroiliitis. Forward bending resulted in a compensatory movement toward the left side with a slight lumbar bulge on the right side. Slight tenderness was noted over the trochanter of the right femur. Based on his clinical findings, the pediatric orthopedist suspected an enthesiopathy in the right hip region (greater trochanter, iliac spines), also noting hamstring shortening on the right side, shortening of the right leg, and limited motion in the lumbar spine. HLA-B27 was positive. Anti-inflammatory therapy was initiated. A diagnosis of chronic recurrent multifocal osteomyelitis (CRMO) was considered based on the radiologic findings.

Radiologic Findings

Initial MRI (▶ Fig. 3.46 **a**) shows a prominent edema-like signal in the right lateral mass of the sacrum. The adjacent sacroiliac joint and ilium appear normal. CT scans (▶ Fig. 3.46 **b–h**) show an irregular, frayed subchondral contour of the right sacrum. Fusion of the synchondrosis between sacral segments 1 and 2 has not (yet?) occurred, in contrast to the opposite side. Sclerotic changes are visible along the margins of S2 (▶ Fig. 3.46 **c, e**). Bone spurs are noted at the capsular attachment on the anterior and inferior aspects of the sacroiliac joint on both the sacral and iliac sides (▶ Fig. 3.46 **h**) and are similar in appearance to traction spondylophytes (arrow in ▶ Fig. 3.46 **h**).

Location

The key radiologic findings are limited to the variant anatomy of the right lateral mass of the sacrum.

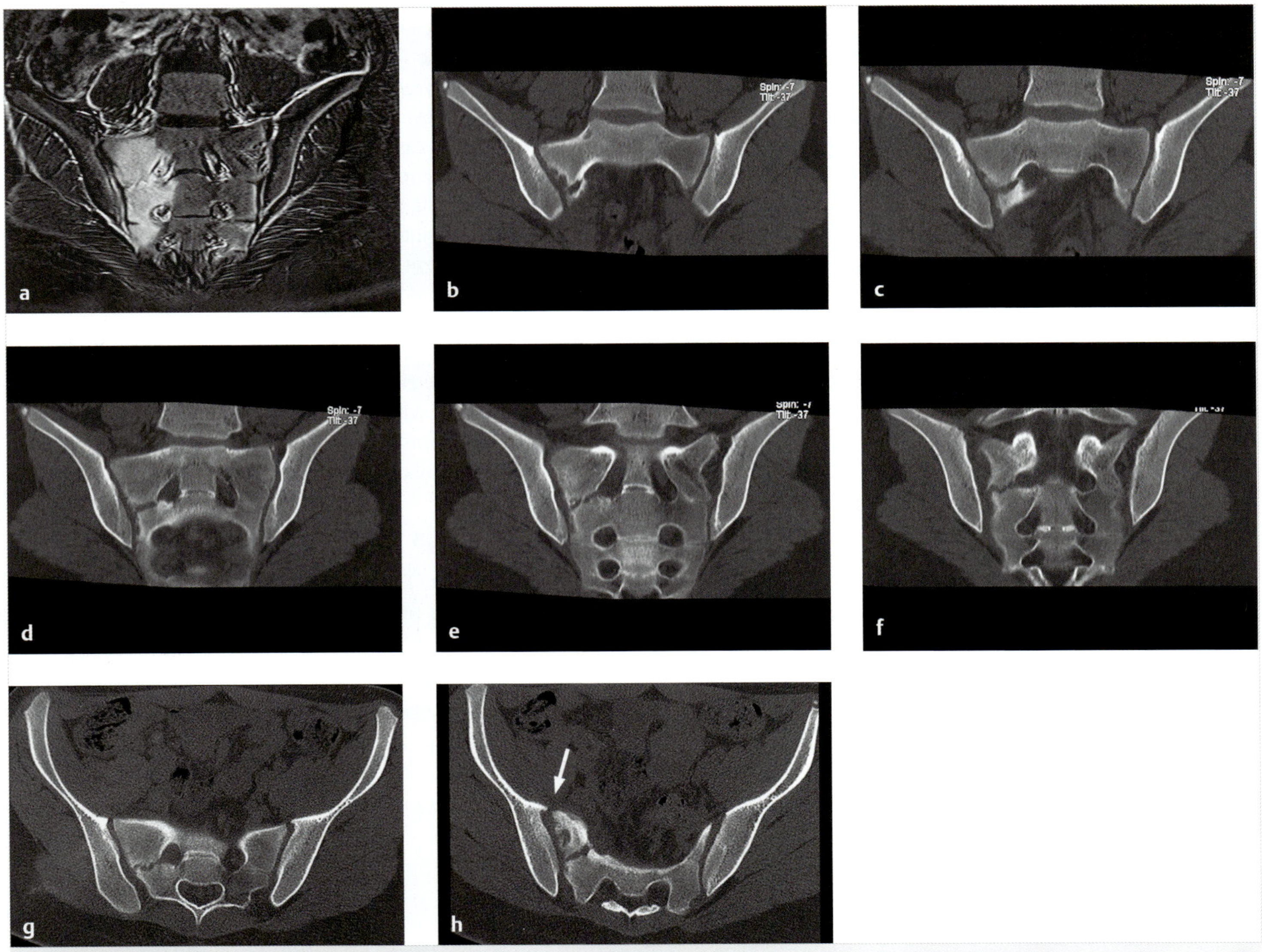

Fig. 3.46 a–h Chronic nonbacterial osteitis (CNO)?

Pathoanatomic Background of the Findings

The pronounced edema-like signal in the right lateral mass and the sclerotic changes without involvement of the sacroiliac joint, when interpreted within the context of the asymmetric nonfusion of S1 and S2, suggest a mechanically induced reactive process.

Assignment to a Possible Basic Entity

▸ **Normal variant or malformation?** The asymmetric nonfusion (so far) of S1 and S2 on the right side would definitely qualify as a normal variant, similar to many other asymmetric fusions of synchondroses (e.g., ischiopubic) and apophyses in the pelvis.[17] Under certain conditions, however, normal variants of this kind may lead to instabilities and may then become symptomatic (see Synopsis and Discussion below).

▸ **Trauma?** The girl stated that her favorite sports activities were horse riding and trampoline jumping. These activities constitute repetitive trauma to a growing posterior pelvic ring with an anatomic variant.

▸ **Inflammation?** The prominent edema-like signal in the right lateral mass and the erosions in its subchondral contours could be attributed to osteomyelitis—for example, if the adjacent sacroiliac joint were also involved (e.g., effusion). But that is not the case. With such pronounced findings, moreover, we would expect laboratory tests to show an elevated CRP level.

▸ **Tumor?** No. An osteoid osteoma would be plausible in a 12-year-old, but there is no CT or MRI evidence of a nidus, see also Case 44. The only other possibility is primary non-Hodgkin lymphoma of bone, but then we would expect to find central sclerosis in the right lateral mass.

Synopsis and Discussion

Given the many differential diagnostic possibilities, the present case is a prime example of the challenges that are addressed in this book.

In consultation we decided on a radiologically symptomatic normal variant or a stress-induced failure of fusion of S1 and S2. The following factors support this conclusion:

- Asymmetric nonfusion (so far) of S1 and S2 on the right side.
- History of high mechanical stresses to the posterior pelvic ring caused by intensive trampoline jumping along with horse riding and school sports. One might ask whether the radiologic findings would have occurred if the girl had engaged only in school sports and riding. In the case of other stress-induced skeletal changes (stress fracture, chronic avulsion trauma, enthesiopathies, etc.), it is known that adding just one stressor to other chronic loads may cause damage to the unconditioned bone or to an attachment between two bones. In our case it is uncertain whether the nonfusion itself was the precipitating factor for the changes or whether the nonfusion resulted from the stress—similar to the chicken-or-egg riddle. Parallels may be drawn with stress fractures of the lower lumbar spine in growing, competitive athletes.
- Reactive osseous changes, especially in the S2 segment (sclerosis, bone spurs at the anteroinferior capsular attachment on both the sacral and iliac sides), which indicate that the sacroiliac attachment is unstable. The edema-like signal in the right lateral mass is satisfactorily explained by the unphysiologic loads.

A diagnosis of CRMO, while plausible, is weakened by the absence of effusion or other reactive changes in the adjacent sacroiliac joint and an absence of inflammatory markers in the blood. It should be added that the term "CRMO" (chronic recurrent multifocal osteomyelitis) for nonbacterial autoinflammatory osteitis chiefly affecting the metaphyses of the long bones, mandible, and clavicles is of limited use today. This is particularly true when only one site is involved and further developments are uncertain—that is, it is not known whether a multifocal, recurrent, chronic process will develop in future. Understood in these terms, "CRMO" is actually a misnomer. We propose that the term CRMO be used only if all parts of the acronym are fulfilled.

In our own case material, approximately 30 to 40% of all the cases formerly diagnosed as CRMO are associated with sterile pustular skin changes (pustulosis palmoplantaris, pustular psoriasis, see Case 82 and Case 84. This indicates purely reactive osteitic bone changes, which are often HLA-B27 associated. Today most cases with the formerly used term CRMO have been replaced by the acronym CNO, which stands for chronic nonbacterial osteitis or osteomyelitis. The only factor supporting this diagnosis in the present case would be the positive detection of HLA-B27, but that proves nothing, since 10% of the healthy population is also HLA-B27-positive. This raises the question of whether the patient might have incipient seronegative spondyloarthritis. But this diagnosis is not at all consistent with the absence of clinical and radiologic signs of sacroiliitis.

The nonspecific clinical manifestations in the present case do not have a definite etiologic explanation, though we personally believe that asymmetric findings in the posterior pelvic ring may often be associated with very nonspecific signs including pseudoradicular symptoms. Another consideration is that children often have an atypical pattern of pain projection.

Final Diagnosis

Asymmetric fusion of S1 and S2 with stress-induced instability of the posterior pelvic ring or right massa lateralis, or conversely, possible stress-induced nonfusion of S1 and S2.

Comments

Even normal variants may become symptomatic when subjected to unusual mechanical loads, especially in the growing skeleton. The nonfusion of two bone segments may be a result of chronic overuse.

Case 44 (▶ Fig. 3.47)

Case description

- Referring physician: radiologist.
- Prior history and clinical question: A 16-year-old girl had a 7-month history of pain in the left side of the pelvis, most noticeable at rest, with some pain radiating to the left leg. She was an active soccer player who claimed to have suffered no notable injuries in the past year. The radiologist interpreted the lesion in the left proximal massa lateralis of S2 as osteoid osteoma and requested a consult because of the rarity of this lesion.

Radiologic Findings

The MR images (▶ Fig. 3.47 **b, d**) show edema-like signal in the S2 segment on the left side. No other contributory findings were noted in any other images. This logically prompted a CT examination for more detailed visualization of the bone. CT revealed an abnormality in the form of a small cancellous bone defect with a small central calcification (see arrows in ▶ Fig. 3.47 **a, c**). The defect is surrounded by osteosclerosis (▶ Fig. 3.47 **c**) and is located just posterior to the S2 foramen (▶ Fig. 3.47 **a**).

Pathoanatomic Background of the Findings

It is reasonable to assume a link between the edema-like signal and the bony CT findings in the left lateral mass. The small osteolytic lesion with central mineralization and marginal sclerosis could be interpreted as osteomyelitic destruction with a sequestrum, but it could just as well be an osteoid osteoma with central mineralization or even ossification of the nidus. Both entities are generally associated with marginal sclerosis and, in their florid stage, with perifocal inflammatory edema.

Assignment to a Possible Basic Entity

▶ **Normal variant or malformation?** No, this interpretation is not supported by the clinical presentation or edema-like signal.

▶ **Inflammation?** Yes in principle, as discussed under Pathoanatomic Background of the Findings. The edema-like signal in both entities reflects a reactive, inflammation-related process.

▶ **Tumor?** Yes, with osteoid osteoma as the only possibility (small tumor, big impact!).

Synopsis and Discussion

The following factors make osteoid osteoma very likely:

- *Pain at rest:* The referring physician did not know if the pain was relieved by aspirin.
- *Age of the patient:* More than 50% of all osteoid osteomas occur in the second decade of life.
- *Location:* From 5 to 20% of all osteoid osteomas are located in the spine and sacrum.
- *Radiology:* A round defect with central mineralization or even ossification rimmed by sclerosis with an edema-like signal is very specific for osteoid osteoma. The "nidus" represents the actual tumor, which produces osteoid that undergoes central ossification and has a rich blood supply. This high perfusion is explained by increased prostaglandin and bradykinin production by the nidus; this increases the intralesional pressure on afferent nerves in the nidus, causing pain. Aspirin suppresses prostaglandin production and reduces or relieves the pain, but only in about 60% of cases. The edema results from increased vascular permeability caused by bradykinin.

Additional cases of osteoid osteoma: Case 74, Case 104, Case 144, Case 146, and Case 149). Osteomyelitis is mainly of academic interest in this context and is not a plausible explanation for the clinical and radiologic findings. Osteomyelitis of the sacrum in an otherwise healthy 16-year-old would be exceedingly rare. Moreover, the lesions generally are not round but have irregular margins.

The tumor does not require diagnostic biopsy. It can be excised in toto or percutaneously ablated, as there is practically no realistic differential diagnosis, especially with regard to a malignant process.

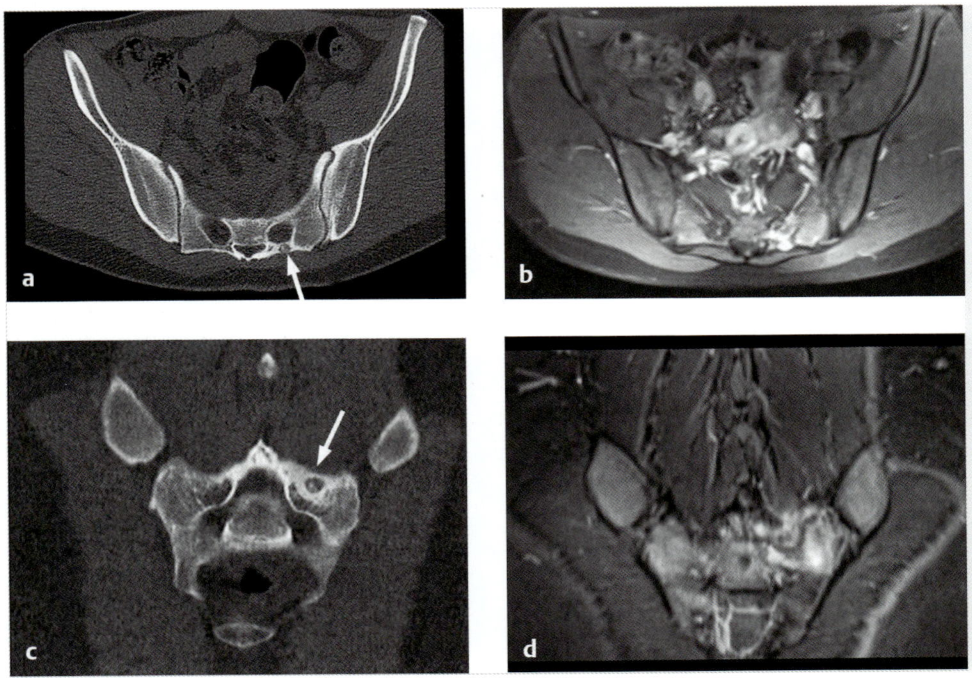

Fig. 3.47 a–d Osteomyelitis?

Final Diagnosis

Osteoid osteoma in the left massa lateralis of the sacrum.

Comments

A small, round osteolytic lesion with central calcification, marginal sclerosis, and perifocal edema-like signal that is causing pain disproportionate to the size of the lesion should always suggest osteoid osteoma, especially when detected in a young, otherwise healthy patient.

Case 45 (▶ Fig. 3.48)

Case description

- Referring physician: radiologist.
- Prior history and clinical question: A 17-year-old girl had a 6-month history of pain in the sacral region. This case was furnished by Prof. Muhle (Vechta, Germany) along with the correct diagnosis for use in this book.

Radiologic Findings

The CT images (▶ Fig. 3.48 **a–e**) show an expansile lesion that has almost completely obliterated the normal bony structures of the sacrum. Faint septa-like densities are visible within the lesion. The lesion is enveloped by a thin shell of periosteal ossification. The interior of the lesion is inhomogeneous in the soft-tissue CT window (▶ Fig. 3.48 **a**), creating the appearance of disseminated small and minute rounded hypodensities interspersed among the septa-like structures. T2w MRI (▶ Fig. 3.48 **f–h**) explains the latter CT findings by showing innumerable small, cystlike spaces with fluid–fluid levels that are oriented parallel to the plane of the table.

Pathoanatomic Background of the Findings

The normal bone of the sacrum has been replaced over a large area by a mass that contains cavities with fluid levels separated by solid septa, some showing osseous density. The process is surrounded on all sides by a very thin shell of periosteal bone, which means that the lesion is less aggressive and does not invade surrounding tissues. This description precisely fits an aneurysmal bone cyst.

Assignment to a Possible Basic Entity

The assignment of the lesion to an aneurysmal bone cyst was made above and does not require any further differentiating considerations.

Synopsis and Discussion

The clinical and radiologic findings in this case are consistent with a primary aneurysmal bone cyst. *Aneurysmal bone cyst* is a benign cystic lesion of bone consisting of blood-filled spaces that are separated by septa composed of fibroblasts, osteoclastic giant cells, and reactive connective tissue. Aneurysmal bone cysts may be primary or secondary. The latter type occurs in benign and malignant bone tumors that have undergone hemorrhagic transformation. Fully half of all cases are diagnosed in the second decade of life (as in our case), and 2% of cases occur in the sacrum. The imaging appearance of aneurysmal bone cyst is that of a soap-bubble lucency with well-defined margins and a thin shell of periosteal ossification where the lesion has completely destroyed the original bone. The internal pathoanatomy of the lesion is reflected precisely in the radiologic findings of small, cystlike, blood-filled spaces separated by connective-tissue septa. The fluid–fluid levels, which are very typical of blood, are explained by the sedimentation of red blood cells, much as in anticoagulated blood (upper portion is hyperintense in T2w images, lower portion is hypointense). While in principle, fluid levels may occur in nearly all tumors and tumorlike lesions, including metastases, a primary aneurysmal bone cyst is by far the most likely diagnosis when fluid–fluid levels are present in more than 70% of the lesion. The septa between the cystlike spaces are well perfused and usually enhance after contrast administration.

Differentiation is required from a *primary bone tumor* such as telangiectatic osteosarcoma, which contains large blood-filled spaces. A definitive diagnosis requires histologic evaluation, which in this case identified the lesion as an aneurysmal bone cyst.

Final Diagnosis

Aneurysmal bone cyst in the sacrum.

Comments

When radiographs or CT scans show an expansile osteolytic lesion surrounded by a thin shell of periosteal ossification, MRI should always be performed to look for fluid–fluid levels. If fluid levels are found in more than 70% of the lesion, this always suggests an aneurysmal bone cyst in a young individual.

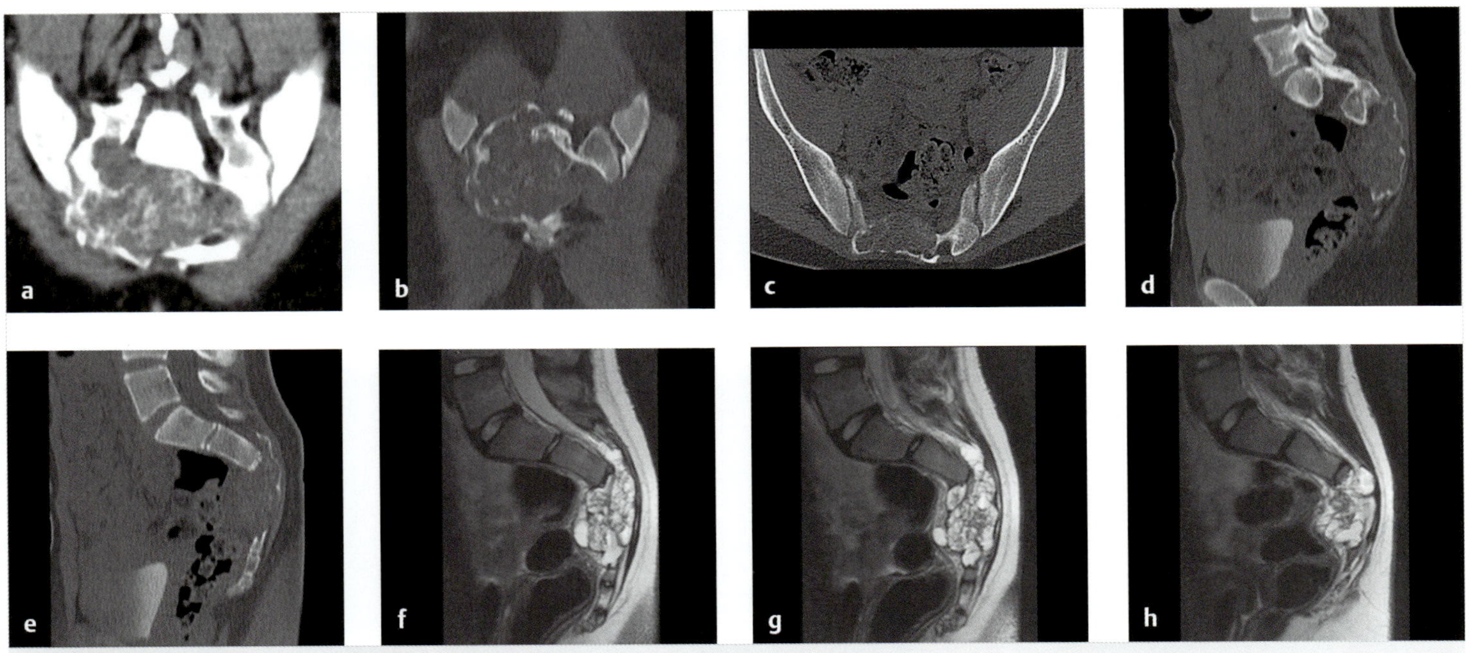

Fig. 3.48 a–h Osteosarcoma or metastatic destruction?

Case 46 (► Fig. 3.49)

Case description

- Referring physician: radiologist.
- Prior history and clinical question: A 65-year-old woman had sciatica-like pain on the right side that was investigated by MRI, which demonstrated significant edema-like signal in the sacrum. Further investigation by CT revealed an unusual bony structure in the sacrum. A correct diagnosis of Paget disease was made. The referring physician wants to know if there is any sign of malignant transformation to Paget sarcoma.

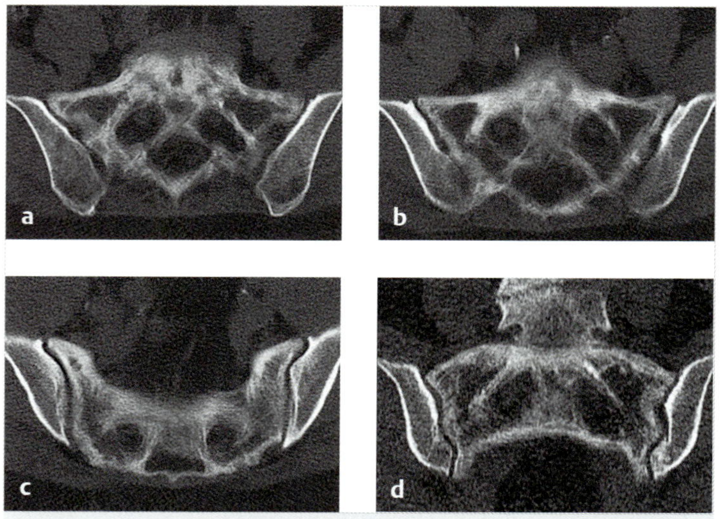

Fig. 3.49 a–d Paget sarcoma?

Radiologic Findings

The CT scans (► Fig. 3.49 **a–d**) demonstrate coarse striations throughout the sacrum. The bone appears enlarged, though it still fits against the ilium. The sacroiliac joints appear normal except for thickening of the iliac subchondral plates and the presence of anterior marginal osteophytes. The sacral foramina have a picture-frame appearance.

Location

The structural changes are confined to the sacrum. The adjacent ilium appears normal.

Pathoanatomic Background of the Findings

Coarse striations, volume expansion, and the picture-frame appearance evoke an engrammatic association with the sclerotic phase of Paget disease (osteitis deformans). In fact they are pathognomonic for that condition.

The differential diagnosis will stop here, as the author of this book cannot think of any other possible entities that could account for these changes.

Synopsis and Discussion

The diagnosis of Paget disease is considered definitive and there is no need for histologic confirmation. Besides the signs noted above, the following arguments support this diagnosis:

- The abnormal structural changes in the bone are confined to one anatomic unit, the sacrum; they have not spread to the adjacent ilium. This would occur only if the sacroiliac joints had been obliterated by degenerative disease or previous sacroiliitis.
- The age of the patient.
- An absence of clinical manifestations consistent with the findings. This factor also excludes malignant transformation, which generally would be associated with pain.

As noted above, there are no signs of malignant transformation such as destruction, a soft-tissue mass, etc. (see also Case 52). The disease is in the sclerotic (probably inactive) phase, so we would not expect an elevated serum alkaline phosphatase unless additional skeletal lesions were present. We therefore advised further investigation by bone scintigraphy. If the bone scan showed no additional (active) lesions in weight-bearing skeletal regions, there would be no indication for pharmacologic treatment with bisphosphonates.

For more details on Paget disease see Case 8, Case 9, Case 12, Case 14, Case 51, Case 83, Case 107, and Case 140.

Final Diagnosis

Paget disease.

Comments

Coarse striations, expansion, and the picture-frame appearance can provide bloodless proof of Paget disease in an asymptomatic patient.

4 Pelvis

4.1 Sclerotic Changes

Case 47 (▶ Fig. 4.1)

Case description

- Referring physician: rheumatologist.
- Prior history and clinical question: A 46-year-old woman presented with steroid-sensitive pain in her spine and peripheral joints. She had clinical manifestations of a fibromyalgia syndrome. No functional abnormalities were noted on musculoskeletal physical examination. The pelvic radiograph showed very dense sclerotic areas around the sacroiliac joints and pubic symphysis. These areas were negative on bone scintigraphy. The patient denied having psoriasis or pustulosis palmoplantaris. The test for HLA-B27 gave a negative result.

Radiologic Findings

The pelvic radiograph shows very dense, homogeneous sclerosis on both the iliac and sacral sides and around the pubic symphysis. While the sacroiliac joints have smooth contours and normal width, the symphyseal contours have a slightly ragged appearance. The upper left edge of the symphysis is approximately 4 to 5 mm higher than the right (▶ Fig. 4.1 **a**). The bone scan shows no pelvic abnormalities (▶ Fig. 4.1 **b**).

Location

The sclerotic areas are distributed about the articular and synchondrotic junctions.

Pathoanatomic Background of the Findings

The sclerotic areas are interpreted as a reactive phenomenon in response to some or other stimulus originating from the sacroiliac joint and the synchondrotic attachment of the pubic bones. The negative bone scan shows that the sclerotic areas are inactive —"the party is over," so to speak.

Assignment to a Possible Basic Entity

▶ **Normal variant or malformation?** Yes, triangular hyperostoses about the sacroiliac joints, also called hyperostosis triangularis ilii, are a common finding in asymptomatic women of childbearing age.[17] Most women with this condition are biparous or multiparous. This also applies to sclerotic areas about the symphysis, especially when associated with hyperostosis triangularis ilii.

▶ **Inflammation?** Given the positive answer above, there is no need to pursue the question of inflammation. The fact that the sclerotic areas are negative on bone scans (see ▶ Fig. 4.1 **b**) and were detected incidentally is also inconsistent with inflammation. The normal width of the sacroiliac joint spaces and their smooth contours exclude a reactive inflammatory process such as enthesitis or synchondritis in a setting of spondyloarthritis.

Synopsis and Discussion

The question from the referring rheumatologist implied that spondyloarthritis might be responsible for the sclerotic changes about the sacroiliac joints and symphysis. In particular, he may have considered a pustular arthro-osteitis or enthesio-osteitis, or SAPHO (synovitis, acne, pustulosis, hyperostosis, osteitis) syndrome, which are often associated with unusual, nonspecific inflammatory (enthesitic) sclerosis (see Case 39, Case 40, Case 48, Case 49, and Case 97). He had doubts, however, because the patient had neither pustulosis palmoplantaris nor psoriasis, did not have a positive family history, and her HLA-B27 test was negative.

Hyperostosis triangularis ilii (formerly called osteitis condensans ilii) results from transient loosening of the anterior and posterior pelvic ring and symphysis due to pregnancy, but is also found in degenerative diseases of the sacroiliac joints. The increased mobility of the pelvic ring in pregnancy, or the loss of the articular cartilage buffer due to degenerative disease, leads to greater pressure loads and stimulates reactive new bone formation around the anteroinferior corner of the ilium (joint),

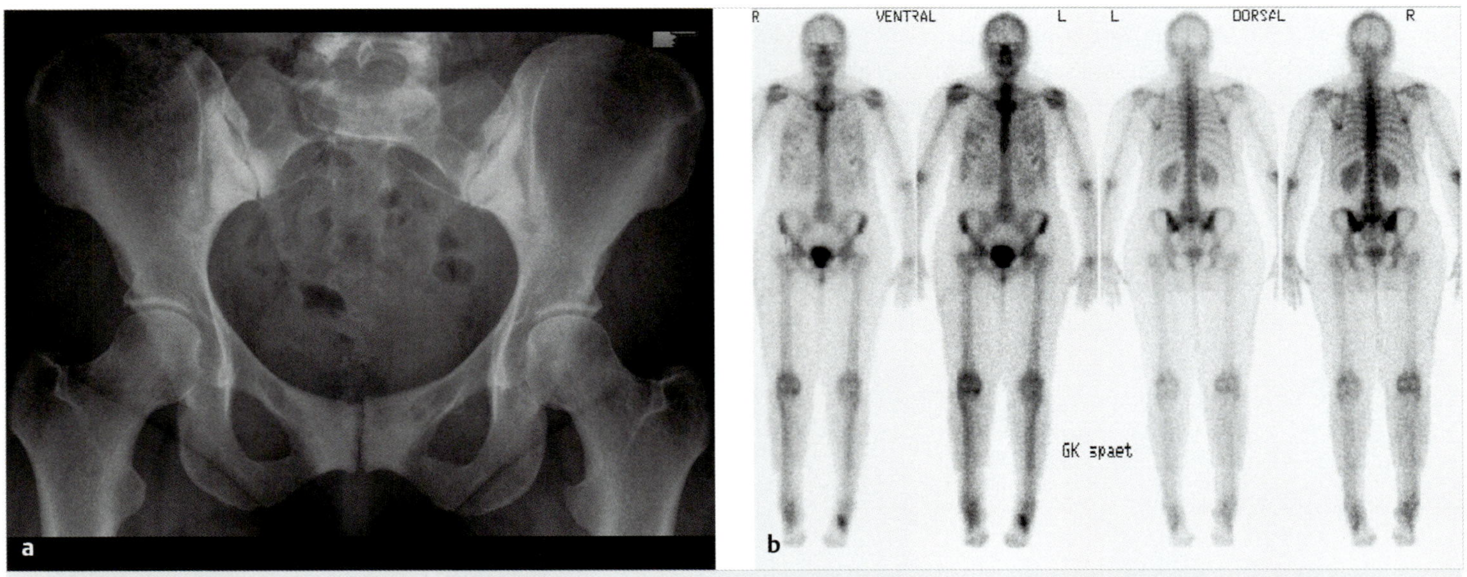

a b

Fig. 4.1 a, b Sacroiliitis in ankylosing spondyloarthritis?

which marks the pressure center of the sacroiliac joints in standing on both legs. As a result, reactive new bone formation develops around the inferior corner of the ilium, eventually leading to triangular hyperostosis. A similar mechanism is operative at the symphysis pubis, which in the present case shows a step-off that further documents transient loosening of the symphysis.

Final Diagnosis

Reactive sclerosis around the sacroiliac joints (hyperostosis triangularis ilii) and symphysis after pregnancy-related loosening of the pelvic ring, considered an incidental finding and a normal variant.

Comments

When sclerotic skeletal changes are detected incidentally around bony junctions, stress-related hyperostosis should be considered first. Any remaining doubts can be resolved by bone scintigraphy, which will be negative in the case of older stress reactions or normal variants.

Case 48 (▶ Fig. 4.2)

Case description

- Referring physician: orthopedist.
- Prior history and clinical question: A 42-year-old woman had a 6-month history of increasing pain in the right hip and upper left thigh. Physical examination showed limitation of motion in the right hip joint. No palpable mass or local warmth was noted in the left thigh. The referring orthopedist stated that no other physical abnormalities were found. Serum inflammatory markers were not elevated. The complaints regressed in response to anti-inflammatory treatment. The orthopedist suspected that the patient had two separate foci of Paget disease.

Radiologic Findings

The radiograph shows massive sclerosis and expansion of proximal portions of the right ilium and left proximal femoral shaft including the metaphysis (▶ Fig. 4.2 **a**). As the CT images demonstrate, the hyperostotic changes originate from the cortex and/or the periosteum, rather than from the narrowed but still-intact medullary cavities (▶ Fig. 4.2 **b–d**). Bone scans (not pictured here) showed markedly increased uptake in the suspicious skeletal regions with no other abnormalities. The nuclear medicine physician interpreted these as showing "chronic osteomyelitis," but bone tumors were also considered.

Location

As noted above, the ossifications originate from the cortex or periosteum, not from the medullary cavity.

Pathoanatomic Background of the Findings

As the bone scan showed, the hyperostotic changes in the right ilium and left femur are active, so this would largely exclude congenital hyperostosis. The most frequent causes of noncongenital hyperostosis are chronic inflammation and primary or secondary bone tumors. It is important to note that the hyperostotic changes do not originate from the medullary cavities but from the cortex and/or the periosteum, also largely excluding a septic bifocal osteomyelitis. This finding also excludes bone tumors such as primary non-Hodgkin lymphoma of bone, which generally arise from or involve the medullary cavities (see also ▶ Fig. 4.3). Exceptions are periosteal osteoid osteoma and osteosarcoma, but the CT scans do not show a nidus of osteoid osteoma, nor do they show spicules or other features suggestive of periosteal osteosarcoma.

We can also exclude Paget disease because the hyperostotic changes in this case are symptomatic; this would be extremely unusual for Paget disease (see Case 8, Case 9, Case 12, Case 14, Case 51, Case 107, and Case 140). Moreover, the changes in the left femur do not involve the epiphysis, where the structural alterations in Paget disease generally originate in long bones. This leaves us with a bifocal, reactive, chronic proliferative bone proc-

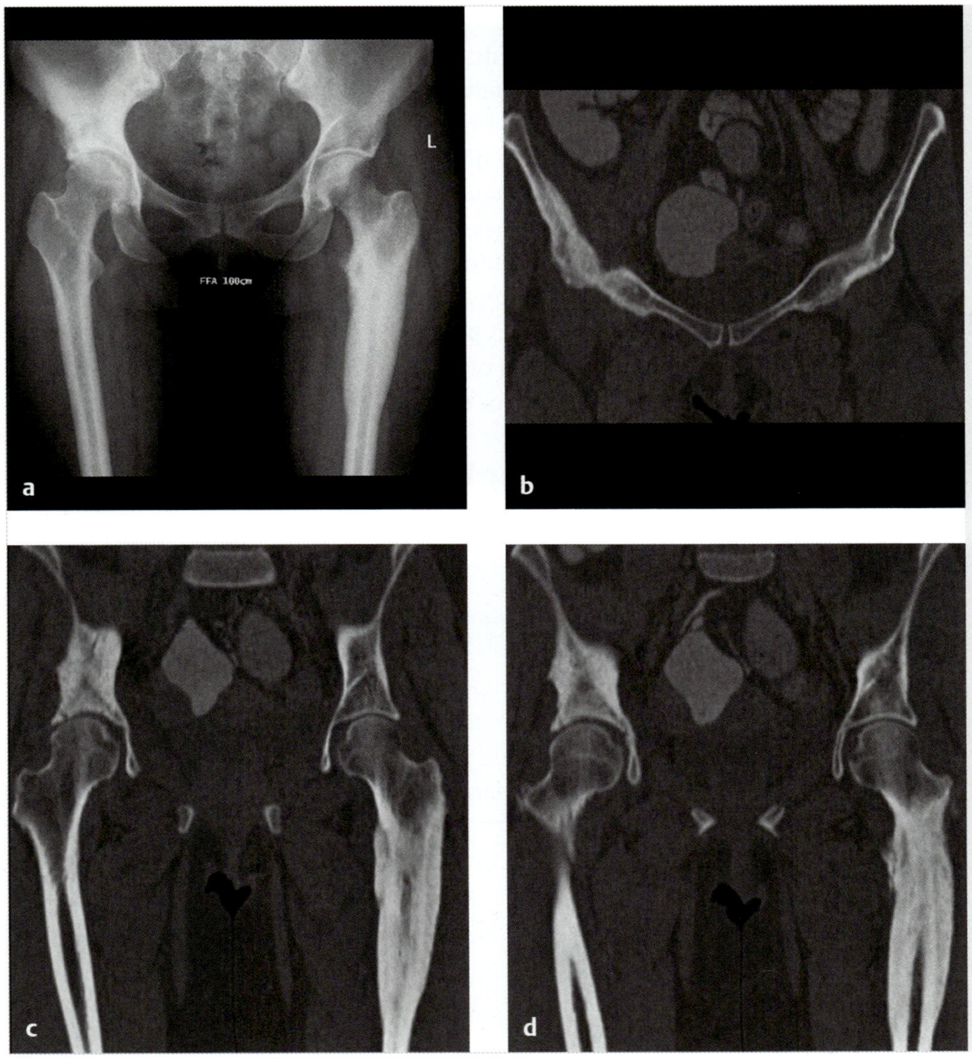

Fig. 4.2 a–d Two foci Paget disease?

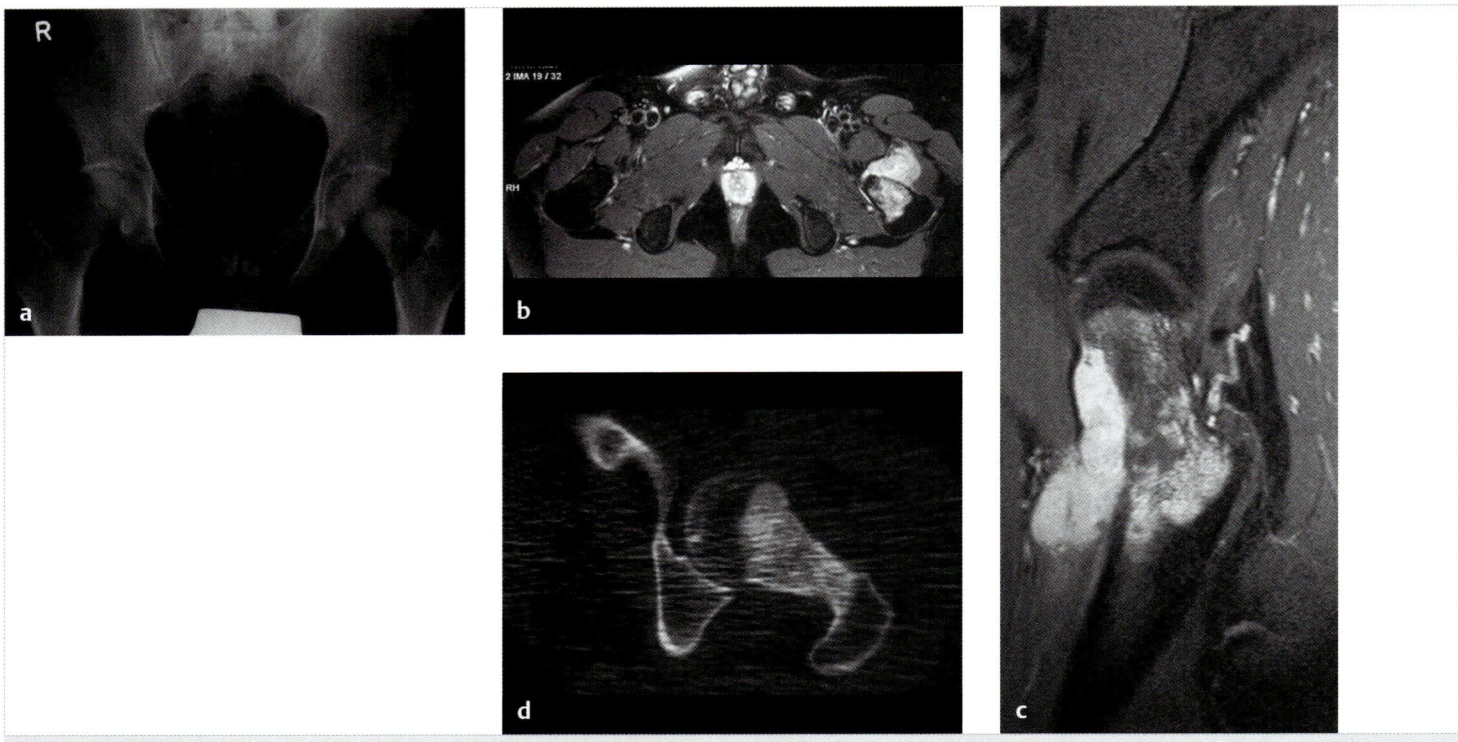

Fig. 4.3 a–d Osteosclerotic osteosarcoma in an 18-year-old male.

ess that appears to arise from the periosteum. These characteristics are suspicious for enthesitis.

Assignment to a Possible Basic Entity

▸ **Inflammation?** Yes, a reactive type. The considerations under Pathoanatomic Background of the Findings would suggest a bifocal enthesitis with proliferative periosteal new bone formation, since current theory interprets the periosteum as an enthesis—that is, a site where soft-tissue structures are attached to bone. These junctions are highly susceptible to systemic reactive inflammatory changes. The areas of cortical thickening on the ilium and femur are also due partly to incipient osteitis.

▸ **Tumor?** Very unlikely, aside from a very unusual bifocal form of non-Hodgkin lymphoma of bone.

Synopsis and Discussion

Based on the considerations above, the most likely diagnosis is a "rheumatic" *enthesitis*, which is a type of seronegative spondyloarthritis. Systemic forms of enthesitis associated with exuberant hyperostosis include spondyloarthritis with pustular skin changes (psoriasis and its variant, pustulosis palmoplantaris). After further consultation with the referring orthopedist, we learned that the patient had none of these skin diseases. Of course, this alone does not positively exclude the presence of a skin disease, which would require a dermatologic consult including biopsy of suspicious areas (see Case 39, Case 40, and Case 49). The orthopedist stated that there was no clinical evidence of another form of spondyloarthritis. We recommended that the patient should see a rheumatologist, but unfortunately she has not followed this recommendation as far as we know. An imaging follow-up at 6 months showed no change in the skeletal abnormalities. This makes a neoplastic process very unlikely and does not suggest a pressing need for histologic evaluation. It should be added that hyperostotic changes in spondyloarthritis do not have a specific histology, so a biopsy would have served only to narrow the differential diagnosis.

Regarding the differential diagnosis of sclerotic changes in the femur, the case in ▸ Fig. 4.3 shows an osteosclerotic *osteosarcoma* in the femoral neck of an 18-year-old male. Unlike Case 48, the sclerotic process is located in the bone, not in or along the periosteum. The MR images show that the lesion has broken through the bone on the anterior side. The morphology of this case and the patient's age suggest an immediate diagnosis of osteosarcoma. The only other possible entity would be a primary non-Hodgkin lymphoma of bone, and that condition should be histologically confirmed or excluded.

Preliminary or Working Diagnosis

Reactive inflammatory bone changes consistent with a proliferative enthesitis in a still-unspecified form of spondyloarthritis.

Comments

If the periosteal component is dominant in active hyperostotic changes, the differential diagnosis should include a rheumatic enthesitis in a setting of spondyloarthritis. CT is the best study for proving the dominance of periosteal new bone formation.

Case 49 (▶ Fig. 4.4)

Case description

- Referring physician: orthopedist.
- Prior history and clinical question: A 26-year-old man complained of chronic pain in the right pelvic region. He had already consulted a number of doctors in various specialties and had undergone several biopsies. The radiologic changes were most commonly interpreted as chronic osteomyelitis and managed with antibiotics. One consulting orthopedist even proposed a hemipelvectomy. The referring orthopedist noted florid psoriatic lesions on whole-body clinical examination (see ▶ Fig. 4.4 **g**) and suspected that they were related to the sclerotic pelvic changes. The engrammatic link of "unusual sclerotic skeletal changes → psoriasis" worked splendidly in this case. The orthopedist requested confirmation.

Radiologic Findings

The pelvic radiograph (▶ Fig. 4.4 **a**) shows a large sclerotic area in the right iliac wing, which also appears expanded. The right sacroiliac joint space is widened and shows irregular contours. Both MRI (▶ Fig. 4.4 **b–d**) and CT (▶ Fig. 4.4 **e, f**) confirm the increased bone volume and show that it is caused by hyperostotic changes that appear to originate from the periosteum. Water-sensitive sequences show marked hyperintensities that are localized mainly to the periosteum on the medial side.

Location

As noted above, the ossifications originate from the cortex or periosteum.

Pathoanatomic Background of the Findings

The changes described above may be interpreted as chronic proliferative changes originating from the periosteum, while the sclerosis in the medullary cavity suggests reactive osteitis. Because periosteum belongs to the entheses, chronic enthesitis in a setting of spondyloarthritis is a possibility.

Assignment to a Possible Basic Entity

▶ **Inflammation?** Yes, but not a chronic bacterial osteomyelitis. That entity would arise from the medullary cavity, which appears

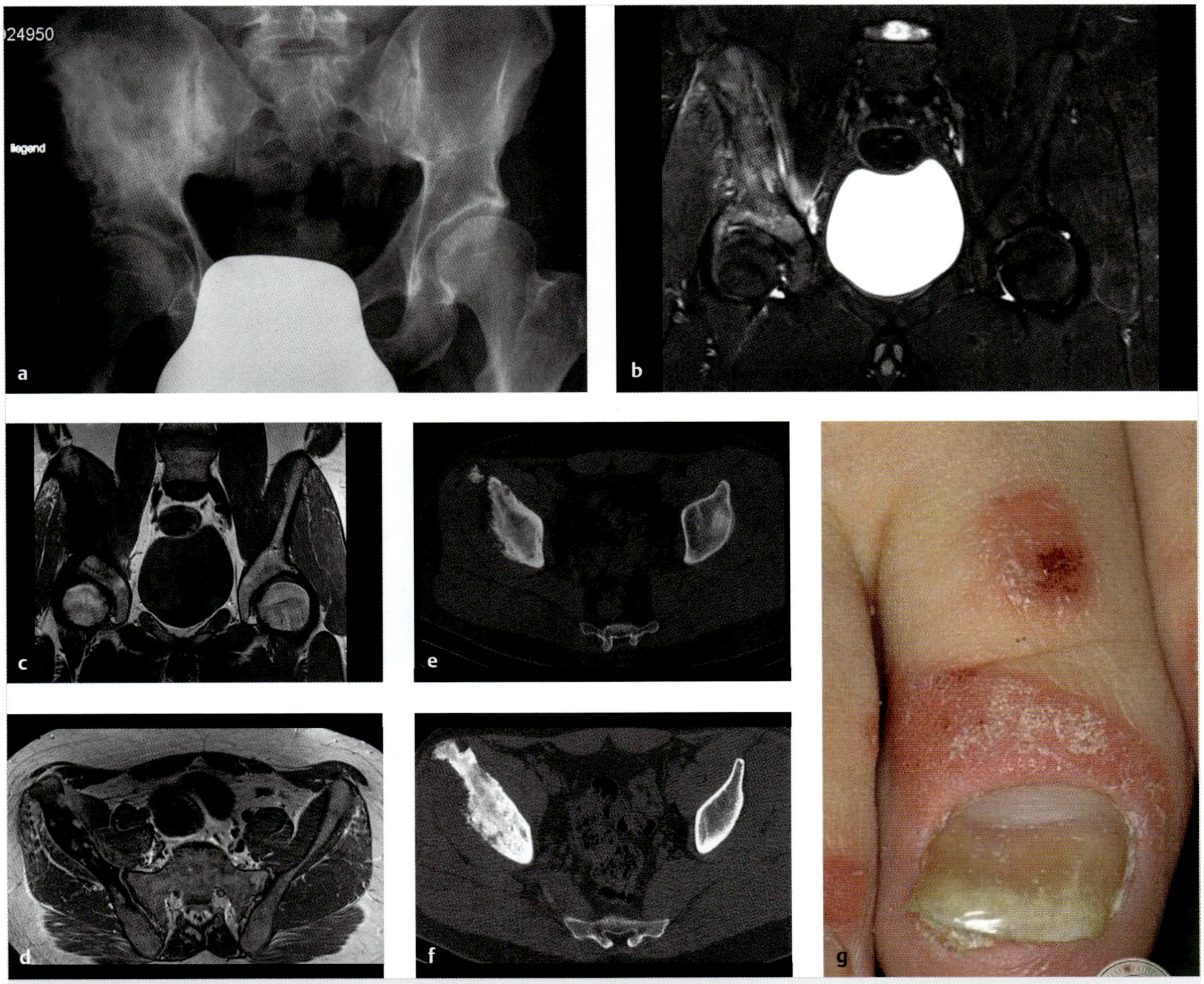

Fig. 4.4 a–g Chronic osteomyelitis?

relatively untouched (see ▶ Fig. 4.4 **e**). A chronic granulating form of osteomyelitis would be expected to produce cavitation and sequestrum formation. The patient would have reported febrile episodes. Based on the considerations under Pathoanatomic Background of the Findings, it should not be difficult to "scroll through" the five known spondyloarthritides and look for corresponding clinical signs. These were found both on and in the patient's skin (see Prior history and clinical question, above).

▶ **Tumor?** No, see under Synopsis and Discussion.

Synopsis and Discussion

Several arguments have already been made against a diagnosis of chronic bacterial (granulocytic) osteomyelitis. The absence of a visible tumor mass over the periosteal ossifications is not consistent with a neoplastic process such as periosteal osteosarcoma. The only remaining possibility is a reactive, chronic proliferative process that originates from the periosteum. Given the presence of florid psoriasis, the disease can be classified and treated (immunosuppressive, anti-inflammatory) as psoriasis-associated enthesitis or periostitis, even without histologic confirmation (see also Case 39, Case 40, Case 48, and Case 97. The role of histology in this group of diseases is discussed in Case 48. A whole-body bone scan should be obtained to define the true extent of the skeletal changes.

Final Diagnosis

Psoriasis-associated enthesitis or periostitis in the right iliac wing.

Comments

When dealing with an unexplained sclerotic process, always look at the skin or check for a history of skin lesions. This can spare the patient the frustration of a fruitless journey that may last for years.

Case 50 (► Fig. 4.5)

Case description

- Referring physician: orthopedist.
- Prior history and clinical question: A 14-year-old girl had nonspecific complaints throughout the pelvic region, but in any case not limited to the left ischium. No palpable abnormalities were found on clinical examination. The pelvic radiograph revealed a dense sclerotic process in the left ischium that was considered suspicious for a tumor. The orthopedist requested further clarification.

Radiologic Findings

The radiograph shows an area of dense, homogeneous sclerosis in the left ischium. The margins of the affected bone are smooth (► Fig. 4.5 **a**).

Pathoanatomic Background of the Findings

A sclerotic process in a young person may reflect a congenital condition, a reactive-reparative process (inflammation, trauma), or an ossified tumor matrix. These three possibilities can be narrowed by investigating the biological activity of the lesion, and this can be accomplished with bone scintigraphy (► Fig. 4.5 **b**).

Assignment to a Possible Basic Entity

► **Normal variant or malformation?** Possibly. The only diagnosis suggested by a circumscribed, uniformly sclerosing process is melorheostosis. Generally this disease is negative on bone scans or shows only slightly increased uptake as in the present case (► Fig. 4.5 **b**).

► **Trauma?** Reparative process involving massive intracancellous callus formation? No, the history is negative for trauma.

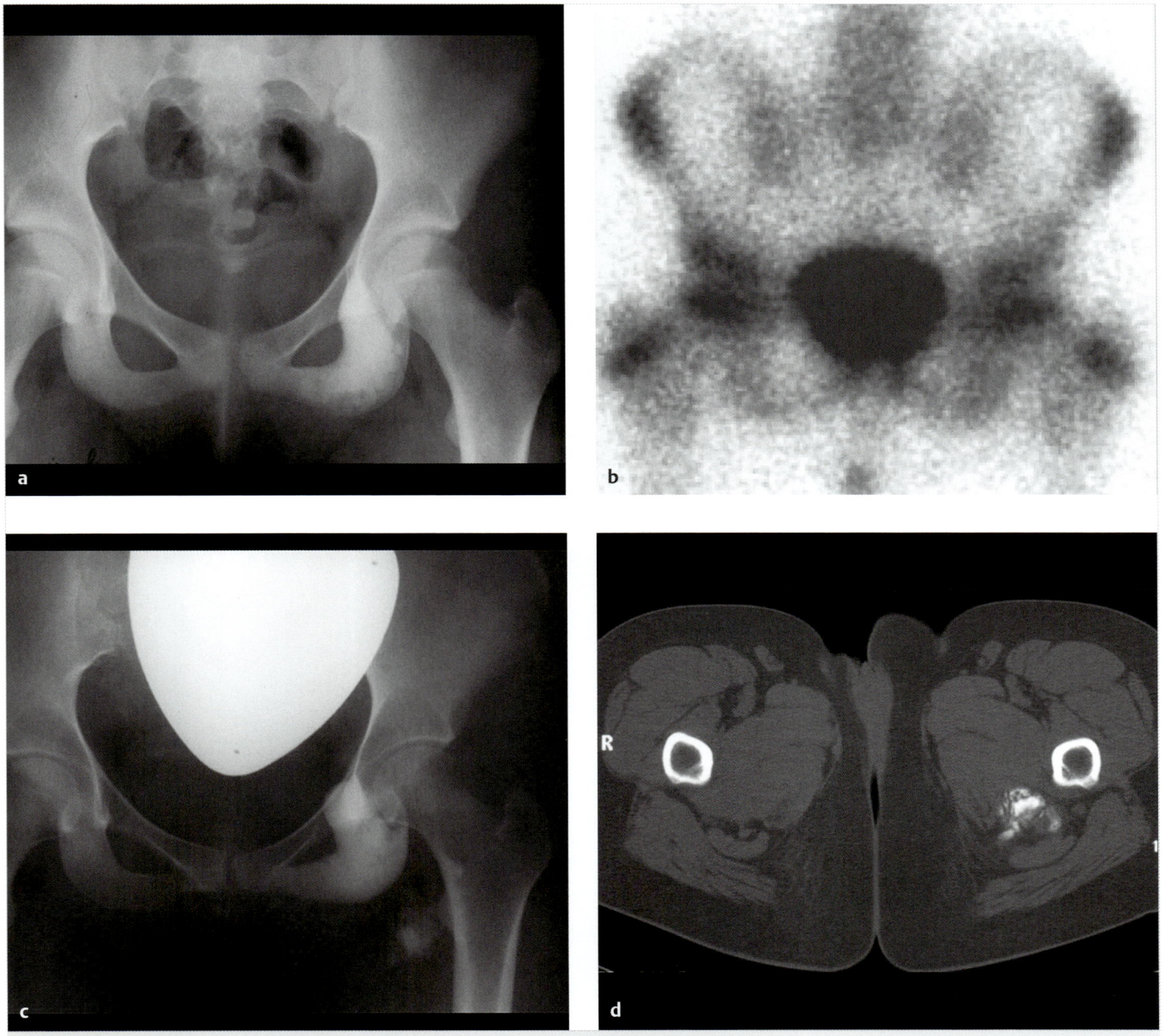

Fig. 4.5 a–d Sclerosing osteosarcoma? The latter two images (c, d) were obtained 7 years later.

▸ **Inflammation?** Unlikely, due to the negative bone scan, negative history, and no visible skin changes.

▸ **Tumor?** No, a bone-forming or osteoid-producing tumor would generally show intense tracer uptake. The nonspecific clinical manifestations do not fit this pattern either. Osteoma is discussed below.

Synopsis and Discussion

After due consideration of all possible basic entities, the only remaining diagnosis is melorheostosis or osteoma. These possibilities are consistent with:

- Patient's age.
- The absence of clinical manifestations that correlate with imaging. It should be added that, based on our own studies, more than half of all patients with melorheostosis, especially when polyostotic, experience pain that is always confined to the area of the positive imaging finding and results from adjacent soft-tissue edema and fibrosis with contractures, etc.[23] (see also Case 99). In our case, however, the radiologic abnormality had no associated clinical symptoms; this suggests an incidental finding.
- The radiologic appearance of very dense, homogeneous sclerosis. The lesion is osteoma-like and purely intraosseous, one of the many possible manifestations of melorheostosis (classic type with "flowing candle wax" sclerosis, osteopathia striata-like type, osteoma-like type, or myositis ossificans-like type).
- The almost negative bone scan (see ▸ Fig. 4.5 **b**).

Based on these facts, a biopsy was unnecessary—especially since neither melorheostosis nor osteoma has a specific histology.

Seven years later the patient presented again, complaining of severe pain in the left groin area and at the back of the thigh, corresponding to the sciatic nerve distribution. The pelvic radiograph now shows multicentric, relatively dense ossification in the soft tissues overlying the lesser trochanter (▸ Fig. 4.5 **c**), which are located directly adjacent to the neurovascular bundle, as CT demonstrates (▸ Fig. 4.5 **d**). Thus, there is additional myositis ossificans-like ossification in the soft tissues on the same side of the body. An initial attempt at total excision of the lesion was unsuccessful due to the very close proximity of the sciatic nerve, but it did reduce pain symptoms for several years. By that time the tumorlike mass had recurred and caused severe pain in the distribution of the sciatic nerve.

Other cases of melorheostosis are illustrated in Case 17 and Case 99.

Final Diagnosis

Melorheostosis of the osteoma type in the left ischium with the development of a myositis ossificans-like lesion in the adjacent soft tissues.

Comments

A uniformly dense, sclerosing mass in or on an otherwise normal bone that is clinically silent and shows little or no scintigraphic uptake is very likely to be melorheostosis or an osteoma. Melorheostosis is the more likely diagnosis in symptomatic cases.

Case 51 (▶ Fig. 4.6)

Case description

- Referring physician: oncologist.
- Prior history and clinical question: A 68-year-old woman with breast cancer underwent staging scintigraphy which showed intense uptake in the pelvis, considered suspicious for metastasis. The patient had no clinical complaints in the pelvic region, and the rest of the checkup showed no evidence of metastases. Her alkaline phosphatase level was elevated to twice normal.

Radiologic Findings

The anterior bone scan of the pelvis (▶ Fig. 4.6 **b**) shows a long segment of intense, homogeneous tracer uptake in the anterior portions of the pelvis, more intense on the right side. The posterior bone scan (not pictured here) also showed increased uptake in the mid- and right sacrum, which had the same intensity as the anterior pelvic regions on the anterior scan. The rest of the whole-body bone scan was negative. The pelvic radiograph (▶ Fig. 4.6 **a**) shows very "white," bone with coarsened trabecular pattern, cortical thickening as well as thickening in the pelvic rim ("rim sign") in the anterior portions of the ilium, in both acetabula, in the right pubic bone, in both ischia, and also in the sacrum and adjacent iliac segments. The pubis and ischium are enlarged.

Pathoanatomic Background of the Findings

There is an active remodeling process in the pelvic bones. This process enlarges the volume of the affected bone and culminates in a bony mass that shows increased radiation absorption.

Assignment to a Possible Basic Entity

▶ **Inflammation?** Yes, if we consider (as we do) Paget disease to be a special abacterial form of bone inflammation. See Case 8 for a more detailed account of this disease; additional cases are Case 9, Case 12, Case 14, Case 51, Case 107, and Case 140.

▶ **Tumor?** No. Metastatic cancer rarely causes a homogeneous structural alteration of bone, and only in its late stages. The otherwise negative whole-body bone scan is also inconsistent with metastasis.

Synopsis and Discussion

The following factors support a diagnosis of Paget disease (osteitis deformans):

- Large area of intense, homogeneous uptake
- "White" bone with coarsened trabecular pattern, cortical thickening as well as thickening in the pelvic rim (rim sign) and enlargement of the pubis and ischium
- Absence of clinical complaints
- Elevated alkaline phosphatase level; see also Case 8
- Age of the patient. (Around 5–7% of the population over age 60 in Central Europe, especially southern England and northern Germany, have Paget disease, usually as an incidental finding!)
- The pelvis is one of the most common sites of occurrence for Paget disease

In contrast to Case 46, the disease has affected the ilium and sacrum simultaneously or has spread from one bone to the other across "fused" sacroiliac joints.

Other differential diagnoses such as late bone metastasis or fibrous dysplasia are unrealistic and do not merit further discussion.

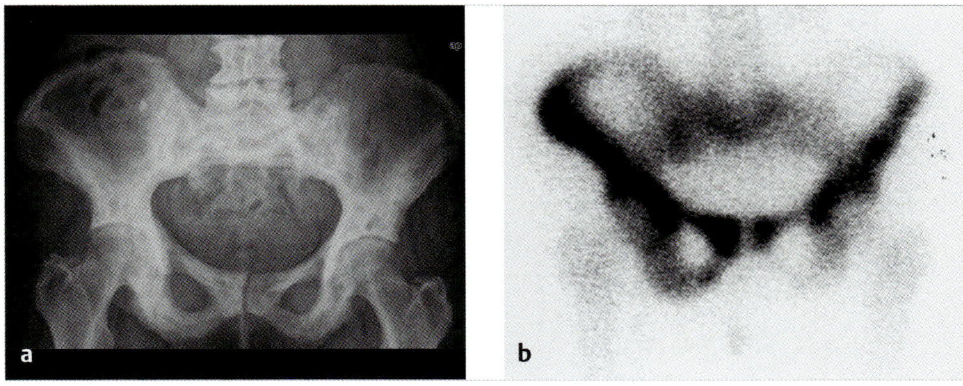

Fig. 4.6 a, b Metastatic breast cancer?

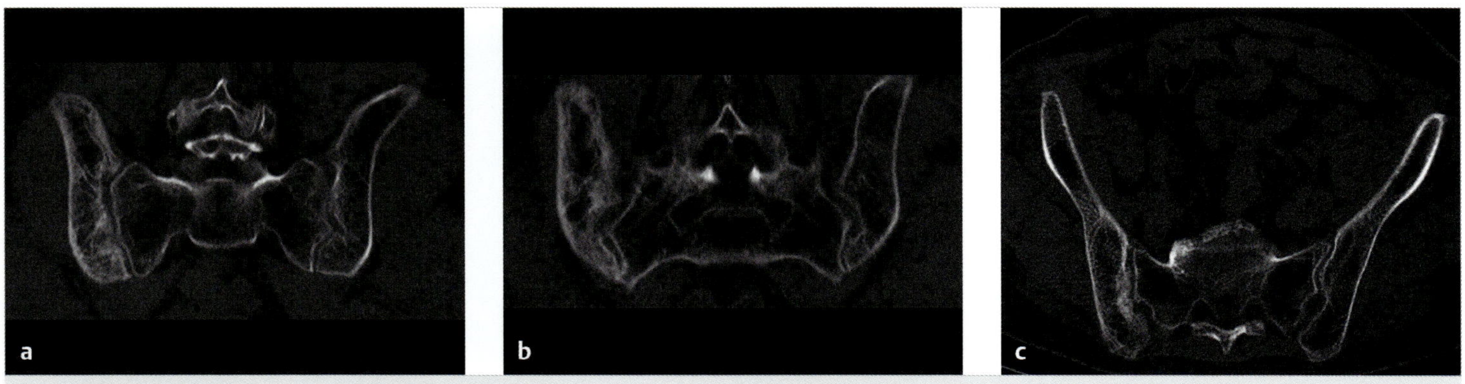

Fig. 4.7 a–c Paget disease in a 77-year-old woman.

▶ Fig. 4.7 shows CT scans from a 77-year-old woman with nonspecific right pelvic pain on weight-bearing. The right posterior portions of the ilium show a coarsened trabecular pattern, cortical thickening, and slight enlargement—signs that are highly specific for Paget disease. The alkaline phosphatase level was normal (relatively small affected bone volume, inactive stage of the disease). The complaints may be interpreted as a result of altered static loads in the right posterior pelvic ring.

Final Diagnosis

Paget disease of the pelvis, detected as an incidental finding and considered to have no pathologic significance.

Comments

There are alternatives to metastasis! Paget disease as a cause of a sclerosing bone process in the pelvis is undoubtedly more likely than metastatic breast cancer confined exclusively to the pelvis.

Case 52 (▶ Fig. 4.8)

Case description

- Referring physician: orthopedist.
- Prior history and clinical question: A 68-year-old man had a 4-week history of increasing right-sided lumbar pain radiating to the right leg. A swelling over the right iliac crest enlarged rapidly over the 4-week period. The patient had a known history of Paget disease of the pelvis. Clinical question: what is causing his present complaints?

Radiologic Findings

The plain radiographs in ▶ Fig. 4.8 **a, b** display typical features of Paget disease in the right ischium and pubis and in the right iliac wing (see also Case 51). The magnified view in ▶ Fig. 4.8 **b** shows a large, central lucent area with smaller opacities projected over the right iliac wing. Subsequent CT and MRI as shown in ▶ Fig. 4.8 **c–f** reveals a grotesque mass about the right iliac wing; it contains bizarre ossifications and shows central bone destruction (▶ Fig. 4.8 **d, f**).

Location

The epicenter of the mass is located in the bone showing pronounced structural alterations.

Pathoanatomic Background of the Findings

Because the epicenter of the mass is located in the bone and has partially destroyed it (▶ Fig. 4.8 **d, f**) and because the patient has Paget disease in the right iliac wing, it is reasonable to assume that the two processes are interrelated, and that an aggressive tumor has developed in the setting of the previous disease.

Assignment to a Possible Basic Entity

In this case there is no need to consider a normal variant, trauma, or inflammation. We are dealing with a secondary, highly aggressive sarcoma in a setting of Paget disease.

Synopsis and Discussion

In approximately 1% of all monostotic and 7 to 10% of all polyostotic cases of Paget disease, a secondary sarcoma develops in the diseased bone structures, with a special predilection for the pelvis and skull. Most patients are known to have had the disease for years. Patients with Paget disease have an approximately 30 times higher risk of developing a sarcoma in adulthood than persons without Paget disease. Sarcoma can arise from all cellular elements that are involved in bone turnover (osteosarcoma from osteoblasts, osteoclastic sarcoma from osteoclasts, and fibrosarcoma from fibroblasts). Osteosarcomas can be recognized by their ossified matrix, as in the present case.

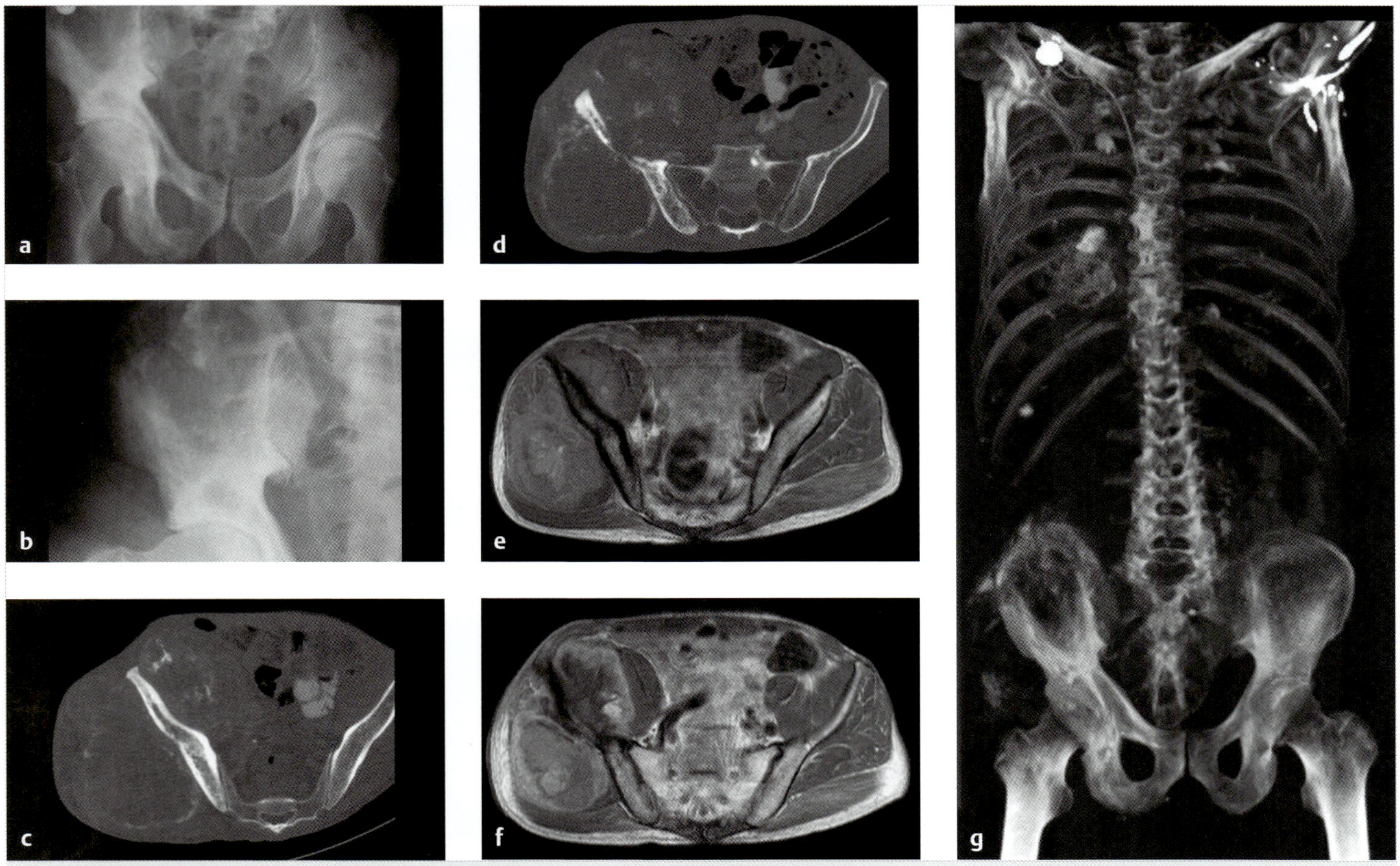

Fig. 4.8 a–g Paget sarcoma?

Sarcomas that occur in a setting of Paget disease tend to be highly aggressive, developing in a matter of weeks. The main clinical signs are pain of sudden onset, which feels new to the patient, and frequently a palpable mass. Most cases have a grave prognosis. The radiologic hallmarks are bone destruction (osteolysis), a paraosseous mass with or without matrix ossification, and a cold lesion within an area of increased uptake on bone scans. The differential diagnosis of osteolytic lesions in Paget disease includes giant cell tumor–like reactive lesions and, rarely, focal osteomalacia due to a bisposphonate overdose (see also under Paget Disease in Freyschmidt 2008).[13]

In rare cases, the radiologic appearance of Paget disease may show rapid, dramatic change with volume expansion and a greater osteolytic component as a result of trauma, for example. This rapid change can mimic the development of a sarcoma. It is helpful in these cases to measure the attenuation values in the lesion. In the absence of sarcoma, fat attenuation will almost always be found in the medullary cavity, indicating that there is no need to proceed with biopsy.

Our radiologic diagnosis of secondary osteosarcoma was confirmed histologically as a "poorly differentiated osteosarcoma with small-cell features." A short time later the patient developed pulmonary metastases (▶ Fig. 4.8 **g**), which resulted in his death.

Final Diagnosis

Osteosarcoma secondary to Paget disease in the right iliac wing.

This case was furnished to us by Prof. Dr. M. Libicher of Schwäbisch-Hall, Germany.

Comments

Pain and a mass in a bone affected by Paget disease, plus the radiologic detection of an osteolytic lesion that is cold on bone scans, are always highly suspicious for a secondary sarcoma.

4.2 Osteolytic Changes and Changes Associated with Decreased Bone Density

Case 53 (► Fig. 4.9)

Case description

- Referring physician: trauma surgeon.
- Prior history and clinical question: Posttraumatic pelvic radiographs in a 26-year-old woman incidentally revealed a coarse defect in the left iliac wing. Tumor? The patient did not have a prior history of surgery.

Radiologic Findings

The pelvic radiograph shows a large elliptical bone defect with well-defined margins in the left ilium (arrows in ► Fig. 4.9 a). The iliac crest bridges the defect laterally and superiorly but appears to form a pseudarthrosis at the junction with the solid anterior portions of the ilium. The findings are unchanged on follow-up radiographs obtained at 1 year (► Fig. 4.9 **b**) and 2 years (► Fig. 4.9 **c**). The lesion is classified as Lodwick type IB (punched-out lesion).

Pathoanatomic Background of the Findings

Any interpretation of the radiographs is somewhat speculative without sectional images. But the fact that the defect remained unchanged in its size, shape, and margins over a 3-year period suggests a congenital anomaly. It is important to know that the bony pelvis, like the calvarium, may have congenital gaps and defects that have no clinical significance and whose etiology is a matter of speculation.

Assignment to a Possible Basic Entity

► **Normal variant or malformation?** Yes, very likely. The absence of change over time strongly supports this interpretation.

► **Inflammation?** No, even a "burned-out" inflammation is excluded by the negative history.

► **Tumor?** Should at least be considered. A Lodwick type IB lesion in the pelvis could represent a focus of Langerhans-cell histiocytosis, for example. While this type of lesion may be clinically silent, it would show some change over a 3-year period such as an increase or decrease in size, marginal sclerosis, additional foci, etc. As in Case 54, we might also consider vanishing bone disease (Gorham–Stout disease, phantom bone, massive osteolysis, disappearing bone, regional angiomatosis), but the absence of radiologic change would make this diagnosis unlikely as well. The patient is too young for a solitary plasmacytoma, which would also produce clinical manifestations. A simple bone cyst is not supported by the absence of lesion expansion and the lack of marginal sclerosis, which a cyst would surely have developed over a 3-year period.

► **Necrosis?** Possibly, but the negative history and location suggest otherwise. To the author's knowledge, avascular necrosis has never been reported in this region. This is because the affected region is not located in a terminal vascular bed.

Synopsis and Discussion

As explained above, the asymptomatic bone defect in the left iliac wing could only be a congenital lesion or an old, burned-out tumor that has taken an atypical course. Aside from simple follow-up radiographs, the patient declined sectional imaging studies and also refused a histologic work-up. The latter decision cannot be faulted, for what would it have accomplished? Remember that this defect has neither a traumatic nor iatrogenic cause. Moreover, the patient had no external scars or focal scleroderma (see Case 11).

Preliminary or Working Diagnosis

Congenital bone defect in the iliac wing.

Comments

A congenital malformation should be considered for an incidentally detected bone defect with no associated periosteal reaction located in the pelvis or skull.

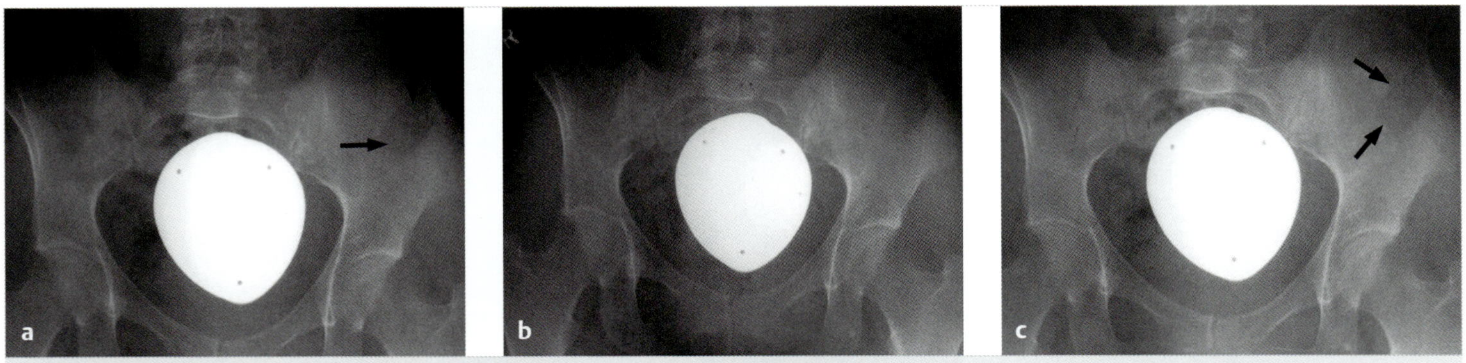

Fig. 4.9 Langerhans-cell histiocytosis? The radiographs were taken in 2004 (a), 2005 (b), and 2006 (c).

Case 54 (▶ Fig. 4.10)

Case description

- Referring physician: rheumatologist.
- Prior history and clinical question: A 29-year-old woman complained of progressive stabbing and burning pains in the right gluteal region radiating to the right thigh. The symptoms began during a (second) pregnancy about 18 months previously. After the delivery she underwent CT and MRI, which revealed "osteolytic changes and demineralization with cortical defects in the right ilium." A biopsy showed "corticocancellous bone tissue with chronic scarring and inflammation, consistent with chronic osteomyelitis." At that point the patient declined further diagnostic studies. Eventually her symptoms worsened until she was unable to walk. The patient stated that she then visited a chiropractor, who gave her an injection and a manual adjustment. She claimed that afterward she was able to walk again. One month before seeing the rheumatologist, she fell onto her buttock and her pain returned. A doctor elsewhere voiced suspicion of a rheumatic disease, and this prompted referral to the rheumatologist. Clinical examination showed no evidence of a rheumatic process. Because the patient was originally from Kazakhstan, the rheumatologist considered tuberculous osteomyelitis with sacroiliitis. He consulted us before ordering another biopsy.

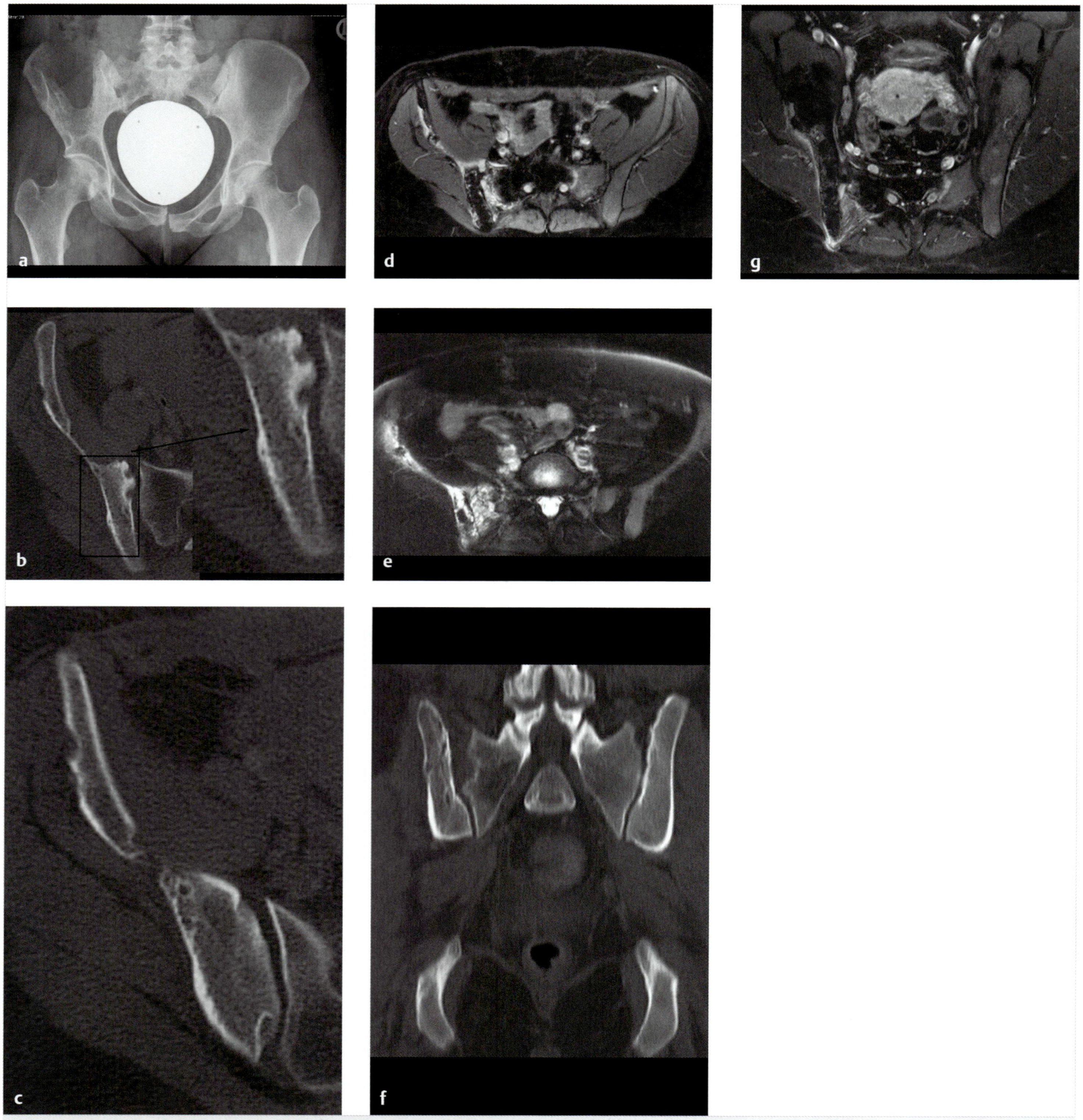

Fig. 4.10 a–g Malignant or inflammatory destructive process?

Radiologic Findings

The current pelvic radiograph (▶ Fig. 4.10 **a**) shows a large defect in the right iliac wing that includes the iliac crest. The defect is surrounded by osteolytic changes with a mixed honeycomb and streaky pattern, which are bordered by a sclerotic zone that is most prominent on the medial side. The symphysis is still widened from the previous pregnancy. The CT scans in ▶ Fig. 4.10 **b, c, f** show subperiosteal and subchondral erosions medial and lateral to the defect. Closer scrutiny of the posterior portions of the ilium in ▶ Fig. 4.10 **b** (magnified view on the right) reveals tortuous, vermiform lucencies in the cancellous bone. Current contrast-enhanced MR images (▶ Fig. 4.10 **d, e, g**) show patchy hyperintensities in and around the bone.

Pathoanatomic Background of the Findings

The key pathoanatomic findings are the large bone defect and the honeycomb lucencies around the defect, which must be interpreted as vascular prints. The destructive changes, therefore, are most likely based on an underlying vascular process.

Assignment to a Possible Basic Entity

▶ **Normal variant or malformation?** No. This is excluded by the clinical presentation and imaging findings.

▶ **Trauma?** No. The process was not initiated by trauma, and pregnancy-related loosening of the pelvic ring could not produce structural changes of this kind.

▶ **Inflammation?** No. A chronic, septic inflammatory process of this size would include osteolytic changes, sequestra, dense sclerosis, and clinical manifestations of fever, soft-tissue abscess formation, etc.

▶ **Tumor or tumorlike lesion?** Yes, probably an angiomatous process that cannot strictly be classified as neoplastic (further details below).

Synopsis and Discussion

As noted above, there is evidence of an angiomatous process that has gradually dissolved the bone. The findings are consistent with vanishing bone disease (Gorham–Stout disease, phantom bone, massive osteolysis, disappearing bone, regional angiomatosis; see also Case 11). This is an extremely rare skeletal disease, difficult to diagnosis histologically, which is characterized by increasing regional resorption of cancellous and cortical bone and their replacement by an aggressively spreading vascular tissue similar to hemangioma or lymphangioma. In recent years the vessels have been identified as mainly lymphatic vessels that may relate to a disturbance of lymphangiogenesis.[33] Later the resorbed bone is replaced by vascularized fibrous tissue, at which point a specific histologic diagnosis can no longer be made. The freely proliferating neovascular tissue incites an active hyperemia that probably upsets the normal balance between osteoclasts and osteoblasts causing a predominance of bone resorption, see neurovascular theory in Case 11, section on "Perfusion disorder?". Today it is known that neither infectious nor malignant or neuropathic factors have causal significance in vanishing bone disease. The main clinical symptom in most patients is a boring pain of gradual onset, as in the present case. Plain radiographs early in the disease show a "patchy osteoporosis" appearing as multiple intramedullary and subcortical lucencies, which in our advanced case are still in direct proximity to the large osteolytic area. Later these foci enlarge and coalesce while new foci appear at the periphery. Then the contours and internal structure of the bone gradually disappear as "demineralization" progresses. The vanished bone areas may reach considerable size, causing grotesque anatomic distortions. Generally the disease is self-limiting and resolves in 1 to 2 years, although some cases may have a fatal termination, especially if complications arise such as chylothorax or severe hemorrhage.[13] Further details on this disease are presented in Case 11.

A second biopsy taken from the conspicuous area of soft-tissue changes on MRI, interpreted with the help of a reference pathologist, revealed lymphangiomatosis and confirmed our impression of vanishing bone disease.

Final Diagnosis

Vanishing bone disease (synonyms: Gorham–Stout disease, phantom bone, massive osteolysis, disappearing bone, regional angiomatosis) in the right iliac wing.

Comments

Vanishing bone disease is a rare entity that should be considered in younger patients with large, painful osteolytic defects and no associated osteoblastic or periosteal reaction.

Case 55 (▶ Fig. 4.11)

Case description

- Referring physician: radiologist.
- Prior history and clinical question: A 24-year-old professional soccer player underwent MRI of the pelvis for investigation of pubalgia. The images incidentally revealed a hyperintense (water-equivalent) lesion in the right iliac wing (▶ Fig. 4.11 **a**). Pelvic stability was investigated further by CT (▶ Fig. 4.11 **b–g**), which showed attenuation values of 10 to 20 HU in the lesion. The patient had no prior history of major trauma and no prolonged episodes of pain in the right iliac wing.

Radiologic Findings

The CT correlate of the MRI finding is an expansile osteolytic lesion with no internal structural features and a solid bony cap over its medial and lateral portions. Linear lucencies, interpreted as vascular channels, radiate from the upper and lower ends of the lesion into the intact cancellous bone (▶ Fig. 4.11 **e, g**).

Location

The expansile osteolytic lesion is located in a region of the iliac wing that is very thin. It is related superiorly and inferiorly to two large vessels.

Pathoanatomic Background of the Findings

The MRI and CT findings indicate a cystic process rather than a solid lesion.

Assignment to a Possible Basic Entity

▶ **Normal variant or malformation?** Not previously described at this location, although this interpretation would be consistent with the negative history and lack of clinical manifestations.

▶ **Trauma?** Yes, in principle, especially in a professional soccer player who is constantly subject to jolts, falls, kicks, etc. that could have caused intraosseous bleeding.

▶ **Tumor or tumorlike lesion?** We might consider a unilocular juvenile bone cyst at an unusual location (only about 2% of all juvenile bone cysts are located in the pelvis).

Synopsis and Discussion

The lesion in the right iliac wing can certainly be interpreted as cystic. But imaging can definitely classify the lesion as a juvenile or unilocular bone cyst only if contrast-enhanced MRI can show an enhancing cyst wall (membrane composed of loose, vascularized fibrous tissue (see Case 132, and ▶ Fig. 7.25 in Case 143) and if the interior of the lesion does not show significant enhancement during the usual examination time. This study was not

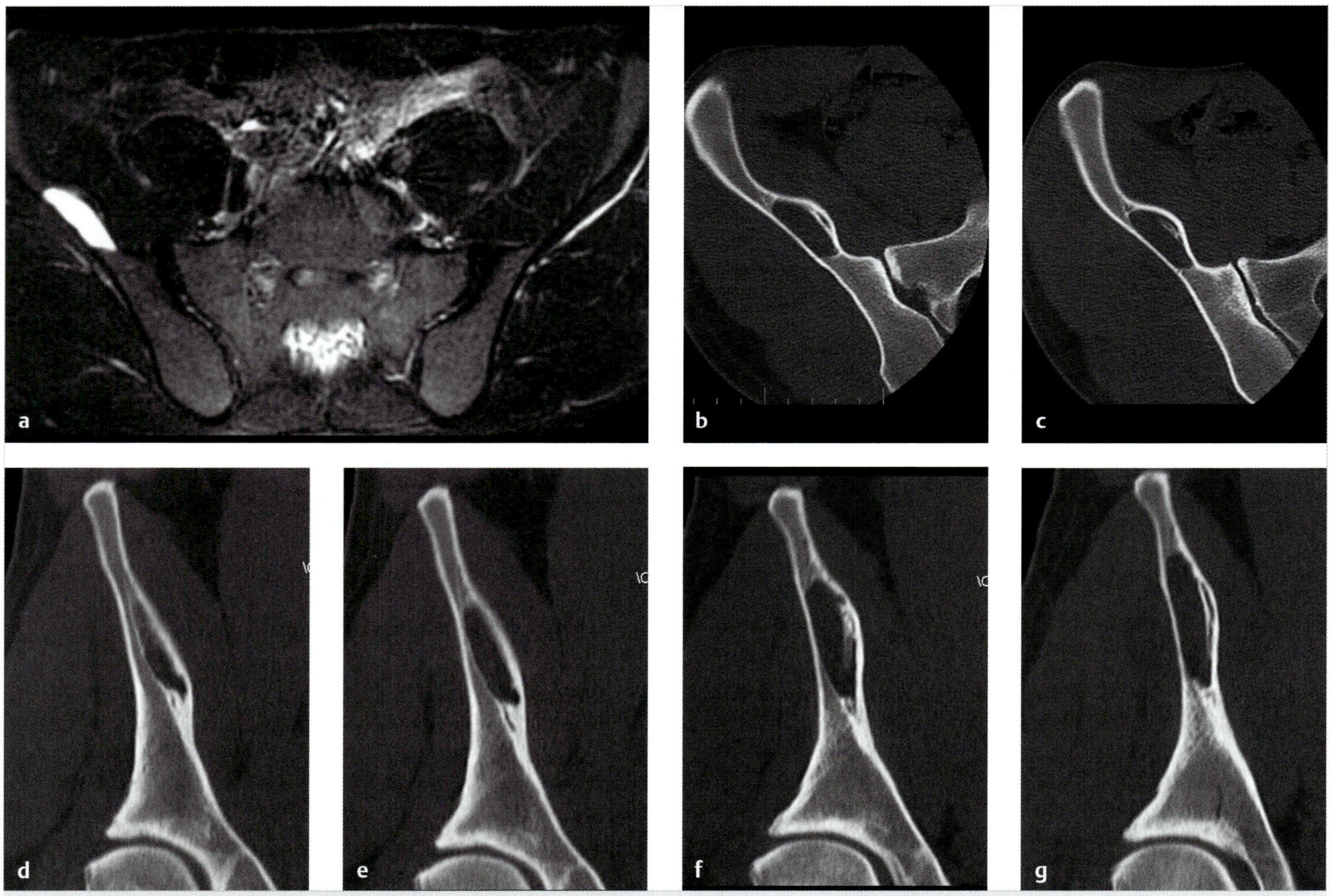

Fig. 4.11 a–g Incidental finding in a soccer player.

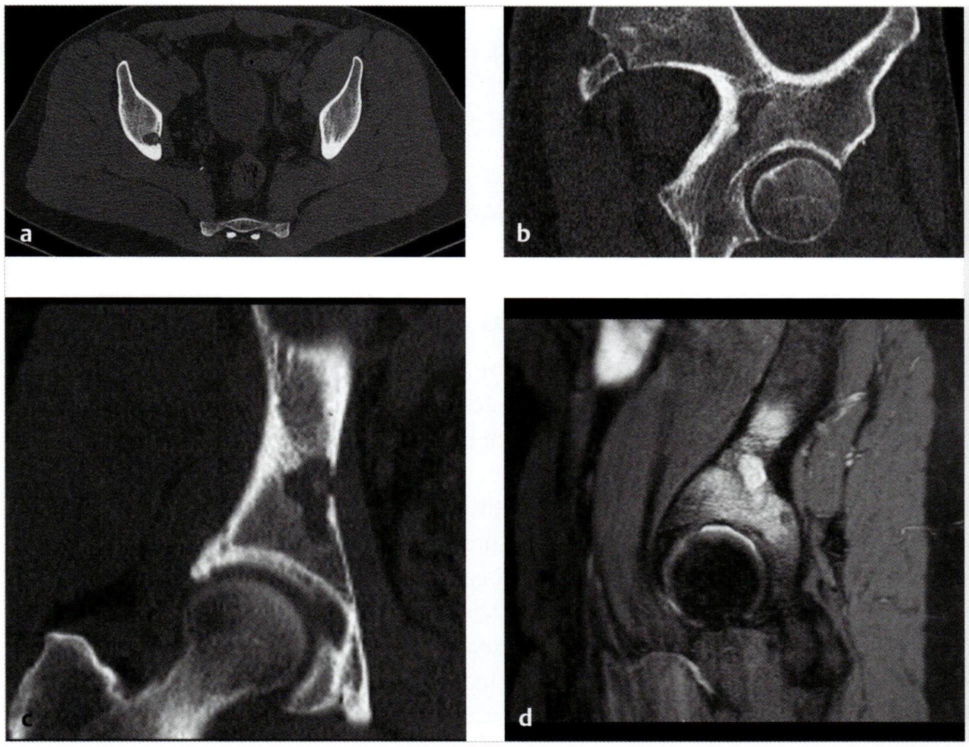

Fig. 4.12 a–d Langerhans-cell histiocytosis in a 41-year-old man.

done in the present case, nor is it strictly necessary, since the lesion is an asymptomatic incidental finding. Given the vascular channels noted at the superior and inferior poles of the lesion, the cyst may well have developed at one time as an asymptomatic sequel to a traumatic intraosseous hemorrhage, since the ilium at the lesion site is very thin. Ultimately we cannot say if the lesion should be classified as a posttraumatic intraosseous cyst or as a juvenile bone cyst that has not yet resolved.

As noted above, a unilocular (juvenile) bone cyst in the pelvis is rare. A bone cyst at that location is more common in older patients, which is not surprising when we consider that the lesion in the present case was a purely incidental finding. Juvenile bone cysts are typically located in the long tubular bones (ca. 81% in the humerus and femur). They become symptomatic only when disrupted due to trauma. On MRI the associated intracystic hemorrhage may produce a fluid level within the otherwise clear intralesional fluid, though it would occupy an uninterrupted area (see ▶ Fig. 7.25) and would not form multiple levels as in an aneurysmal bone cyst.

A histologic examination or even prophylactic dissection would be unnecessary in our case if the patient remains free of complaints.

▶ Fig. 4.12 illustrates the case of a 41-year-old man with a focus of Langerhans-cell histiocytosis or eosinophilic granuloma in the right lower ilium. The patient had an approximately 6-month history of pain in that area, which was initially interpreted as "sciatica-like" and treated with anti-inflammatory drugs. The lesion had a "geographic" shape on CT scans (▶ Fig. 4.12 **a–c**) with a small central "sequestrum." This prompted us to classify the lesion as a typical eosinophilic granuloma or focus of Langerhans-cell histiocytosis (see also Case 9 and Case 24. Unfortunately, MRI was also performed (▶ Fig. 4.12 **d**) and water-sensitive sequences showed significant edema-like signal which caused us to question our diagnosis of Langerhans-cell histiocytosis. The edema-like signal also suggested an osteoblastoma. A CT-guided percutaneous biopsy finally confirmed a focus of Langerhans-cell histiocytosis.

Final Diagnosis

Old posttraumatic cyst in the right iliac wing. The differential diagnosis includes an "old juvenile bone cyst" as an incidental finding. The lesion does not compromise stability.

Comments

Cystic pelvic lesions detected incidentally in young patients who engage in contact sports may result from intraosseous hemorrhage, especially if large vascular structures are found in close proximity to the lesion.

Case 56 (▶ Fig. 4.13)

Case description

- Referring physician: radiologist.
- Prior history and clinical question: Staging CT of the abdomen in a 67-year-old man with lung cancer demonstrated an expansile lesion in the left iliac wing. There was no history relating to that region. The patient had been on anticoagulant therapy for many years for coronary heart disease. The radiologist wants to know the cause of the expansile lesion.

Radiologic Findings

The left iliac wing is expanded in its middle third. That region is traversed by a thin, laterally convex bony plate (arrow in ▶ Fig. 4.13 **f**). Anatomically it represents the former inner cortex of the iliac wing; this is evident on comparison with the opposite side. The current inner (medial) cortex is convex toward the medial side and undulating. Between it and the interior bony plate there are slightly rarefied bone trabeculae with enlarged medullary cavities.

Location

The expansile process is located just medial to the normal medullary cavity of the left iliac wing, but it forms an anatomic unit with it. It is not juxtaosseous or even extraosseous, but is subperiosteal in its location.

Pathoanatomic Background of the Findings

The medial and lateral "compartments" of the lesion contain cancellous bone that is somewhat rarefied medially. This does not indicate a destructive process

Assignment to a Possible Basic Entity

▶ **Normal variant or malformation?** This question is justified given the absence of clinical symptoms, but there are no reports of this normal variant in the literature.

▶ **Trauma?** Yes, with subperiosteal hemorrhage. The hematoma has displaced the periosteum medially, and a neocortex has formed. The original cortex has atrophied over time and is represented by the thin, laterally convex bony plate inside the lesion. The blood has been reabsorbed with healing, and cancellous bone with an almost normal medullary cavity has developed within the space formerly occupied by hematoma.

▶ **Inflammation?** No clinical manifestations.

▶ **Tumor?** Yes, if this category includes pseudotumors and tumorlike lesions.

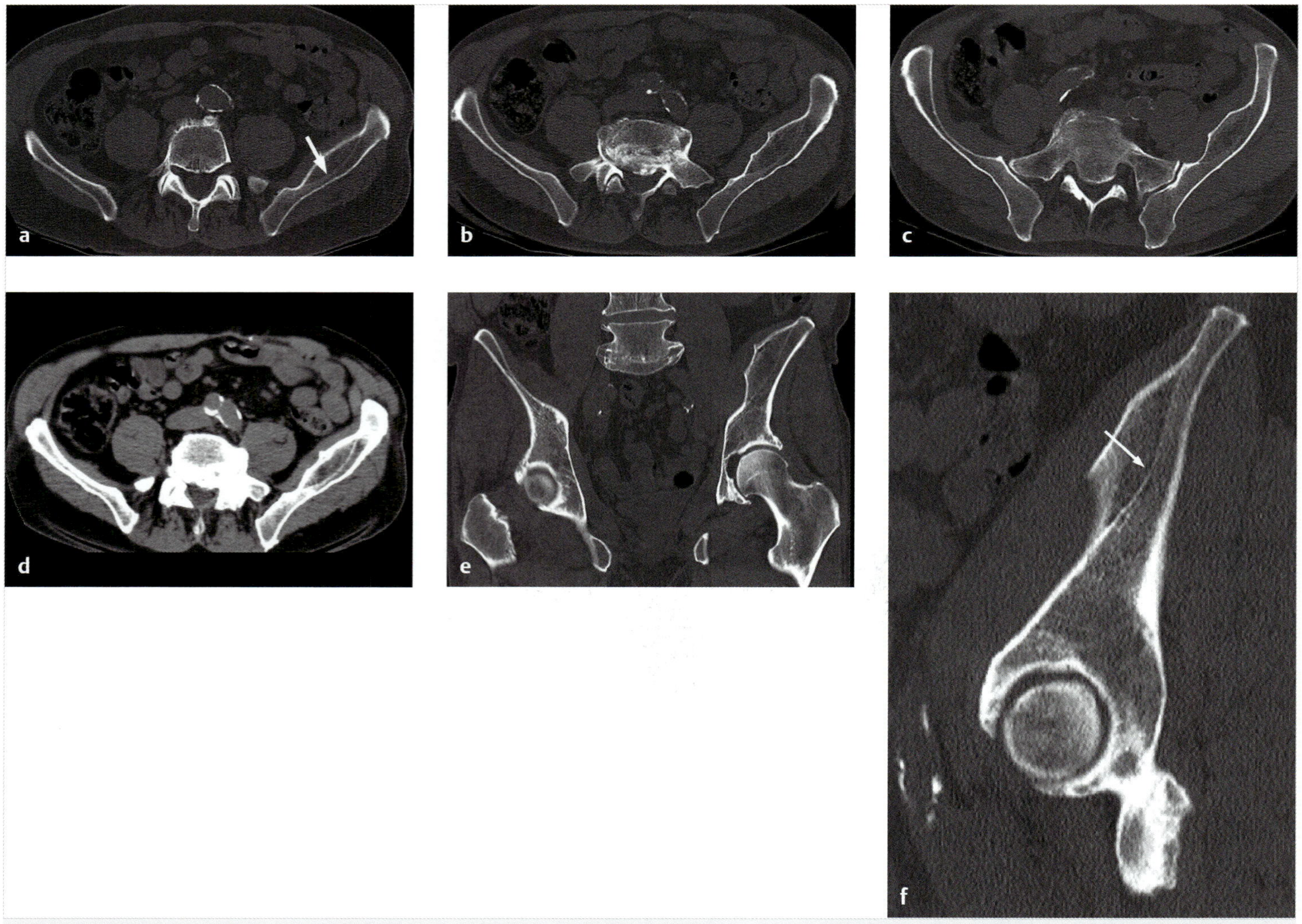

Fig. 4.13 a–f Incidental finding in a lung cancer patient on anticoagulant therapy. The last image shown here (f) is a sagittal reformatted CT scan.

Synopsis and Discussion

A subperiosteal hemorrhage with the development of a pseudotumor can be diagnosed from the radiologic findings. The patient could not recall pelvic trauma, but the anticoagulant medication increased the risk of subperiosteal bleeding. Even minor trauma, not remembered by the patient, would be sufficient to cause a subperiosteal or intraosseous hemorrhage. Such an event may take a more or less silent course, depending on pain perception and processing by the individual patient, and could heal, leaving a pseudotumor behind.

Pseudotumors of this kind are also called *hemophilic pseudotumors*, which present as an intraosseous or subperiosteal expansile process.[34] They are known to occur in hemophilia A and B. Approximately 1 to 2% of all hemophiliacs develop a hemophilic pseudotumor, most commonly in the bones of the hands, feet, and pelvis. But anticoagulant medication also predisposes to this complication. Hemophilic pseudotumors may enlarge. A "chronic expanding hematoma" is one that increases in volume for more than 1 month after the initial hemorrhage.[35]

Final Diagnosis

Old subperiosteal hemorrhage in the left ilium of a patient on anticoagulant medication (hemophilic pseudotumor).

Comments

A rare lesion can be correctly diagnosed by interpreting radiologic findings in relation to anatomic structures.

Case 57 (▶ Fig. 4.14)

Case description

- Referring physician: orthopedist.
- Prior history and clinical question: A 12-year-old boy had a 4-month history of pain in the left hip. The pain was attributed to primary limb length shortening on the left side. A cystic mass was detected incidentally in the left iliac wing, and an open biopsy yielded the following report: "The material may have been sampled from the margin of a simple bone cyst; no evidence of malignancy." It should be added that the pathologist could not make a more specific diagnosis because apparently he did not have representative material. But adding "no evidence of malignancy" is superfluous and reminds us of the old practice of branding every histologic finding with the stereotypic phrase "no evidence of tuberculosis or malignancy." (As if these entities were the only possibilities!) The orthopedist referred the case to us for evaluation.

Radiologic Findings

The pelvis has an atypical shape with a medial shift of the linea terminalis, imparting an asymmetrical heart shape to the pelvis (▶ Fig. 4.14 **a**). The hip joint is approximately 2 cm higher on the left side than on the right. A multicentric or loculated osteolytic mass is noted in the left iliac wing (▶ Fig. 4.14 **a**). The MR images (▶ Fig. 4.14 **b–g**) show fluid-equivalent signal intensities in the mass with numerous septa that are devoid of signal. They give the lesion a loculated appearance. The mass extends inferiorly to the acetabulum and posteriorly to the retroarticular space of the left sacroiliac joint. No fluid–fluid levels are seen.

Pathoanatomic Background of the Findings

The blisterlike expansion of the left iliac wing and fluid-equivalent signal intensities indicate a cystic rather than solid mass.

Assignment to a Possible Basic Entity

▸ **Normal variant or malformation?** No known precedents in this form. Because the boy has no other clinical skeletal abnormalities, a syndrome with cyst formation (e.g., basal cell nevus syndrome) cannot be considered.

▸ **Trauma?** No history; see also Case 55.

▸ **Inflammation?** No clinical manifestations.

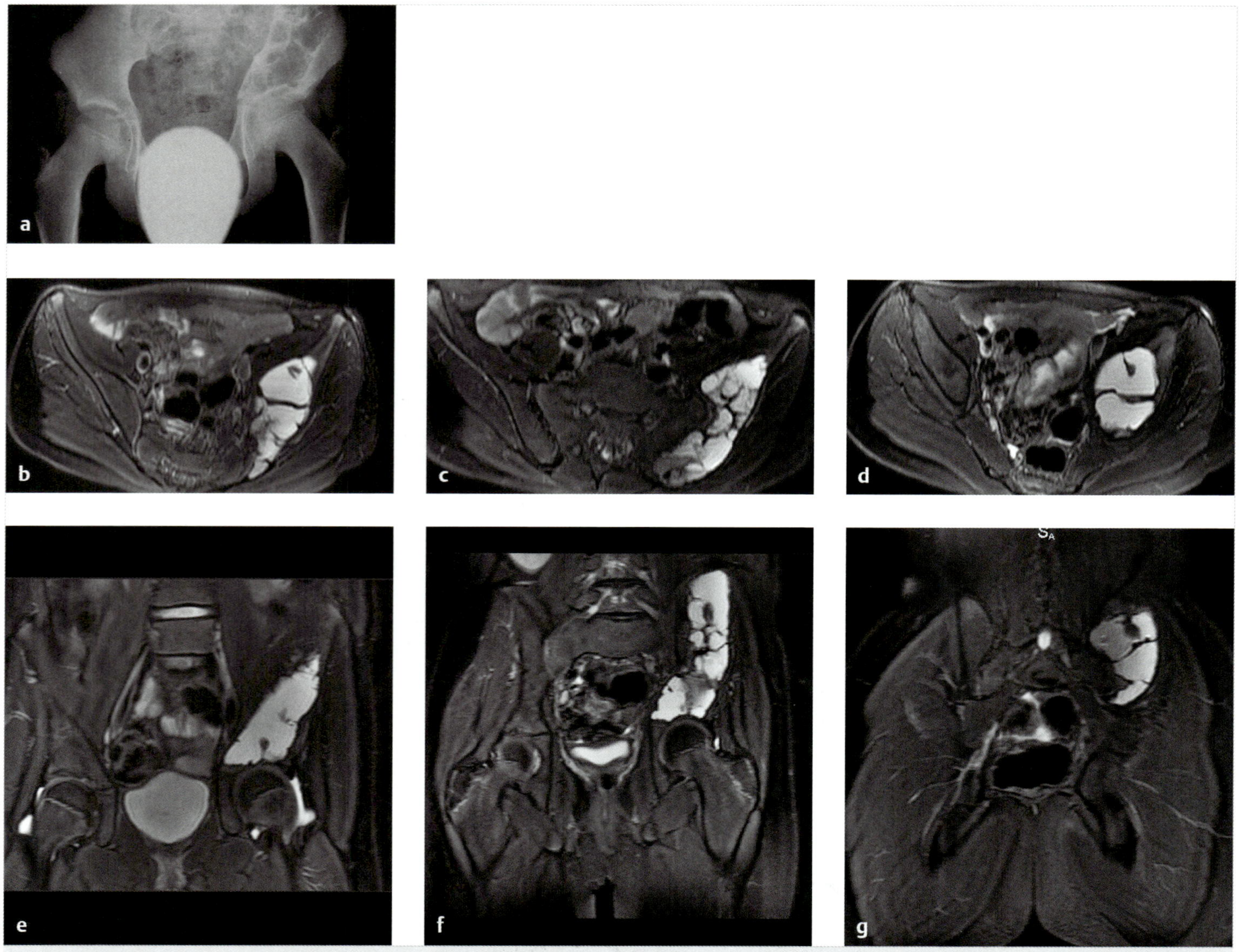

Fig. 4.14 a–g Incidental radiologic finding in a patient with clinical shortening of the left leg.

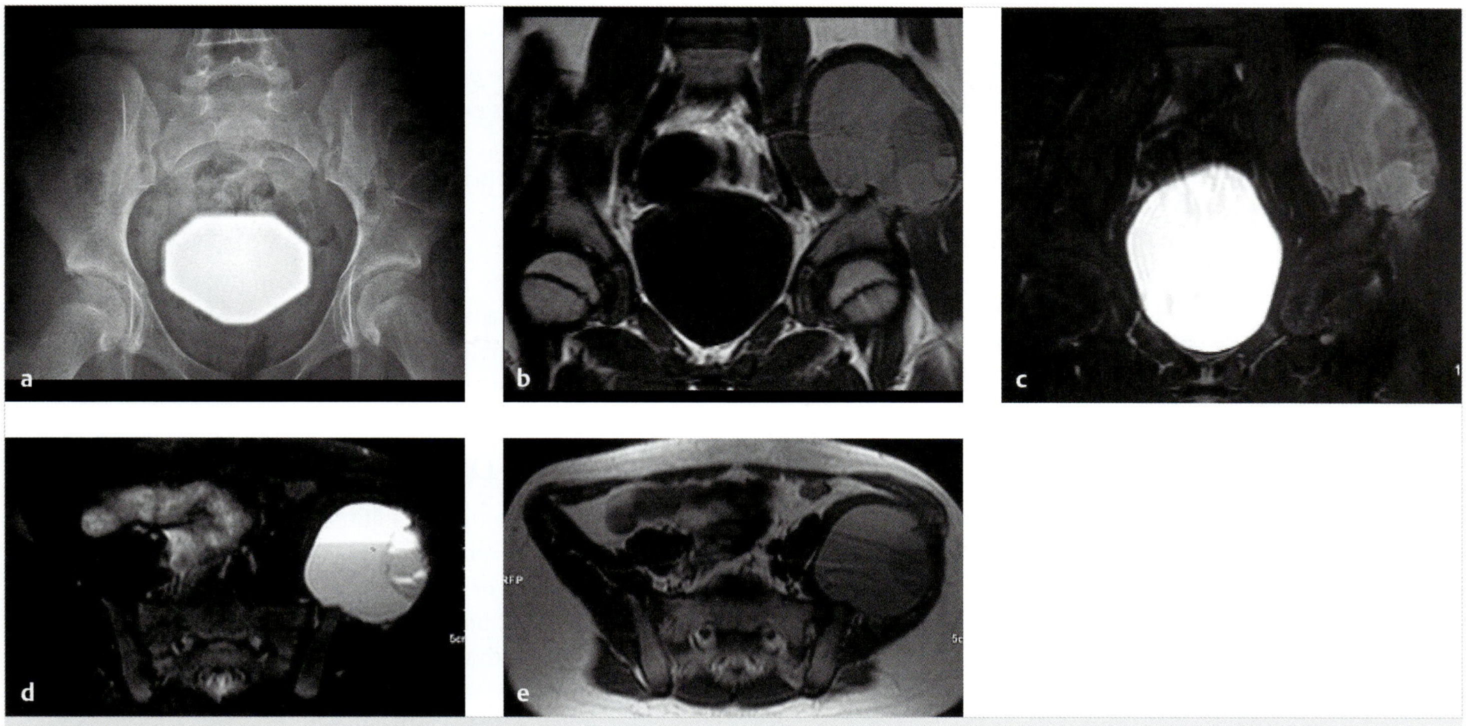

Fig. 4.15 a–e Juvenile bone cyst in an 11-year-old girl.

▶ **Tumor?** Yes, a tumorlike lesion in the form of a bone cyst.

Synopsis and Discussion

We are dealing with a loculated cystic mass in the left iliac wing that has already caused significant growth disturbance with one hip joint higher than the other. This explains the limb length shortening on the left side, which may have led to the complaints. The pelvic radiograph raises the following possibilities:

- Juvenile bone cyst (synonyms: unilocular juvenile bone cyst, solitary bone cyst, simple bone cyst)
- Aneurysmal bone cyst
- Fibrous dysplasia, although a uniform ground-glass appearance is not seen

The MR images exclude an aneurysmal bone cyst because they do not show the fluid levels specific for that lesion; see example in Case 45. Since the lesion is completely filled with fluid, even a mostly liquefied area of fibrous dysplasia is extremely unlikely.

Juvenile bone cysts are generally asymptomatic in the absence of trauma. When a bone cyst is traumatized, the thin wall may rupture causing intralesional hemorrhage (see different case in ▶ Fig. 4.15). Only then does the lesion become painful. This means that the history is generally short. On the other hand, patients with an aneurysmal bone cyst have a longer pain history.

The lesion was treated surgically as it threatened the stability of the hip joint. When opened it discharged a clear amber-colored fluid; no palpable septa were found. Apparently the "septa" seen on MRI were sectional views of bony ridges projecting from the wall into the lesion. The working diagnosis of juvenile bone cyst was confirmed histologically. Actifuse, a synthetic bone substitute, was instilled into the cyst cavity.

▶ Fig. 4.15 **a–e** shows another unusually large juvenile bone cyst in an 11-year-old girl. In this case trauma had fractured the cyst wall causing an intralesional hemorrhage with a fluid level demonstrated by MRI in the supine patient (▶ Fig. 4.15 **d**). The detection of a cyst lining of 1 to 2 mm thickness after contrast administration (▶ Fig. 4.15 **e**) is not consistent with an aneurysmal bone cyst.

Final Diagnosis

Unusually large juvenile bone cyst in the left iliac wing with associated growth disturbance of the left hemipelvis.

Comments

It is not possible to distinguish among a juvenile bone cyst, aneurysmal bone cyst, and fibrous dysplasia on plain pelvic radiographs alone. MRI after contrast administration is best for detecting liquid contents with a cyst lining of 1 to 2 mm thickness. Histologic confirmation (e.g., by biopsy) may be problematic if the surgeon misses the cyst lining and samples only peripheral bone.

Case 58 (▶ Fig. 4.16)

Case description

- Referring physician: orthopedist.
- Prior history and clinical question: An expansile lesion was detected incidentally in the left iliac wing of a 41-year-old man (▶ Fig. 4.16 **a**). The orthopedist requested that we determine etiology and assess the need for biopsy.

Radiologic Findings

The radiograph shows a blisterlike expansion of the bone in the upper third of the left iliac wing, corresponding to a Lodwick IA classification. The lesion contains scattered trabecula-like bone structures (▶ Fig. 4.16 **b–d**) and is bounded by solid cortex on all sides. A soft-tissue window was not used, so we cannot measure or estimate the attenuation values in the lesion. But the bone-window images do show that fine calcifications or ossifications are present at the very periphery of the lesion (▶ Fig. 4.16 **b**).

Pathoanatomic Background of the Findings

Given the lack of attenuation values and soft-tissue window images, we can only speculate as to the internal composition of the lesion. It probably consists of multiple components such as connective tissue, fine woven bone, fat, and possible liquid material.

Assignment to a Possible Basic Entity

▶ **Trauma?** No. The patient denied pelvic trauma, so a posttraumatic lesion appears extremely unlikely.

▶ **Inflammation?** No history.

▶ **Tumor?** Yes. The Lodwick IA classification indicates a slow-growing process. The presumed multicomponent structure suggests fibrous dysplasia, but an old, simple, unhealed bone cyst would also be possible. We might even consider an old lipoma with regressive changes.

Synopsis and Discussion

We cannot offer a definitive solution for this case because the CT examination was incomplete. The absence of symptoms (incidental finding), the age of the patient, the site of occurrence, and the peripheral calcifications or ossifications could indicate regressive changes in fibrous dysplasia. See also Case 7, Case 73, and Case 133. In the case of an unhealed, simple juvenile bone cyst, it would be unlikely that the cyst, given its exposed location, could have gone decades without becoming traumatized, fractured and symptomatic. Finally, an intraosseous lipoma would be plausible only if a preponderance of fatty tissue had been detected in the lesion.

To be noncommittal, we could simply describe the process as a "benign fibro-osseous lesion of indeterminate origin." This also

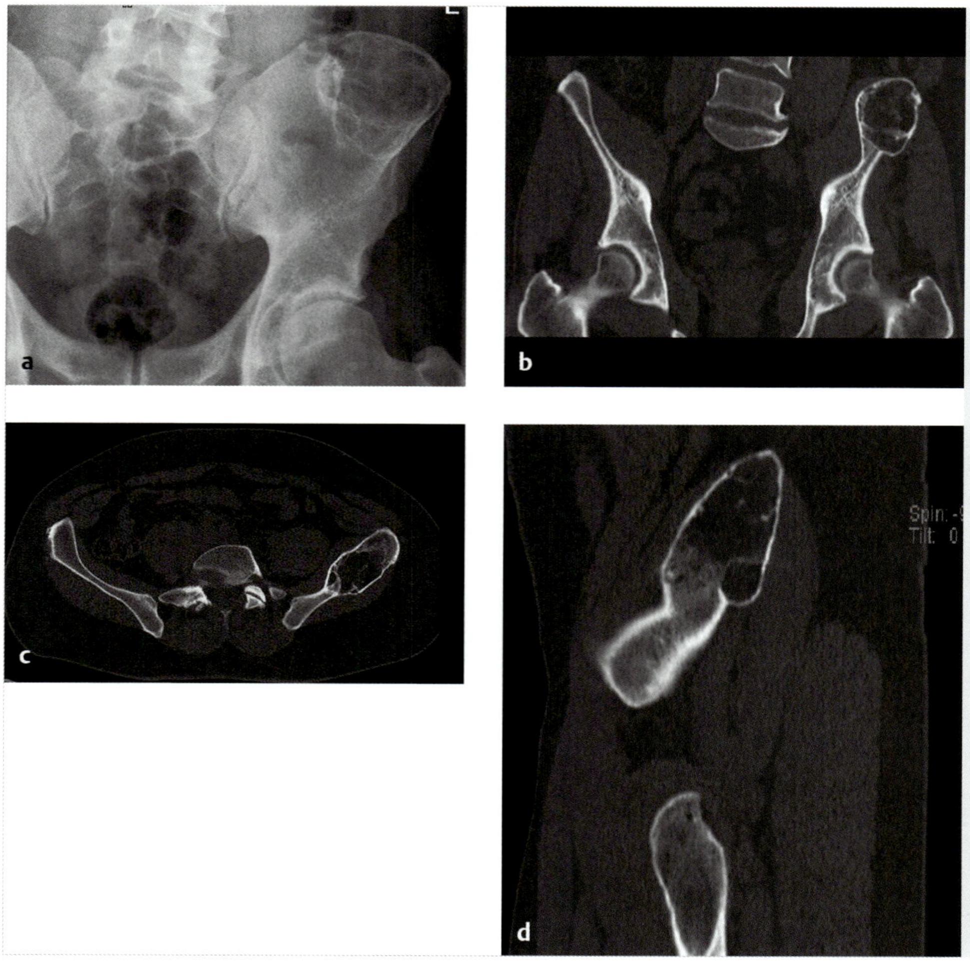

Fig. 4.16 a–d Incidental finding. Biopsy?

implies that a histologic examination would probably be inconclusive, leaving us with a "don't touch me" lesion or "leave me alone" lesion.

Much ado about nothing? No, imaging with a soft-tissue window and densitometry could definitely have supplied a more precise lesion classification, to which the patient and treating orthopedist are entitled. We know from experience that uncertainty often motivates patients and their doctors to proceed with invasive procedures.

Radiologic Working Diagnosis

Benign fibro-osseous ("leave me alone") lesion in the left iliac wing. Possible etiologies:

- Fibrous dysplasia with regressive changes
- Old juvenile bone cyst
- Lipoma with regressive changes

Comments

CT examinations of bony lesions should always be combined with attenuation measurements to fully utilize the capabilities of CT technology!

Case 59 (▶ Fig. 4.17)

Case description

- Referring physician: pediatrician.
- Prior history and clinical question: An 8½-year-old boy had been clinically normal except for delayed speech development and hearing impairment since kindergarten. He showed marked improvement in response to speech therapy. When subjective hearing loss worsened 1 year previously, he was seen by an otolaryngologist who performed a paracentesis and drainage of the middle-ear on the right side. Reportedly, the procedure was not possible on the left side. Finally the patient was referred to a different ear, nose and throat (ENT) facility, where a left-sided mass was found arising from the floor of the auditory canal. Imaging studies were then performed. It should be added that the general clinical examination showed no other abnormalities.

Radiologic Findings

The medial portions of the left petrous bone show bubbly expansion and opacification (▶ Fig. 4.17 **a, b**). T2w axial MRI (▶ Fig. 4.17 **c**) shows innumerable cystlike hyperintensities in the left petrous bone. The left jugular foramen is not defined. (Further details on the ear canal, tympanic cavity, and inner ear are omitted here.)

The MR images showed additional abnormalities in the right occipital condyle and cervical spine (▶ Fig. 4.17 **c–e**), which prompted whole-body MRI. Water-sensitive sequences revealed disseminated focal hyperintensities throughout the spine and pelvis (▶ Fig. 4.17 **f–j**), in the left intertrochanteric region, in the distal femoral medullary cavities, in one rib, and in one fibula. CT images showed disseminated osteolytic lesions at corresponding sites (▶ Fig. 4.17 **k–o**).

Location

The lesions are located predominantly in the axial skeleton, but whole-body MRI shows additional lesions in the long bones, that is, wherever cancellous bone occurs. None of the lesion has penetrated the cortex.

Pathoanatomic Background of the Findings

The disseminated skeletal foci represent proton-rich lesions that have caused extensive lucencies in the affected cancellous bone.

Assignment to a Possible Basic Entity

▶ **Normal variant or malformation?** Naturally this question must be asked of a child who is healthy except for hearing impairment. If the answer is yes, we would have to consider a syndromic condition. But the clinical presentation suggests otherwise, with the physical examination and laboratory tests showing no evidence of a malformation.

▶ **Trauma?** No trauma is recalled.

▶ **Inflammation?** No clinical manifestations.

▶ **Tumor?** The predilection of the lesions for red marrow suggests a disseminated process associated with proliferating tissue. The possibilities would include all cell lines occurring in red marrow (e.g., lymphoma, leukemia) as well as granulomatous diseases such as sarcoidosis and Langerhans-cell histiocytosis. A disseminated vascular process should also be considered.

Synopsis and Discussion

The clinical presentation (hearing impairment in an otherwise healthy child) excludes systemic diseases such as *leukemia*. Because the chest radiograph was normal, *sarcoidosis* is also eliminated. A diagnosis of *Langerhans-cell histiocytosis* confined to one organ (bone) is consistent with the age and lack of clinical symptoms but does not explain the fully intact cortex. As a rule, foci of Langerhans-cell histiocytosis will disrupt the cortex at some location, with histiocytic tissue sometimes penetrating the cortex and extending into the soft tissues.

Another possibility is *cystic angiomatosis*. This diagnosis is consistent with the absence of systemic signs and absence of complaints relating to the skeletal lesions (aside from hearing loss). A biopsy was obtained from the left petrous bone. The first pathologist favored a "burned-out inflammation or otitis" based on heavy fibrosis in the biopsy material. He excluded Langerhans-cell histiocytosis based on the absence of typical markers such as S 100 and CD 1A. A bone tumor reference pathologist placed special emphasis on a vascular component found in the specimens. He described "greatly dilated vascular cavities, some resembling incomplete vein walls, embedded in a fibrotic connective-tissue medullary stroma," which he interpreted as a vascular malformation. This diagnosis is fully consistent with the imaging findings. Case 32, Case 33, and Case 34 illustrate cystic angiomatosis and review the essential aspects of this disease.

Here we shall note a new aspect of angiomatosis. Recent studies by Bruder et al[33] cast doubt on the traditional view of angiomatosis as true vascular, multicentric neoplasia, because the proliferation rate is less than 1% and the endothelial cells are consistently negative for GLUT1 and only minimally positive for WT1. This suggests that at least some lesions previously classified histologically as angiomatosis comprising multiple hemangiomas are, in fact, vascular malformations (usually venous). It is difficult to distinguish between a hemangioma and vascular malformation by light microscopy. This is also consistent with our observations in 22 cases. The complex classification of vascular malformations and angiodysplasias is beyond our present scope, and detailed accounts may be found in monographs.[13,18] Pathoanatomically, we can picture the lesions as cavities in bone that contain vascular malformations. This model also explains the MRI and CT findings: the lesions are hyperintense (but not cystic!) in water-sensitive MRI sequences (see Case 33, Case 134, and Case 154) because the flow in the vessels is apparently very slow in venous and lymphatic malformations, as opposed to high-flow arteriovenous malformations. The CT appearance of the cavities is that of a focal, multicentric or confluent effacement of trabecular structures.

Since the boy was relatively free of complaints (see above), treatment that would inhibit vascular proliferation (angioneogenesis) was withheld. A year later he was free of complaints except for unilateral hearing loss.

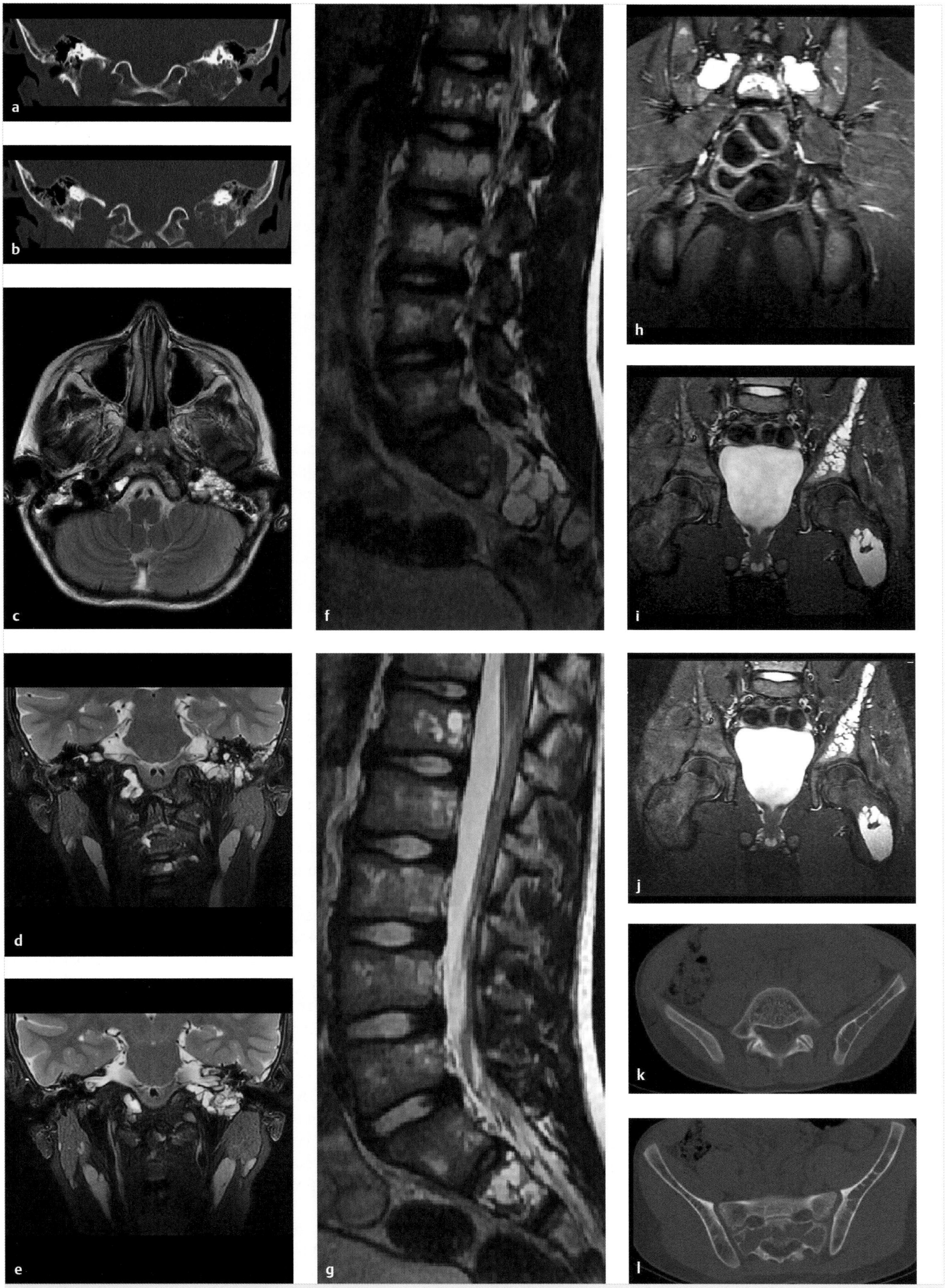

Fig. 4.17 a–o 8½ year-old boy with hearing loss: cysts in the left petrous bone?

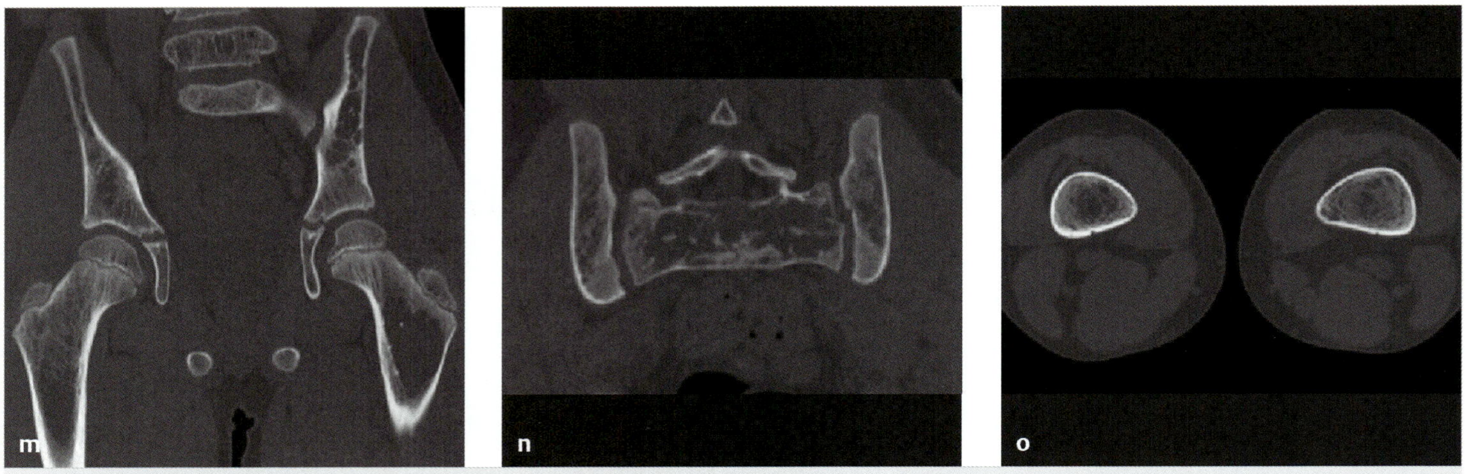

Fig. 4.17 a–o Continued.

Final Diagnosis

Cystic angiomatosis or hemangiomatosis in the form of a vascular malformation with disseminated skeletal involvement that includes the petrous bones.

Comments

Disseminated osteolytic lesions that are hyperintense in water-sensitive sequences in a young patient with no systemic symptoms may represent (hem)angiomatosis.

Case 60 (▶ Fig. 4.18)

Case description

- *Referral:* self-referred by the patient.
- *Prior history and clinical question:* A 68-year-old woman complained of nonspecific lower abdominal and lumbar pain. She was otherwise in good health, athletically active, and led a healthy lifestyle. Laboratory tests were normal. Abdominal MRI to investigate the lower abdominal complaints showed altered signal intensity in the right lateral mass of the sacrum, which had not been present on previous abdominal MRI 1 year earlier. That finding remained constant through the latest examination (▶ Fig. 4.18 **a–d**). The patient asked about the etiology and the need for biopsy.

Radiologic Findings

The T1w image in ▶ Fig. 4.18 **a** shows slight hypointensity in the posterior portion of the right lateral mass, which is hyperintense to its surroundings in the T2w image (▶ Fig. 4.18 **d**). The lesion shows moderate enhancement after contrast administration (▶ Fig. 4.18 **b, c**).

Two weeks later we ordered CT scans (▶ Fig. 4.18 **e, f**) for a more detailed bone evaluation. The scans showed negative attenuation values (up to –220 HU) in the region of the MRI abnormality. It should be added that bone scintigraphy with SPECT images in the region of interest was normal and that glucose PET-CT (^{18}F-FDG whole-body PET-CT) was negative.

Pathoanatomic Background of the Findings

Regardless of the MRI result, it is significant that CT showed fat attenuation in the lesion in the right lateral mass. This virtually excludes a solid tumor. The fatty structure is asymmetric relative to the opposite side, meaning that less cancellous bone is present in that area.

Assignment to a Possible Basic Entity

▶ **Normal variant or malformation?** No, the lesion developed during the past year.

▶ **Trauma?** The patient could not recall trauma. She does engage in gymnastics and Nordic walking, but not to excess.

▶ **Inflammation?** No clinical manifestations or laboratory markers.

▶ **Tumor?** No, the CT findings and negative PET-CT scan are not consistent with a tumor.

▶ **Necrosis?** Very likely (see below).

Synopsis and Discussion

The lesion in the right lateral mass is definitely benign for several reasons:

- It was detected incidentally.
- It was negative on ^{18}F-FDG whole-body PET-CT.
- It was negative on bone scintigraphy with SPECT.
- It is composed of fat.

The key to a correct radiologic classification of the equivocal MRI finding lies in the CT examination, which demonstrated fat or fatty structures throughout the affected area. *Fat is the radiologist's friend*, as it virtually excludes a tumor. Of course, this does not apply to lesions that contain fatty elements (e.g., some renal cell carcinomas, angiomyolipomas, etc.).

But how can we reconcile the MRI and CT findings? It is reasonable to assume that circumscribed bone marrow necrosis, or perhaps the necrosis of pre-existing focal hematopoietic hyperplasia, took place in the region of interest (see also ▶ Fig. 2.12 in Case 5). If the necrotic area is not completely deprived of a blood supply (not located in a terminal vascular bed), that would explain the contrast-enhanced findings. Saponifying processes are probably

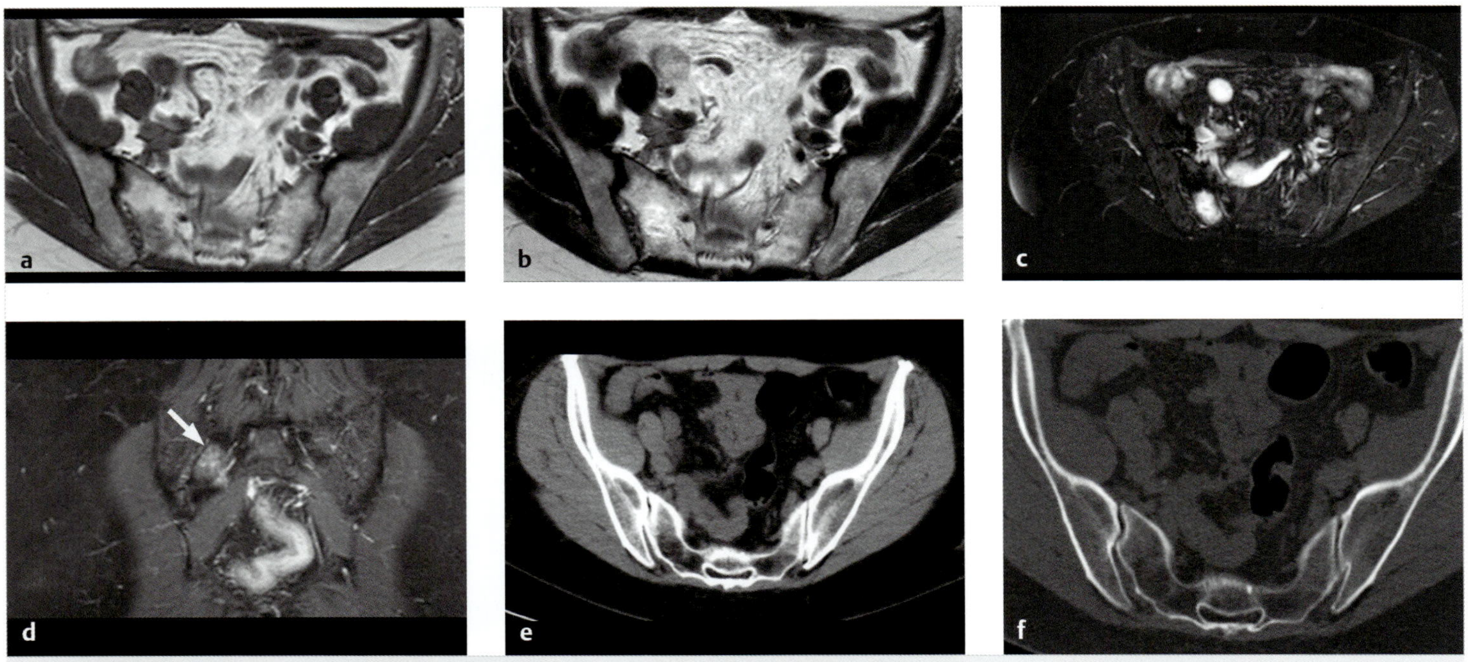

Fig. 4.18 a–f Incidental finding on abdominal CT: biopsy?

responsible for the increased signal intensity in T2w images. This could also explain the "paradoxical" finding of less fat on MRI and more fat on CT. This case also demonstrates that CT is more reliable than MRI in defining fatty tissue.

We did not see a need for biopsy confirmation. Whether the clinically silent lesion should be followed is a matter of discretion. As a postscript, the lesion was followed for more than a year at the patient's request and remained unchanged over that period.

Final Diagnosis

Circumscribed bone marrow necrosis in the right lateral mass that healed with fatty replacement.

Comments

A CT examination is essential for investigating skeletal MRI findings that are equivocal or lack a plausible explanation. If CT shows predominant fat attenuation, the equivocal MRI finding should be classified as benign.

4.3 Unusual Fractures

Case 61 (▶ Fig. 4.19)

Case description

- *Referral:* self-referred by the patient.
- *Prior history and clinical question:* The patient claimed an approximately 6-week history of low back pain radiating to the right leg. Until several years previously, he participated in competitive sports.

Radiologic Findings

Imaging shows a small osteolytic lesion with sclerotic margins in the right posterior ilium. A lucent track, which resembles a gaping fracture line, extends medially downward from the osteolytic focus to the adjacent sacroiliac joint. The joint appears normal, especially on its sacral side, in all CT sections (▶ Fig. 4.19 **a, d–f**) and on MRI (▶ Fig. 4.19 **b, c**). Caudal to the bony lesion is a circumscribed area of edema-like signal within the bone (▶ Fig. 4.19 **b, c**). MR images of the lumbar spine (not pictured here) clearly demonstrated a mediolateral disk herniation at the L5–S1 level on the right side.

Location

The changes described above are located entirely within the cancellous bone and occupy an area of the posterior pelvic ring that is subject to large physiologic loads (anterior superior corner of the ilium).

Pathoanatomic Background of the Findings

It is clear that, particularly in ▶ Fig. 4.19 **f, a** small triangular bone fragment has separated from the surrounding bone. Lateral to the fragment is a bone defect that may be interpreted as an area of resorption or destruction.

Assignment to a Possible Basic Entity

▶ **Normal variant?** No known precedent.

▶ **Trauma?** Very likely. The patient was a competitive athlete, and it would not be unusual for a stress fracture to develop in the anterior superior corner of the posterior ilium leading to necrosis and separation of a small triangular bone fragment. Accordingly, the small osteolytic focus in the coronal reformatted CT image (▶ Fig. 4.19 **a**) would represent a resorption zone lateral to the fragment seen in the magnified axial view (▶ Fig. 4.19 **f**). The marginal sclerosis suggests an older process, which would be consistent with the patient's history. The edema-like signal, lateral and caudal to the main focus, could reflect a certain instability of the bone fragment. It should not be interpreted as the cause of the pain. Many ill-defined hyperintensities in water-sensitive sequences (edema-like signal, not bone marrow edema, see Ill-Defined Hyperintensity in Chapter 1) are known to have no clinical relevance.

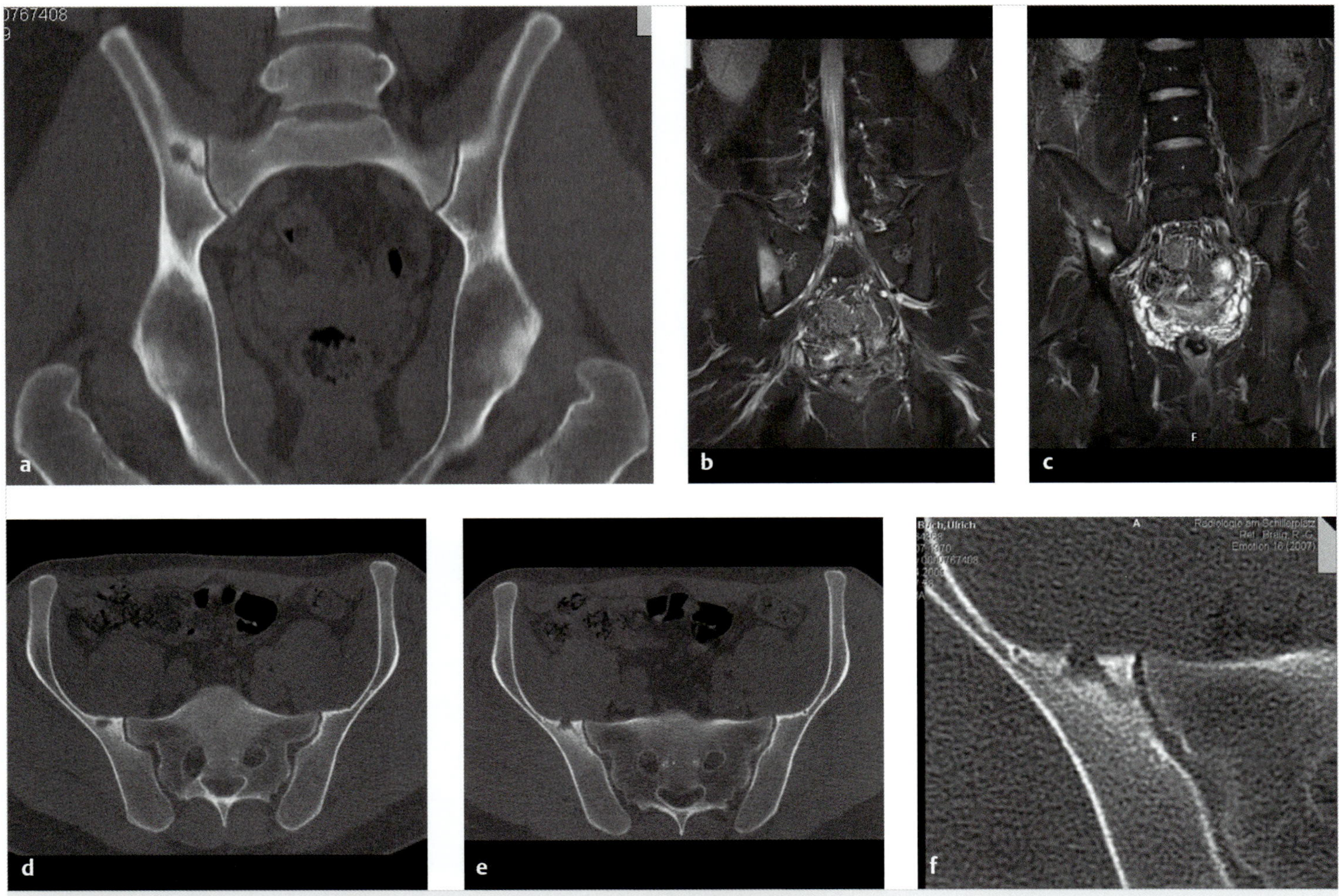

Fig. 4.19 a–f Low back pain on the right side, equivocal finding in the right ilium. Tumor?

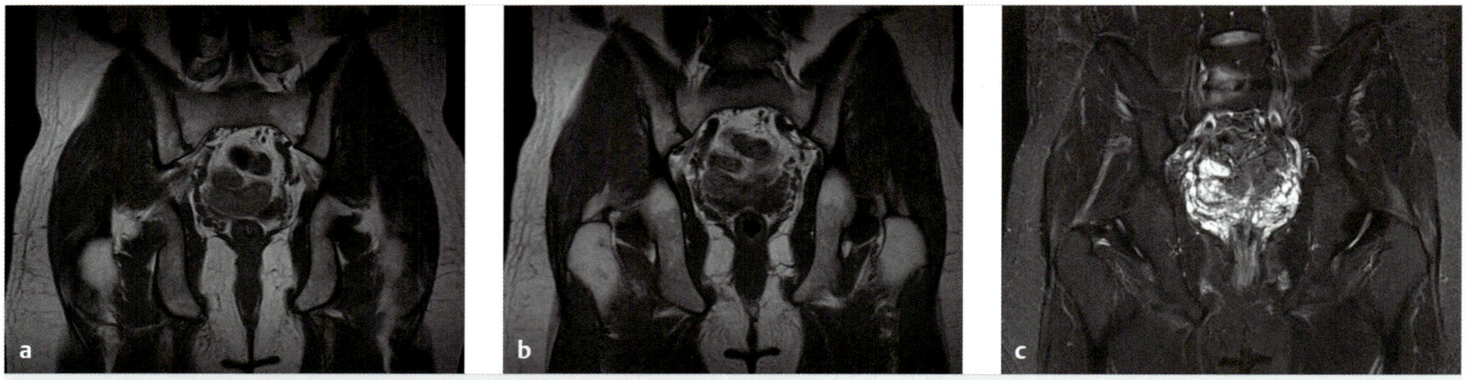

Fig. 4.20 a–c MRI follow-up of the patient in ► Fig. 4.19 at 2 years.

► **Inflammation?** No, the location at a peripheral site in the ilium of an adult would be extremely unusual.

► **Tumor?** No, it is difficult to conceive of a tumor (eosinophilic granuloma, non-Hodgkin lymphoma?) that would cause necrosis and separation of a bone fragment.

► **Necrosis?** To a degree; see under Trauma? above. To the author's knowledge, the occurrence of primary necrosis has not previously been described in this region, which is not a terminal vascular bed. The patient is not known to have any diseases or other factors (e.g., corticosteroid use) that would predispose to osteonecrosis.

Synopsis and Discussion

The osteolytic lesion is probably an incidental finding, as the 6-week pain history is more consistent with a radicular process relating to a herniated nucleus pulposus at L5–S1. When specifically questioned, the patient claimed that his symptoms resolved within days after taking a nonsteroidal anti-inflammatory drug. This also points to a radicular cause.

In summary, the history of competitive sports participation suggests a previous stress fracture that did not heal completely and caused necrosis leading to the separation of a small bone fragment. Because the marginal sclerosis appears to be of long standing (see section on Trauma? above), it is reasonable to assume an earlier onset of clinical manifestations, perhaps several years ago.

Follow-up MRI at 2 years documented complete consolidation of the stress fracture (► Fig. 4.20).

Working Diagnosis

Old, unhealed stress fracture in the anterior superior corner of the ilium.

Comments

The clinical relevance of an imaging abnormality can be determined only by considering the patient's history. In this case the patient had two radiologic findings (herniated disk plus a bony lesion of the ilium) with only one dominant clinical complaint: low back pain with radicular symptoms. The radiologist must now consider what diagnosis is congruent with these findings, aided by consultation with the referring clinician whenever possible.

Case 62 (▶ Fig. 4.21)

Case description

- *Referring physicians:* trauma surgeon and internist (endocrinologist).
- *Prior history and clinical question:* A 66-year-old woman presented with diffuse skeletal and muscle pain that rendered her unable to walk. She lived alone. An internist diagnosed hepatopathy of unknown cause. She reportedly suffered recurrent bone fractures following trivial trauma. We ordered laboratory tests which showed a greatly elevated alkaline phosphatase level.

Radiologic Findings

The plain radiographs (▶ Fig. 4.21 **a, b**) show a "butterfly" pattern of fractures in the anterior pelvic ring with progressive displacement from May to December of 2009 and associated callus formation that is exuberant for the age of the patient. The bones of the posterior pelvic ring show structural alterations that CT (abdominal examination in May, 2009) identifies as large fracture gaps with surrounding reactive-reparative sclerosis in the sacrum (▶ Fig. 4.21 **d–f, h–k**). The images in ▶ Fig. 4.21 **g–i** demonstrate a fracture of the right pubic ramus; highly structured ossifications are projected anterior and lateral to the fracture site (see also ▶ Fig. 4.21 **l**). A radiograph of the right foot taken in May of 2009 (▶ Fig. 4.21 **c**) shows a broad, incomplete fracture at the base of the fifth metatarsal. Axial CT scans of the bony thorax (▶ Fig. 4.21 **m, n**) show rib fractures that are unhealed despite callus formation. CT scans of the spine (not pictured here) did not show spinal fractures.

Location

The principal fractures are located in the anterior *and* posterior pelvic ring and at the anterior and posterior bends of the rib cage.

Pathoanatomic Background of the Findings

Unhealed fractures in skeletal regions exposed to large mechanical loads (anterior and posterior pelvic ring, bends of the rib cage, base of the fifth metatarsal) in patients without a significant trauma history are always suspicious for insufficiency fractures, or fractures occurring in structurally weakened bone as in osteomalacia. The ossifications about the right pubic fracture may be heterotopic ossifications due to hemorrhage.

Assignment to a Possible Basic Entity

▶ **Trauma?** No.

▶ **Systemic disease?** Yes. The main possibilities are osteoporosis, osteomalacia, hyperparathyroidism, and fibrogenesis imperfecta ossium.

Synopsis and Discussion

We may rule out *osteoporosis* as the principal cause of the multiple fractures, because the patient had no fractures at sites that are typical for age-related osteoporotic fractures (the spine).

Fibrogenesis imperfecta ossium is a generalized bone disease with an acquired defect of collagen synthesis in the bone, probably with an enzymatic basis. This disease affects only the collagen fibers of lamellar bone. As in osteomalacia, patients suffer from increasing bone pain and fractures. The bone becomes radiologically denser due to widening and thickening of the blurred trabecular structure, and lucencies may be found among the denser areas. The result is an overall patchy appearance, which is not seen in the present case. Patients often suffer from spinal fractures. Ultimately the diagnosis can be established only by microscopic examination in polarized light. The alkaline phosphatase level may be elevated while other laboratory values are normal.

A diagnosis of *primary hyperparathyroidism* is not consistent with the radiologic findings (no subperiosteal resorption in the tubular bones of the foot, no brown tumors) or the clinical presentation (no cognitive impairment, cardiac arrhythmia, mental status change, or elevated serum calcium or parathormone levels).

The only realistic diagnosis is *osteomalacia*, which is supported by the following findings:

- Insufficiency fractures, which in this case may be called Looser zones or pseudofractures and are distinguished by bilaterally symmetrical fracture lines of variable width, often with abundant but undifferentiated callus. Histologically they are incompletely consolidated fractures that are united by unmineralized or slightly mineralized osteoid and connective tissue. The insufficiency fractures in osteomalacia typically show a bilateral symmetrical distribution in the anterior, lateral, and posterior (more heavily stressed) bends of the ribs, in the anterior and posterior pelvic ring, and in the metatarsals.
- The life situation of the patient. The patient is an elderly woman who lives alone, is rarely exposed to sunlight, and has poor nutrition, especially with regard to vitamin D and calcium. Osteomalacia may exacerbate pre-existing senile osteopenia or osteoporosis, but we do not consider this to be the main cause of the severe fractures.
- Pseudotumor development at the site of the pubic fracture caused by hemorrhage and heterotopic ossification. We have seen many such cases in recent years that were managed surgically due to lack of awareness of the possible cause, namely a systemic bone disease.
- The low serum level of vitamin D and the elevated alkaline phosphatase level.

Regarding the mechanism of insufficiency fractures in the pubis, it should be noted that insufficiency fractures usually develop first in the posterior pelvic ring (sacrum and/or ilium). The resulting instability in the posterior pelvic ring places greater stresses on the anterior pelvic ring, allowing insufficiency fractures to develop in the already weakened bone. Insufficiency fractures of the posterior pelvic ring are characterized on bone

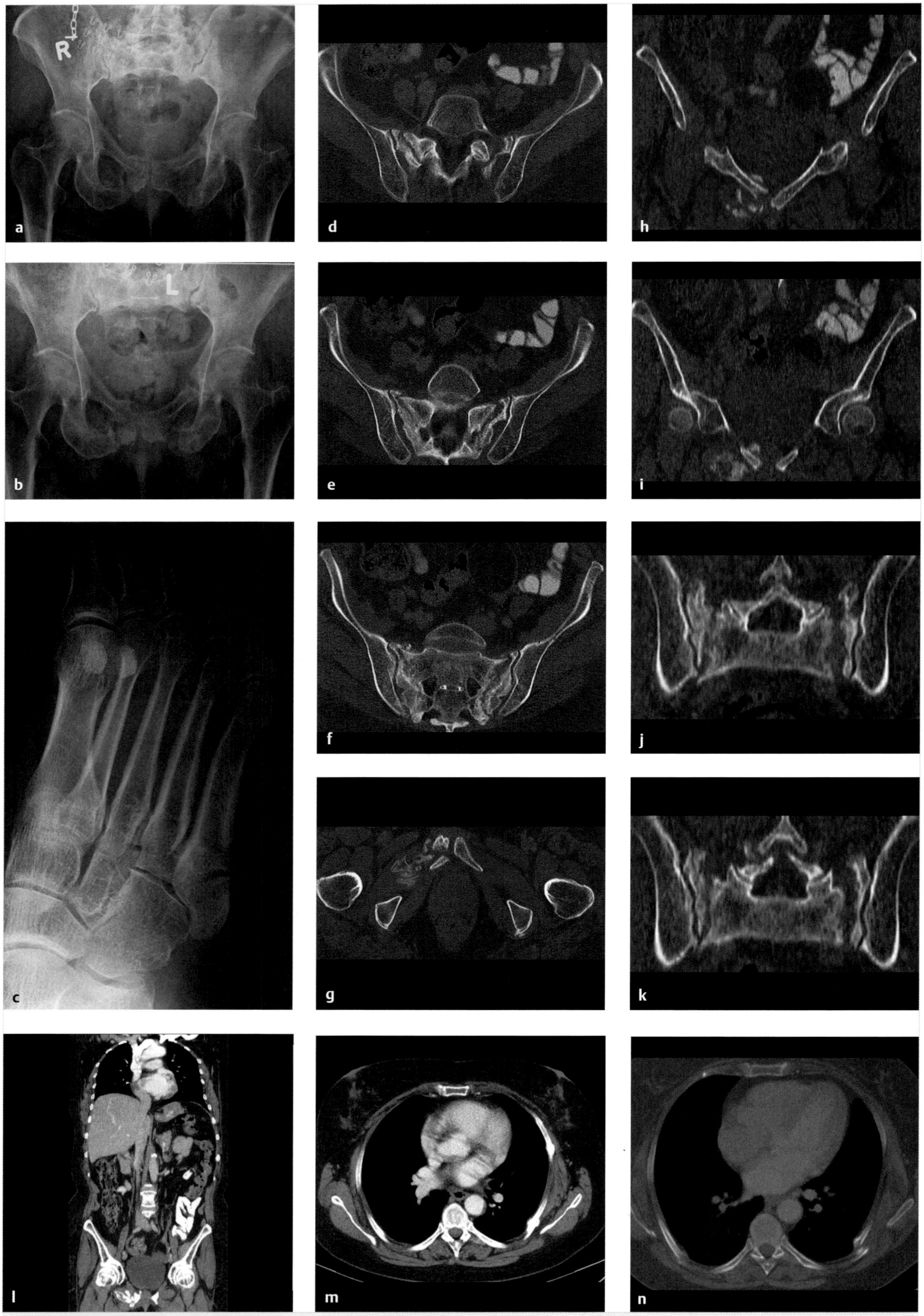

Fig. 4.21 a–n Recurrent bone fractures.

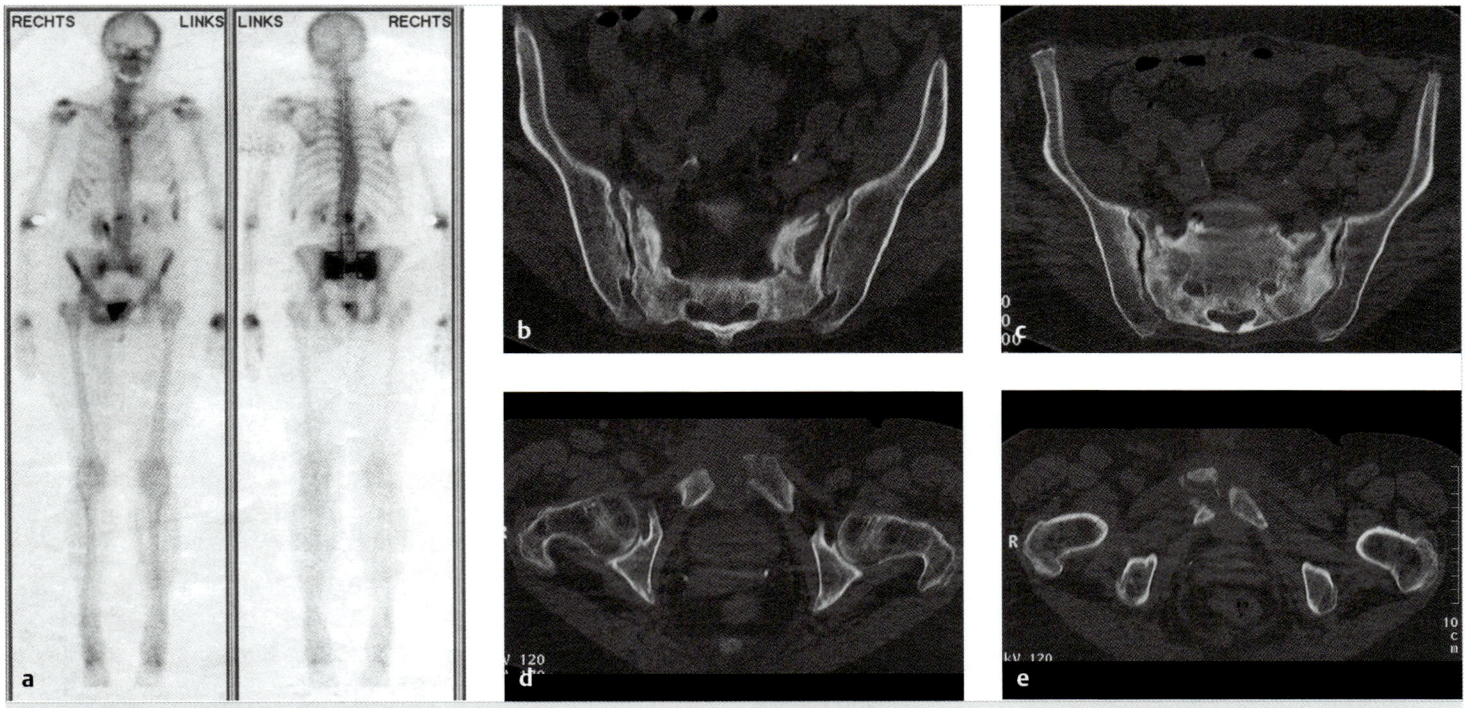

Fig. 4.22 a–e "Honda sign" in an elderly woman.

scintigraphy by intense bilateral uptake in the posterior pelvic ring, called the "Honda sign" (▶ Fig. 4.22).

The patient was placed on vitamin D and calcium replacement therapy, and shortly thereafter her skeletal and muscle pain resolved and the numerous fractures consolidated.

▶ Fig. 4.22 illustrates the case of another elderly woman who lived in a poorly managed nursing home and developed severe osteomalacia with insufficiency fractures of the anterior and posterior pelvic ring. The bone scan in this case showed high uptake in the anterior and posterior pelvic ring with a positive Honda sign. This finding plus the prior history of severe, diffuse bone and muscle pain made the case easy to diagnose. Subsequent CT scans were obtained mainly to document the fracture lines and degree of displacement.

▶ Fig. 4.23 shows the case of a 45-year-old woman with very severe osteoporosis and osteomalacia and associated insufficiency fractures in the posterior pelvic ring, left iliac wing, and anterior pelvic ring. The patient had a 15-year history of rheumatoid arthritis and had been taking 75 mg of prednisolone daily for 8 years. She underwent a total right hip replacement for avascular necrosis of the femoral head and a femoral neck fracture after a fall. The incipient insufficiency fractures were considered trauma-related and the patient was released to the care of her family doctor. Later she was readmitted for excruciating skeletal pain, predominantly in the pelvis. The patient was unable to walk. Her alkaline phosphatase level was elevated to several times normal, and her 25-hydroxyvitamin D_3 level was very low. With suitable replacement therapy, her complaints quickly improved and the fractures healed. The unusual gross insufficiency fracture in the left iliac wing probably occurred at a structural weak point in the iliac wing, that is, at a relatively large, oblique intraosseous vascular channel that occurs physiologically in that area.

Final Diagnosis

Osteomalacia with severe insufficiency fractures in the anterior and posterior pelvic ring and a pseudotumor in the right groin.

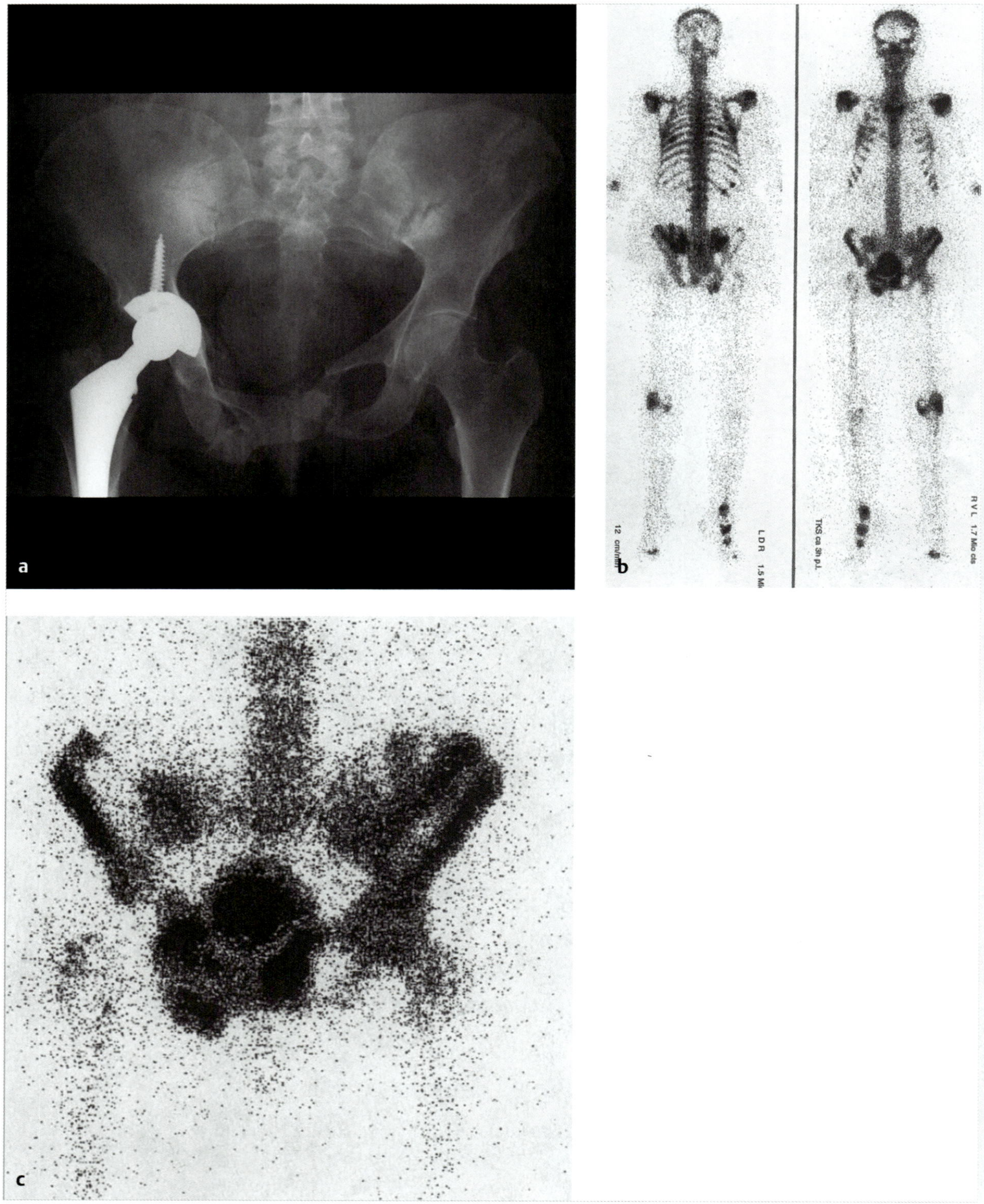

Fig. 4.23 a–c Pelvic insufficiency fractures in a 45-year-old woman.

Comments

The differential diagnosis of diffuse skeletal and muscle pain in older women with a recent fracture history should always include osteomalacia or an osteomalacic component of osteoporosis.

Case 63 (▶ Fig. 4.24)

Case description

- *Referral:* father of the patient.
- *Prior history and clinical question:* A 25-year-old man had an approximately 3-week history of pain, swelling, and local warmth in his left groin. He reported a previous episode of very severe pain that occurred while he was playing soccer. He stated that he was an avid soccer player, and that in the past 6 months he had experienced repeated attacks of left groin pain when kicking into the air. MRI of the left groin (▶ Fig. 4.24) was inconclusive, and a tumor was included in the differential diagnosis (due to intense enhancement). An excisional biopsy was proposed. The concerned father requested a consult.

Radiologic Findings

The MR images in ▶ Fig. 4.24 show an intensely enhancing mass in the left groin with rounded hypointense structures at its center.

Location

The lesion demonstrated by MRI is located in the region of the anterior inferior iliac spine.

Pathoanatomic Background of the Findings

The intense enhancement of the mass in the left groin indicates a rich blood supply. The tapered proximal and distal "extensions" of high signal intensity and the medial margin outlining the iliopsoas contour suggest a former fluid origin. The central hypointensities *may* be ossifications.

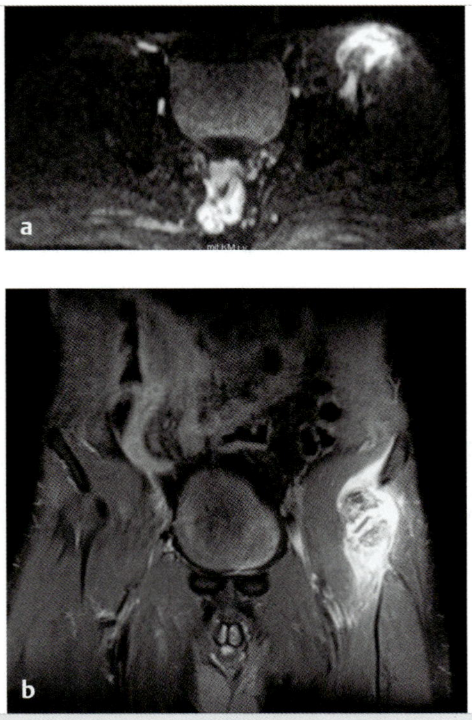

Fig. 4.24 a, b Soccer player with a tumor in the left groin?

Assignment to a Possible Basic Entity

▶ **Trauma?** Yes, because the patient is an amateur soccer player and often misses the ball when kicking. It should be noted that this action of "kicking into the air" may lead to avulsion trauma or true avulsion fractures of the anterior inferior iliac spine. CT scans should be obtained for further investigation and documentation. The scans that we ordered (▶ Fig. 4.25 **a, b**) show the classic features of a shallow avulsion fracture of the anterior inferior spine.

▶ **Tumor?** No, because the medial margin of the lesion, its oblong shape, and its sharply tapered poles are not consistent with a tumor. Tumors tend to develop in a concentric pattern and do not necessarily follow fascial planes, as blood would typically do.

Synopsis and Discussion

This case is actually classic when the imaging findings are interpreted within the context of the history and clinical presentation. It is unnecessary to proceed with biopsy, which might even lead an inexperienced pathologist to diagnose osteosarcoma based on the presence of immature fibroblastic tissue with frequent mitoses, slight nuclear irregularities at the center, and osteoid formation in the intermediate zone of the lesion.

An avulsion fracture is defined as a structural failure of the bone at the attachment of a tendon or aponeurosis in response to forcible traction. The injury may be caused by a single, massive traction event or by multiple repetitive events. Generally there is considerable deep tissue bleeding, which may lead to heterotopic ossification or myositis ossificans (for details on pathogenesis see Case 29, Case 30, and Case 156). With repetitive trauma, this process is often multicentric and may be encountered in various stages of maturity. Accordingly, the imaging spectrum ranges from highly vascularized soft tissue to fully mature bone, as in the present case. The peripheral ossifications are always more solid and mature than the central myositis ossificans. Between them is an intermediate zone. The result is an overall trizonal structure, which incidentally is reversed in periosteal osteosarcoma (which has a solid, heavily ossified base and a periphery com-

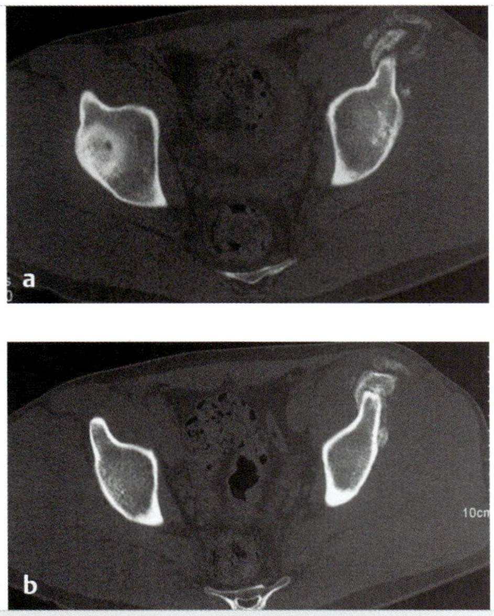

Fig. 4.25 a, b CT scans supplement the images in ▶ Fig. 4.24.

posed of nonossified osteoid). In soccer players, especially adolescents, the anterior inferior iliac spine is second only to the ischial tuberosity as a site of predilection for fracture-separations and avulsion fractures. It provides attachment for the rectus femoris muscle.

Final Diagnosis

Metachronous avulsion fracture of the anterior inferior iliac spine with the development of traumatic myositis ossificans.

Comments

Cases with equivocal MRI findings close to a muscular attachment should be investigated further by CT, which allows the simple, unequivocal detection of an avulsion fracture.

Case 64 (▶ Fig. 4.26)

Case description

- Referring physician: pathologist.
- Prior history and clinical question: Six months previously a 16-year-old boy experienced sudden pain in the left ischium during a "casual" soccer game, accompanied by intermittent numbness at the back of the left thigh and lower leg. Clinical examination showed no palpable abnormalities in the pelvic region. The patient had a normal gait and no neurologic abnormalities. He had a history of anorexia nervosa. The radiologic findings raised suspicion of myositis ossificans, and the differential diagnosis included paraosseous osteosarcoma. This prompted a wide biopsy, but the reference pathologist found no traces of myositis ossificans or paraosseous osteosarcoma in the specimens. As an experienced bone pathologist he suspected the correct diagnosis and requested a radiology consult for confirmation.

Radiologic Findings

The plain radiographs (▶ Fig. 4.26 **a, b**) show a bony figure capped by two peripheral, crescent-shaped ossifications located below and slightly to the left ischial tuberosity. The adjacent ischium bears a wide defect (relative to the opposite side) that is congruent with the larger, proximal bony figure. Other bony contours and structures appear normal, aside from the fact that the epiphyseal and apophyseal plates have not yet closed. This is still normal for a 16-year-old but somewhat unusual. The MR images in ▶ Fig. 4.26 **c–j** (T1w TSE SENSE) show definite edema-like signal in the muscles surrounding the bony figures and in the ischium.

Location

The ossifications are in close proximity to the former apophysis of the ischium. The largest, proximal ossification is congruent with an adjacent defect in the ischium.

Pathoanatomic Background of the Findings

The normal trabecular structure, most apparent in the larger ossified figure, and the close relationship of the ossified figure to the ischial defect (described under Location) would suggest a bony avulsion fracture.

Assignment to a Possible Basic Entity

▶ **Normal variant or malformation?** Apophyseal plate closure may be extremely variable, especially in the pubis and ischium,[17] and the long persistence of apophyses is not uncommon (see details below).

▶ **Trauma?** Yes, the history shows a definite temporal relationship between soccer trauma and the onset of pain. Given the relationship described under Pathoanatomic Background of the Findings, it is logical to classify at least the larger ossifications as an avulsion fracture of the ischial tuberosity, which is a severe avulsion injury. The crescent-shaped bony figures distal to it are discussed under Synopsis and Discussion below.

▶ **Tumor or tumorlike lesion?** Because the ossifications correspond to anatomic structures and, as detailed below, the ischial tuberosity is the most common site of pelvic avulsion fractures in adolescents, it would be unreasonable to consider a neoplastic process such as paraosseous osteosarcoma. If myositis ossificans is considered a type of tumorlike bone lesion, it is conceivable, and consistent with the trauma history, that histology might show corresponding findings in and around the lesions.

Synopsis and Discussion

Based on the discussions above, it is reasonable to conclude that the images depict an avulsion fracture of the ischial tuberosity. Arguments in favor of this diagnosis:

- There is a definite temporal relationship between soccer trauma and clinical manifestations.
- According to studies by Rossi and Dragoni,[36] the ischial tuberosity is the most common site for avulsion fractures of the pelvis in adolescent athletes. Avulsions at the attachments of the following muscles are particularly common in soccer (running and kicking) and sprinting:
  - Adductor magnus
  - Quadriceps femoris
  - Semimembranosus
  - Semitendinosus
  - Long head of biceps femoris
- The largest of the three bony figures "fits" into the defect in the tuberosity; theoretically it could be pushed back into the defect.
- The bony figures have cancellous trabeculae, proving that they are not amorphous ossifications composed of tumor osteoid.

The crescent-shaped bony figures distal to the largest fragment may represent earlier metachronous avulsions or a variant or abnormal ossification that has been displaced by avulsion of the large fragment. Abnormal ossification is supported by a history of anorexia nervosa, which can interfere with normal bone development. The open growth plates in this 16-year-old would be a further argument, though it should be added that ossification and adaptation processes in the pelvic apophyses are subject to considerable variation. Viewed in its entirety, the case can be explained purely on the basis of radiologic findings; there is no need for biopsy. The pathologist was able to exclude myositis ossificans.

Perhaps the treating physicians were misled by the confusing MRI findings. A CT examination should have been ordered to provide a better spatial understanding of the anatomic relationships and a more accurate evaluation of the bony (trabecular) structures. On the other hand, a careful interpretation of the radiograph in this case would have led to a correct interpretation of the MRI findings.

Final Diagnosis

Avulsion fracture of the ischial tuberosity.

Comments

Equivocal musculoskeletal findings on MRI in young patients can be clarified by supplementary CT, or at least by plain radiographs, to help avoid unnecessary biopsies and reduce the anxiety of patients and their parents.

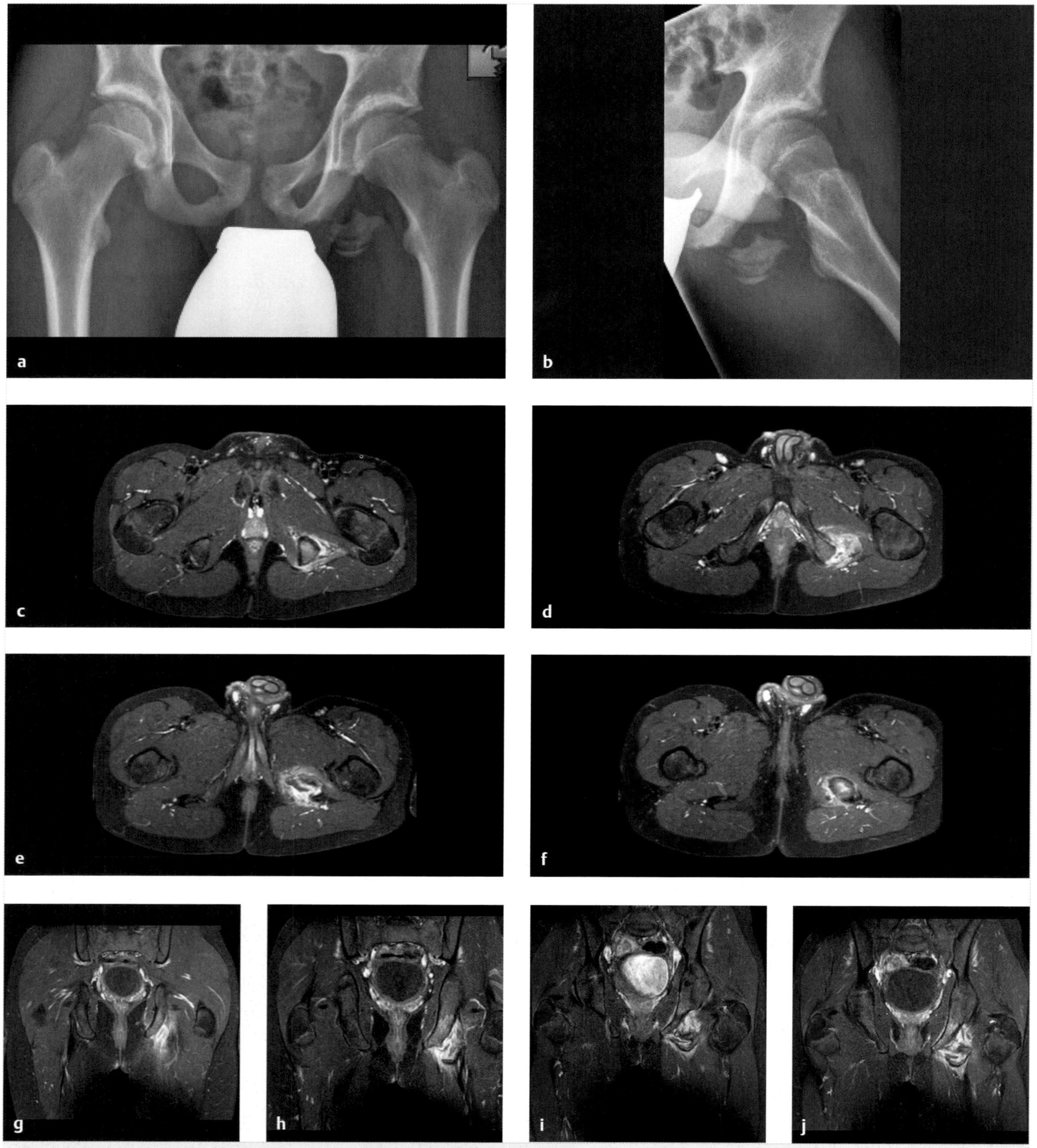

Fig. 4.26 a–j Soccer player with a tumor in the left ischium?

4.4 Bone Lesions with a Predominantly Extraosseous Component

Case 65 (▶ Fig. 4.27)

Case description

- Referring physician: orthopedist.
- Prior history and clinical question: A 29-year-old man presented with rapidly increasing pain and swelling in the right gluteal region.

Radiologic Findings

CT demonstrates a broad-based ossified lesion on the right ilium that communicates directly with the medullary cavity with no intervening cortex (▶ Fig. 4.27 **b**). The attenuation values inside the lesion are like those in the adjacent medullary cavity (▶ Fig. 4.27 **b, f**). The lesion is surrounded peripherally by a grotesque soft-tissue mass that is inhomogeneously dense on CT and less dense on average than the muscles (▶ Fig. 4.27 **c–f**). Scattered calcifications are visible within the mass (arrows in ▶ Fig. 4.27 **d**). MRI (▶ Fig. 4.27 **a**, T2w fat-suppressed image) shows a fine linear hyperintensity that directly abuts the ossified mass. The large mass is hypointense to muscle and is encircled by an irregular, hyperintense rim of nonuniform thickness.

Location

The ossified lesion on the ilium is in direct contact with the medullary cavity of the underlying bone, that is, the medullary cavities of the exostotic lesion and the ilium communicate with each other.

Pathoanatomic Background of the Findings

It is not difficult to describe the lesion on the ilium as an exostosis. Because the medullary cavities of the "parent" bone and exostosis communicate with each other and the exostosis is bordered by a thin film of hyperintense material that is isointense to cartilage, we are dealing with a cartilaginous exostosis (osteochondroma). By its volume alone, the surrounding grotesque soft-tissue mass appears to be sarcomatous tissue that is rimmed by hyperintense tumor cartilage. But is this necessarily true?

Assignment to a Possible Basic Entity

▶ **Trauma?** Perhaps there was some kind of crush injury to the hard exostosis that caused bleeding into the gluteal muscles. The patient did not report this type of injury, however, and we would expect to find cavities with fluid levels in a large intramuscular hemorrhage.

▶ **Inflammation?** This question can relate only to the large mass, and chronic trauma might be considered as a cause. But then the patient would have had much more dramatic symptoms, and a mass of this size would show some degree of necrosis and liquefaction.

▶ **Tumor?** Yes, the very size of the lesion suggests a malignant cartilaginous tumor, in this case an exostotic chondrosarcoma.

Synopsis and Discussion

The above arguments strongly support a diagnosis of exostotic chondrosarcoma that has developed from a cartilaginous exostosis. Now, there are large cartilaginous exostoses that are inherently benign. What are the differentiating criteria? The following

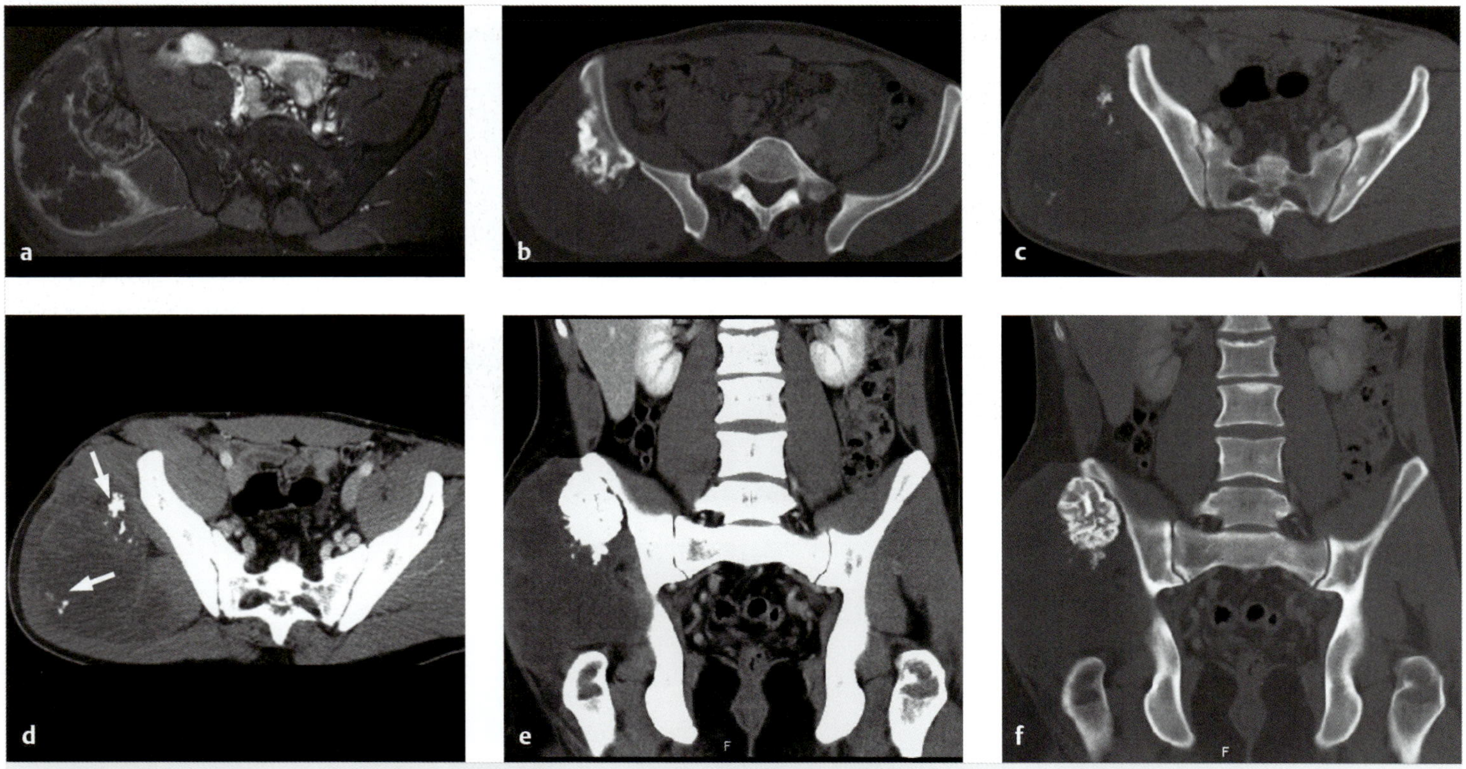

Fig. 4.27 a–f Palpable mass in the right gluteal region.

findings and arguments indicate a high probability of chondrosarcoma[18]:

- Mature exostosis with enchondral ossification topped by thick cartilaginous structures. If the cartilage cap is thicker than 3 cm, the probability of chondrosarcoma is high and the tumor should be surgically removed. If the cartilage cap is 2 cm or less in thickness, the tumor may be left alone and followed, although we recommend prophylactic removal in patients under 40 years of age. In our case the thick cartilage cap, which was certainly pre-existing, has been destroyed by the sarcomatous tissue, leaving only a thin cartilage film on the ossified exostosis (▶ Fig. 4.27 **a**) and a peripheral cartilage film bordering the hypointense mass. Perhaps the sarcomatous tissue split apart the previously homogeneous cartilage mass, displacing the peripheral portions outward.
- Small, irregular ossifications of tumor cartilage located in a cartilaginous or fibrous mass distant from the ossified base (▶ Fig. 4.27 **d**).
- Lesion located in or near the trunk.
- A recent history of tumor enlargement accompanied by pain. In rare cases these symptoms may also be caused by bursitis over the lesion.
- If the patient has hereditary osteochondromatosis, there is an increased risk of developing a chondrosarcoma in one of the exostoses (5–7% of all patients with a cartilaginous exostotic disease develop chondrosarcoma). This does not apply in our case.

▶ Fig. 4.28 **a–g** shows a (benign) cartilaginous exostosis or osteochondroma, also located on the iliac wing (25-year-old woman with occasional right gluteal pain). The exostosis is attached to the ilium by a narrow base that communicates directly with the medullary cavity of the iliac wing with no interposed cortex (▶ Fig. 4.28 **b**). Thus the tumor is defined. The head of the exostosis is covered by a thin layer of tumor cartilage, as demonstrated by MRI (▶ Fig. 4.28 **c, f, g**). This cartilage cap is only a few millimeters thick. We attribute the increased density in the subcutaneous fat (▶ Fig. 4.28 **e**) to a kind of sustained compression. Sometimes a bursa develops over the head of the exostosis and may become inflamed. The bursitis cannot always be identified as such on MRI, and ultrasound is better for this purpose.

Final Diagnosis

Large exostotic chondrosarcoma on the right iliac wing.

Comments

Unusually large tumors, especially of cartilaginous origin, are always suspicious for chondrosarcoma. But other definite criteria are available for making a radiologic diagnosis of exostotic chondrosarcoma.

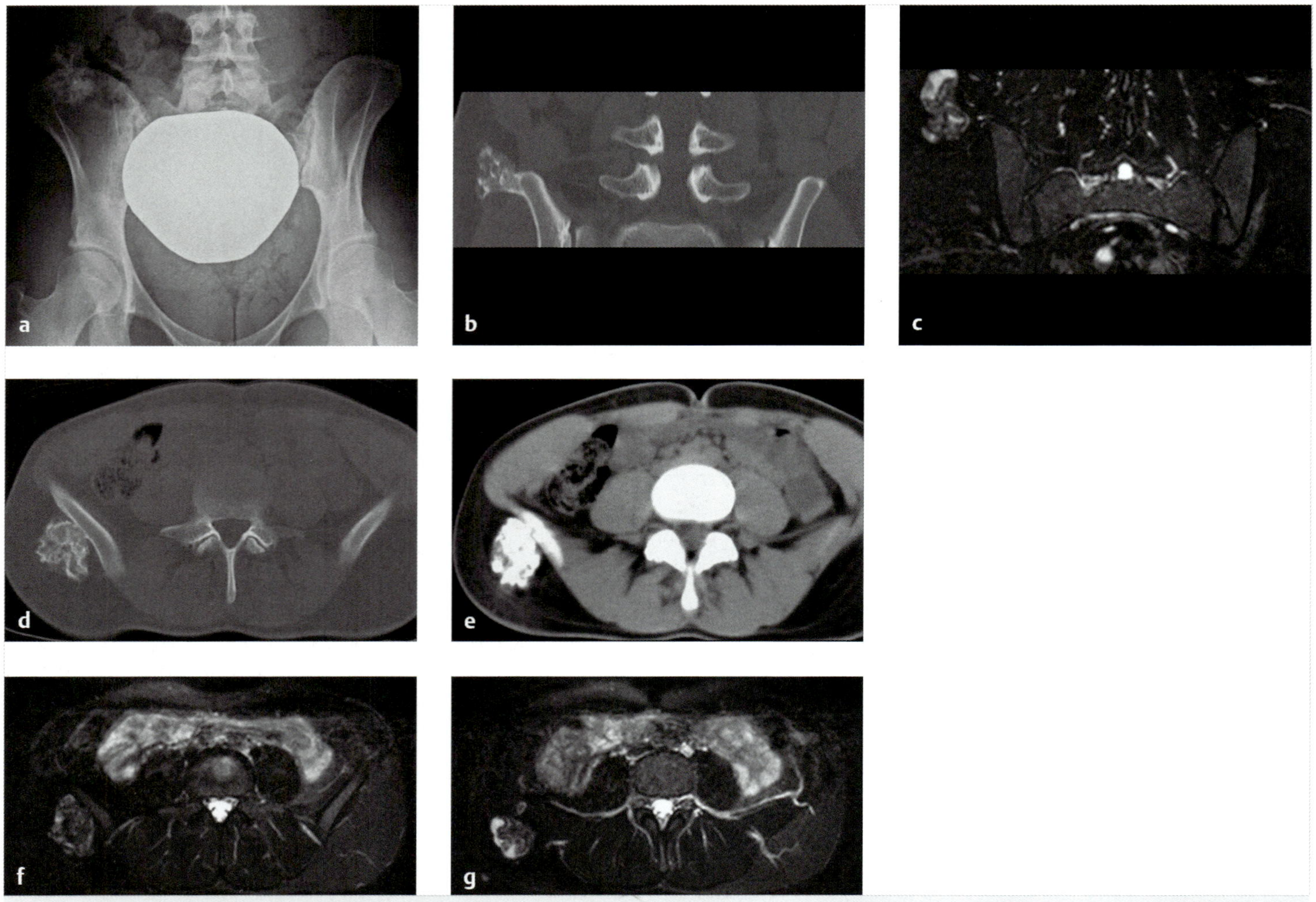

Fig. 4.28 a–g Osteochondroma in a 25-year-old woman.

4.5 Soft-Tissue Mineralization

Case 66 (▶ Fig. 4.29)

Case description

- Referring physician: nephrologist.
- Prior history and clinical question: This patient, already on long-term dialysis, was 24 years old when the images shown here (▶ Fig. 4.29) were obtained. His hyperphosphatemia due to chronic renal failure had not been treated for reasons not detailed here. The patient recently developed swellings about the shoulder, hip, and several metacarpophalangeal joints. The nephrologist wanted to know the cause of the joint swellings.

Radiologic Findings

Radiographs show extensive mineralized masses of calcific density ("calcifications") about the hip joints, especially on the right side (▶ Fig. 4.29 **a**), on the ulnar side of the right fourth metacarpophalangeal joint (▶ Fig. 4.29 **b**), and above the olecranon (▶ Fig. 4.29 **c**). There were also grotesque calcifications about the shoulder joints (not pictured here). Coarsening of the trabeculae is noted in the bones of the hand, and the bony margins of the terminal tufts are ill defined (▶ Fig. 4.29 **b**).

Location

The "calcified" conglomerates are located in juxta-articular soft tissues, especially the bursae.

Pathoanatomic Background of the Findings

Given the prior history and the findings in the hand skeleton, the "calcifications" may be interpreted as metastatic calcifications due to the precipitation of calcium phosphate and calcium carbonate or oxalate. When the calcium phosphate product is greater than 70, precipitation occurs in the soft tissues, most notably about the joints and blood vessels. This is most commonly observed in renal osteopathy and hypervitaminosis D.

Assignment to a Possible Basic Entity

The fact that the patient is on long-term dialysis and is having problems with his phosphate metabolism narrows the differential diagnosis to one of the possible basic entities (such as normal variant, trauma, inflammation, or tumor) and focuses our attention on his metabolic problem.

Synopsis and Discussion

Localization of the tumorlike calcifications to periarticular soft-tissue structures, especially the bursae, facilitates the diagnosis of soft-tissue calcifications in a setting of *renal osteopathy*, which is also confirmed by the radiograph of the hand (coarsened trabecular pattern, subperiosteal resorption, cortical striation and terminal tuft resorption due to osteomalacia and secondary hyperparathyroidism). These calcifications typically occur at interstitial sites in the vessel walls, in cartilage, and in periarticular soft tissues. The images in ▶ Fig. 4.29 **a–c** reflect one stage of the process; later images showed grotesque enlargement and thickening of the calcifications. The calcifications completely disappeared within 1 year following renal transplantation and parathyroidectomy.

From a clinical standpoint, the differential diagnosis should also include unusual amyloid deposition but the patient had no radiologic signs of β 2-microglobulinemia (erosive destructive changes in the carpus).

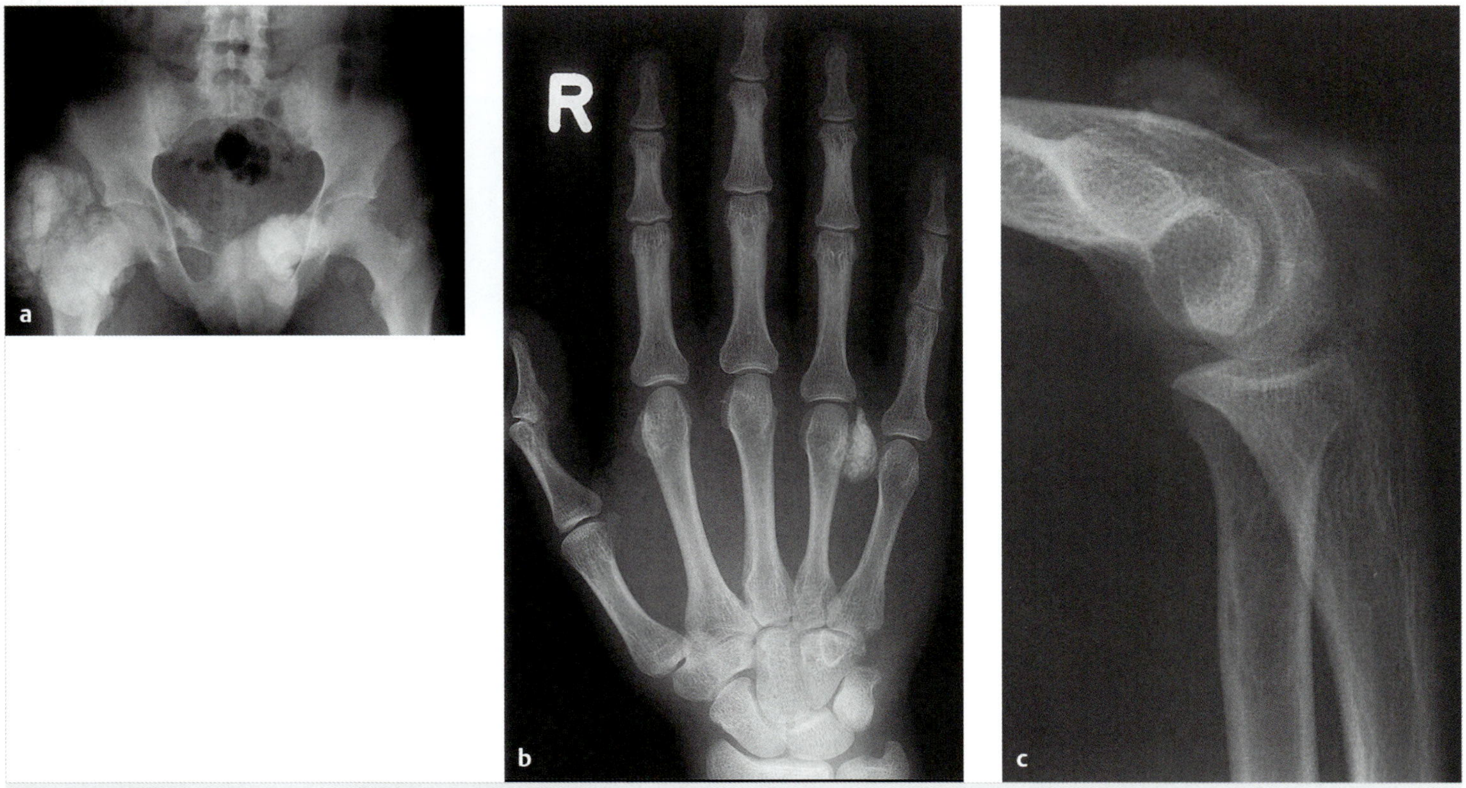

Fig. 4.29 a–c Unexplained joint swellings in a dialysis patient.

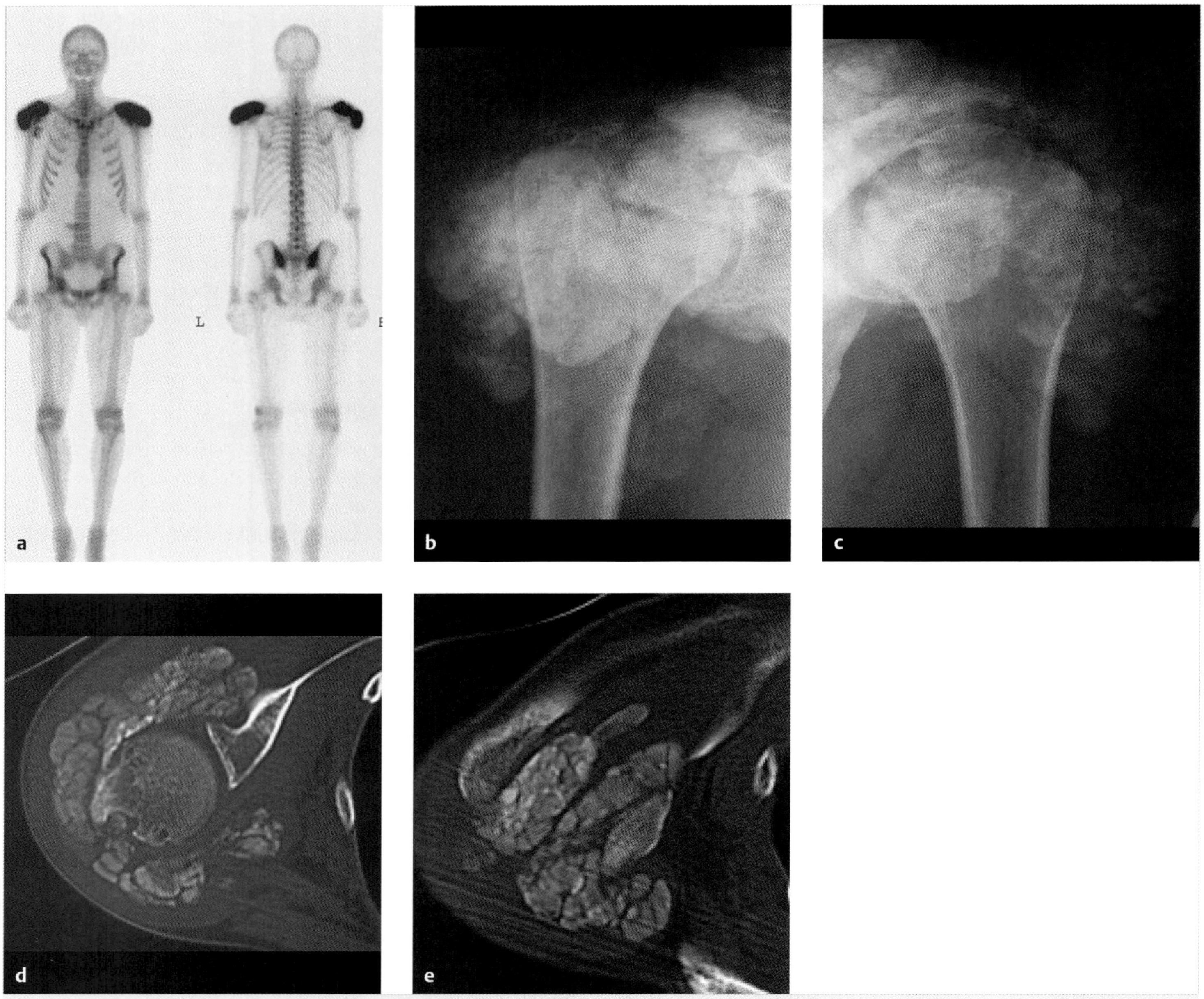

Fig. 4.30 a–e Soft-tissue calcifications in a patient with renal osteodystrophy.

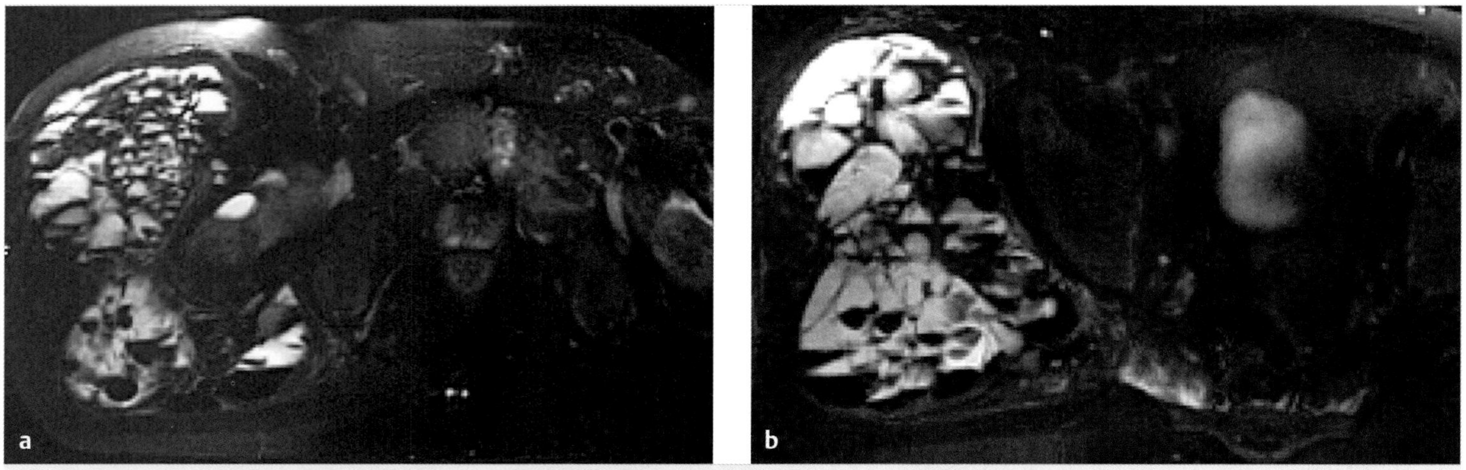

Fig. 4.31 a, b MRI of the right hip in a 31-year-old man on long-term dialysis.

The tumorlike calcinosis shown here should not be confused with tumoral calcinosis or, more precisely, *pseudotumoral calcinosis*, which is a hereditary disease.

▶ Fig. 4.30 shows a bone scan, radiographs, and CT scans from a 33-year-old man with grotesque soft-tissue calcifications in the shoulder region, who had been on dialysis for 12 years and had significant renal osteopathy. The areas of increased uptake in the shoulders resemble the epaulettes of a military uniform or the shoulder pads of a football player.

The calcifications may also produce sedimentation effects, as shown by MR images in a 31-year-old man on long-term dialysis (► Fig. 4.31). This patient also had extensive renal osteopathy.

Final Diagnosis

Tumorlike periarticular soft-tissue calcifications in renal osteopathy.

Comments

Periarticular, tumorlike, soft-tissue calcifications in dialysis patients generally indicate hyperphosphatemia in renal osteopathy or hypervitaminosis D.

4.6 Hip Region

Case 67 (▶ Fig. 4.32)

Case description

- Referring physician: rheumatologist.
- Prior history and clinical question: A 31-year-old woman complained of pain in the metacarpophalangeal joints, knees, and hips. She had been diagnosed 11 years earlier with status post-Perthes disease and treated surgically, but no further information was available on this condition. She gave no history of health problems in childhood or puberty. The metacarpophalangeal joint pain raised suspicion of hemochromatosis, but the referring rheumatologist excluded that disease based on normal iron metabolism markers and genetic testing. Rheumatoid serology and inflammatory markers were normal.

Radiologic Findings

The femoral heads appear flattened and the femoral necks shortened. Due to the flattened shape of the femoral heads, the acetabula are relatively shallow and do not form a normal, medially convex curve (▶ Fig. 4.32 **a**). The joint spaces show central narrowing on both sides. An osteophyte is noted on the right femoral head, and the left femoral head shows subchondral, cystlike lucencies. The heads of the metacarpals (▶ Fig. 4.32 **b**) are consistently flattened, similar to the femoral heads. Sclerotic foci and small rounded lucencies are noted, especially in the second and third metacarpals of the right hand. The metacarpophalangeal joint spaces are of normal width, and the opposing joint contours of the proximal phalanges appear normal. All other articular structures, including the carpal joints, also appear normal.

Location

The pathologic findings are concentrated on the epiphyses.

Pathoanatomic Background of the Findings

The flattening and structural irregularities of the femoral and metacarpal heads suggest a congenital growth disturbance of the epiphyses.

Assignment to a Possible Basic Entity

▶ **Normal variant or malformation?** Yes. This is supported by the multiple sites of occurrence of anatomically deformed epiphyses (epiphyseal dysplasia).

▶ **Perfusion defect with necrosis?** This question is appropriate with regard to the hip joints. But if we place the hip and metacarpal deformities under one heading (osteonecrosis), as it is tempting to do, it would be difficult to imagine multiple osteonecrotic foci in all the metacarpal heads.

Synopsis and Discussion

In retrospect, the diagnosis of status post-Perthes disease made 10 years ago at a different institution is not reasonable because it is not consistent with the radiologic findings in the metatarsal heads 10 years later. The late sequelae of avascular necrosis of the femoral heads in childhood may have imaging features similar to epiphyseal dysplasia (flattened heads, shallow acetabula, subchondral structural changes), but generally the clinical history would show evidence of long-term pain. Moreover, Perthes disease is very rare in girls.

Viewed in themselves, the deformities of the metatarsal heads might well be attributed to hemochromatosis (see ▶ Fig. 7.45 **d** in Case 155). But the following arguments do not support hemochromatosis as the cause of the metacarpophalangeal joint changes, quite apart from the genetic and laboratory test results:

- The disease occurs very rarely in females.
- There are no cartilage calcifications to indicate secondary chondrocalcinosis.
- The carpal joints are not involved.

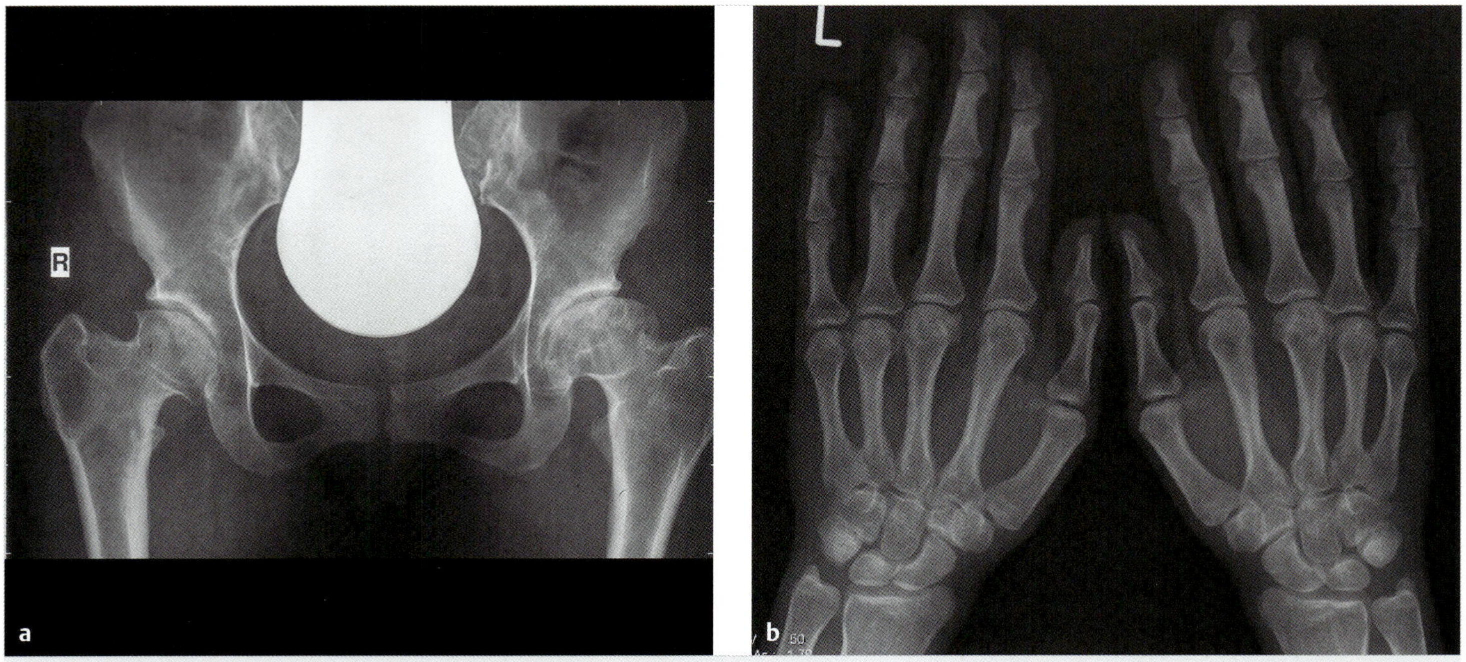

Fig. 4.32 a, b Old Perthes disease? Hemochromatosis?

- There are no anatomic changes in the bases of the phalanges that oppose the deformed metacarpal heads. This proves that the deformities are not based on a disease arising from the joint.

Thus, a synoptic review of all the findings definitely points to a systemic epiphyseal dysplasia (known also as multiple epiphyseal dysplasia or Fairbank disease), a skeletal disease with an autosomal dominant mode of inheritance. It is a genetically heterogeneous dysplasia based on a nonallelic mutation. Its clinical presentation is variable but is relatively constant within families. It most commonly affects the epiphyses of the hip, knee, ankle, and shoulder joints. Typical clinical signs are as follows[37]:

- Prominent, usually painful joints with limited mobility, a waddling gait
- Normal or moderately short stature with normal body proportions
- Frequent pronounced thoracic kyphosis, back pain

Classic radiologic signs are as follows:

- Irregularities of the epiphyses and later in the joint contours of tubular bones (hips, knees, ankles, hands, and feet). In middle and late childhood the epiphyses become flat (Ribbing type) or small (Fairbank type).
- Variable flattening of vertebral bodies and irregular endplates, especially in the thoracic spine
- Normal metaphyses with minimal shortening of tubular bones

The disease is usually manifested after 2 years of age but occasionally goes unnoticed until early adulthood. Common differential diagnoses are hypoparathyroidism, pseudoachondroplasia, and (in the hip joint) Perthes disease.

Our case, while not classic, is nevertheless clear-cut. The anomalies represent a very potent preosteoarthritic condition.

Final Diagnosis

Epiphyseal dysplasia of the metacarpal and femoral heads with secondary acetabular dysplasia—not prior avascular necrosis of the femoral heads. (Synonyms for epiphyseal dysplasia: multiple epiphyseal dysplasia, Fairbank disease, Ribbing disease, dysostosis epiphysealis multiplex.)

Comments

Besides prior avascular necrosis (Perthes disease), the differential diagnosis of deformed femoral heads and acetabula should include dysplasias, which can be confirmed or excluded by imaging additional joints (e.g., hands, knees).

Case 68 (▶ Fig. 4.33)

Case description

- *Referring physicians:* orthopedist and radiologist.
- *Prior history and clinical question:* A 48-year-old man complained of occasional left hip pain after jogging. Maximum passive flexion and internal rotation did not reproduce the pain. The orthopedist asked about a possible bone tumor (biopsy: yes or no?), and the radiologist requested interpretation of the sectional imaging findings in the left hip (normal variant?).

Radiologic Findings

CT images (▶ Fig. 4.33 **d, e**) show a circumscribed osteolytic lesion with marginal sclerosis at the anterior femoral head–neck junction. It correlates on MRI with a slightly inhomogeneous, hyperintense figure (▶ Fig. 4.33 **a–c**). There is also a mild associated hip effusion. The offset between the femoral head and femoral neck is absent, that is, the anterior contour of the femoral neck is not posteriorly convex at the head–neck junction. Thus we do not see the usual tapering of the femoral neck relative to the head.

Location

The radiologic findings are located precisely where the joint capsule is closely apposed to the bone, and also where the distance between the acetabular margin and femoral neck is shortest at high degrees of flexion and internal rotation. This area is also called the "vulnerable zone."

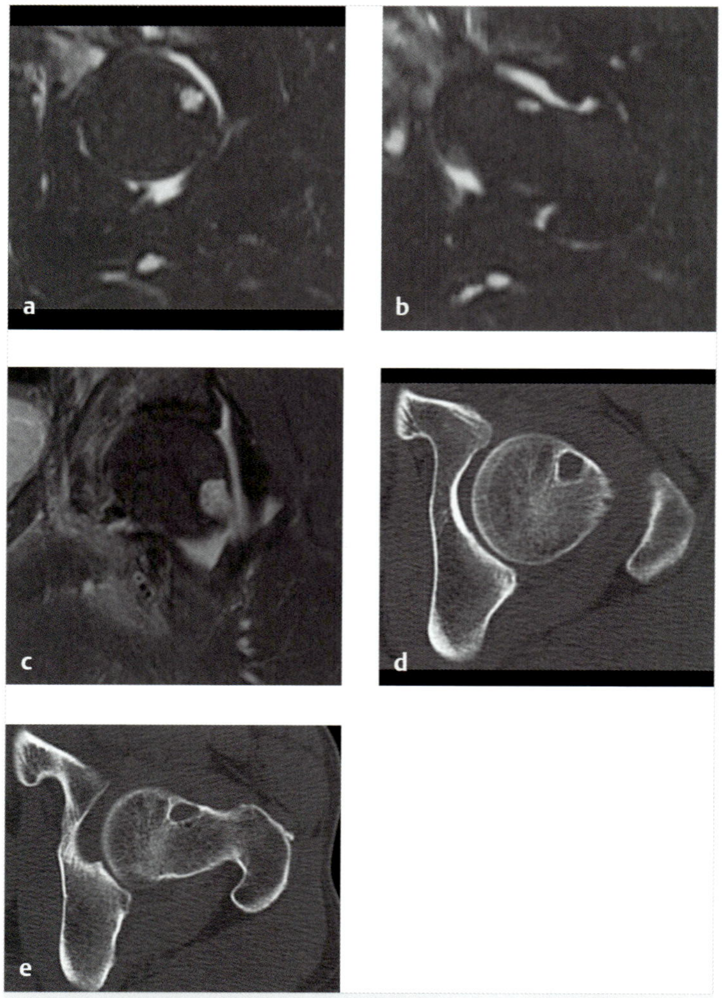

Fig. 4.33 a–e Cyst or normal variant?

Pathoanatomic Background of the Findings

Given the location of the finding, it is not difficult to characterize it as stress-induced—for example, circumscribed bone resorption based on mucoid degeneration of the subchondral bone.

Assignment to a Possible Basic Entity

▶ **Normal variant or malformation?** This question is justified because this type of finding, called a herniation pit (where synovial and cartilage tissue herniate into the bone), is often noted incidentally on pelvic radiographs. Histologically the pit contains connective tissue with loose myxoid, necrotic bone, cartilage, and fluid. This is definitely pathologic, of course, but when such a finding is detected incidentally, in many healthy individuals it can also be correctly classified as a normal variant. It should be added that histology has apparently been investigated only in symptomatic hips. On the other hand, a herniation pit is very often found in cam-type hip impingement; some authors attribute this to constant impingement of the convex-shaped femoral neck against the acetabular rim. Reportedly this also causes frictional wear and/or avulsion of the acetabular cartilage and/or labrum. In the present case, the complete MRI series (not pictured here) showed no pathologic changes in the labrum. A recent study[38] found no relationship between the presence of a herniation pit and femoroacetabular impingement. It is likely that only long-term results over a period of 10 to 20 years would show whether a herniation pit with or without hip impingement is an early indicator of later osteoarthritis.

▶ **Trauma?** As a chronic stress-related phenomenon, yes.

▶ **Tumor?** No. This answer follows from the discussion under Normal variant or malformation above.

▶ **Regressive change?** Yes, if an intraosseous ganglion is considered as a stress-induced regressive change.

Synopsis and Discussion

Given the lack of clinical symptoms, the finding in the proximal anterolateral quadrant of the femoral neck can be classified as a herniation pit.

▶ Fig. 4.34 **a–c** shows radiographs and CT of a herniation pit (arrows in ▶ Fig. 4.34 **a**) in a different patient. Again, the radiolucency with marginal sclerosis was noted as an incidental finding.

Final Diagnosis

Herniation pit, which probably did not cause the patient's complaints.

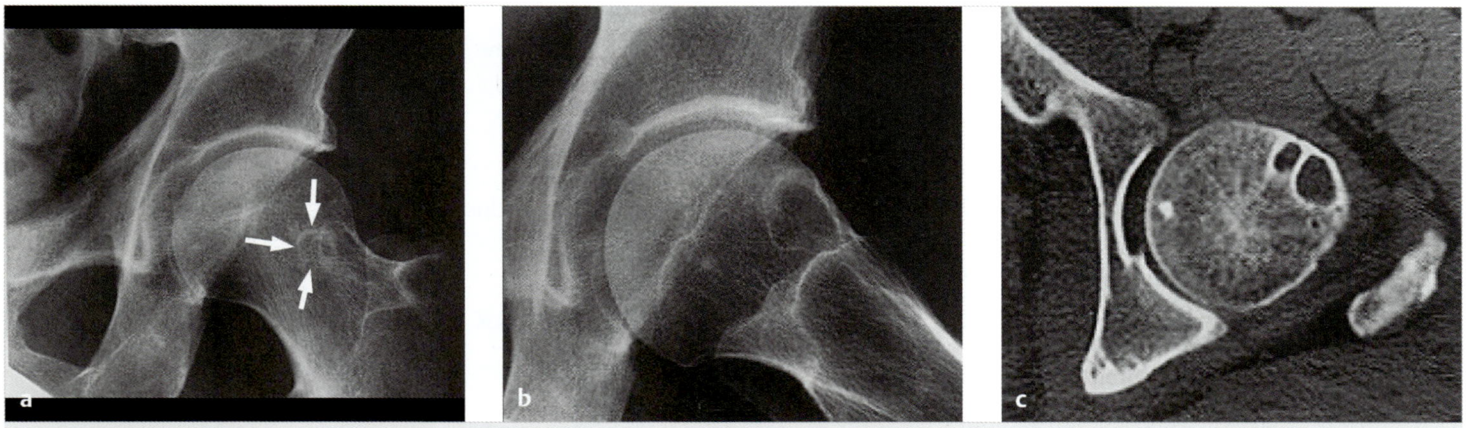

Fig. 4.34 a–c Herniation pit in another patient.

Comments

Herniation pits may be observed as an incidental finding and normal variant or in association with cam-type hip impingement. The latter is proven clinically by forcible flexion and internal rotation.

Case 69 (▶ Fig. 4.35)

Case description

- Referring physician: pathologist.
- Prior history and clinical question: A 53-year-old man had a 1-year history of right hip pain, most noticeable after prolonged exercise and while sitting. On clinical examination, a stabbing pain was elicited by strong passive flexion and internal rotation of the hip. MRI revealed a tear in the acetabular labrum (▶ Fig. 4.35 **a, c**). The orthopedist confirmed the labral tear arthroscopically and took a sample from the proximal anterior femoral neck (specifically, the anterosuperior quadrant of the femoral neck) because he could not confidently classify the finding at that location by radiography or MRI. He suspected an enchondroma. The pathologist found a pleomorphic fibro-osseous lesion (connective tissue with loose myxoid, small lymphocytic inflammatory foci, and necrotic bone), which he could not positively identify. He was not satisfied to report "no evidence of malignancy" and requested a consult.

Radiologic Findings

The T2w MR images show a multicentric lesion of inhomogeneous signal intensity in the anterior (anterosuperior) femoral neck. Fine hyperintensities are visible among irregular signal voids. The anterior labrum is torn, and a joint effusion is present. The femoral neck bulges anteriorly, eliminating the usual offset between the femoral head and neck. The radiographs (arrows in ▶ Fig. 4.35 **d, e**) show multicentric lucencies in the anterolateral femoral neck, that is, in the "vulnerable zone" (see Case 68).

Location

The lesion in question is located in the "vulnerable zone," see Case 68.

Pathoanatomic Background of the Findings

The location of the lesion makes it easy to classify as a stress-induced, reactive phenomenon. This interpretation is supported by its multicentric structure.

Assignment to a Possible Basic Entity

▸ **Normal variant or malformation?** The combined presence of the labral tear and femoral neck lesion is suggestive of hip impingement with a herniation pit, especially since the anatomy of the femoral neck predisposes to that condition.

▸ **Inflammation?** The lymphocytic inflammation described by the pathologist is purely reactive, and the overall finding does not result from osteomyelitis, for example. An inflammatory process would also produce different clinical findings.

▸ **Tumor?** No. What kind of tumor would occupy an eccentric location on the femoral neck margin? An eccentric chondroma,

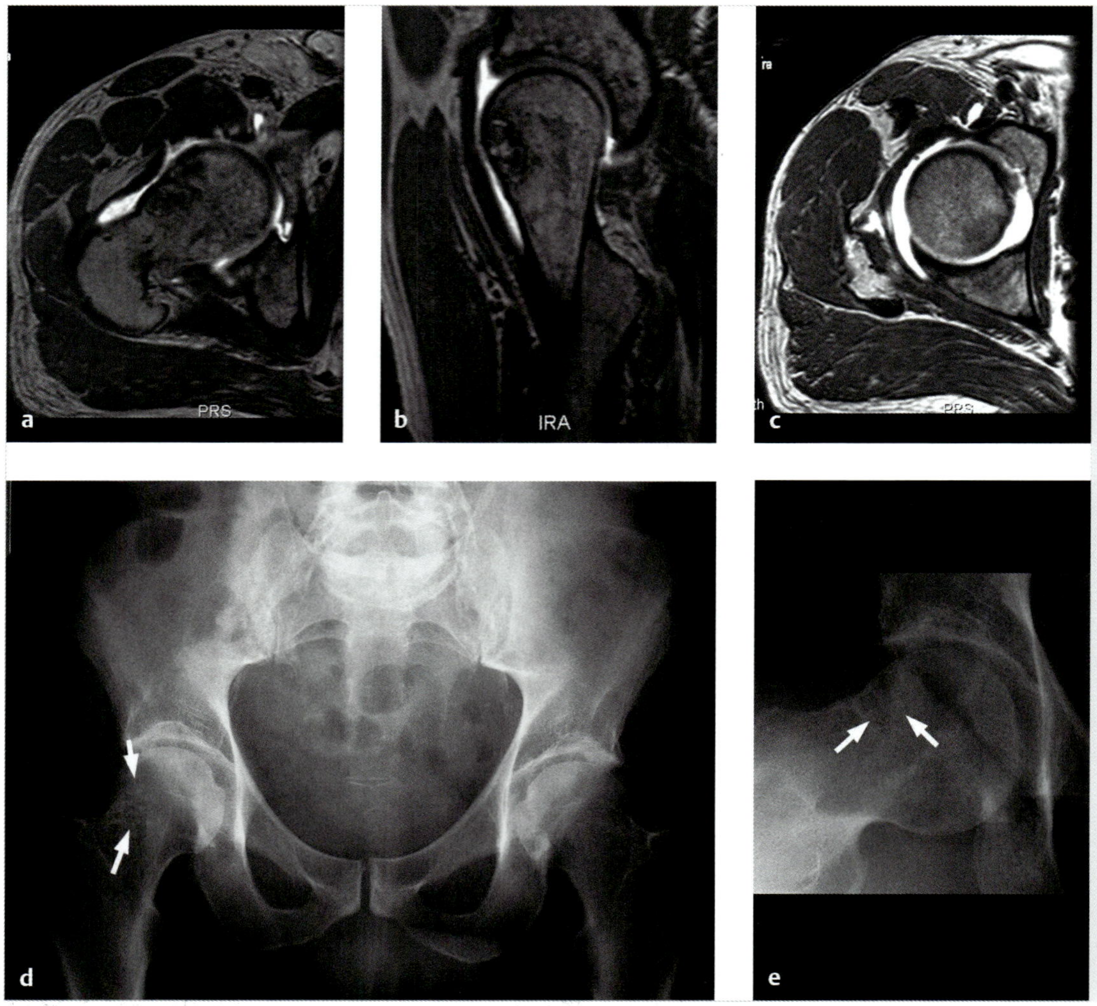

Fig. 4.35 a–e Cartilage-forming tumor?

see Case 70? If the multiple lucencies on the radiograph were interpreted as cartilage lobules, they would show markedly increased signal intensity on MRI. But this is not the case. The multicentric pattern on MRI is also inconsistent with chondromyxoid fibroma.

▶ **Regressive change?** See under Case 68.

Synopsis and Discussion

In contrast to Case 68, the herniation pit is symptomatic and apparently results from cam-type hip impingement.

Final Diagnosis

Multicentric herniation pit of the right femoral neck, most likely occurring within the context of hip impingement and a labral tear.

Comments

When a labral tear is confirmed radiologically and arthroscopically in a cam-type hip impingement syndrome, an osteolytic lesion in the "vulnerable zone" probably represents a symptomatic herniation pit.

Case 70 (▶ Fig. 4.36)

Case description

- *Referring physicians:* orthopedist and radiologist.
- *Prior history and clinical question:* An 11-year-old boy presented with right hip pain and could walk only on crutches. He responded well to nonsteroidal anti-inflammatory medication. The orthopedist thought that the radiograph indicated a cyst. The radiologist believed it was a solid tumor.

Radiologic Findings

The radiographs show an eccentric osteolytic lesion with a partially sclerotic margin located in the medial portion of the right femoral head (▶ Fig. 4.36 **a, b**) corresponding to a Lodwick Grade I C osteolytic lesion (the medial cortex is disrupted, and the margin with the epiphyseal plate is poorly defined and probably disrupted). MRI, especially the T1w images, shows a definite absence of medial cortex on the femoral head. The lesion shows marked contrast enhancement (▶ Fig. 4.36 **e, f**), and ▶ Fig. 4.36 **f** shows penetration to the epiphyseal plate. The lesion contains small "cystic" cavities with fluid levels (▶ Fig. 4.36 **g, h**), and joint effusion is present. The water-sensitive sequences (▶ Fig. 4.36 **d, g–i**) and contrast-enhanced images show markedly increased, edema-like signal intensity in both the femoral head and neck.

Location

The lesion has its epicenter in the proximal femoral epiphysis.

Pathoanatomic Background of the Findings

The findings indicate a solid tumor (contrast enhancement!) that has invaded the joint and epiphyseal plate from the femoral head and is associated with significant edema in the adjacent bone. The joint effusion most likely results from tumor ingrowth into the joint but may also represent a "sympathetic" effusion, or both. The small cavities within the lesion may be circumscribed hemorrhagic areas with fluid levels, that is, secondary aneurysmal bone cysts.

Assignment to a Possible Basic Entity

▶ **Inflammation?** No clinical manifestations. Also, we would expect to find reactive sclerosis around the lesion.

▶ **Tumor?** Yes, one whose epicenter is the capital femoral epiphysis and is associated with edema and joint effusion. It contains

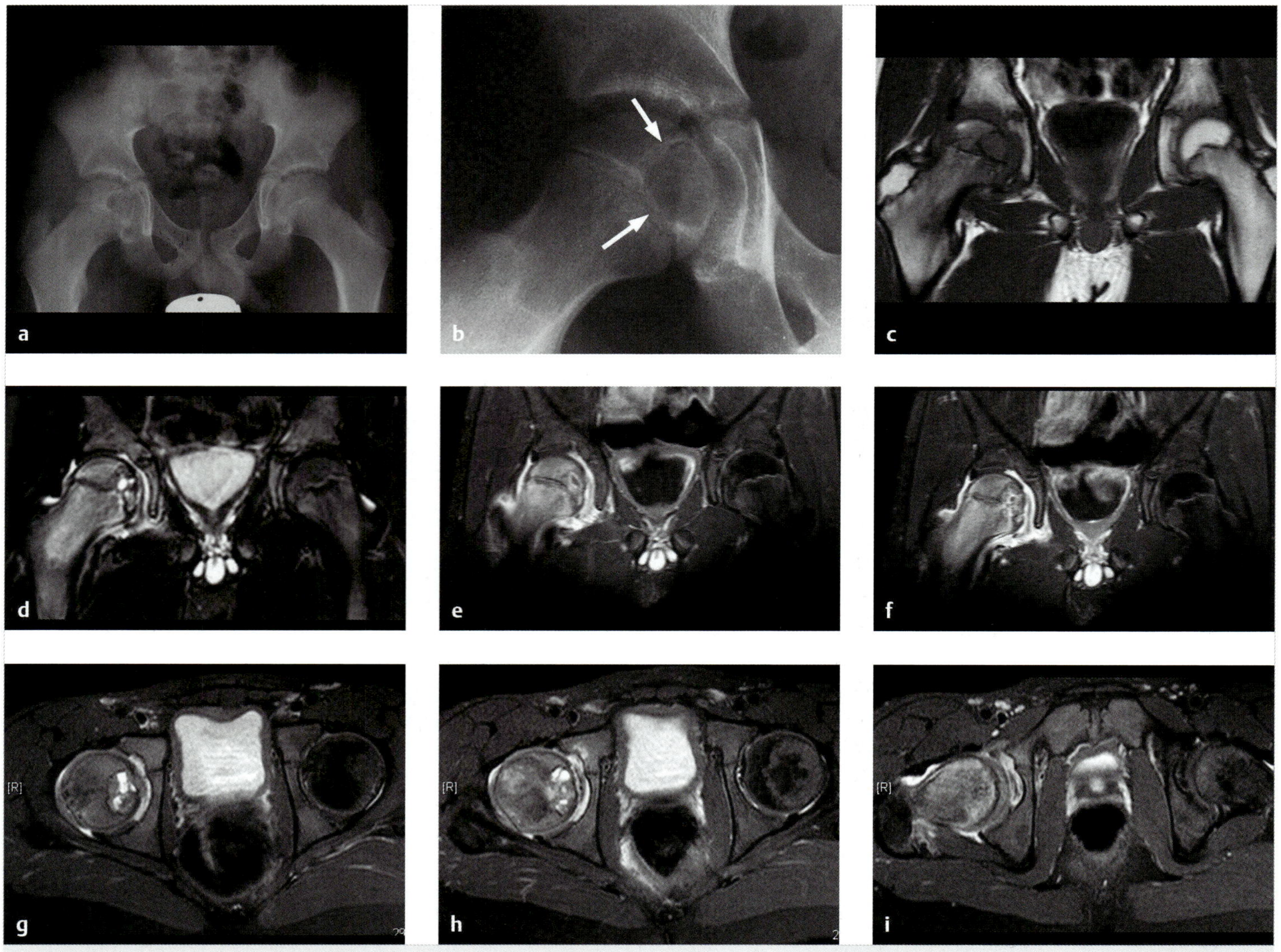

Fig. 4.36 a–i Epiphyseal cyst?

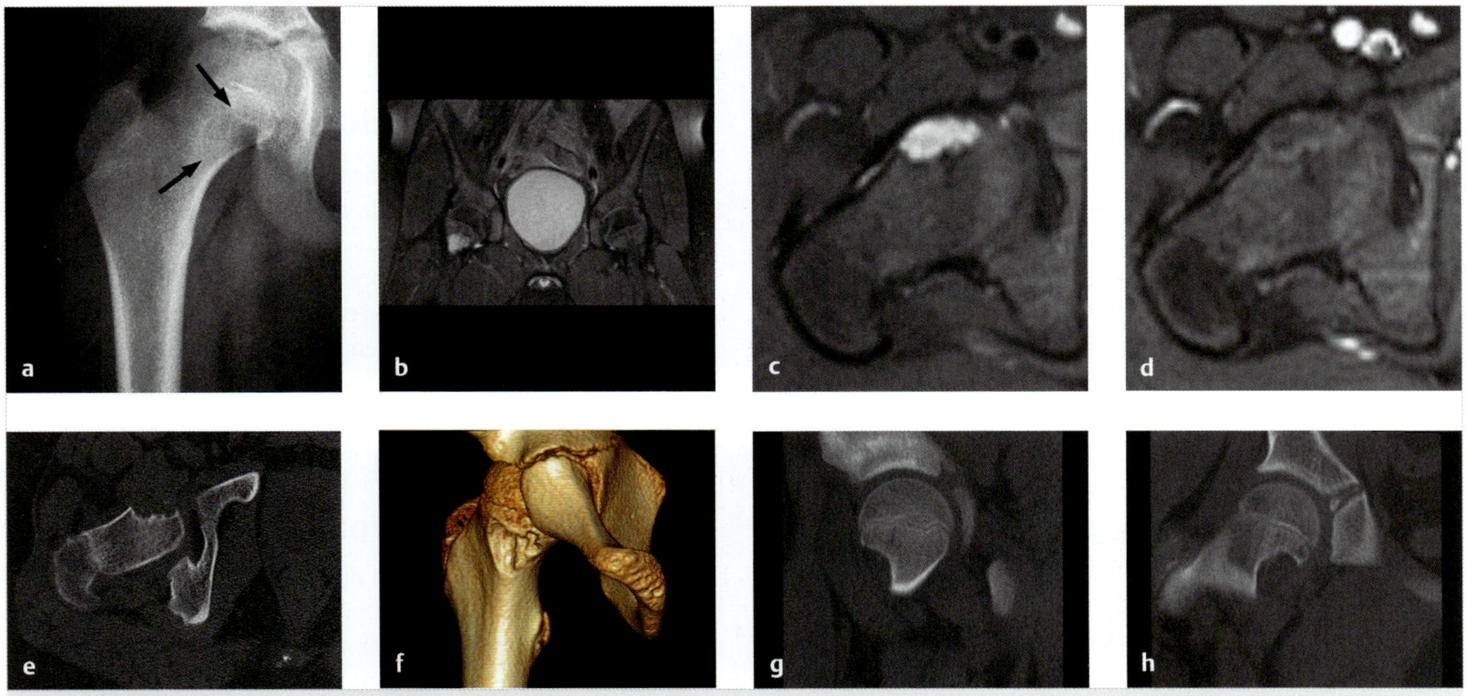

Fig. 4.37 a–h Enchondroma or fibrous dysplasia?

small cavities with fluid levels consistent with secondary aneurysmal bone cysts, as described above.

► **Avascular necrosis?** No, primary avascular necrosis of the femoral head would be associated with signs of fragmentation.

Synopsis and Discussion

Given the age of the patient, the site of occurrence, and the morphology of the osteolysis, there is a high probability that the lesion is a chondroblastoma. The lesion and its location have all the essential elements of chondroblastoma:

- More than 80% of cases occur in the second decade of life.
- The femoral head, with 9% of cases, is the fourth most common site of occurrence after the humeral head (ca. 17%) and the epiphyses of the knee (34%).
- In 50% of cases the tumor occurs in both the epiphysis and the metaphysis (as in our case). In approximately 45% of cases it is confined to the epiphysis or apophysis, but is always close to the growth plate. Only about 5% of tumors occur in the metaphysis. Approximately 75% of chondroblastomas have an eccentric location in the epiphysis.
- The cortex is involved in around 80% of cases.
- In approximately 60% of cases the interior of the tumor shows trabeculation and/or matrix calcification. We cannot confirm the latter in our case because CT scans were not obtained.
- Secondary aneurysmal bone cysts occur in a full one-fifth of cases.
- The majority of cases investigated to date by MRI have shown marked perifocal edema (along with synovitis), attributed in part to the high prostaglandin level in the tumor. Today, perifocal edema provides a highly reliable differentiating criterion from epiphyseal enchondroma (rare, see below) and giant cell tumor. Most chondroblastomas have a rich vascular supply.

The radiologic diagnosis was confirmed histologically.

► Fig. 4.37 **a–h** illustrates the case of a 10-year-old boy with a metaphyseal enchondroma in the right proximal femur (see arrows in ► Fig. 4.37 **a**). The lobular arrangement of the lesion is subtly displayed in the MR images in ► Fig. 4.37 **b, c** (T2w) and ► Fig. 4.37 **d** (contrast-enhanced). No perifocal edema was found. Our differential diagnosis included chondromyxoid fibroma, a herniation pit at an atypical site (too far medially), and finally eosinophilic granuloma. Because the boy was symptomatic, a biopsy was performed. We were surprised by the diagnosis of enchondroma.

Final Diagnosis

Chondroblastoma in the right proximal femoral epiphysis.

Comments

A well-perfused osteolytic lesion in an epiphysis with marked perifocal edema in a young patient is strongly suspicious for chondroblastoma.

Case 71 (► Fig. 4.38)

Case description

- Referring physician: orthopedist.
- Prior history and clinical question: A 42-year-old woman had a 2-year history of increasing right hip pain. She was otherwise healthy and showed no abnormalities on physical examination. A subsequent pelvic radiograph (► Fig. 4.38 **a**) displayed multiple "cysts" in the femoral head and neck and in the acetabulum. The hip joint space was narrowed relative to the left side. Unusual presentation of hip osteoarthritis or a tumor?

Radiologic Findings

The pelvic radiograph shows multicentric lucencies in the acetabulum, femoral head, and proximal femoral neck with narrowing of the joint space (► Fig. 4.38 **a**). Corresponding MR images (► Fig. 4.38 **b, c**) demonstrate a well-perfused synovial process with a nodular structure. The CT scans in ► Fig. 4.38 **d, e** clearly display the deep defects in both articulating bones. Calcifications are not visible within the defects or holes.

Location

Intra-articular focus with spread to the articulating bones.

Pathoanatomic Background of the Findings

The findings indicate an active, proliferative, nodular or villous synovial process that is destroying the adjacent bony structures. The concomitant destruction of articular cartilage has led to joint space narrowing.

Assignment to a Possible Basic Entity

► **Inflammation?** Possibly, since any chronic inflammatory synovial process can first erode and then destroy the adjacent bone.

► **Tumor?** Yes in principle, for even tumors that spread along the surface of the synovial membrane (e.g., hemangioma, primary synovial sarcoma) or tumorlike lesions (osteochondromatosis, pigmented villonodular synovitis [PVNS]) can destroy the adjacent bone.

Synopsis and Discussion

As noted above, the differential diagnosis is broad, ranging from an inflammatory or granulomatous synovial process to a malignant tumor of the synovial membrane:

1. We may be dealing with an inflammatory rheumatoid process. *Gout* may produce changes similar to those in our case, except that the bone defects arise mostly from medullary tophi and not from inflamed synovium (see Case 136). *Rheumatoid arthritis* would involve multiple joints, especially in the hands and feet, and would produce bilateral changes. The same applies to a very rare granulomatous articular process, namely multicentric reticulohistiocytosis (see Case 123). Our patient had complaints only in her right hip, however.
2. *Hemangioma* or a *posttraumatic vascular malformation* can produce the same radiologic features as in our case, but gener-

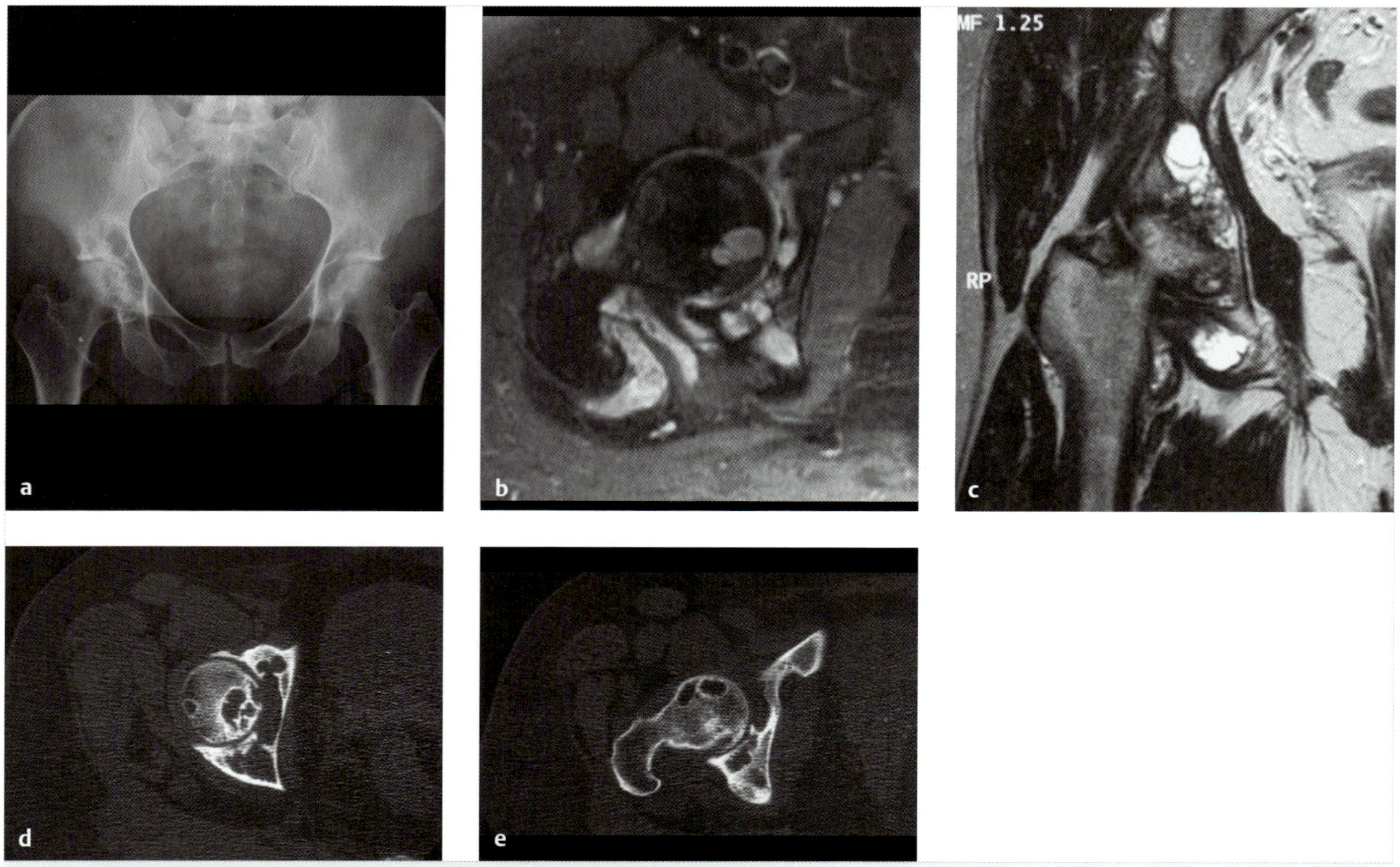

Fig. 4.38 a–e Unusual subchondral cyst or tumor?

ally they are associated with severe and recurrent hemarthrosis. In the case of an arteriovenous malformation, we know from experience that the larger vessels are directly visualized in postcontrast CT or MRI; this did not occur in our case.

3. If osteochondromatosis were present, T2w MRI would show intra-articular loose bodies with high signal intensity in the thickened synovial membrane, while CT might show calcified chondromatous bodies.
4. The most likely diagnosis is *PVNS* for the following reasons:
   - The relatively long history is consistent with PVNS.
   - The process is solitary.
   - The radiograph and sectional images show large cystlike lucencies in the cancellous bone with destruction of the subchondral plate in *both articulating bones*. The sectional images clearly show that the destructive process originates from the synovial membrane. An "apple-core sign" is often present in the femoral head and neck (see Case 72) though it is absent in our case. Fine linear and focal hypointensities in the proliferative synovial process caused by iron deposition from recurrent intrasynovial hemorrhages are not clearly visible in the images reproduced here (for technical reasons) but can be seen in the originals. There is no periarticular osteoporosis like that which may occur in bacterial or rheumatoid arthritis.
   - The cartilage destruction and the cartilage-damaging effect of iron deposits have led to degenerative changes with joint space narrowing.

The diagnosis of PVNS is very likely but still requires histologic confirmation, as in the present case. PVNS is a chronic, generally monoarticular joint disease characterized by heavy villous formation and synovial proliferation, which is usually destructive to adjacent bone. Histology reveals severe, villous histiocytic and vascular proliferation.

Final Diagnosis

PVNS (synonym: diffuse synovial giant cell tumor) of the right hip joint.

Comments

Monoarticular cystlike lucencies in both articulating bones of one knee, hip, or ankle joint suggest villonodular synovitis in patients with a long pain history.

Case 72 (▶ Fig. 4.39)

Case description

- Referring physician: orthopedist.
- Prior history and clinical question: A 33-year-old man, otherwise in good health, had a 1-year history of increasing pain and frequent locking in the left hip joint. He stated that he could restore mobility to the locked joint by painfully rotating and flexing it. The orthopedist ordered a radiograph that appeared to show a destructive neoplastic process and requested further clarification.

Radiologic Findings

The radiograph (▶ Fig. 4.39 **a**) shows erosion of the femoral head and neck. The changes are most pronounced in the lower portions of the head. With some imagination, one can see an "apple-core sign" of circumferential femoral erosion,[39] which is displayed even more clearly on CT (▶ Fig. 4.39 **e–h**). MRI (▶ Fig. 4.39 **b–d**) shows a joint effusion containing innumerable close-packed, hyperintense globular bodies, which partially take the place of the eroded bone. These globules are not calcified, as the CT images show. Scans with a soft-tissue window (▶ Fig. 4.39 **g**, **h**) clearly demonstrate the joint effusion.

Location

Intra-articular.

Pathoanatomic Background of the Findings

The images reveal a bone-eroding intra-articular process with associated effusion. In addition, clustered hyperintense globules are visible in water-sensitive sequences.

Assignment to a Possible Basic Entity

▸ **Inflammation?** Unlikely. The rice-body synovitis that occurs in chronic inflammatory joint diseases, especially rheumatoid arthritis, consists of much smaller granular structures (see below).

▸ **Tumor or tumorlike lesion?** Yes. The signal intensity of the intra-articular globules suggests that they are composed of nonmineralized cartilage. This is also consistent with their nonvisualization on CT. The globular structures occur mainly in areas that were formerly occupied by bone. But it is unlikely that these bodies alone could have exerted enough pressure to erode the bone. The pathogenesis of the bone erosion more likely relates to a proliferative synovial process (see below). In summary, we are probably dealing with a cartilaginous synovial process—synovial osteochondromatosis or osteochondromatosis, known also as Reichel disease.

▸ **Avascular necrosis?** No. Necrotic bone has a crumbly, amorphous appearance.

Synopsis and Discussion

The clinical manifestations (joint locking) and radiologic findings are fully consistent with *synovial osteochondromatosis*. This is a rare, tumorlike disease of the synovial membrane believed to result from an abnormal differentiation of joint-forming mesenchyme with the transformation of fibroblasts into chondroblasts, giving rise to a tumorlike proliferation of cartilage. The current WHO classification of bone tumors (Lyon 2013) places synovial osteochondromatosis under benign chondrogenic tumors. The disease can be divided into three phases:

1. Early phase with active synovitis and no loose bodies

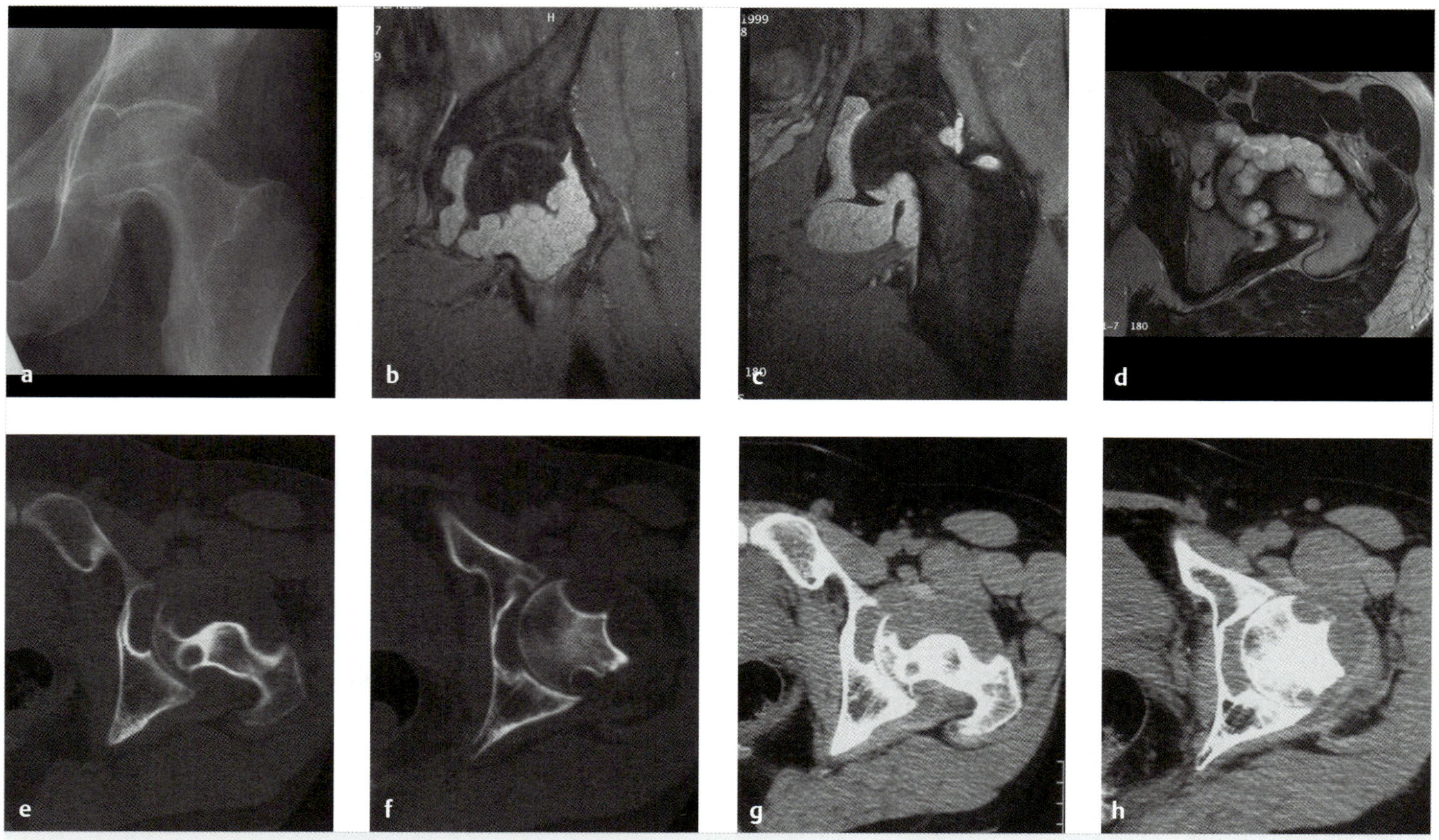

Fig. 4.39 a–h Tumor in the left femoral neck?

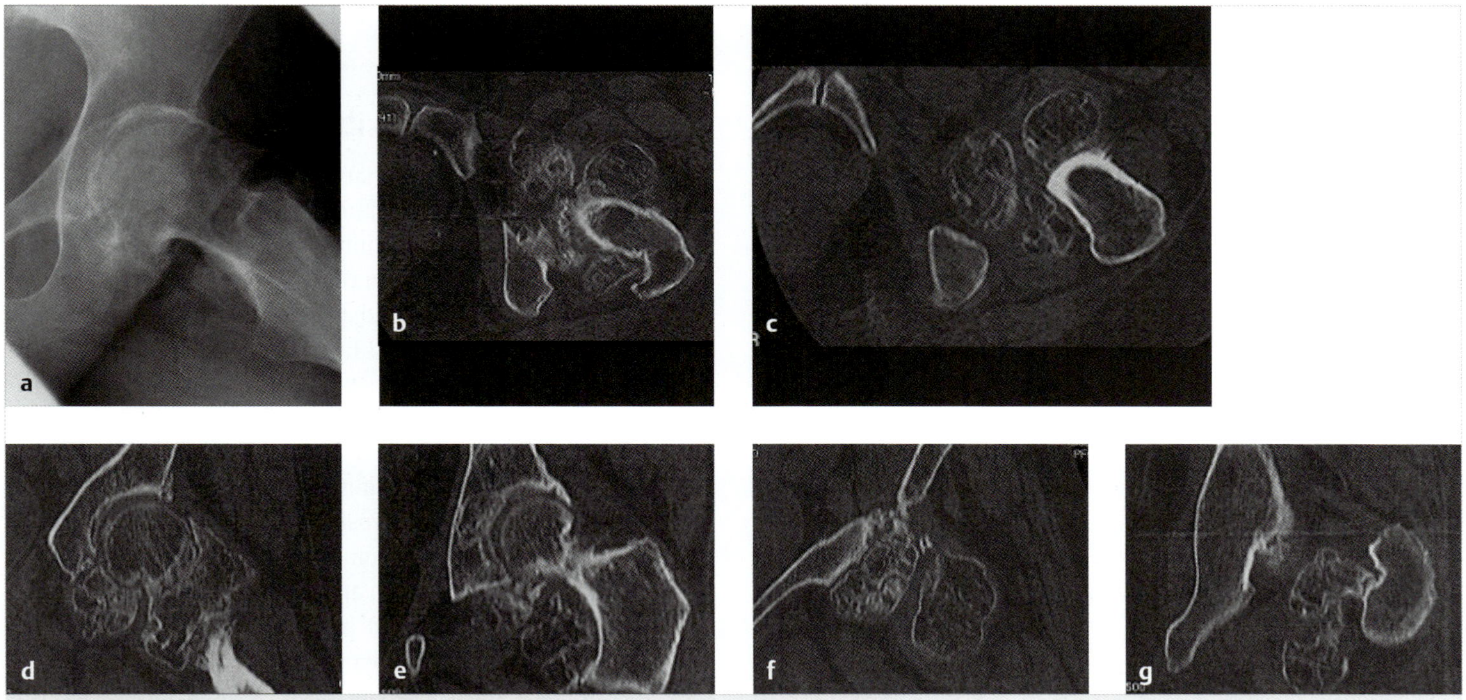

Fig. 4.40 a–g Synovial osteochondromatosis in a 64-year-old woman.

2. Transitional phase with nodular synovitis and the formation of loose bodies
3. Loose bodies (without active synovitis), the largest of which calcify and become visible on radiographs

Chondromas usually occur in large numbers in the synovial membrane and are arranged in chains or grapelike clusters. Over time they detach from the synovial membrane and travel into the joint space, where they become intra-articular loose bodies that cause catching or locking, as in osteochondritis dissecans. There is also an extra-articular form of synovial osteochondromatosis that occurs in bursae or tendon sheaths and tends to undergo malignant transformation to chondrosarcoma. The disease is predominantly monoarticular and most commonly affects males between 20 and 40 years of age, as in our case. Sites of predilection are, in order of frequency, the knee, elbow, hip, shoulder, and ankle joints, followed by the carpal and phalangeal joints. The clinical presentation is marked by limited motion or locking of the affected joint. Micronodular and macronodular forms are distinguished radiologically. Micronodular chondroma chains are not visible on plain radiographs unless contrast medium is injected into the joint. The macronodular form presents on radiographs and CT scans as calcified rice-grain to pea-sized spheres, as illustrated for the wrist in Case 127. On MRI, uncalcified chondromas in an effusion are not visible in T1w images but appear as bright globules in T2w images, as in the present case. Bone erosion is absent in most cases. We attribute the “apple-core sign” in our case to prior nodular synovitis (much as in villonodular synovitis) combined with pressure-induced erosion.

Clinical differentiation is mainly required from osteochondritis dissecans. The latter condition is distinguished radiologically by the presence of a crater associated with the osteochondral fragment.

The differential diagnosis also includes rice-body synovitis, in which small fibrin granules (just a few millimeters in diameter) have intermediate T1w signal intensity and low T2w signal intensity relative to muscle. Their hypointensity on T2w images helps to identify them in an effusion. If the rice bodies are very protein-rich, they appear hyperintense to the effusion on T1w images.

The case was treated surgically and confirmed histologically.

The case of a 64-year-old woman with mature synovial osteochondromatosis is shown in ▶ Fig. 4.40. The ossified chondromas have apparently coalesced and matured enough to develop actual bone marrow. Since indeterminate soft-tissue structures were found among the chondromas on MRI, a secondary synovial sarcoma was suspected but was not confirmed histologically.

Final Diagnosis

Synovial osteochondromatosis of the hip joint.

Comments

In rare cases synovial osteochondromatosis may cause erosion of the adjacent bone, producing an apple-core sign in the proximal femur.

Case 73 (▶ Fig. 4.41)

Case description

- Referring physician: radiologist.
- Prior history and clinical question: A 48-year-old woman was hospitalized for pyelonephritis and diabetes mellitus. Tests included abdominal CT, which showed fine erosive changes in the anterior femoral neck on each side. When questioned, the patient stated that abduction of the hip was painful. A subsequent pelvic radiograph showed a radiolucent zone in the right femoral neck, which necessitated further investigation by MRI. The radiologist wanted to know the etiology of the lucent zone in the right femoral neck (cyst?).

Radiologic Findings

The radiographs (▶ Fig. 4.41 **a, b**) show a unilateral radiolucent zone in the right femoral neck (arrows in ▶ Fig. 4.41 **b**), which is isointense to fat on T1w MRI (▶ Fig. 4.41 **c**). It is hyperintense on postcontrast and fat-suppressed images but does not differ significantly from the signal intensity on the contralateral side. On CT scans (▶ Fig. 4.41 **e, f**) the area is hypodense to muscle but slightly hyperdense to fat (▶ Fig. 4.41 **f**). The surrounding cortical bone appears normal in the bone-window view. The CT scans also show shallow anterior "erosions" in the femoral necks. The offset between the femoral head and neck appears reduced on plain radiographs (see also Case 68 and Case 69).

Pathoanatomic Background of the Findings

Looking at the lucent zone in the femoral neck and comparing it with the contralateral side, we find that its signal characteristics (on MRI) and attenuation values (on CT) are consistent with hematopoietic bone marrow. The "erosions" in the anterior femoral necks are discussed below.

Assignment to a Possible Basic Entity

▶ **Normal variant or malformation?** Yes, regarding the lucent area in the femoral neck. This interpretation is supported by the attenuation values and signal intensities, which show a similar but less pronounced pattern on the opposite side. Moreover, the anterior and posterior cortex adjacent to the area of interest appear intact. As in the proximal humerus, the femoral neck contains lucent zones that may be symmetrical or asymmetrical. The zones contain bone marrow, that is, hematopoietic and fatty marrow. The hematopoietic marrow is well perfused and therefore enhances after contrast administration. It is difficult to say whether the symmetrical "erosions" in the anterior femoral necks—which we classify as somewhat atypical herniation pits (see Case 68 and Case 69) with an associated cortical defect—resulted from the reduced offset between the femoral head and neck with anterior prominence of the femoral neck, or whether they are simply a normal variant with no clinical or prognostic significance. In any case, the clinical presentation (pain only on abduction, not on forcible flexion and internal rotation) suggests that the finding is not relevant in terms of current hip impingement.

▶ **Trauma?** The patient gave no history of trauma on either side.

▶ **Inflammation?** No clinical manifestations or radiologic signs of inflammation, even in the hip joint.

▶ **Tumor?** There is no evidence of a tumor or a tumorlike lesion such as a cyst. Contrast-enhanced MRI alone is inconsistent with a cyst.

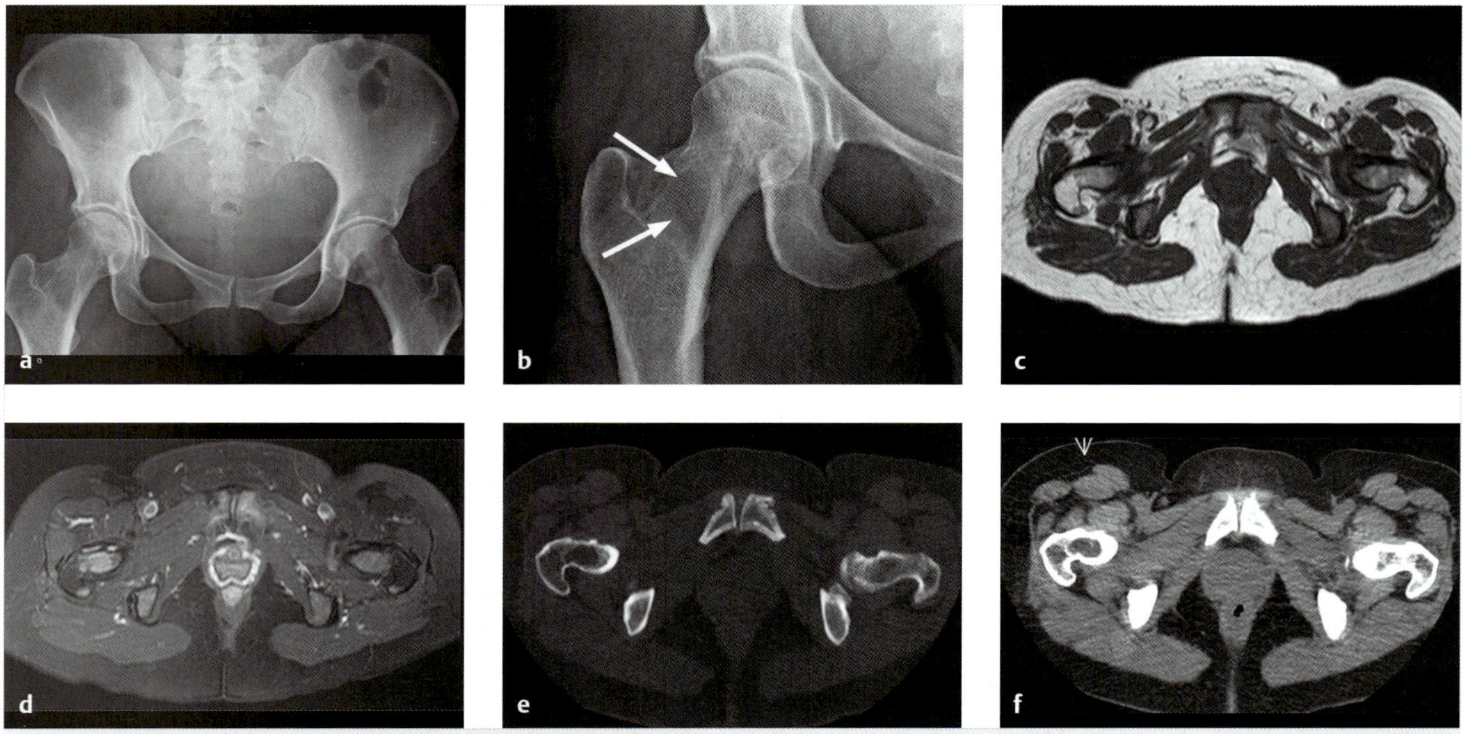

Fig. 4.41 a–f Tumor in the right femoral neck and erosion of the anterior femoral necks?

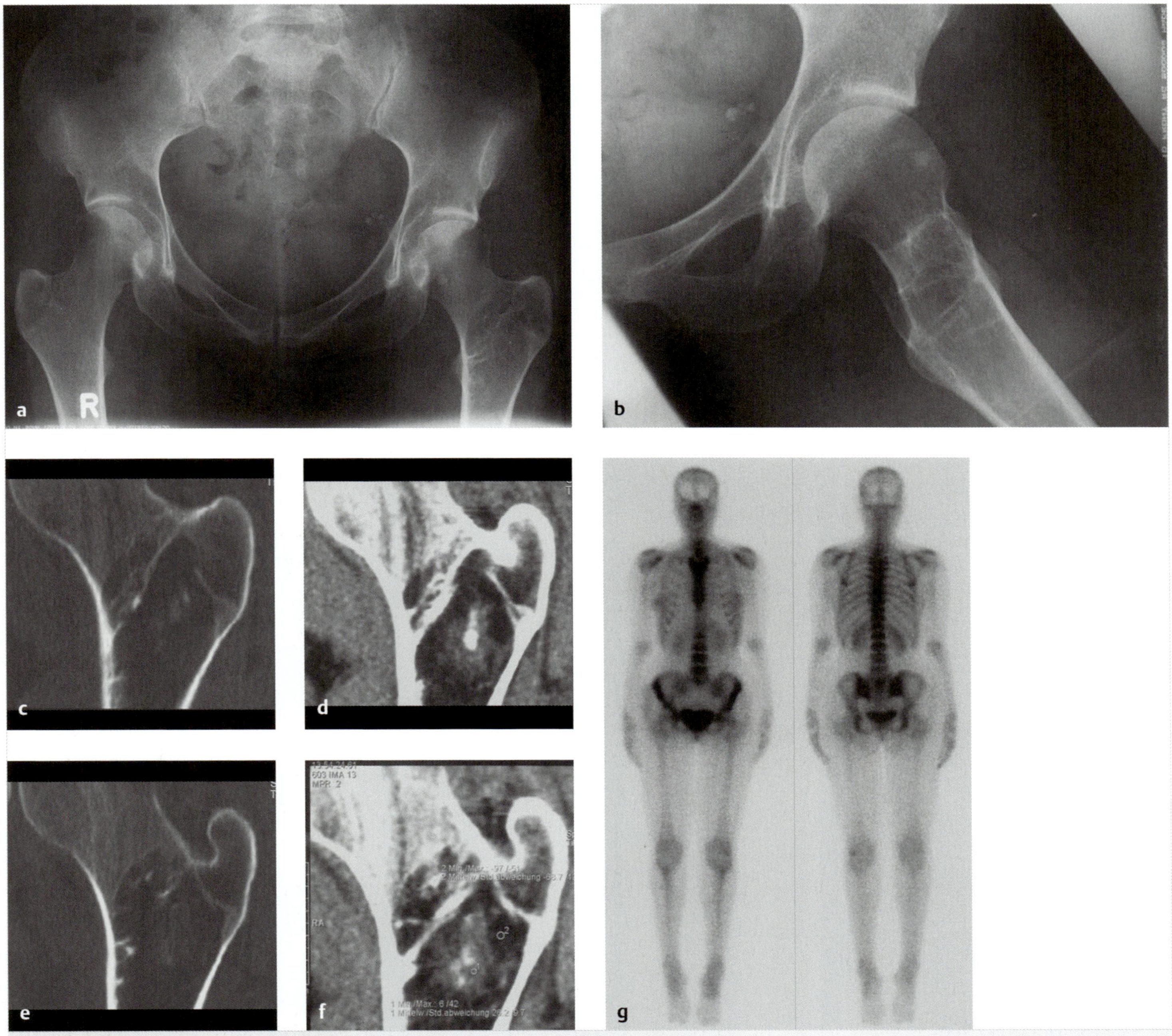

Fig. 4.42 a–g Lipoma or extreme normal variant in the intertrochanteric region of a 33-year-old woman.

Synopsis and Discussion

The lucent area in the right femoral neck is a normal variant that may have arisen in one of two ways:

- An area containing little or no cancellous bone but filled with fatty and red marrow has always been present as a normal variant.
- Hematopoietic hyperplasia, which may occur in any bone with a medullary cavity, was once present in the affected area and caused a secondary rarefaction or disappearance of trabecular bone.

Given the fact that sectional images show a similar but less pronounced finding on the opposite side and the patient has no clinical manifestations of a tumor or tumorlike process on the right side, it is appropriate to classify the finding as a normal variant. It is not an unusual finding in asymptomatic individuals and, at a more proximal site, in osteoporosis patients.

The second apparent abnormality—an erosion in the anterior border of each femoral neck—is not clinically relevant at present. It may be a kind of herniation pit with otherwise normal anatomy of the femoral head and neck, making it a normal variant, or it may be interpreted as a feature accompanying or resulting from the relative prominence of the femoral necks.

▶ Fig. 4.42 illustrates the case of a 33-year-old woman in whom extreme "rarefaction" or absence of trabeculation was noted incidentally in the left intertrochanteric region. Sectional imaging (MRI, CT) showed no evidence of active bone destruction, and the bone scan (▶ Fig. 4.42 **g**) was negative. CT density measurements in the affected region showed negative attenuation values (HU) in large portions of the "lesion," indicating fat. This in itself excludes a malignant tumor such as sarcoma (fat is the radiologist's friend!). The very dense central calcifications probably represent calcified necrotic fat. This suggests that the lesion is a harmless lipoma (see also Case 133 and Case 135). It may also be an extreme normal variant in which intertrochanteric cancellous bone was absent and has been replaced by fat, which underwent central necrosis. The area of fatty replacement is large enough to cause a central perfusion defect. When seen at follow-up 5 years later, the patient was still asymptomatic and the imaging findings (not pictured here) were unchanged.

Final Diagnosis

- Normal variant of sparse trabeculae in the right femoral neck as an incidental finding
- Bilateral herniation pits

Comments

The normal variant of sparse trabeculae, occurring predominantly in the femoral neck but also in the humeral head, can mimic a tumor mass. The absence of active bone destruction and reactive changes on sectional imaging and the detection of similar changes on the contralateral side make further investigation (e.g., biopsy or follow-ups) unnecessary in an asymptomatic patient.

Case 74 (▶ Fig. 4.43)

Case description

- Referring physician: radiologist.
- Prior history and clinical question: A 13-year-old boy complained of increasing pain in the right hip, especially at night. He walked with a pronounced limp. The radiograph (▶ Fig. 4.43 **a, b**) was interpreted as negative, and MRI added no information. Since the boy was an avid athlete, his symptoms were attributed to overuse or an "occult" stress fracture, but abstinence from sports did not relieve his complaints. Question: Do the symptoms have a different cause?

Radiologic Findings

The radiographs (▶ Fig. 4.43 **a, b**) show slight demineralization of the right proximal femoral epimetaphysis. Water-sensitive MRI sequences (▶ Fig. 4.43 **c–e**) show definite edema-like signal in the right intertrochanteric region and in the greater trochanter in addition to a joint effusion. The T1w image (▶ Fig. 4.43 **f**) shows only decreased signal intensity in the area of edema-like signal. Further details are covered below.

Pathoanatomic Background of the Findings

The following interpretation refers exclusively to ▶ Fig. 4.43 **a–f**. The demineralization apparently results from the intraosseous edema-like signal (osteoclast stimulation), which in turn incited the intra-articular effusion. The effusion (e.g., in arthritis) is definitely not the cause of the other two findings, for then we would also expect to find edema-like signal in the femoral head *and* acetabulum. The cause of the three radiologic findings (osteopenia, edema-like signal, effusion), presumably bone-related, is not defined in this series of images.

Assignment to a Possible Basic Entity

▶ **Trauma?** This question is justified because the boy is athletically active. He cannot recall a significant current or prior injury, although chronic trauma is a possibility. Imaging to date has shown no evidence of an eccentric stress fracture or other injury, however.

▶ **Inflammation?** No. The bone shows no destructive changes, and arthritis is not a possibility (see above).

▶ **Tumor?** Yes. Finding this type of pain (present at night, not exercise-related) in a 13-year-old boy is strongly suggestive of an

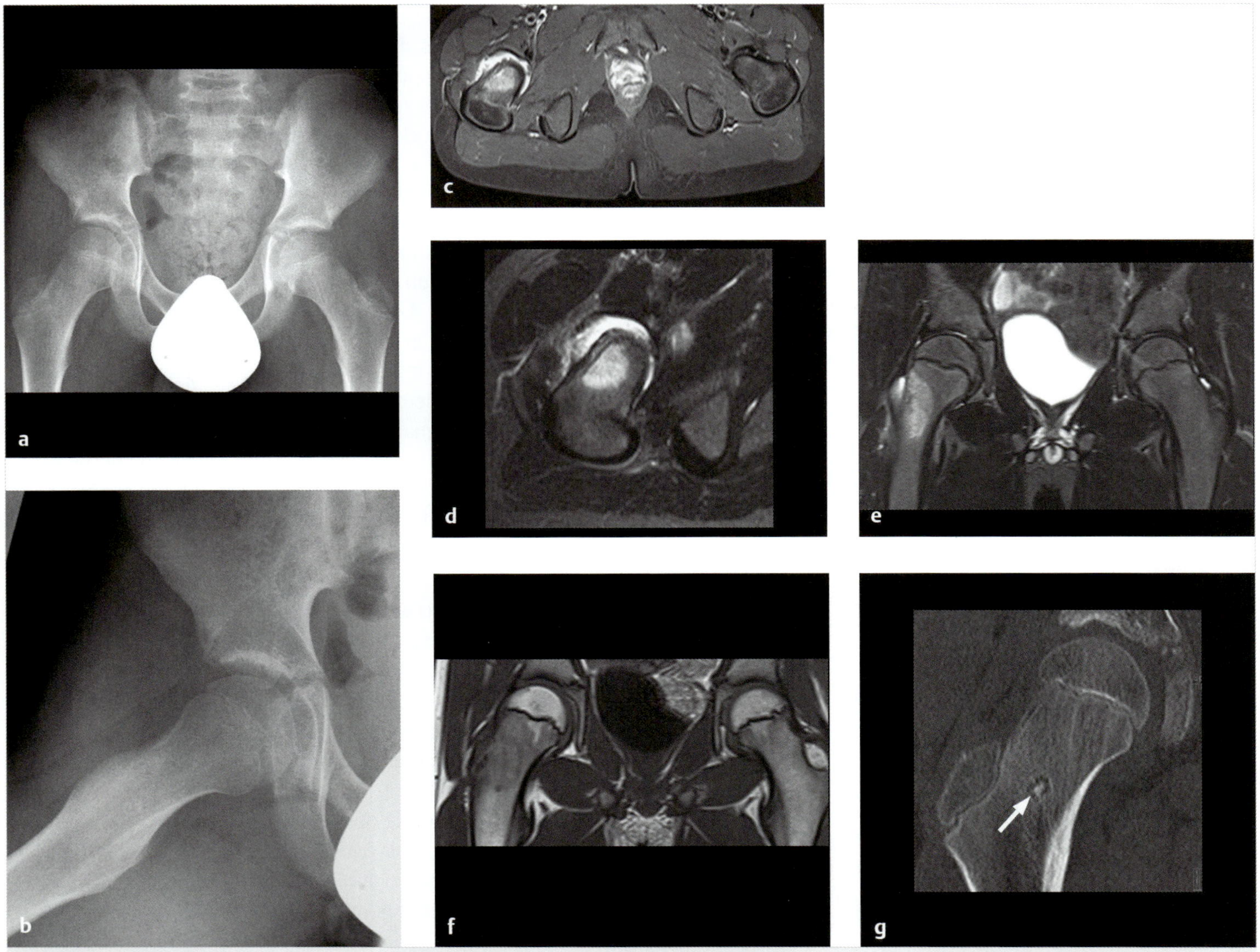

Fig. 4.43 a–g Occult stress fracture in the right femoral neck?

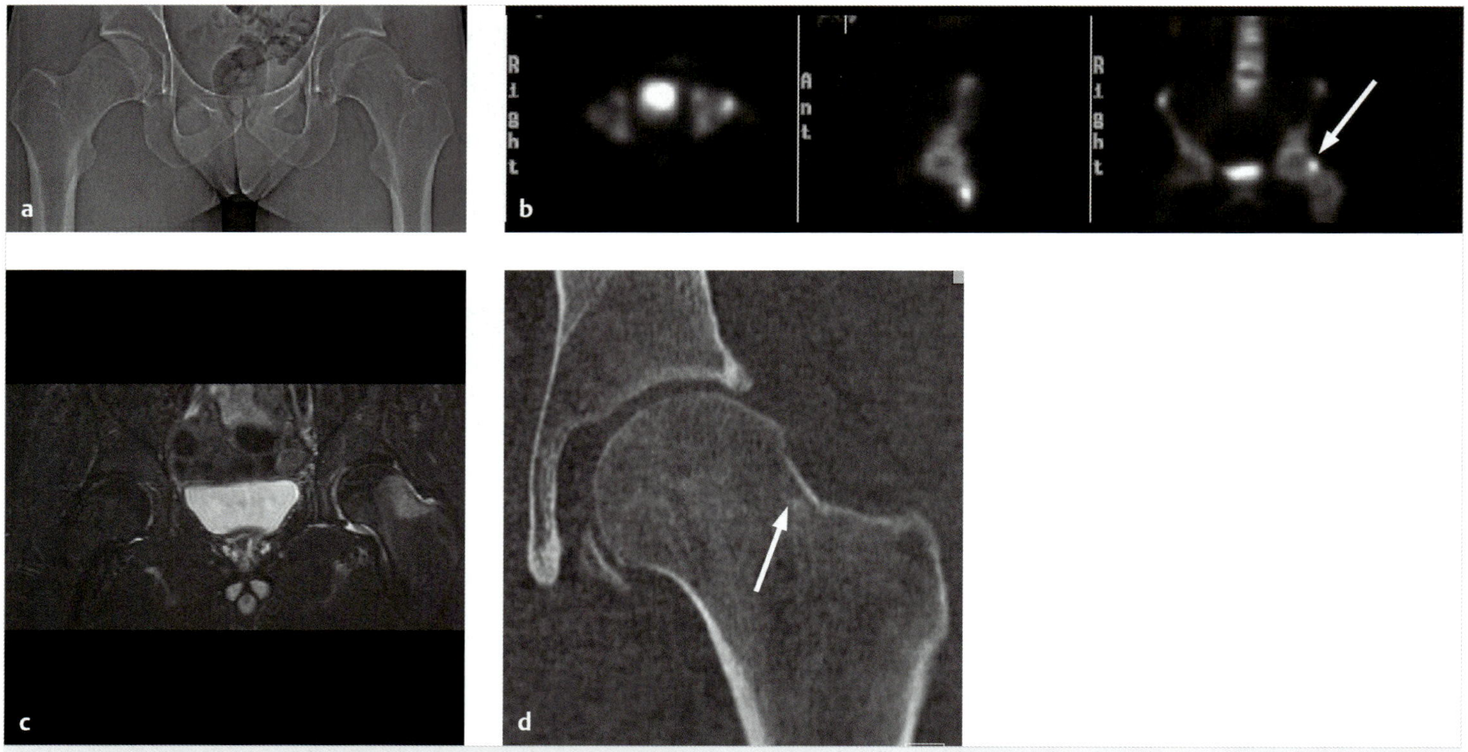

Fig. 4.44 a–d Osteoid osteoma in the femoral neck in a 26-year-old man.

osteoid osteoma that has not yet been detected by imaging (see Synopsis and Discussion below for more details.)

Synopsis and Discussion

It is clear that the plain radiographs, MRI, and especially the clinical presentation (patient age, pain characteristics, location) provided definite evidence of an osteoid osteoma, but there was still a need for imaging proof. The author of this book strongly recommended supplemental CT scans and an aspirin test. The boy's parents initially rejected this advice due to concerns about radiation exposure and aspirin side effects. But as the symptoms worsened in the following months, they finally consented to a CT examination, which revealed the unmistakable calcified nidus of an *osteoid osteoma* located at the approximate center of the edema-like signal (arrow in ▶ Fig. 4.43 **g**). The tumor was surrounded by mild reactive osteosclerosis, especially on the proximal and lateral sides. In addition, the volume of the femoral neck was increased in its upper lateral portion.

Approximately 30% of osteoid osteomas occur in the femur, with a predilection for the femoral neck. Boys in the second decade of life are predominantly affected (ca. 50% of cases). The typical radiology and pathophysiology of osteoid osteoma are illustrated in Case 44. Diagnosis relies critically upon detecting the nidus, which generally consists of an osteolytic area up to 1 cm in diameter with central calcification. Bone scans display it as a hot spot surrounded by a variable degree of increased uptake (the "double density" sign). A lesion in the axial skeleton is often detectable only by SPECT or SPECT/CT fusion imaging (see Case 144). *The best modality for directly visualizing the tumor, and especially its typical central calcification, is CT.* Experience has shown that MRI fails to detect the nidus in many cases. If the nidus has already been localized by scintigraphy, just a few low-dose CT scans are often sufficient to demonstrate and confirm the tumor.

Based on the clinical presentation and probabilities, a *stress fracture* was considered in the present case, but we know from experience that this diagnosis can often be established only by high-resolution computed tomography (HRCT). The presumptive diagnosis of a stress fracture based on MRI in the present case was more or less plucked out of thin air, since a fracture line was not visualized.

A radiologically similar case is illustrated in ▶ Fig. 4.44. The 26-year-old man had extreme, non–exercise-related pain in the left hip region that was dramatically relieved by aspirin. This raised appropriate suspicion of osteoid osteoma. The radiograph (CT scout view in ▶ Fig. 4.44 **a**) showed no definite abnormality, but the SPECT images in ▶ Fig. 4.44 **b** showed increased uptake throughout the hip region with a central hot spot on the lateral femoral neck (double-density sign). MRI (▶ Fig. 4.44 **c**) shows definite edema-like signal in the central and lateral portions of the femoral neck, but a nidus was not detectable in any of the varied sequences. An initial CT series (not pictured here) with a 2-mm slice thickness could not detect the presumed nidus, but this was finally accomplished using a 1-mm slice thickness (see arrow in ▶ Fig. 4.44 **d**). This case also demonstrates that radiologists must employ every means at their disposal if they strongly suspect an osteoid osteoma based on the clinical presentation and previous imaging studies but a nidus has not yet been positively identified. As with the case shown in ▶ Fig. 4.43, the nidus was removed by percutaneous CT-guided enucleation. Both patients were free of complaints on the day after surgery.

▶ Fig. 4.45 also illustrates the technical problems involved in the radiologic diagnosis of osteoid osteoma. The patient, a 23-year-old woman, complained of increasing pain in her right hip, also present (and worse) at night. Clinical examination was unremarkable. MRI before and after intra-articular contrast injection detected a lesion of the acetabular labrum, but that lesion did not explain the clinical manifestations. This radiologic diagnosis was irrelevant, therefore. Meanwhile 6 months had passed and the

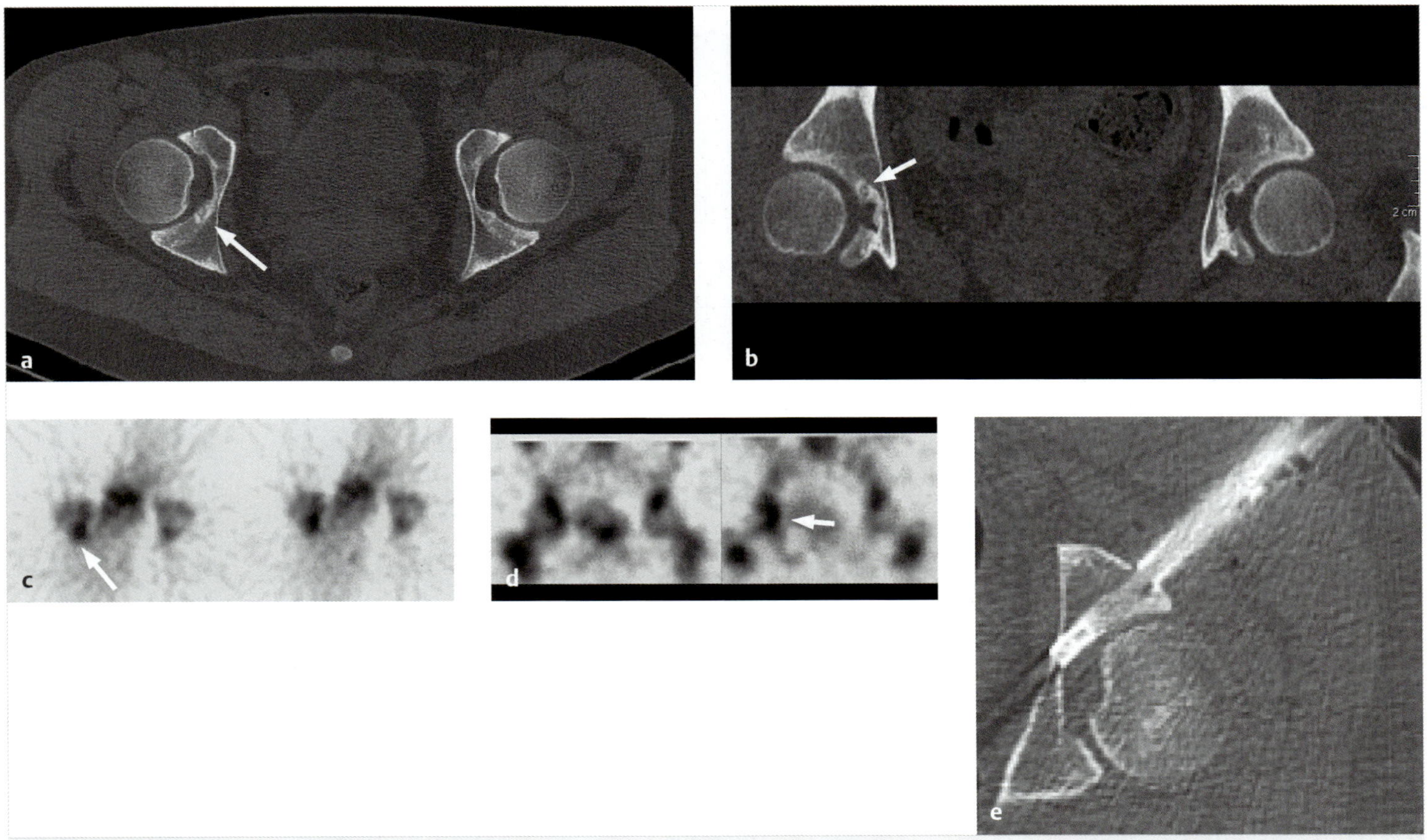

Fig. 4.45 a–e Small osteoid osteoma in the acetabulum in a 23-year-old woman.

pains were increasing. Nonsteroidal anti-inflammatory drugs were no longer beneficial, and the patient was placed on opioid analgesics. Finally the desperate patient came to us for advice. Her clinical presentation immediately raised suspicion of osteoid osteoma. To verify its presence and location, we ordered a bone scan with SPECT images, which showed focal increased uptake at the center of the right hip (arrows in ▶ Fig. 4.45 **c, d**). This focus was demonstrated in both axial (▶ Fig. 4.45 **c**) and coronal images (▶ Fig. 4.45 **d**). Previous HRCT had shown a very subtle abnormality in the right acetabulum (arrows in ▶ Fig. 4.45 **a, b**), but ultimately it was indistinguishable from a structural variation. We were now certain that the lesion was a "mini-osteoid osteoma" with a calcified nidus owing to the congruence of the CT and SPECT findings. The nidus was successfully removed by percutaneous CT-guided enucleation (Dr. J. Wiens, Wolfsburg), and 2 days later the patient was free of complaints.

Final Diagnosis

Osteoid osteoma in the right femoral neck.

Comments

If the clinical presentation is suspicious for osteoid osteoma (hallmark: small tumor with a disproportionately large effect), the radiologist should make every effort to demonstrate the tumor so that it can be removed, preferably by a minimally invasive procedure.

Case 75 (▶ Fig. 4.46)

Case description

- *Referral:* self-referral by the patient.
- *Prior history and clinical question:* A 72-year-old man presented with moderate, exercise-related "rheumatic" pain in his left hip region. CT and bone scans performed at a different institution raised suspicion of a burned-out osteoid osteoma in the left lesser trochanter. A Brodie abscess was also considered. The patient read about osteoid osteoma on the Internet and questioned the diagnosis based primarily on his age.

Radiologic Findings

Whole-body multiphase bone scintigraphy (not pictured here) showed slightly increased tracer uptake in the left lesser trochanter in the early phase. The late-phase image showed higher uptake comparable to that in the osteoarthritic right knee. A double-density sign was not observed (see Case 74). CT demonstrates a productive bony process anterior to the left lesser trochanter at the attachment of the iliofemoral ligament (▶ Fig. 4.46 **a–d**). The process has a central rounded lucency with fine extensions, one each passing through the medial and lateral contour of the cortex. No calcification is visible in the central lucency. Other areas of the pelvic skeleton show marked sites of fibro-ostotic bone proliferation about the symphysis (▶ Fig. 4.46 **d**), in the ischia (▶ Fig. 4.46 **c, d**), and on the iliac spines, iliac crest, and acetabula (not pictured).

Location

The productive bony process is located precisely at the attachment of the iliofemoral ligament to the intertrochanteric line. The iliofemoral ligament is the strongest ligament in the human body.

Pathoanatomic Background of the Findings

Considering the location of the productive bone lesion at the attachment of the iliofemoral ligament, along with the other productive bone changes located at pelvic entheses, the most likely interpretation of the radiologic finding is a fibro-ostotic process with central resorptive changes. Other possibilities are an ossified tumor matrix of periosteal osteoid osteoma and reactive-reparative new bone formation in response to an inflammatory process or stress fracture.

Assignment to a Possible Basic Entity

▶ **Normal variant or malformation?** This definitely does not apply for the main lesion in front of the the lesser trochanter. When dealing with productive fibro-ostotic (enthesiopathic) changes, it is important to determine whether they are appropriate for age, since they are found on pelvic CT scans in the majority of older individuals.

▶ **Trauma?** The patient could not recall old or acute trauma. He is not active athletically and does not take long hikes, so we cannot point to chronic (repetitive) stress as the cause of the process. It should be added, however, that the radiologic features are altogether consistent with a stress fracture (see Case 61).

▶ **Inflammation?** No. Chronic osteomyelitis with a Brodie abscess, for example, normally arises from the medullary cavity and not from the bone surface, and it presents radiographically as a lucency within a larger sclerotic area. The usual clinical hallmark is non–exercise-related pain.

▶ **Tumor?** The patient is too old for a cortical osteoid osteoma, although that diagnosis would be consistent with lesion morphology. Osteoid osteoma is extremely rare past 60 years of age, and we have no instances of it in our large case collection. Other bone-producing tumors such as periosteal osteosarcoma are not consistent with the location or the nonspecific bone scan, which would be very "hot" in the case of osteosarcoma.

▶ **Regressive process?** Yes, see below.

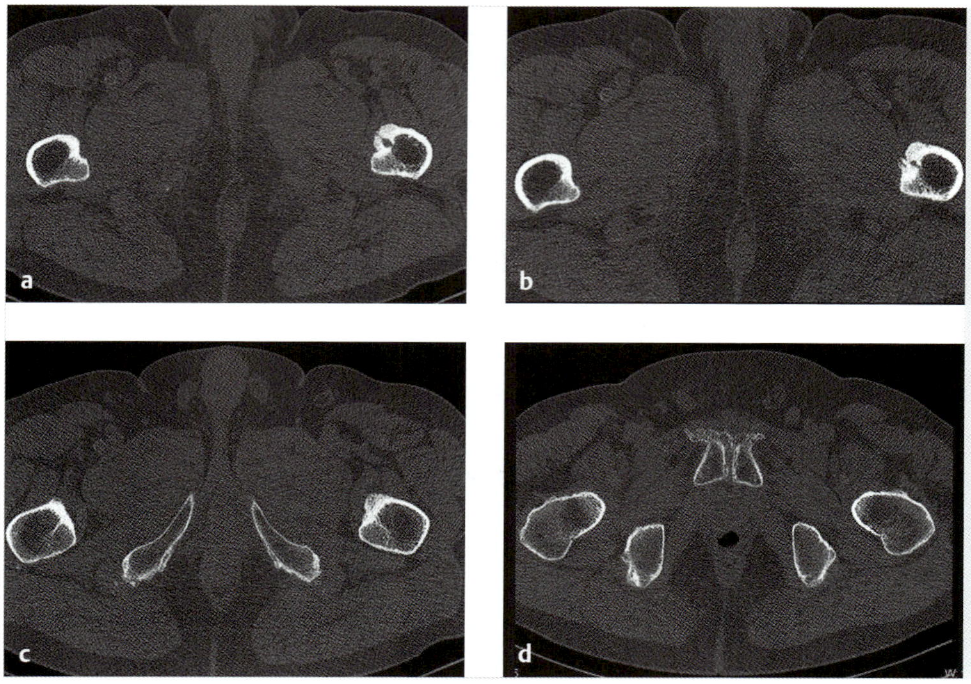

Fig. 4.46 a–d Osteoid osteoma or Brodie abscess?

Synopsis and Discussion

Based on the above considerations, productive fibro-ostosis in the form of a *degenerative enthesiopathy* is the most likely diagnosis. The following findings support this conclusion:

- Unimpressive clinical findings with exercise-related pain
- Location at the attachment of the iliofemoral ligament, which is the strongest ligament in the human body
- Detection of additional sites of enthesiopathic proliferation in the pelvis
- Relatively low uptake in the multiphase bone scan
- Follow-up after more than 1 year shows identical clinical and radiologic findings (not pictured here)

The radiologic lesion in itself would be consistent with a "burned-out" periosteal osteoid osteoma, but that interpretation contradicts the clinical presentation and the patient's biological data (see above).

A stress fracture is extremely unlikely because the patient has no stress.

Other typical cases of degenerative enthesiopathic changes are found in Case 101, Case 102, Case 103, Case 104, and also in ▶ Fig. 4.47, which shows another example of degenerative enthesiopathy at the attachment of the pectineus and/or vastus medialis muscle, but with the interesting differential diagnosis of a double lesser trochanter. The 58-year-old man complained of occasional pain in the left proximal thigh. The patient had a known history of recurrent bursitis over the trochanters. The radiograph and CT scans (▶ Fig. 4.47 **a–e**) show a hyperostotic process on the cortex below the left lesser trochanter. The structure on the actual cortical hyperostosis, which resembles the head of an osteochondroma, is composed of mature bone with its own medullary cavities, which do not communicate with the medullary cavity of the parent bone. This excludes an osteochondroma from the differential diagnosis. The cortical hyperostosis extends several centimeters proximally and distally, which suggests insertional tendinopathy over a broad area. We therefore interpreted the finding as productive fibro-ostosis due to degenerative enthesiopathy. This diagnosis is also consistent with the patient's history. The structure on the cortical hyperostosis that looks like an osteochondroma may be interpreted either as an ossified accessory bursa or myositis ossificans resulting from recurrent muscular bruising. The symptoms resolved with anti-inflammatory therapy, and follow-up at slightly more than 1 year showed no further change (▶ Fig. 4.47 **e**). Since we noted that the medial thigh muscles appeared thicker and denser on the left side than on the right (▶ Fig. 4.47 **a**), we also considered—mostly for academic reasons—a double lesser trochanter with productive fibro-ostotic changes relating to an anatomically faulty or variant origin of the medial thigh muscles. Proving this, however, would have required MRI, which the patient unfortunately declined.

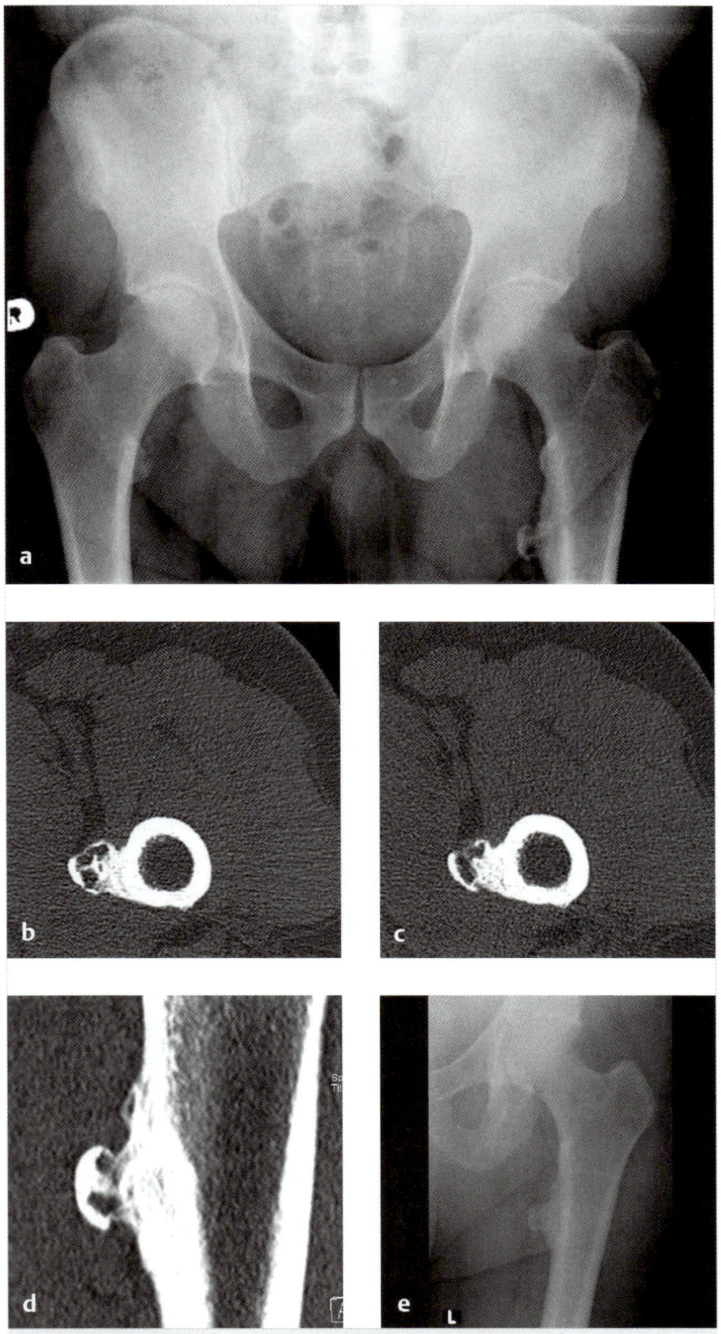

Fig. 4.47 a–e Double lesser trochanter?

Comments

When a radiologic finding is detected by a particular modality (e.g., CT) and is open to varying interpretations, a correct diagnosis can be made by obtaining additional radiologic, clinical, localizing, and biological data. In interpreting the above cases with similar radiologic findings, we followed the principle of Ockham's razor, see Chapter 1, since other diagnostic possibilities would have required going to extraordinary hypothetical lengths.

Final Diagnosis

Productive fibro-ostosis due to degenerative enthesiopathy at the attachment of the iliofemoral ligament.

Case 76 (▶ Fig. 4.48)

Case description

- Referring physician: orthopedist.
- Prior history and clinical question: A 32-year-old man had a 3-week history of left hip pain, which was also present at night and worsened with exercise. He claimed that the pain had a sudden onset. He could not recall trauma to the hip. Question: Early avascular necrosis of the femoral head?

Radiologic Findings

T1w MRI (▶ Fig. 4.48 **a**) shows considerable loss of normal medullary cavity signal on the left side, while the T2w image and subtraction image show very high signal intensity in the left femoral head and neck (▶ Fig. 4.48 **b**). Radiographs taken 9 weeks later ▶ Fig. 4.48 **c, d**) show markedly decreased density in the left femoral head and neck. The remaining trabecular structures are ill-defined, similar to the “eraser or India-rubber sign” in osteomalacia.

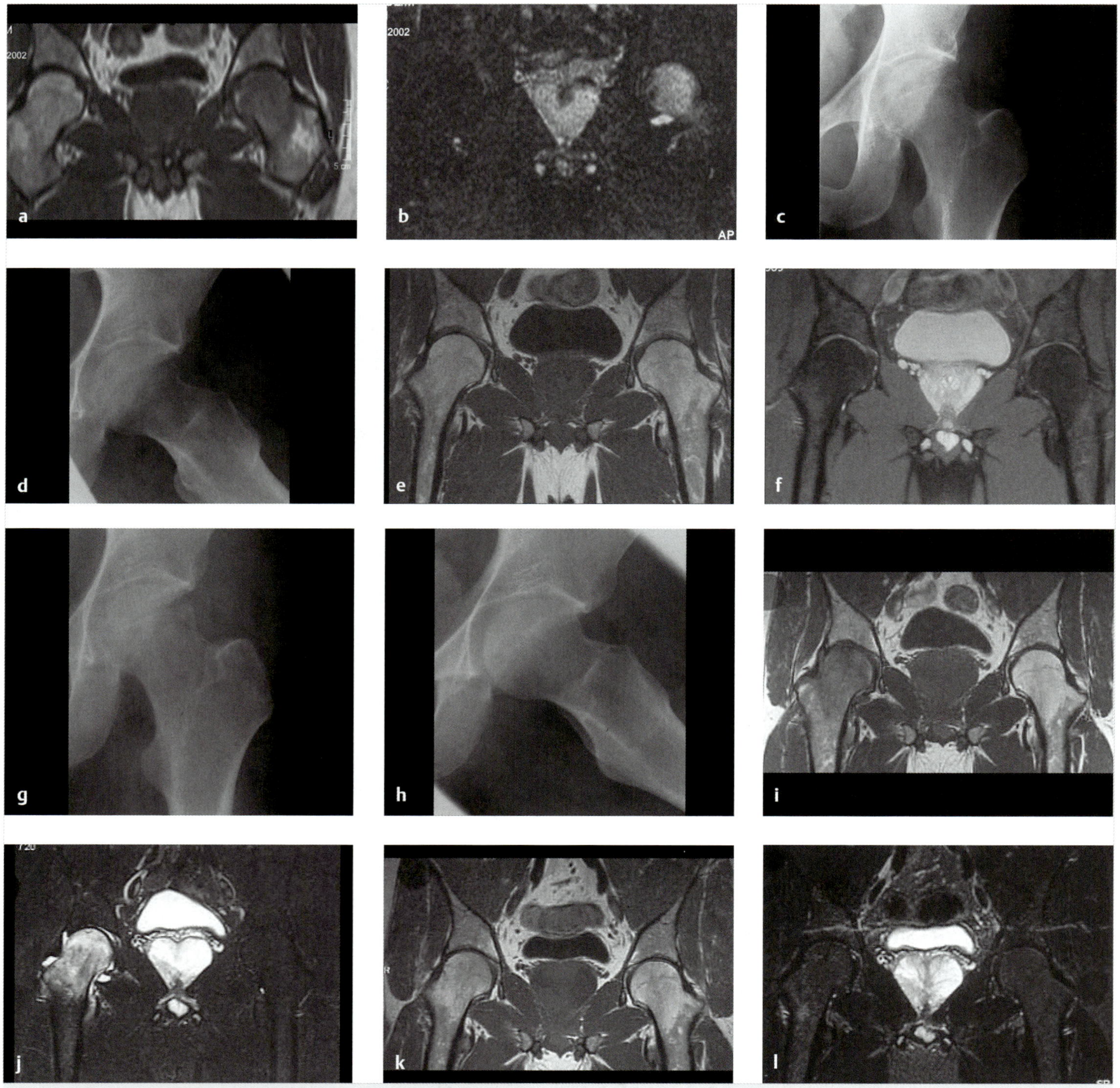

Fig. 4.48 Incipient avascular necrosis of the left femoral head? The first two images (**a, b**) were taken in September 2002, followed by two in December of that year (**c, d**). Later images were acquired at follow-up in January 2003 (**e, f**), at follow-up in March 2003 (**g, h**), at follow-up in October 2006 (**i, j**), and at follow-up in April 2007 (**k, l**).

Pathoanatomic Background of the Findings

The signal changes in the left femoral head and neck indicate a proton-rich process that is uniformly distributed in these anatomic structures. The decreased radiographic density probably results from secondary osteoclast stimulation, and the ill-defined trabeculae from increased osteoid formation by stimulated osteoblasts.

Assignment to a Possible Basic Entity

► **Normal variant or malformation?** No, the clinical and radiologic findings indicate a definite pathologic process, which excludes a normal variant. A corresponding malformation is not known to occur at this location.

► **Trauma?** The history elicited no evidence of acute or chronic trauma.

► **Inflammation?** No clinical manifestations (fever, elevated inflammatory markers, effusion, etc.).

► **Tumor?** No, there is no evidence of bone destruction or new bone formation (see also under Pathoanatomic Background of the Findings above).

► **Perfusion defect?** Yes, see Synopsis and Discussion below.

Synopsis and Discussion

The clinical presentation (pain of sudden onset) and radiologic appearance (signs of edema and osteomalacia) indicate a disease process associated with edema formation, demineralization, and increased osteoid formation in the proximal femoral epimetaphysis. Since we have eliminated trauma, inflammation (e.g., coxitis, osteomyelitis), and tumor (osteoid osteoma, etc. do not fit the history), we are left with idiopathic, (probably) *transient bone marrow edema with osteoporosis of sudden onset.* We recommended that the referring orthopedist treat the patient with a bisphosphonate (Fosamax for osteoclast inhibition and pain relief) and non-weight-bearing on the affected hip (crutch walking only) for at least 6 weeks. Non-weight-bearing is intended to prevent fracturing, especially at the subchondral level, with the development of secondary osteonecrosis. We also recommended therapeutic exercises plus training on a bicycle ergometer and swimming. After 6 weeks, weight-bearing was incrementally increased by 10 kg/week according to pain tolerance.

By 6 months the patient was able to bear full weight on the hip with no complaints. MRI follow-up at 4 months had already confirmed the complete resolution of edema (► Fig. 4.48 **e, f**). Radiographic follow-up at 6 months documented complete regression of osteoporosis. This course identified the condition as transient edema with transient osteoporosis. Four years later the same symptoms appeared on the contralateral side, where MRI showed pronounced edema-like signal (► Fig. 4.48 **i, j**). It also showed a small, subchondral, distally convex linear signal void, probably representing a fracture line (► Fig. 4.48 **i, j**). Vande Berg et al.[40] ascribe no prognostic significance to this finding as long as it is less than 4 mm wide and less than 12.5 mm long (see also Freyschmidt 2008).[13] The same treatment regimen was followed as before, and by 5 months all clinical symptoms and MRI changes had resolved (► Fig. 4.48 **k, l**). Radiographs in this instance showed no osteoporosis. The overall course can now be classified as *migrating transient bone marrow edema with and without osteoporosis.*

The initial findings on the left side prompted consideration of *early avascular necrosis of the femoral head,* but the following facts did not support this diagnosis:

- *Clinical presentation:* With idiopathic avascular necrosis, the pain would have a gradual and insidious onset. This usually aggravates the further course of the disease, as the patient continues to bear weight on the affected side for some time.
- *Radiology:* The MRI abnormalities are generally confined to the femoral head. There is a double-line sign with little or no surrounding edema-like signal (edema, inflammation, etc.).

Based on current understanding, a fundamental difference between transient edema and avascular necrosis of the femoral head is that transient bone-marrow edema apparently results from *hyperperfusion* while avascular necrosis results from *deficient blood flow.* Transient bone-marrow edema may give rise to necrosis if the patient continues to use the hip and a subchondral fracture leads to circulatory impairment due to vascular injuries and compression. This does not mean, however, that transient edema is the same as early avascular necrosis of the femoral head.

Final Diagnosis

Migrating transient bone-marrow edema in both proximal femoral epimetaphyses.

Comments

When clinical and radiologic findings have excluded other causes (tumor, inflammation, etc.), a presumptive diagnosis of transient bone-marrow edema should be made without delay. Non-weight-bearing should be strictly enforced to prevent a subchondral fracture and secondary osteonecrosis.

Case 77 (▶ Fig. 4.49)

Case description

- Referring physician: orthopedist.
- Prior history and clinical question: A 55-year-old woman was seen 11 years after undergoing treatment for breast cancer (surgery and postoperative radiation to the chest wall, chemotherapy, and antihormonal therapy). She now complained of pain in both hips, and the orthopedist suspected hip impingement based on his clinical examination. The patient was referred for MRI, which showed abnormalities in the left femoral head and both trochanters. Given the patient's history, the lesions were interpreted as bone metastases. The orthopedist doubted this interpretation and requested a consult.

Radiologic Findings

MRI shows a subchondral abnormality in a triangular segment of the left femoral head. It is hypointense—like the muscles—in the T1w image (▶ Fig. 4.49 **a**) and hyperintense in a water-sensitive sequence (▶ Fig. 4.49 **e, g**). It enhances markedly after intravenous contrast administration (▶ Fig. 4.49 **b**). A similar MRI pattern is found in both greater trochanters (▶ Fig. 4.49 **c, d, f**).

Location

The lesion in the femoral head is located in a terminal vascular bed. The changes in the greater trochanters are located at the attachments of the gluteal muscles and piriformis to the greater trochanter, that is, at entheses.

Pathoanatomic Background of the Findings

The geometry of the lesion in the femoral head, located in a terminal vascular bed, suggests a vascular process that may have either of two causes:

- Impaired venous drainage leading to edema formation and capillary leak, which could explain the contrast enhancement
- Hyperperfusion like that in transient edema (see Case 76)

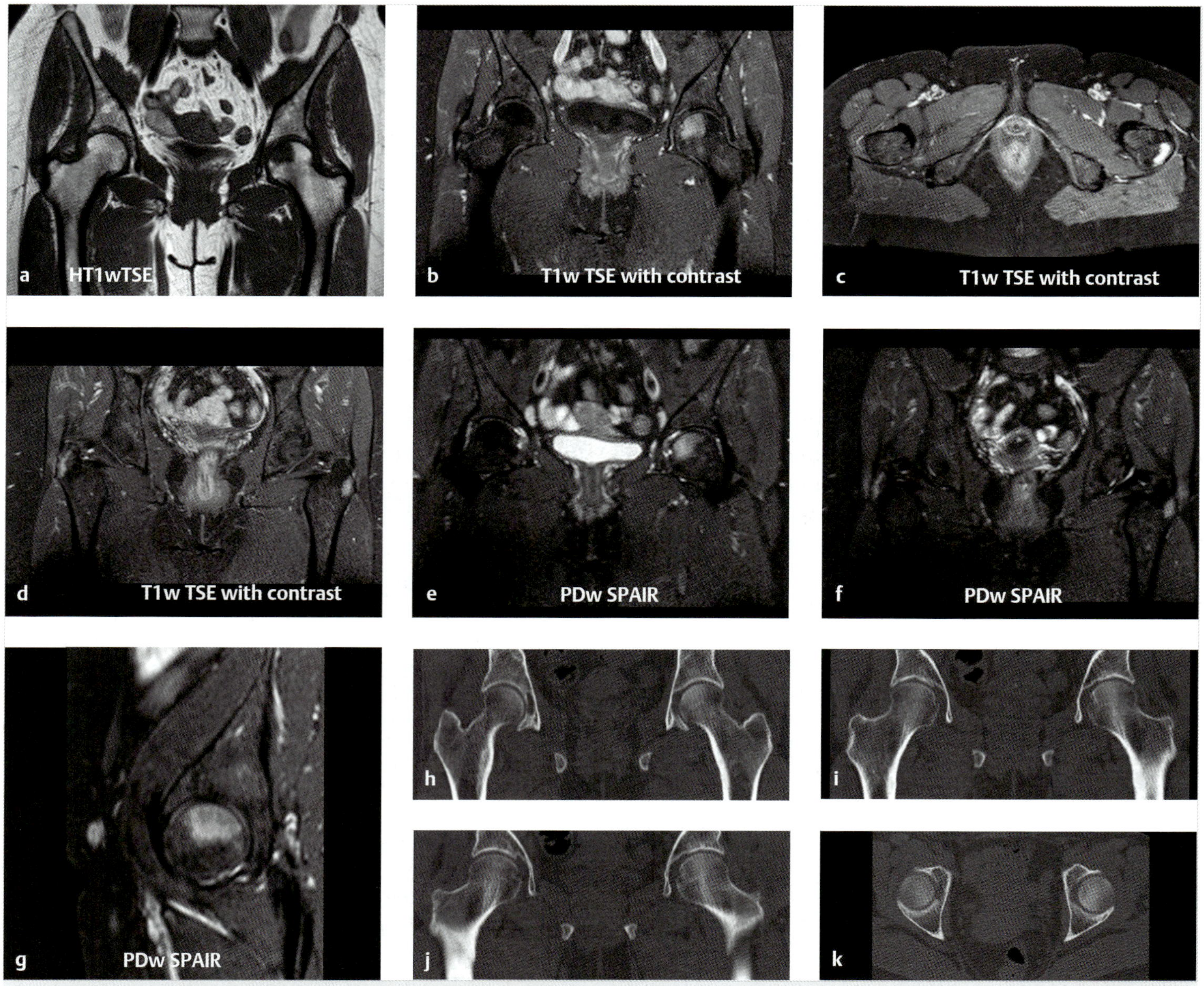

Fig. 4.49 a–k Breast cancer patient: metastases? The last four images were taken 6 weeks later (h–k).

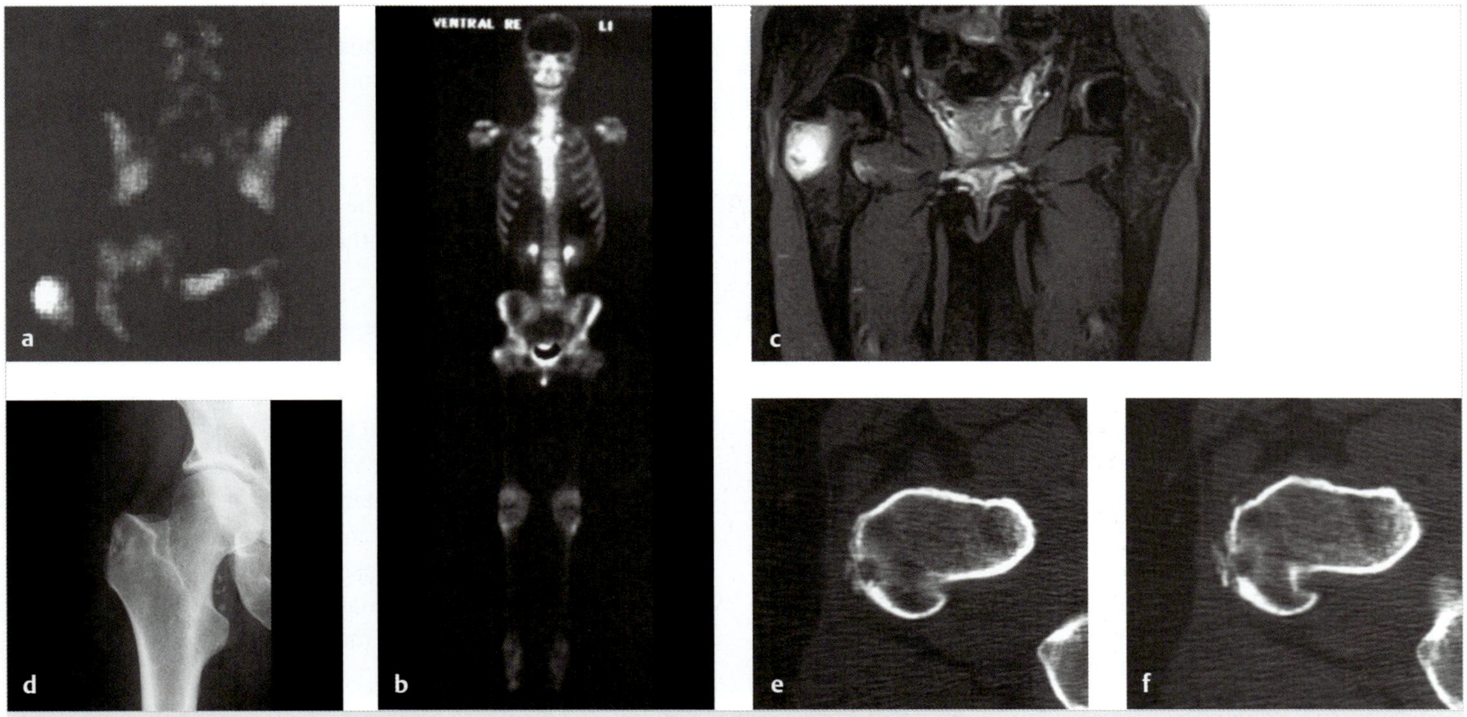

Fig. 4.50 a–f Trochanteric lesion in a 58-year-old breast cancer patient. Metastasis?

The findings in the greater trochanters probably represent reactive osteitis in a setting of insertional tendinopathy or degenerative enthesiopathy.

Assignment to a Possible Basic Entity

► **Normal variant or malformation?** No, there are no precedents in this form.

► **Trauma?** The patient gave no history of acute trauma. The findings in the trochanters might conceivably result from chronic subthreshold trauma to the fibro-osseous junctions, which are at an exposed location.

► **Inflammation?** Not in reference to the femoral head. There is no clinical correlate and no evidence of destructive changes. The changes in the greater trochanters may, however, represent reactive osteitis.

► **Tumor?** No. A metastatic lesion generally shows concentric (centrifugal) growth producing a round shape. But the lesion in our case has a triangular shape. The elongated shape and subchondral location of the changes in the greater trochanters are also inconsistent with metastasis.

► **Perfusion defect?** In the femoral head, yes (see Pathoanatomic Background of the Findings).

Synopsis and Discussion

The radiologic location and geometry of the findings do not support a diagnosis of three metastases (one in the left femoral head and one each in the greater trochanters). Moreover, it is highly unlikely that bone metastases would develop exclusively in both hips after 11 disease-free years following primary treatment for breast cancer.

On our recommendation, CT scans of both hips were obtained 6 weeks later (► Fig. 4.49 **h–k**). The CT images show a subtle geometric pattern of reactive-reparative sclerosis in the femoral head at the site of the MRI abnormality but show no evidence of fragmentation like that in typical osteonecrosis, for example. The greater trochanters also exhibit no destructive changes but do show typical, slightly productive fibro-ostotic changes (► Fig. 4.49 **i, j**).

Ultimately, only a perfusion defect could account for the lesion in the left femoral head. This does not explain the mild clinical features, however (see above), which are more suggestive of degenerative insertional tendinopathy (degenerative enthesiopathy) on the greater trochanters.

► Fig. 4.50 illustrates the case a 58-year-old woman with a history of breast cancer (treated 1 year earlier) who had suffered severe right hip pain for several weeks. Extreme tenderness was noted over the right greater trochanter. A radiologist known to the patient recommended an ^{18}F-FDG PET scan (► Fig. 4.50 **a**), which showed a hypermetabolic focus in the area of the right trochanter. The finding was considered suspicious for metastasis ("What else could it be?"). Whole-body bone scintigraphy to detect or exclude additional metastases showed intense uptake in the right greater trochanter with no other abnormalities (► Fig. 4.50 **b**). Procurement of a simple radiograph was withheld due to concerns about radiation exposure, and MRI, deemed to be more specific, was ordered instead. It showed a hyperintense focus in the right trochanter. The overall impression was that of a "typical metastasis from known breast cancer." Her gynecologist did not believe that a metastasis fitted the prior history of a very small primary tumor, and he requested a consult. We obtained a long-overdue radiograph (► Fig. 4.50 **d**), which showed an osteolytic area with calcifications at the border of the greater trochanter. Calcifications were also noted medial to the femoral neck. The overall impression is calcifying bursitis of the iliopectineal bursa and the bursae around the greater trochanter. The trochanteric bursitis had eroded the adjacent bone, similar to the complicated bursitis of the greater tuberosity shown in Case 101. The lesson from this case is: *Never use an imaging modality whose interpretation is still evolving for the initial investigation of clinical symptomatology!* Even an erosive bursitis with reactive osteitis needs glucose! Scintigraphy cannot increase the specificity of a glucose PET scan, because bone scintigraphy gives information on bone turnover while glucose PET supplies information on glucose metabolism and energy consumption. MRI was added in this case but did not provide a more specific solution because it measures proton density and relaxation times. A simple radiograph could have steered the investigation in a more rational direction by supplying concrete information on bone status, as X-rays provide direct visualization of bone. We then clarified the radiographic findings by adding circumscribed low-dose CT (10 scans at a 2-mm slice thickness), which clearly demonstrated bone erosion by calcifying bursitis (▶ Fig. 4.50 **e, f**). This case reaffirms that calcifications which can advance the diagnosis are detected most accurately and easily by radiography and/or CT. A major advantage of radiography, besides its expediency, is the fact that the radiologist can call upon well-established memory engrams when reading the films (see also Chapter 1).

The "high radiation risk" of radiographs and CT should not justify the use of modalities that do not employ ionizing radiation when those modalities are still more or less in the clinical testing stage and yield too many false-positives. Stoking or exploiting radiation fears may lead to disastrous misinterpretations.

Final Diagnosis

Transient perfusion defect in the left femoral head; insertional tendinopathy (degenerative enthesiopathy) of the greater trochanters.

Comments

Radiologic skeletal abnormalities in a patient with a tumor history should not be hastily interpreted as metastases, especially if the tumor biology and history (e.g., a very long disease-free interval) suggest a low probability of metastasis. There are diagnoses other than "metastasis," and they can be discovered when the morphology and location of radiologic abnormalities are systematically interpreted. It is also important to consider the emotional response of patients and family members to a diagnosis of metastasis.

5 Shoulder Girdle and Thoracic Cage

5.1 Clavicle

Case 78 (▶ Fig. 5.1)

Case description

- Referring physician: orthopedist.
- Prior history and clinical question: A 21-year-old man was examined radiologically for multiple injuries. A radiograph of the left clavicle showed a defect in the inferior border just lateral to the head of the clavicle (the medial or sternal end of the clavicle). Before ordering biopsy, the orthopedist wanted to know what the defect might represent.

Radiologic Findings

A semicircular defect is visible in the inferior border of the clavicle just lateral to the clavicular head (see arrows in ▶ Fig. 5.1 **a**). A subsequent whole-body bone scan (▶ Fig. 5.1 **b**) appears normal. Slightly increased uptake in the manubriosternal synchondrosis is considered appropriate for age.

Location

The defect is located at the attachment of the costoclavicular ligament. This was also seen in CT scans, which are not reproduced here because the case can be solved without them (see Assignment to a Possible Basic Entity below). A similar but very subtle finding was also noted on the contralateral side.

Pathoanatomic Background of the Findings

The tissue structure replacing the bone is not associated with increased bone turnover (negative bone scan)—that is, it does not incite a perifocal reaction, and it does not form a matrix (e.g., bone, cartilage, ossifying connective tissue).

Assignment to a Possible Basic Entity

▶ **Normal variant or malformation?** Yes. The very fact that the defect was detected incidentally and was negative on the bone scan suggests a normal variant. When we consider its location (see above), it is reasonable to assume that we are dealing with a normal variant.

▶ **Trauma, inflammation, tumor?** The negative history and negative bone scan exclude these basic entities from a realistic differential diagnosis.

Synopsis and Discussion

The apparent defect in the undersurface of the clavicle, just lateral to the medial end of the clavicule (clavicular head), is called a "ligament groove" in the literature and corresponds to the attachment of the costoclavicular ligament.[17] This attachment site generally appears radiographically as a more or less pronounced irregularity in the contour of the bone. In extreme cases it forms an actual groove and appears as a well-defined defect, especially when the shoulder girdle has been subjected to particularly high mechanical stresses. This is not necessarily an insertional tendinopathy in the form of a rarefying fibro-ostosis, as this would show at least slightly increased tracer uptake on the bone scan. Similar findings are known to occur in the femoral neck (see Case 69 and Case 73), the ischia, at the pectoralis attachment (see images in Case 102, Case 103, and Case 104), and at other sites.

Final Diagnosis

Ligament groove at the attachment of the costoclavicular ligament, considered a normal variant.

Comments

The key to the correct interpretation of a radiologic finding often lies in its location.

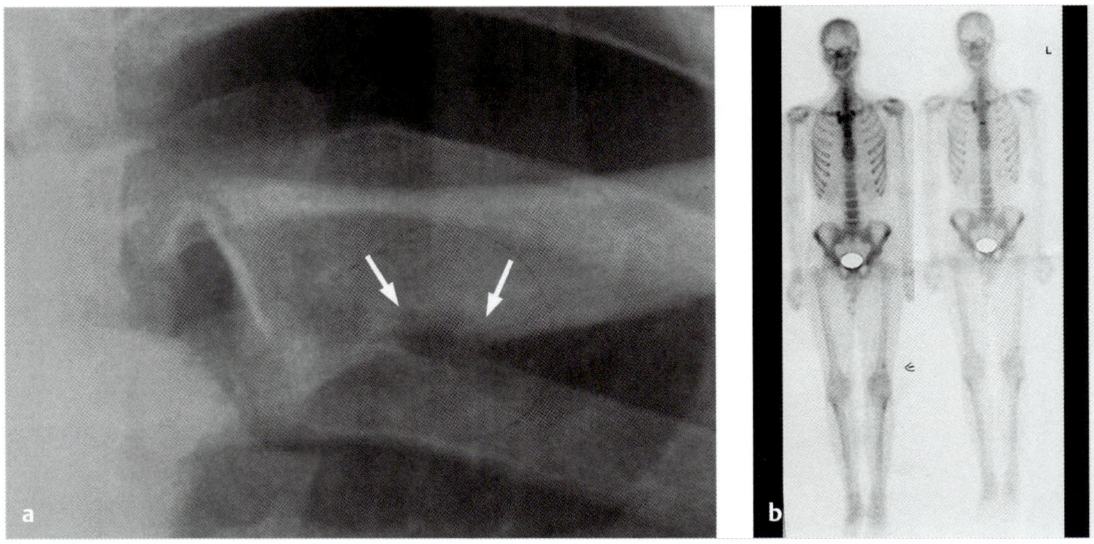

Fig. 5.1 a, b Tumor? Excisional biopsy?

Case 79 (▸ Fig. 5.2)

Case description

- Referring physician: radiologist.
- Prior history and clinical question: A 37-year-old woman, otherwise healthy, felt a lump in her left supraclavicular fossa. She stated that many years ago she had suffered head and neck sprains in a motor vehicle accident but could recall no further details. The radiologist wanted to know the origin of the finger-shaped structure at the junction of the neck and shoulder. Malformation?

Radiologic Findings

The radiograph in ▸ Fig. 5.2 shows a finger-shaped bony structure that follows the lateral border of the trapezius muscle and widens from above downward in a trapezoidal pattern. A kind of pseudarthrosis is noted at the center of the structure. The acromial end of the clavicle shows pencil-like tapering and is surrounded by a club- or cuff-shaped ossification.

Location

As stated above, the ossified structure follows the lateral border of the trapezius muscle. The peripheral end of the left clavicle has vanished. In terms of vascular anatomy, this area represents a terminal vascular bed with a critical blood supply. The finger-shaped ossification on the lateral side of trapezius appears connected to the lateral cuff-shaped structure by the clavicular attachment of the trapezius muscle.

Pathoanatomic Background of the Findings

The oblong structure at the lateral junction of the neck and shoulder is composed of solid bone with a cortex and medullary cavity, causing it to resemble a finger. The bony cuff around the tapered peripheral clavicle is also composed of solid bone.

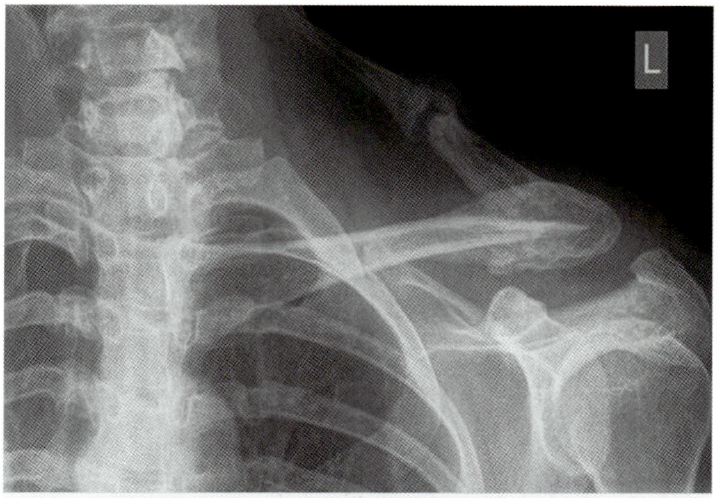

Fig. 5.2 Malformation?

Assignment to a Possible Basic Entity

▸ **Normal variant or malformation?** A kind of accessory bone called the os omovertebrale (Latin *om* = shoulder) located at the junction of the shoulder and lateral neck has been described in the literature.[17] It is known to occur in Klippel–Feil syndrome. The finger-shaped bony structure could very well be an os omovertebrale, but the cervical vertebrae that appear in the radiograph do not show any gross signs of Klippel–Feil syndrome such as blocking. Could this be due to trauma?

The ossifications could be a result of old myositis ossificans (heterotopic ossification) caused by trauma. This would be consistent with the patient's history.

▸ **Inflammation or tumor?** This diagnosis would not be consistent with the clinical presentation or radiologic findings.

Synopsis and Discussion

The finger-shaped structure most likely represents a mature form of myositis ossificans traumatica. The pseudarthrosis is explained by its location, which is the site that undergoes the greatest deformation when the arm is raised and lowered. A diagnosis of myositis ossificans traumatica is also supported by the changes in the peripheral clavicle: The trauma probably caused a fracture of the peripheral clavicle or an acromioclavicular joint separation, leading to the development of avascular acro-osteolysis or acronecrosis (see also Case 93), which is a fairly common result of trauma to the peripheral clavicle. The "licked candy stick" appearance is considered proof of acro-osteolysis or acronecrosis. The club-shaped ossification around the tapered peripheral end of the clavicle probably also represents a mature myositis ossificans.

▸ Fig. 5.3 **a–c** illustrates another case of heterotopic ossification (myositis ossificans traumatica) in the shoulder girdle. The 62-year-old patient suffered a serious shoulder injury with rupture of the left acromioclavicular joint, as documented on the post-traumatic radiograph in ▸ Fig. 5.3 **c**. With a 10-kg weight held in each hand, the distance between the superior border of the coracoid process and the inferior border of the clavicle is two times greater on the left side than on the right—a sure sign of a Tossy stage III acromioclavicular joint rupture. At follow-up 1 year later, a radiograph of the left acromioclavicular joint (▸ Fig. 5.3 **b**) showed bone formation between the left clavicle and coracoid process that followed the exact course of the coracoclavicular ligament and represented heterotopic ossification or myositis ossificans traumatica. This case has another distinctive feature, however: the examining orthopedist noticed a ridgelike or barlike ossification at the superior border of the right scapula (arrow in ▸ Fig. 5.3 **c**), which he could not identify. That feature was most likely a congenital (variant) ossification of the *transverse scapular ligament*, which shows a familial occurrence (Giordano 1962, cited in Freyschmidt's "Köhler/Zimmer" 2001).[17,41]

Final Diagnosis

Posttraumatic myositis ossificans in the lateral portions of the trapezius muscle and surrounding an area of acro-osteolysis (avascular necrosis) at the peripheral end of the clavicle.

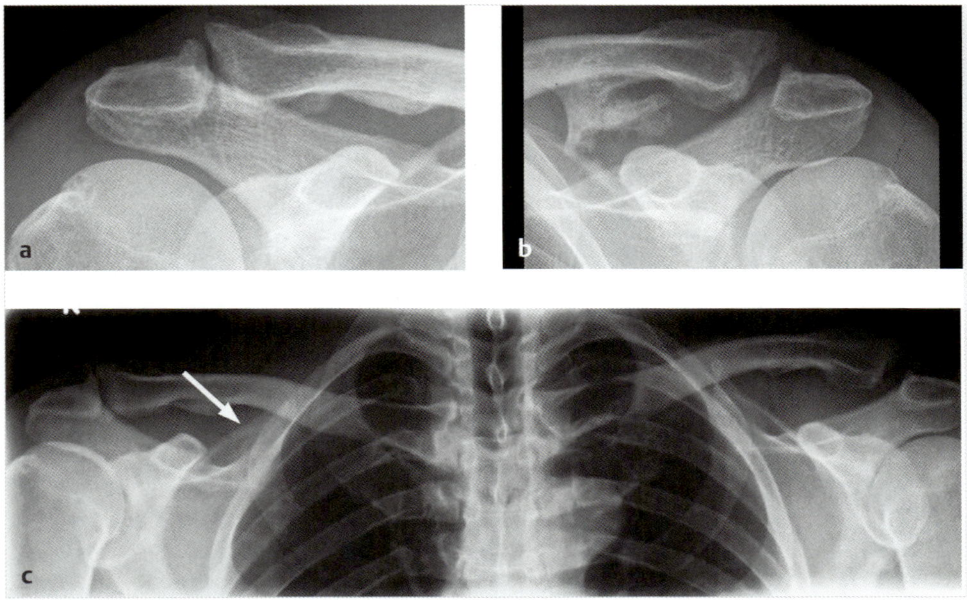

Fig. 5.3 a–c Posttraumatic myositis ossificans in a 62-year-old man.

Comments

Linking together the three key radiologic findings in this case (soft-tissue ossifications in the lateral portion of the trapezius and around the peripheral end of the clavicle, plus acro-osteolysis at the peripheral end of the clavicle) based on their topographic relationship to one another and to the patient's history is sufficient to identify this condition as myositis ossificans and distinguish it from an os omovertebrale.

Case 80 (▸ Fig. 5.4)

Case description

- Referring physician: pediatrician.
- Prior history and clinical question: A 3-year-old girl presented with a painful, palpable, erythematous swelling over the left clavicle. The swelling correlated radiographically with an area of gross bone destruction.

Radiologic Findings

The radiograph (▸ Fig. 5.4 **a**) demonstrates gross bone destruction in the medial half of the left clavicle. The defect is bridged by a cuff of new bone formation The CT scan (▸ Fig. 5.4 **b**) displays the spatial relationships and shows the soft-tissue swelling over the affected site.

Location

The destructive process has destroyed the entire medial portion of the clavicle. Its epicenter is in the medullary cavity, indicating that it may have originated from that area.

Pathoanatomic Background of the Findings

The attenuation values of approximately 50 HU measured in the destructive process may stem from a solid tumor.

Assignment to a Possible Basic Entity

▸ **Inflammation?** The clinical presentation is suspicious for a nonbacterial inflammatory process, given the absence of systemic signs. One possibility is chronic nonbacterial osteomyelitis (CNO; see Case 82 and Case 153), which is typically manifested in the clavicle and often has few systemic signs. This diagnosis is unlikely, however, because CNO generally runs a slower course in which bone destruction and proliferation, predominantly involving the cancellous bone, occur simultaneously and thus produce concurrent radiologic changes.

▸ **Tumor or tumorlike lesion?** The bone destruction affecting the full thickness of the bone and the cuff of periosteal new bone formation are consistent with Langerhans-cell histiocytosis or eosinophilic granuloma.

Synopsis and Discussion

The young age, minimal systemic signs, local clinical findings, and radiologic pattern of change in the left clavicle are fully consistent with an osseous focus of Langerhans-cell histiocytosis (eosinophilic granuloma). Other cases that started with a single- organ involvement are presented in ▸ Fig. 2.17 in Case 9, ▸ Fig. 3.13 and ▸ Fig. 3.14 in Case 24 and ▸ Fig. 4.12 in Case 55). Langerhans-cell histiocytosis is classified as a tumorlike disease of bone.

The differential diagnosis includes the following:

- *CNO* (see section Inflammation? above).
- *Primary bone tumor* such as Ewing sarcoma or osteolytic osteosarcoma. This can ultimately be excluded only by biopsy. These entities, while rare, do occur in the clavicle (Langerhans-cell histiocytosis in approximately 4% of cases, Ewing sarcoma in 2%, osteosarcoma in less than 1%).

The diagnosis in the present case was confirmed by biopsy.

To aid in the differentiation of lytic clavicular lesions, two cases of fibrous dysplasia are illustrated in ▸ Fig. 5.5: a 39-year-old man (a, b) and a 22-year-old man (c). The lesions are only slightly

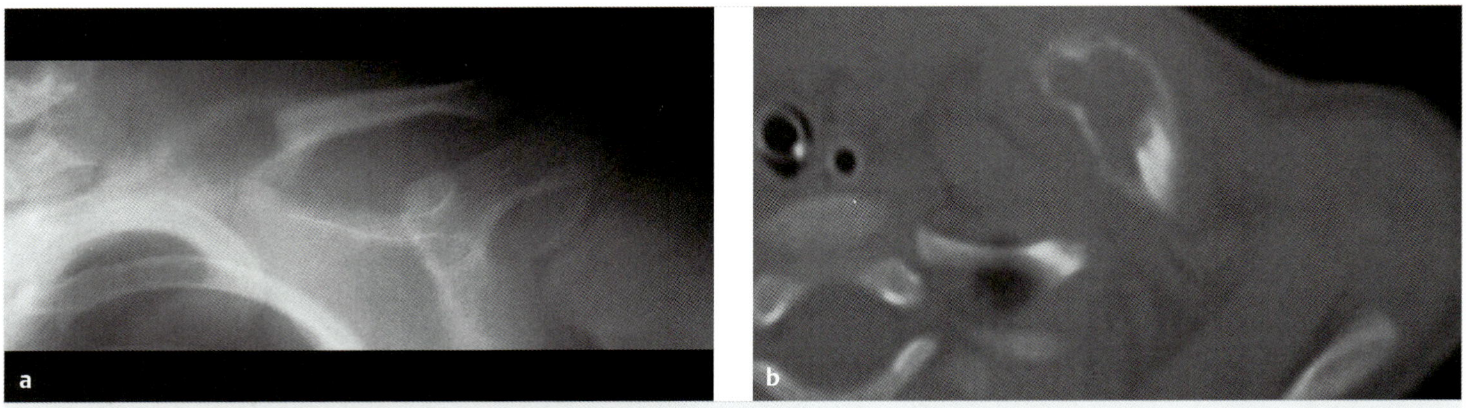

Fig. 5.4 a, b Osteomyelitis? Tumor?

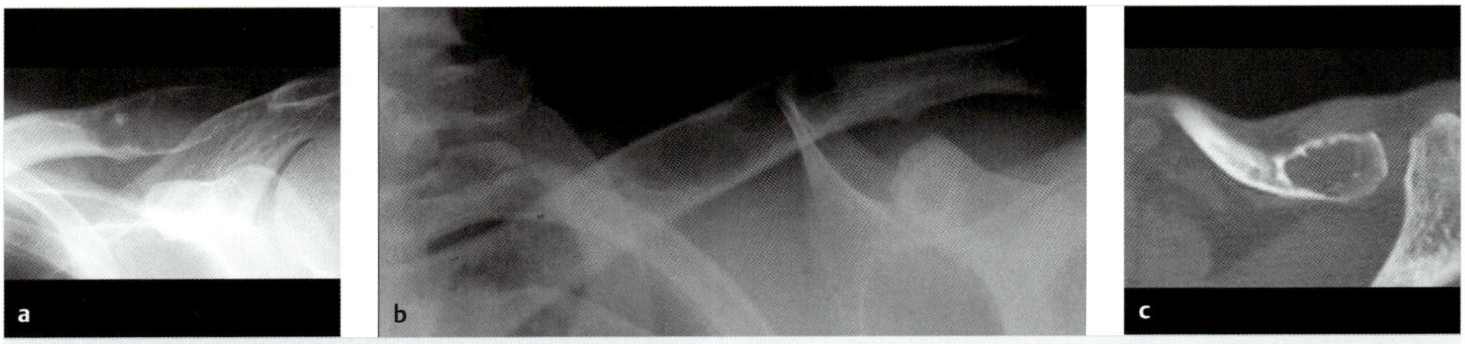

Fig. 5.5 a–c Two cases of fibrous dysplasia for comparison.

expansile, corresponding to Lodwick grade IB, and show some degree of ground-glass opacity; they were detected incidentally. Age, radiology, and lack of clinical manifestations support a diagnosis of fibrous dysplasia (see also Case 7, Case 20, Case 36, Case 37, Case 112, and Case 139); biopsy is unnecessary. Unilocular or simple bone cysts are excluded from the differential diagnosis because they practically never occur in the clavicle. The ground-glass appearance noted above is also inconsistent with this diagnosis. In any case, the differential diagnosis of a "unilocular or simple bone cyst" is meaningless from an oncologic standpoint. Surgical procedures are unnecessary in both cases, provided the lesions are clinically silent.

Final Diagnosis

Focus of Langerhans-cell histiocytosis in the clavicle.

Comments

Langerhans-cell histiocytosis (eosinophilic granuloma) should be the first diagnosis considered in a small child with an osteolytic lesion in the clavicle that has no systemic manifestations but very aggressive radiologic features. On the other hand, well-circumscribed lytic lesions with a Lodwick grade I pattern that are detected incidentally in young adults are more consistent with fibrous dysplasia.

Case 81 (▶ Fig. 5.6)

Case description

- Referring physician: radiologist.
- Prior history and clinical question: A 64-year-old man had a tense, painful swelling above the right acromioclavicular joint. The patient claimed to have had shoulder problems for many years. MRI of the right shoulder showed unusual "cystic" structures in the region of the acromioclavicular joint and adjacent clavicle. Ganglia?

Radiologic Findings

T1w MRI (▶ Fig. 5.6 **a**) reveals a slightly inhomogeneous, hypointense mass in the region of the right acromioclavicular joint. The mass shows multicentric, inhomogeneous high signal intensity in water-sensitive sequences (▶ Fig. 5.6 **b–h**). ▶ Fig. 5.6 **d** clearly shows that some of the hyperintense lesions are located in the peripheral portions of the clavicle and ▶ Fig. 5.6 **e–h** demonstrates that they are located partly above and partly below the acromioclavicular joint, which is no longer delineated. The rotator cuff shows marked degenerative changes. Effusion is present in the glenohumeral joint. The contralateral side, imaged a few days later (▶ Fig. 5.6 **i–k**), shows regressive changes in the acromioclavicular joint plus degenerative changes in the rotator cuff.

Location

The pathologic changes described above have their epicenter in the region of the destroyed acromioclavicular joint.

Pathoanatomic Background of the Findings

The multicentric hyperintense lesions are proton-rich and probably correspond anatomically to loculated synovial or bursal spaces.

Assignment to a Possible Basic Entity

▶ **Trauma?** No history of acute trauma, but possibly chronic trauma.

▶ **Inflammation?** Yes (see Pathoanatomic Background of the Findings above).

▶ **Tumor?** No, at least not a solid tumor.

▶ **Regressive change?** Yes, the rotator cuff is damaged and may well be responsible for the other changes.

Synopsis and Discussion

This case, involving *gross cystic changes in the right acromioclavicular joint*, appears to be extremely rare. In a search of the radiologic literature, we found only one publication,[42] a retrospec-

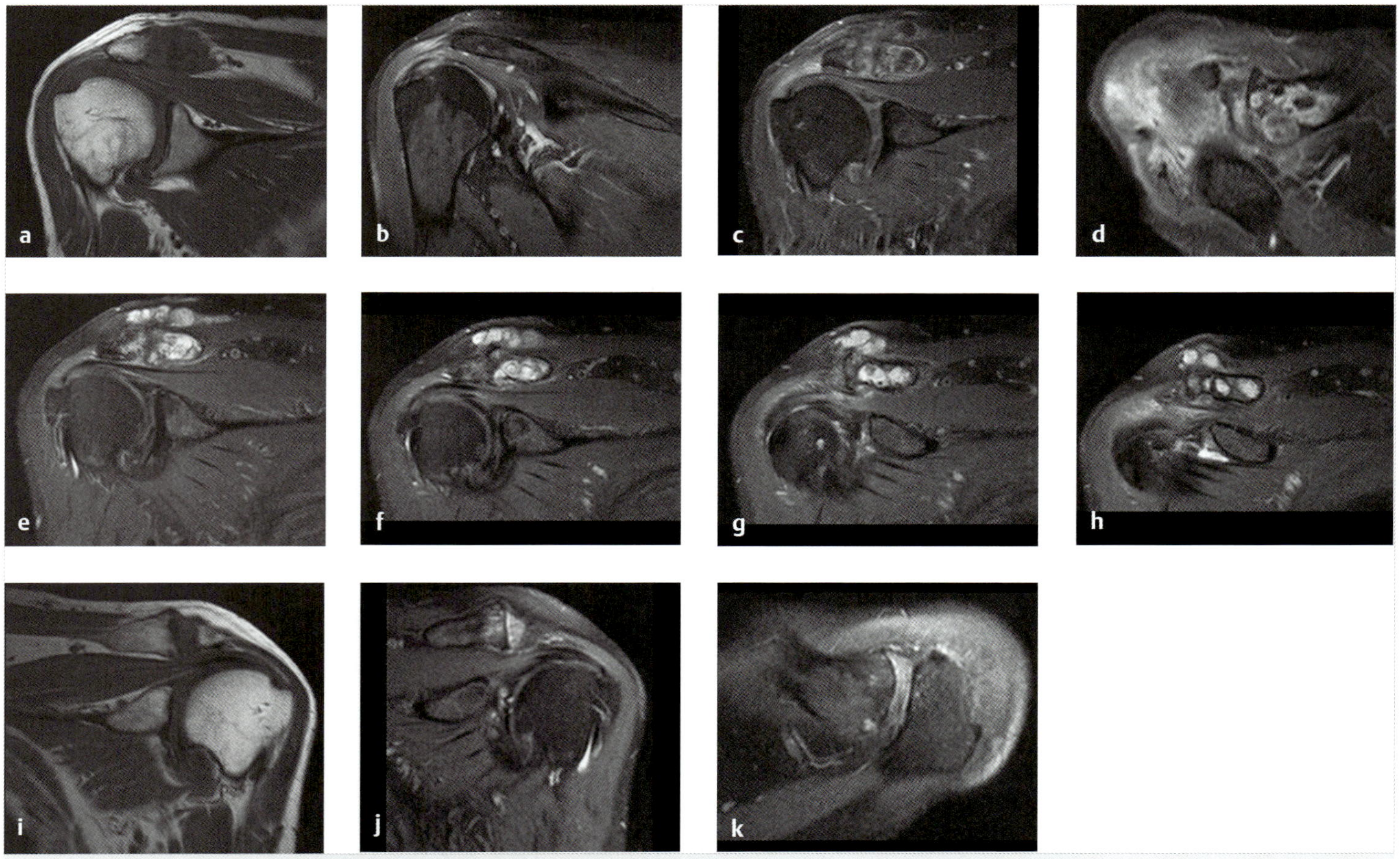

Fig. 5.6 a–k Soft-tissue tumor?

tive review of nine cases, which was helpful in understanding our case. These authors related the pathogenesis of acromioclavicular joint cysts to a large rotator cuff tear, allowing effusion to extend from the glenohumeral joint through the tear into the acromioclavicular joint, eroded inferiorly by impingement, and then perforated outward from that joint. Resorptive changes in the adjacent bones of the acromioclavicular joint are probably pressure-induced. The inhomogeneity of the cystic changes can be explained by primary or secondary chondrocalcinosis or by small deposits similar to rice bodies. Histologically, the cystic lesions were apparently synovial cysts, known also as ganglia. All but one of the patients reviewed by Vogel et al[42] were over 60 years of age.

To prove the spatial connections between the glenohumeral joint on the one hand and the cystic structures in the acromioclavicular joint and its surroundings on the other, we would have liked to inject radiographic contrast medium into the palpable pseudotumor or glenohumeral joint, but the patient declined. This arthrogram would have shown leakage of contrast medium from the glenohumeral joint into the subdeltoid-subacromial bursa and from there into the acromioclavicular joint—a phenomenon known as the Geyser sign.[42] Reportedly this sign confirms a longstanding full-thickness rotator cuff tear. Craig (1984) [43] describes the pathogenic mechanism as follows: The muscle belly of the supraspinatus tendon lies directly below the acromioclavicular joint. Only a thin layer of fat and the bursa separates the joint space from the rotator cuff. On elevation of the arm, the rotator cuff glides directly beneath the anterior acromion, the coracoacromial arch, and the acromioclavicular joint. A positive Geyser sign requires inferior capsular erosion of the acromioclavicular joint. This erosion may result from a gradually enlarging osteophyte on the acromioclavicular joint due to posttraumatic or degenerative change, or there may be mechanical erosion of the undersurface of the acromioclavicular joint by friction from the humeral head—or both. When the patient tries to elevate the arm, the humeral head may engage against the anterior acromion and acromioclavicular joint, increasing the impingement effect. If the rotator cuff tear enlarges, this weakens the function of the external rotators more than that of the internal rotators, and the greater tuberosity is shifted medially and superiorly, causing further trauma to the undersurface of the acromioclavicular joint. The articular cysts may also be interpreted as arthroceles (similar to a Baker cyst).

The differential diagnosis includes *synovial chondromatosis* (see Case 72), which could also explain the rotator cuff tear, but the clinical presentation (patient age, long history, coexisting degenerative changes on the contralateral side) is more consistent with acromioclavicular cysts resulting from leakage in the rotator cuff and in the undersurface of the acromioclavicular joint.

Preliminary Diagnosis

Arthrocele-like acromioclavicular joint cysts with pseudotumor-like extension into the adjacent extra-articular soft tissues and clavicle secondary to a longstanding rotator cuff tear.

Comments

A glenohumeral joint effusion may spread through a rotator cuff tear and perforated into the acromioclavicular joint, producing a pseudotumor in that joint.

Case 82 (▶ Fig. 5.7)

Case description

- *Referring physicians:* radiologist, surgeon.
- *Prior history and clinical question:* A 21-year-old woman had a 3-year history of a recurrent, moderately painful swelling over the left clavicle. She had no significant systemic signs. Her C-reactive protein level and erythrocyte sedimentation rate were slightly elevated. Radiologic findings raised suspicion of osteomyelitis or a neoplasm (e.g., Ewing sarcoma).

Radiologic Findings

The radiograph suggests that medial and central portions of the clavicle have been resorbed and replaced by radiolucent new bone, which appears to have twice the width of the original clavicle (▶ Fig. 5.7 **a**). Scintigraphy shows greatly increased uptake in the affected region (▶ Fig. 5.7 **b, c**). The CT scans in ▶ Fig. 5.7 **d–f** show inhomogeneous new bone formation and soft-tissue swelling on the anterior and posterior sides of the clavicle.

Pathoanatomic Background of the Findings

Findings indicate an active or florid process that has destroyed the original clavicle and replaced it with irregular periosteal new bone. Further differentiation between, say, a neoplastic or chronic inflammatory process cannot be made based on imaging findings alone.

Assignment to a Possible Basic Entity

▶ **Inflammation?** Very likely, occurring in a primary chronic form. This is supported by the clinical presentation (long history, slightly elevated inflammatory markers) and radiologic findings (large volume of new bone, no gross sequestra as in acute osteomyelitis).

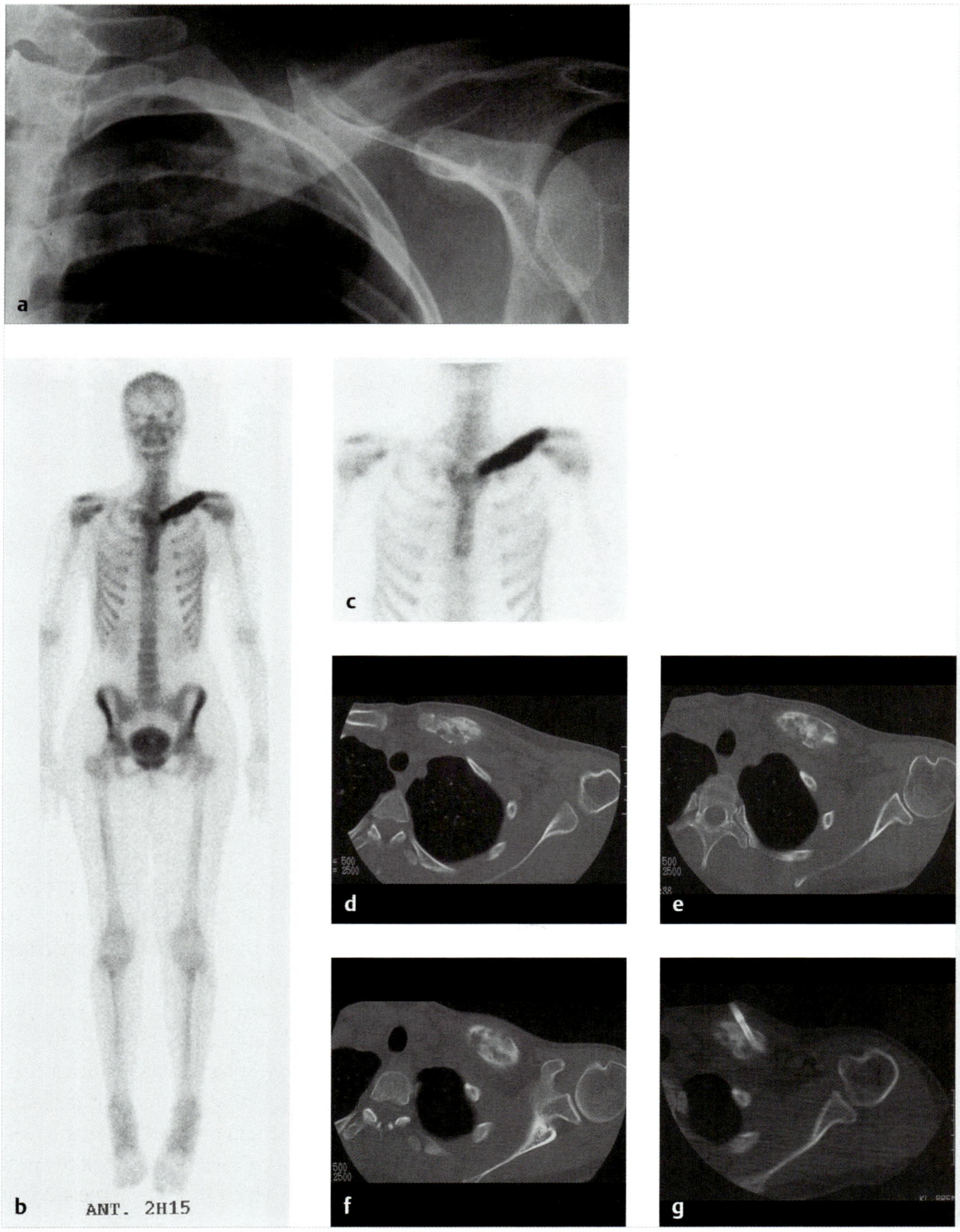

Fig. 5.7 a–g Osteomyelitis or a small- and round-cell tumor?

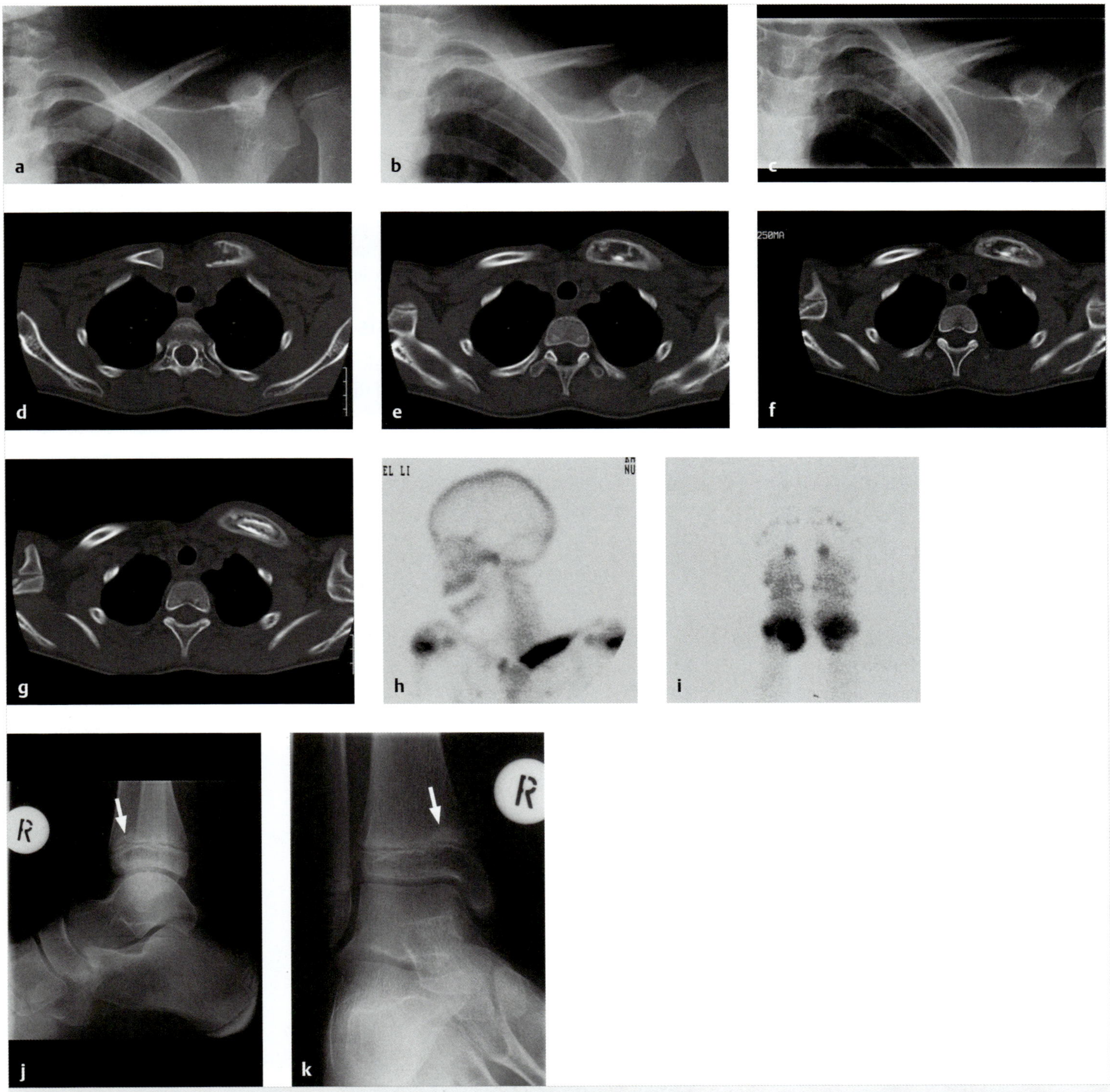

Fig. 5.8 a–k Pustular enthesio-osteitis in an 11-year-old girl.

▶ **Tumor?** Possibilities would include a small and round-cell tumor (e.g. Ewing-sarcoma), a bone-forming tumor (e.g., osteosarcoma, osteoblastoma) or a tumorlike lesion as in the reparative phase of Langerhans-cell histiocytosis (see also Case 80).

Synopsis and Discussion

When we consider the location of the process along with the clinical and radiologic findings, we are most likely dealing with a primary, chronic nonbacterial osteitis or osteomyelitis (CNO). This is known to occur as pustular arthro-osteitis (known more precisely as pustular enthesio-osteitis, PEO) in a setting of pustulosis palmoplantaris, but that condition is most common in children and adolescents. We may also be dealing with an early stage of chronic recurrent multifocal osteomyelitis (CRMO), but we cannot realistically make this diagnosis at present because we do not yet know whether additional foci are present. CNO or CRMO is not a bacterial osteomyelitis but an autoimmune disease characterized by a nonspecific, reactive inflammation of the bone (osteitis) that is currently included in the category of rheumatoid diseases. It is frequently associated with pustulosis palmoplantaris. We tend to regard CNO or CRMO as a special form of pustular arthro-osteitis or enthesio-osteitis (see also Case 39, Case 40, Case 48, Case 49, Case 84, Case 97, and Case 145). The osseous changes in pustular arthro-osteitis or enthesio-osteitis occur predominantly at the entheses, or zones of attachment of tendons, ligaments, joint capsules, and periosteum to bone. Osteitis develops in the underlying bone. Imaging shows a mixed pattern of bone destruction and proliferation, which is best appreciated on radiographs and CT scans. Since the entheses are predominantly affected, the term *pustular enthesio-osteitis* (PEO) would be more appropriate than pustular arthro-osteitis (PAO). We feel that the more widely used term "SAPHO" is too vague and potentially misleading (see Case 40).

In the present case, further questioning of the patient about her history showed that she did have pustulosis palmoplantaris. This made it an easy matter to classify the clavicular changes as pustular arthro-osteitis or enthesio-osteitis.

At the urging of the surgeon, a CT-guided percutaneous biopsy was finally performed (▶ Fig. 5.7 **g**). It yielded a nonspecific, nongranulocytic osteitis and a sterile smear, which confirmed our presumptive diagnosis.

▶ Fig. 5.8 illustrates a case that could still be classified as CRMO but ultimately represents pustular enthesio-osteitis, as we later learned that the 11-year-old girl had a severe pustular form of psoriasis. Her symptoms began with a painful swelling over the left sternoclavicular region with no pronounced systemic signs. The radiograph (▶ Fig. 5.8 **a**) was interpreted as negative. The swelling regressed over the next 3 weeks but recurred 6 weeks later. A radiograph at that time (▶ Fig. 5.8 **b**) showed definite destruction of the medial portions of the clavicle, and new bone formation was apparent at 5 months (▶ Fig. 5.8 **c**). CT (▶ Fig. 5.8 **d–g**) showed a shell or cuff of periosteal new bone around the area of clavicular destruction, which formed a visible bulge. Scintigraphy at that time showed significant tracer uptake in the left clavicle (▶ Fig. 5.8 **h**) and abnormal uptake in the right tibial metaphysis (▶ Fig. 5.8 **i**). Radiographs showed only a minor structural irregularity proximal to the anteromedial epiphyseal plate (arrows in ▶ Fig. 5.8 **j, k**). Langerhans-cell histiocytosis and CRMO were finally included in the differential diagnosis, although the tibial finding was considered to be more consistent with CRMO. Finally an open excisional biopsy was performed, which indicated a nongranulocytic and thus nonbacterial osteitis. Nevertheless, the patient was still placed on long-term antibiotic therapy, which was of no benefit. Anti-inflammatory therapy was finally instituted and provided significant symptomatic relief. Further details on CRMO including its diagnostic criteria are presented in Case 153.

Final Diagnosis

Pustular arthro-osteitis (PAO) or pustular enthesio-osteitis (PEO) with involvement of the left clavicle.

Comments

Mixed destructive and proliferative changes in the clavicle of a young patient should raise suspicion of CNO or, if pustulosis palmoplantaris is present, of pustular arthro-osteitis (PAO) or enthesio-osteitis (PEO). The presence of additional lesions at other sites (e.g., the spine or the metaphyses of long bones) is more suggestive of CRMO.

5.2 Scapula

Case 83 (▶ Fig. 5.9)

Case description

- Referring physician: radiologist.
- Prior history and clinical question: A 67-year-old man with prostate cancer underwent a staging whole-body bone scan (▶ Fig. 5.9 **b**) which showed increased uptake along the superior margin of the left scapula, extending from the superior angle into the acromion. A less pronounced area of intense uptake was also noted in the inferior angle. The corresponding radiograph (▶ Fig. 5.9 **a**) showed enlargement of the superior margin and acromion with a coarsened trabecular pattern. Question: Is this an unusual presentation of metastasis or something else? On repeated questioning, the patient denied having any complaints.

Radiologic Findings

See the case description above.

Pathoanatomic Background of the Findings

There is definitely an active bone remodeling process that has led to enlargement and a coarsened trabecular pattern.

Assignment to a Possible Basic Entity

▶ **Normal variant or malformation?** No, there is no normal variant involving a structural transformation in the upper portions of the scapula.

▶ **Tumor?** No, the geometry of the changes (elongated pattern, not rounded, coarsened trabecular pattern) is not consistent with a tumor or metastasis.

▶ **Perfusion disorder?** No, there is no known precedent in this anatomic region, and a perfusion disorder would not explain the coarsened trabecular pattern.

▶ **Regressive change?** No, what is there in the upper scapular margin that could undergo degenerative changes? There are attachments for muscles and tendons in that area, but degenerative enthesiopathy would not cause such intense tracer uptake or radiographic coarsened trabecular pattern and enlargement with smooth outer margins. Degenerative enthesiopathy would be more likely to cause a rarefying or productive fibro-osteitis with jagged outer margins.

Synopsis and Discussion

All of the above considerations suggest an inflammatory, nonbacterial, chronic bone remodeling process. The lack of clinical manifestations excludes a purely reactive process as in psoriasis or pustulosis palmoplantaris (see Case 84). The only remaining inflammatory osseous process is Paget disease (osteitis deformans) in the active late lytic stage or intermediate stage, although this would be a very unusual site of occurrence (sites of predilection are the pelvis, femur, tibia, and skull). But rare sites of involvement by Paget disease generally occur in the polyostotic form, not in a monostotic form. Even so, the following findings in our case support this diagnosis:

- Age of the patient. Most cases of Paget disease are diagnosed after about 60 years of age, although the disease may develop much earlier. The bone remodeling disorder spreads from the initial focus at a rate of approximately 1 cm/year.
- The absence of any symptoms.
- Typical elongated distribution of highly abnormal tracer uptake on bone scans. This is not characteristic of a metastasis.
- Coarsened trabecular pattern and enlargement of the affected bone area.

We also attributed the small focus in the inferior angle (▶ Fig. 5.9 **b**) to Paget disease based on radiographic findings. Further investigation was unnecessary. Serum alkaline phosphatase was only slightly elevated. Based on the international guidelines, treatment is not indicated.

▶ Fig. 5.10 **a–e** illustrates another case of Paget disease in the scapula, though it is just one of many lesions. This rare site of occurrence is found almost exclusively in the polyostotic form. Additional foci were present in the spine, pelvis (▶ Fig. 5.10 **d**), and left distal femur (▶ Fig. 5.10 **e**). The 65-year-old man was virtually asymptomatic, and the findings were noted incidentally on a whole-body bone scan (▶ Fig. 5.10 **a, b**). His serum alkaline phosphatase level was six times higher than normal. Note the elongated and/or diffuse pattern of tracer uptake in the scapula and

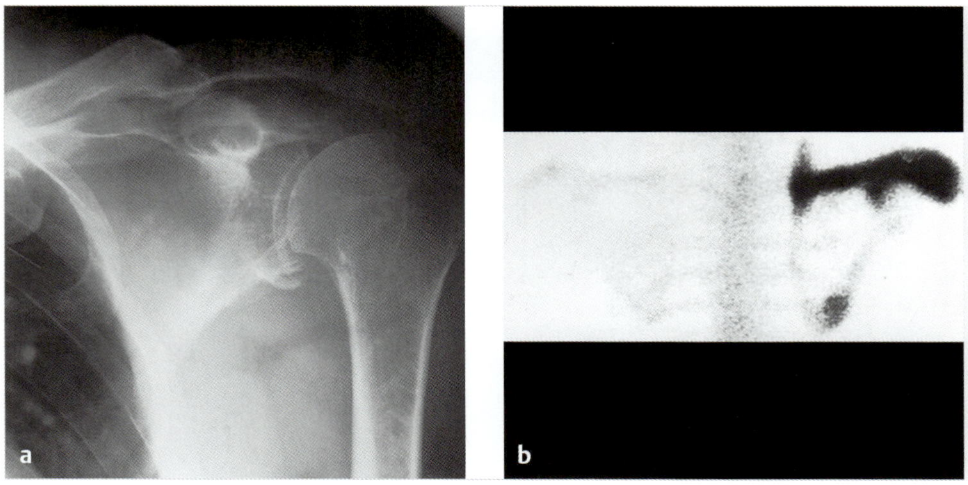

Fig. 5.9 a, b Metastases from prostate cancer?

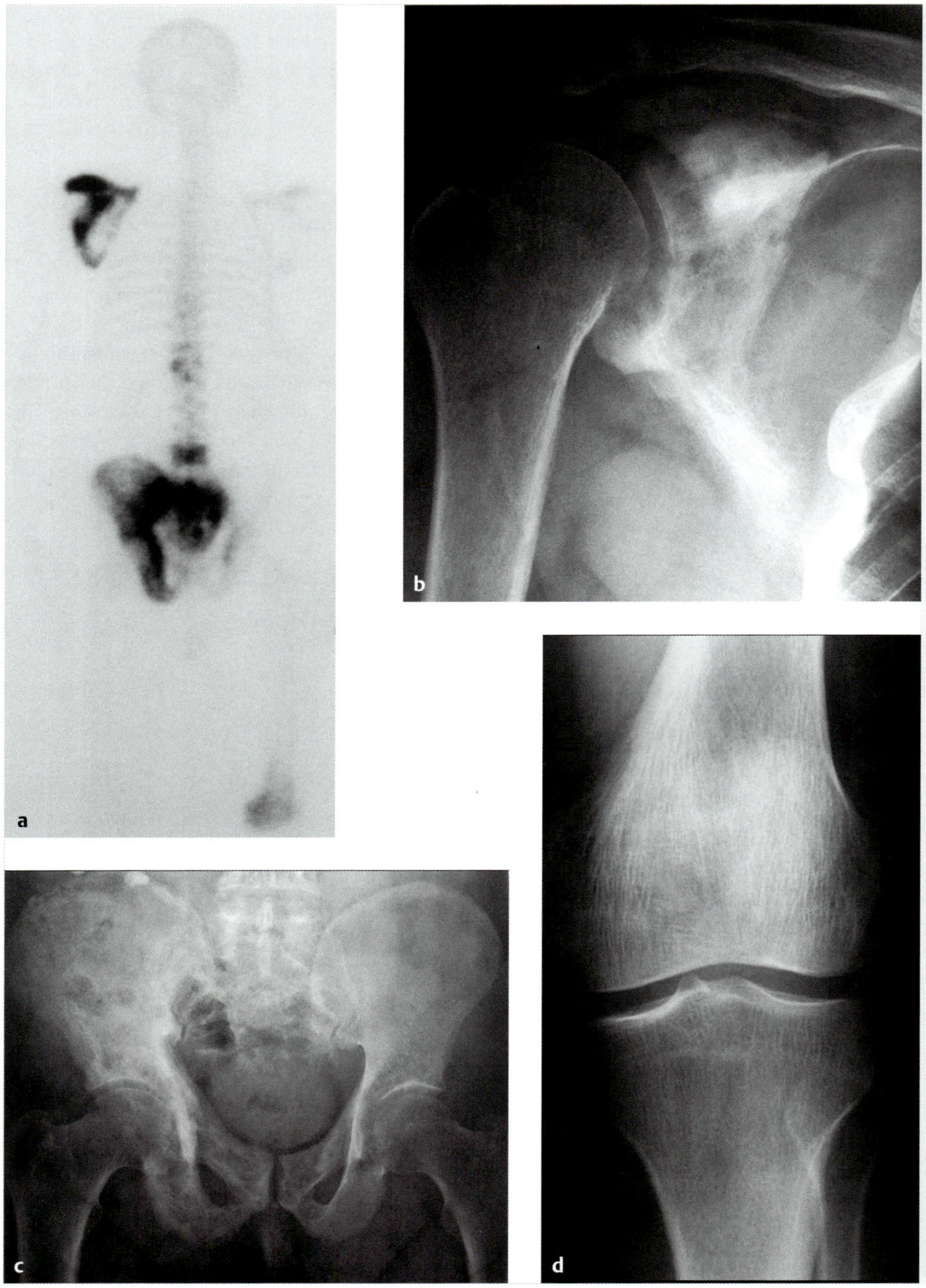

Fig. 5.10 a–e Paget disease of the scapula, spine, and pelvis in a 65-year-old man.

pelvis, which is so typical of active Paget disease. Radiographs of the scapula (▶ Fig. 5.10 **c**) and pelvis (▶ Fig. 5.10 **d**) show a mixed to early, active sclerotic stage of disease, with the distal femur showing a late sclerotic, less active stage (▶ Fig. 5.10 **e**). Other examples of Paget disease are presented in Case 8, Case 9, Case 12, Case 14, Case 46, Case 51, Case 107, and Case 140.

Final Diagnosis

Rare occurrence of Paget disease (osteitis deformans) in the scapula.

Comments

An elongated, continuous pattern of tracer uptake in an older patient generally signifies Paget disease.

Case 84 (▶ Fig. 5.11)

Case description

- *Referral:* self-referral by the patient.
- *Prior history and clinical question:* A 31-year-old woman had an approximately 2-year history of pustulosis palmoplantaris (PPP) (▶ Fig. 5.11 **f**) with a fluctuating course. Symptoms began with pain in the left scapula, accompanied later by pain in the lower lumbar spine. A whole-body bone scan (▶ Fig. 5.11 **e**) showed massive tracer uptake in the upper half of the left scapula with slightly increased uptake also noted around the manubrium sterni and in the L5 and S1 vertebrae. CT scans of the left scapula (▶ Fig. 5.11 **a, b**) showed an extensive sclerotic process, which apparently originated from the periosteum, mainly on the costal side. MRI (▶ Fig. 5.11 **c, d**) showed edema-like signal intensity, especially at paraosseous sites. A radiograph of the lumbar spine (not pictured here) showed predominantly marginal sclerosis in the lower portions of L5 and upper portions of S1. The intervertebral space was obliterated, and the upper and lower vertebral endplates showed slightly irregular margins. A biopsy was taken from the scapula and interpreted histologically as Garré osteomyelitis. Long-term antibiotic therapy was instituted at that point and was followed by some regression of the paraosseous edema-like signal, while clinical complaints persisted. Finally an orthopedist recommended a scapulectomy as a last resort. The patient found that very strange and asked us for a second opinion.

Radiologic Findings

The imaging findings are described above. It should be added that CT and MRI showed thinning and partial resorption of the scapular cortex, predominantly on the costal side. No destructive changes were found in the cancellous bone.

Location

Periosteal new bone formation and paraosseous edema-like signal were found predominantly on the costal side of the scapula,

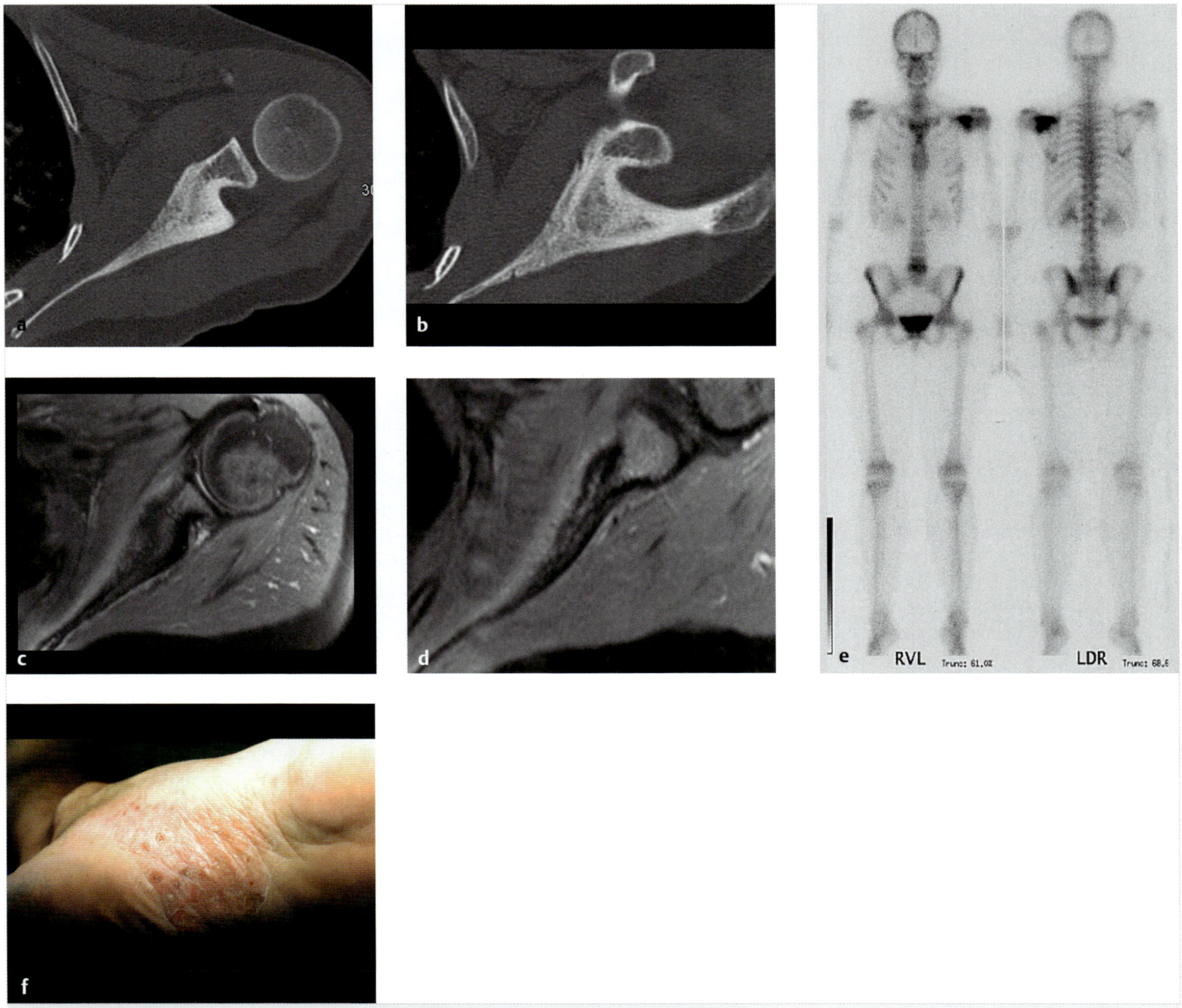

Fig. 5.11 **a–f** Garré osteomyelitis?

suggesting that the epicenter of the changes may lie at the enthesis, or zone of soft-tissue attachment to the bone (subscapularis muscle).

Pathoanatomic Background of the Findings

The findings indicate a mixed destructive and proliferative process whose distribution suggests a chronic active inflammation, very likely arising from entheses on the costal surface of the scapula.

Assignment to a Possible Basic Entity

► **Inflammation?** As stated above, the imaging findings are fully consistent with an inflammatory process. Since it appears to originate from the enthesis, the sclerosis in the scapula would correspond to a reactive inflammation (osteitis). An inflammatory process is also consistent with the changes in L5/S1 (spondylodiskitis) and the relatively subtle scintigraphic changes around the manubrium sterni,

► **Tumor?** No, there is no evidence of a tumor mass. When all pathologic findings are considered together, the scintigraphic and radiographic changes in the lumbar spine do not suggest a tumor such as lymphoma or osteosarcoma and are more consistent with an inflammatory process.

Synopsis and Discussion

The radiologic findings in the left scapula were apparently viewed in isolation and investigated by biopsy in the hope of establishing a clinically useful diagnosis. Histology indicated "Garré osteomyelitis," a catch-all diagnosis for an indeterminate sclerosing osseous process. Garré published a report of his eponymic disease over 100 years ago (1893), and thus before the discovery of X-rays and the establishment of modern microbiology and antibiotic therapy, describing the condition as an acute onset of "fever and swelling of the extremities, pain and marked expansion of the soft tissues that suggests impending abscess formation." He continued, "Instead, the infiltration gradually regresses while fever subsides more quickly, leaving behind only a variable degree of bone expansion while the patient makes gradual progress toward recovery." He published all of this under the title "On Special Forms of Acute Infectious Osteomyelitis."[16] Garré was describing an acute infectious osteomyelitis that heals with bone expansion; he made no mention of sclerosis. That term stems from radiographic terminology used in relation to bone. We have no idea who, ignorant of the original paper, coined the term "Garré chronic sclerosing osteomyelitis," or who then uncritically copied this altered term again and again over the years, but it would make an interesting subject for a dissertation on the history of medicine. From a modern-day perspective, osteomyelitis like that described by Garré would usually be called chronic osteomyelitis arising from an acute osteomyelitis that was treated improperly or too late, or was inherently resistant to antibiotics. Osteomyelitis associated with significant sclerosis, enlargement of the affected bone area, and mild, nonacute clinical symptoms is known as plasma cell osteomyelitis or a Brodie abscess. This differs from reactive forms of osteitis, which are not the same as osteomyelitis because they do not originate from bone marrow due to bacterial colonization. They are reactive processes resulting from an autoimmune disorder, for example, or from an enthesitis like that occurring in seronegative spondyloarthritis.

In the present case, the scapular change was just one manifestation of a systemic disease: pustular arthro-osteitis or enthesio-osteitis (PAO, PEO), known also as *SAPHO*, see Case 40. This is indicated by the following findings:

- Clinical presence of pustulosis palmoplantaris (PPP) accompanied by pain in the left scapula and later in the lumbar spine
- Oligolocular pattern of increased uptake on the whole-body bone scan
- Periosteal enthesitic new bone formation and associated osteitis on CT scans
- Paraosseous edema-like signal on MRI
- Spondylodiscitic changes in L5/S1

These findings are sufficient to make a diagnosis of PAO or PEO and initiate treatment with anti-inflammatory and/or immune-modulating therapy; biopsy is unnecessary. It is important to recognize that pustulosis palmoplantaris is a variant of psoriasis and that psoriasis is not limited to the skin but is a systemic disease that may produce musculoskeletal involvement, cardiovascular changes (hypertension, coronary heart disease), etc. When anti-inflammatory and immune-modulating therapy was instituted in the present case, along with local treatment of the pustulosis palmoplantaris, the clinical and radiologic findings in our patient showed substantial improvement.

For comparison, ► Fig. 5.12 illustrates the case of a child with an *osteosarcoma* in the scapula. The dominant radiographic finding was sclerosis (► Fig. 5.12 **a**) while CT (► Fig. 5.12 **b**) showed fine destructive foci in the scapula with an extensive paraosseous tissue component and spiculations. Sclerosis results from ossification of the osteoid matrix formed by the tumor cells. The de-

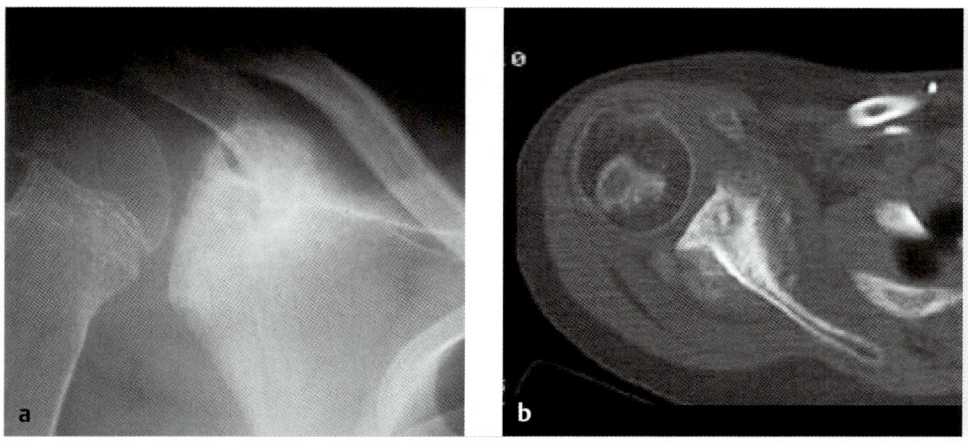

Fig. 5.12 a, b Osteosarcoma of the scapula in a child.

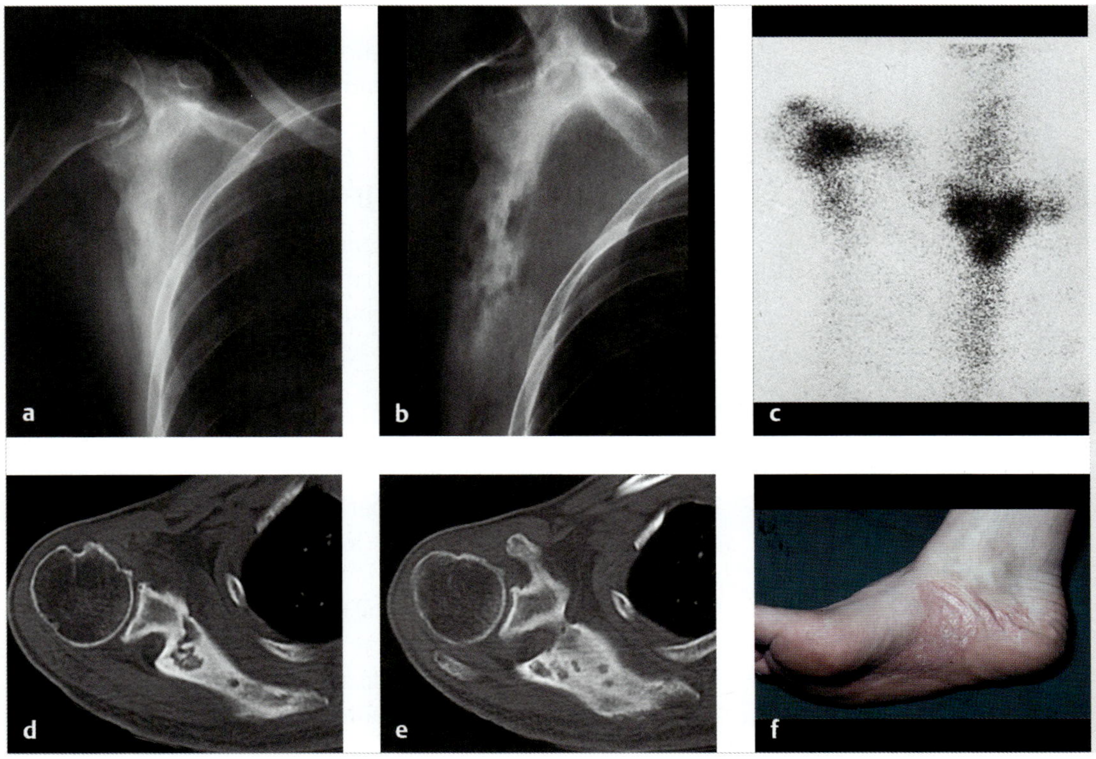

Fig. 5.13 a–f Pustular arthro-osteitis or enthesio-osteitis in a 54-year-old woman.

structive mass lesion and demonstrable matrix ossification clearly distinguish the radiologic features of this case from the case in ▶ Fig. 5.11.

Another case of PAO or PEO, in a 54-year-old woman, is illustrated in ▶ Fig. 5.13 **a–f**. The unusual feature of this case is the presence of small cavities that contain sequestra, which are suggestive of infectious osteomyelitis (▶ Fig. 5.13 **b, d, e**). But the whole-body bone scan showed a bull's head sign in the sternoclavicular region (▶ Fig. 5.13 **c**) and the patient had classic PPP (▶ Fig. 5.13 **f**). These findings were diagnostic, eliminating the need for biopsy. Treatment consisted of immunomodulating therapy with methotrexate, and later cyclosporine, and by 2 years the previously pain-wracked patient was free of complaints. On our advice she later quit smoking, which her dermatologist believed had triggered and/or perpetuated the PPP. A radiologic follow-up at 10 years showed only residual sclerosis of the scapula.

Final Diagnosis

Pustular arthro-osteitis or enthesio-osteitis (PAO, PEO) with involvement of the left scapula and lumbosacral junction.

Comments

Pustular arthro-osteitis or enthesio-osteitis can be diagnosed noninvasively when the radiologic findings are considered within the context of the clinical presentation. Caution is advised with rare (catch-all) diagnoses such as Garré osteomyelitis, especially if they were described correctly in the old medical literature but were later distorted and misinterpreted.

Case 85 (▶ Fig. 5.14)

Case description

- Referring physician: surgeon.
- Prior history and clinical question: A 36-year-old man complained of pain over his swollen right shoulder. He was known to have a multiple exostosis disease, and numerous exostoses had been removed in previous years. The surgeon requested an investigation of the exostoses on the right shoulder.

Radiologic Findings

The CT-pictures in ▶ Fig. 5.14 **a–c,e,g–i** show a bizzare ossified mass around the scapula. The paired images in ▶ Fig. 5.14 (c/d, e/f, and i/j) represent an attempt to compare the CT and MR images, respectively, in the same approximate projections. The imaged exostoses or osteochondromas originate from the base of the acromion (exostosis 1) and, at a lower level, from the growth zones in the costal surface of the scapula (exostosis 2). The CT image of the grotesquely large lower exostosis (exostosis 2) shows a solid and mature central component that is surrounded by fine calcifications, especially on the lateral side (c, e) that are not in contact with the solid portion. Similar calcifications separate from the main body of the exostosis are also visible in ▶ Fig. 5.14 **e, g**. These calcifications are embedded in soft-tissue masses that surround the solid main body of the exostosis and correspond to active, uncalcified tumor cartilage. This is most clearly appreciated on the MR images (▶ Fig. 5.14 **d, f, j**). ▶ Fig. 5.14 **d** shows that portions of the lobulated cartilage cap are up to 3 cm thick.

Pathoanatomic Background of the Findings

The uncalcified cartilage represents the growth zone of the exostoses. A cartilage cap that is 3 cm thick in an adult will almost always contain elements of chondrosarcoma. This answers our standard questions regarding assignment to a basic entity.

Synopsis and Discussion

Patients with an exostosis disease have a 5 to 7% lifetime risk that one of the exostoses will degenerate to chondrosarcoma, usually grade I. There are several signs indicating the development of a *secondary chondrosarcoma:*

- Exostoses located in or near the trunk of the body
- Very large tumor
- Enlargement of the exostosis in adulthood
- Pain, unless caused by an inflamed accessory bursa over the exostosis
- Cartilage cap more than 3 cm thick (a thickness of 2–3 cm makes chondrosarcoma very likely)
- Ossifications located in the tumor cartilage and separate from the actual body of the exostosis (they signal a higher-grade pro-

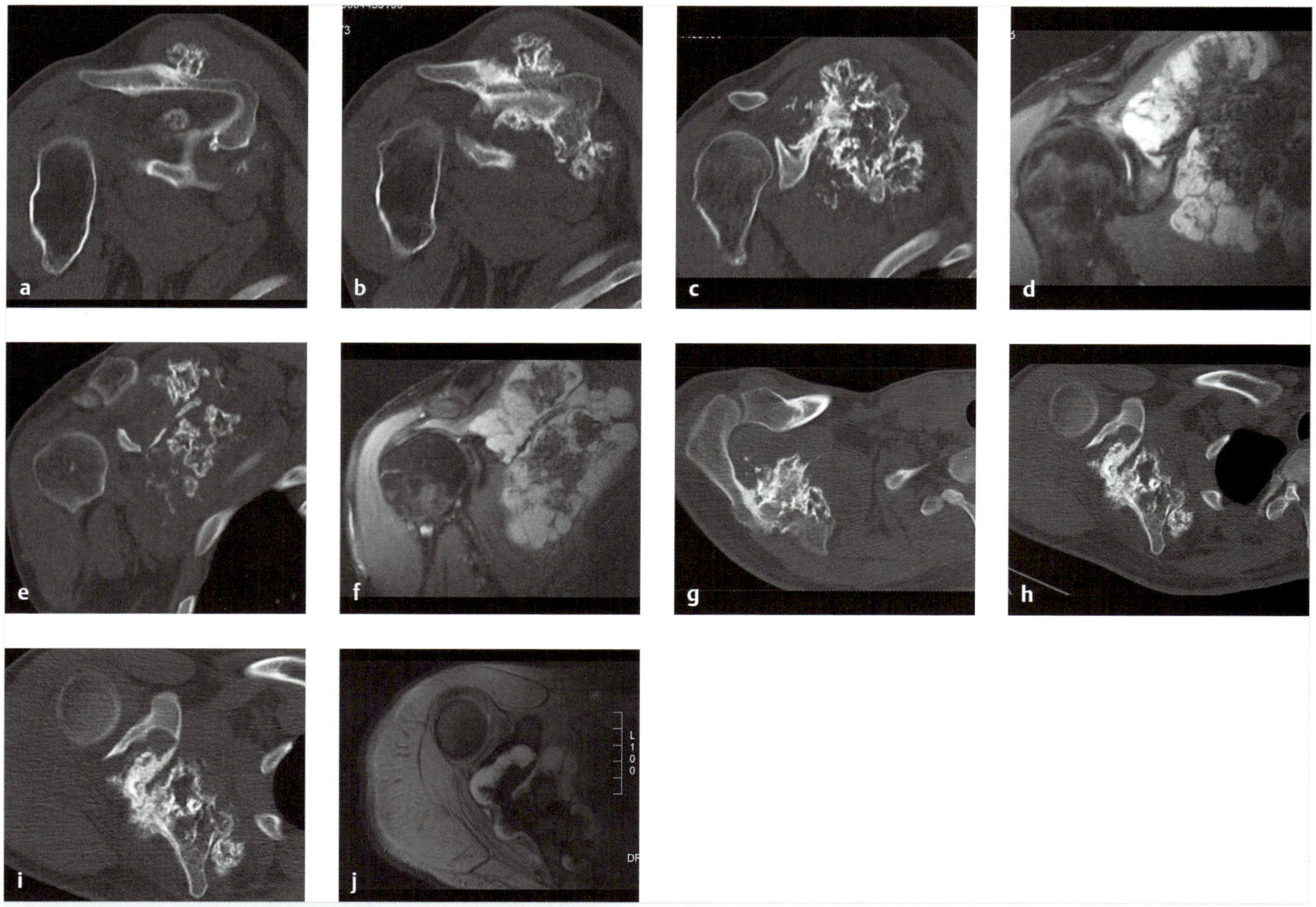

Fig. 5.14 a–j Chondrosarcoma?

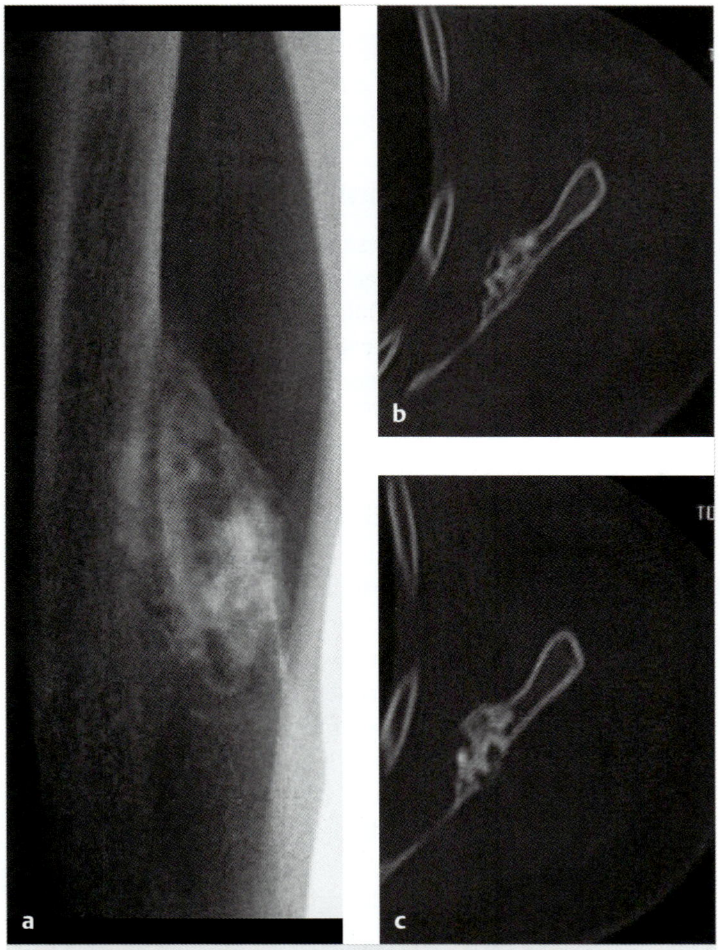

Fig. 5.15 a–c Enchondroma protuberans in a 32-year-old woman.

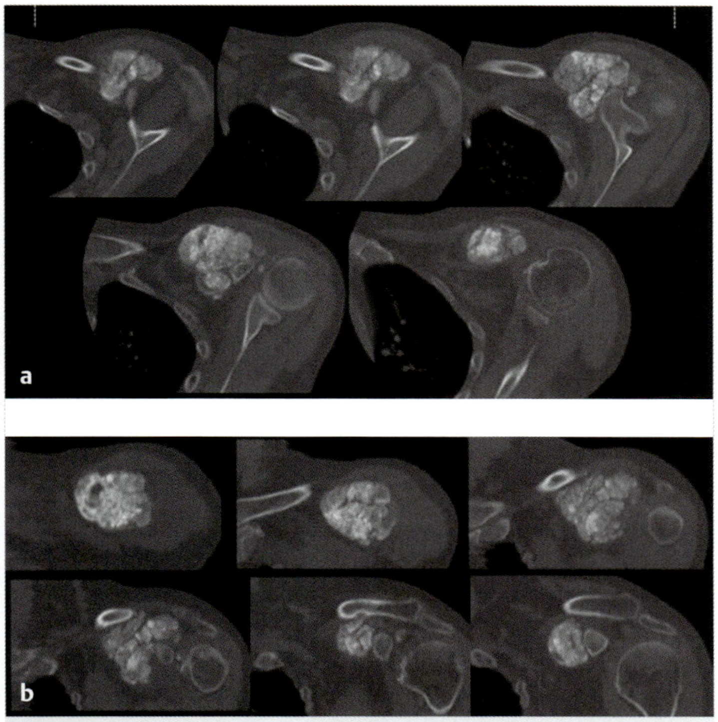

Fig. 5.16 a, b Pseudotumoral calcinosis in a 45-year-old woman.

liferation of tumor cartilage, which hinders solid enchondral ossification)

Both of the latter two criteria are considered definite signs that a secondary chondrosarcoma has formed. Osteochondromas or exostoses with these signs require careful histologic examination with serial sections, as they generally have an inhomogeneous structure. This is also why biopsies are obsolete.

For comparison, ▶ Fig. 5.15 illustrates a harmless *enchondroma protuberans* (an exophytic enchondroma arising from the medullary cavity) in a woman age 32 years at the time of initial diagnosis. The lesion was detected incidentally on a chest radiograph (magnified view in ▶ Fig. 5.15 **a**). A spot film taken 5 years later (not pictured here) showed that the lesion was unchanged. The CT scans (▶ Fig. 5.15 **b, c**) clearly demonstrate how the cartilage-forming tumor grows outward from the medullary cavity, but not like an osteochondroma, which has an extraosseous body and always maintains an open communication with the medullary cavity. Enchondroma protuberans occurs predominantly in small, flat bones, which apparently offer too little room for an actively growing tumor.

To aid further in the differential diagnosis of a large mass of osseous density, ▶ Fig. 5.16 shows the case of a 45-year-old woman with *pseudotumoral calcinosis* in the infraclavicular fossa. The pseudotumor appears as a calcified mass with a coarse nodular structure that is located below the left clavicle and has eroded its inferior surface. The painless pseudotumor must have formed in the past 3 years, since a chest radiograph 3 years earlier showed no significant calcifications in that area and the patient first noticed the mass in recent months. A calcinotic pseudotumor in its early stages is composed macroscopically of an initially soft and later solid mass surrounded by a firm capsule. The cut surface is yellowish or dirty white in color, and its multicystic structure gives it a honeycomb appearance. Some of the cysts are separated by very thick septa. The cysts contain a white to grayish-white liquid or flaky calcified material that is composed chemically of calcium phosphate and/or calcium carbonate. Metaplastic ossifications may also develop. The disease is often bilateral and occurs on extensor surfaces; its etiology is unknown. A familial incidence has been described. Some patients also have hyperphosphatemia with normocalcemia and decreased renal phosphate excretion. This probably accounts for sporadic reports of successful treatment with phosphate binders. Males in the first and second decades are most commonly affected, though the disease may occur at any age. It appears that most patients have no clinical complaints despite the sometimes grotesque tumor mass. Nerve compression may occasionally occur. The only effective treatment at present is surgical excision.

Final Diagnosis

Secondary chondrosarcoma, which developed in the largest exostosis in the scapula (osteochondroma) in a setting of cartilaginous exostosis disease.

Comments

Large, painful exostoses that are located near the trunk and have a thick cartilage cap with fine, undifferentiated ossifications are always suspicious for a secondary (exostotic) chondrosarcoma, especially in patients with cartilaginous exostosis disease, and should be excised in toto. Biopsy is obsolete due to the inhomogeneous structure of this tumor.

Case 86 (▶ Fig. 5.17)

Case description

- Referring physician: surgeon.
- Prior history and clinical question: An 18-year-old male noticed persistent pain after bumping his left shoulder. He consulted a trauma surgeon, who took a radiograph of the left shoulder (not pictured here, as it added little information). The radiograph was considered suspicious for a fracture. CT scans were then obtained, which raised suspicion of a bone cyst.

Radiologic Findings

The CT images (▶ Fig. 5.17 **a, c, e, g, i, j**) show a lucent area in the upper scapula. It appears expanded and is separated from surrounding soft tissues by an eggshell-like layer of periosteal new bone. Since the differential diagnosis would definitely include an aneurysmal bone cyst, we ordered MRI (▶ Fig. 5.17 **b, d, f, h**). That study did not show the expected fluid–fluid levels (see Case 45), thereby excluding an aneurysmal bone cyst. The MR images after intravenous (IV) contrast administration (▶ Fig. 5.17 **d, f, h**) show mostly peripheral rim enhancement with no central enhancement. The center of the lesion shows irregular high T2-weighted (T2w) signal intensity (i.e., it is proton-rich).

Pathoanatomic Background of the Findings

The structure of the expansile lesion as revealed by MRI is most consistent with a tumor that has undergone central necrotic change.

Assignment to a Possible Basic Entity

▶ **Trauma?** No, because imaging does not show a fracture, hematoma, etc.

▶ **Inflammation?** No, the history does not indicate an inflammatory process.

▶ **Tumor?** Yes (see under Synopsis and Discussion below).

Synopsis and Discussion

As noted above, the CT images suggest an *aneurysmal bone cyst* due to the eggshell-like periosteal bone formation. MRI was then performed to document the fluid levels that are so typical of aneurysmal bone cyst (see Case 45). When MRI showed no fluid levels anywhere in the lesion, it effectively excluded that diagnosis.

MRI showed too many solid components for a *simple (juvenile) bone cyst*. The somewhat ragged-looking periosteal bone formation was also highly atypical of a simple bone cyst, as was the site of occurrence in the scapula. In the statistics available to us, we did not find a single case of a simple bone cyst occurring in the scapula.

The only remaining possibility was an otherwise unidentified *tumor that had undergone necrotic ("cystic") degeneration*. Further investigation by biopsy identified the lesion, surprisingly, as a partially necrotic non-Hodgkin lymphoma. Staging examinations showed no additional sites of involvement, so the lesion was diagnosed as primary non-Hodgkin lymphoma of bone.

Subtotal necrosis is very unusual for a non-Hodgkin lymphoma from both a histologic and radiologic standpoint. Non-Hodgkin lymphoma of bone usually presents as a Lodwick grade III lesion or less commonly as a Lodwick grade II lesion. It is associated with reactive sclerosis in 50% of cases. The unusual radiologic appearance can be explained only by extensive necrosis of the very large tumor, which gave the initial impression of a cystic mass.

The most unusual feature of this highly unusual case is the history: The young man claimed to have first experienced pain after receiving a bump to the shoulder. In the past we had seen this almost exclusively with simple bone cysts that fractured and then

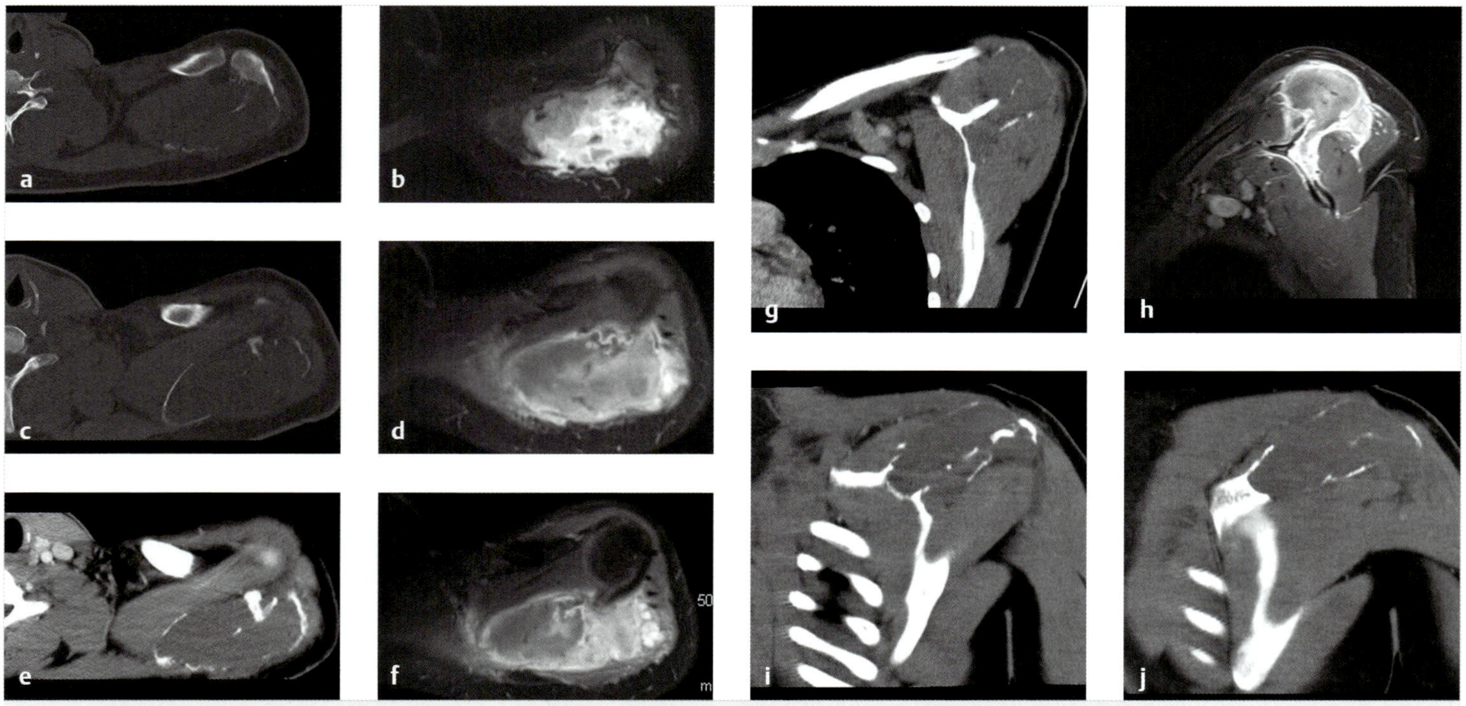

Fig. 5.17 a–j Bone cyst?

became symptomatic due to trauma. This type of history plus an expansile osteolytic lesion in the humerus or femur, for example, always suggests a simple bone cyst.

Final Diagnosis

Partially necrotic primary non-Hodgkin lymphoma in the scapula.

Comments

Very large tumors tend to undergo necrotic changes and can mimic a primary cystic lesion on CT scans. Supplemental MRI in these cases can supply more detailed information on the structure of the lesion.

Case 87 (▶ Fig. 5.18)

Case description

- Referring physician: orthopedist.
- Prior history and clinical question: A 64-year-old woman had an approximately 6-month history of increasing pain in her right shoulder. The range of motion in the right shoulder joint was significantly decreased due to pain. A radiograph (not pictured here) showed a conspicuous lucent area in the right scapula. The orthopedist wanted to know its cause.

Radiologic Findings

The CT scans in ▶ Fig. 5.18 **b** show a subtotal lytic area in the scapula that involves a portion of its anterior contours. The subscapularis muscle is thickened. T2w MRI (▶ Fig. 5.18 **a**) shows a hyperintense mass that has replaced the bone. The humeral head shows patchy areas of increased signal intensity. Postcontrast images (not pictured here) showed marked enhancement.

Pathoanatomic Background of the Findings

Based on its enhancement characteristics, the bone-replacing process in the scapula most likely represents a solid aggressive tumor. This eliminates any further considerations on assigning the lesion to a basic entity.

Synopsis and Discussion

Given the age of the patient, the differential diagnosis consists mainly of solitary plasmacytoma and some type of sarcoma (e.g., fibrosarcoma, malignant fibrous histiocytoma, undifferentiated chondrosarcoma). The patchy hyperintensities in the humeral head are interpreted as a trophic phenomenon based on the long pain history and decreased loading of the bone. The lesion was investigated by CT-guided percutaneous biopsy, which identified it as a *solitary plasmacytoma*. One year after the conclusion of local treatment (radiation), the patient was found to have generalized disease. An expansile osteolytic process in the shoulder girdle (especially the scapula and clavicle) of an older patient most commonly represents a solitary plasmacytoma.

For comparison, ▶ Fig. 5.19 shows an *eosinophilic granuloma* (focus of Langerhans-cell histiocytosis) in the inferior angle of the left scapula in a 2-year-old child. This tumor is an aggressive Lodwick grade II lesion. Approximately 4% of all eosinophilic granulomas are located in the scapula, and 4% of all Ewing sarcomas also occur in that bone. Unlike cranial lesions that show typical punched-out defects with possible sclerotic margins and a small sequestrum, lesions in the shoulder girdle require histologic evaluation.

Final Diagnosis

Solitary plasmacytoma in the scapula.

Comments

Expansive osteolytic lesions in the scapula and clavicle in older patients are usually solitary plasmacytomas. Similar lesions in children are more likely to be eosinophilic granuloma.

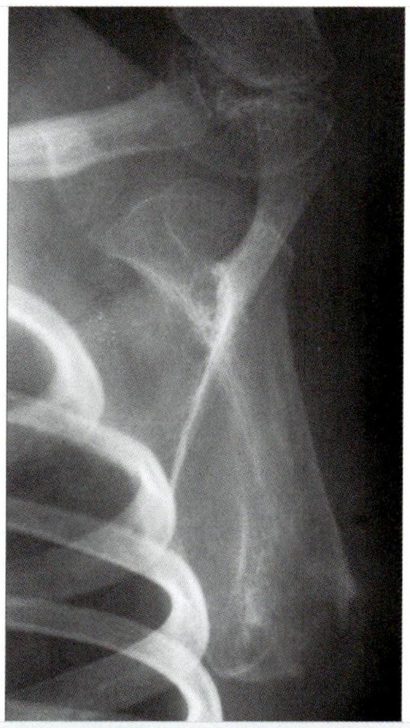

Fig. 5.19 Eosinophilic granuloma in the inferior angle of the scapula.

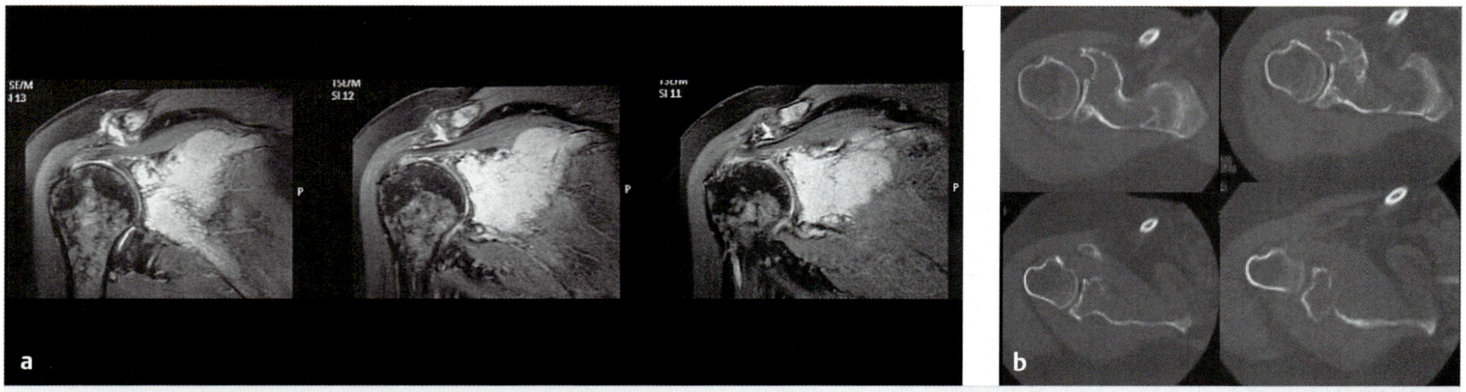

Fig. 5.18 a, b Tumor?

5.3 Ribs

Case 88 (▶ Fig. 5.20)

Case description

- Referring physician: radiologist.
- Prior history and clinical question: A chest radiograph showed thickening and increased density of the right fifth rib in an otherwise healthy 44-year-old man. The radiologist considered this finding to be suspicious for melorheostosis and asked for confirmation.

Radiologic Findings

The right fifth rib appears generally denser than the other ribs on the plain radiograph (▶ Fig. 5.20 **a, b**). Lumpy thickening is noted in the region of its lateral bend.

Location

The representative CT scans shown here (▶ Fig. 5.20 **c, d**) prove that the hyperostotic changes are located both inside and outside the rib.

Pathoanatomic Background of the Findings

The newly formed bone in and on the fifth rib is extremely compact and has smooth margins. It appears to have been present for some time and is similar in density to an osteoma.

Assignment to a Possible Basic Entity

▶ **Normal variant or malformation?** The fact that this is an incidental finding strongly suggests dysplasia with increased bone density. The longitudinal distribution of the hyperostosis with involvement of the whole rib also suggests a dysplastic process.

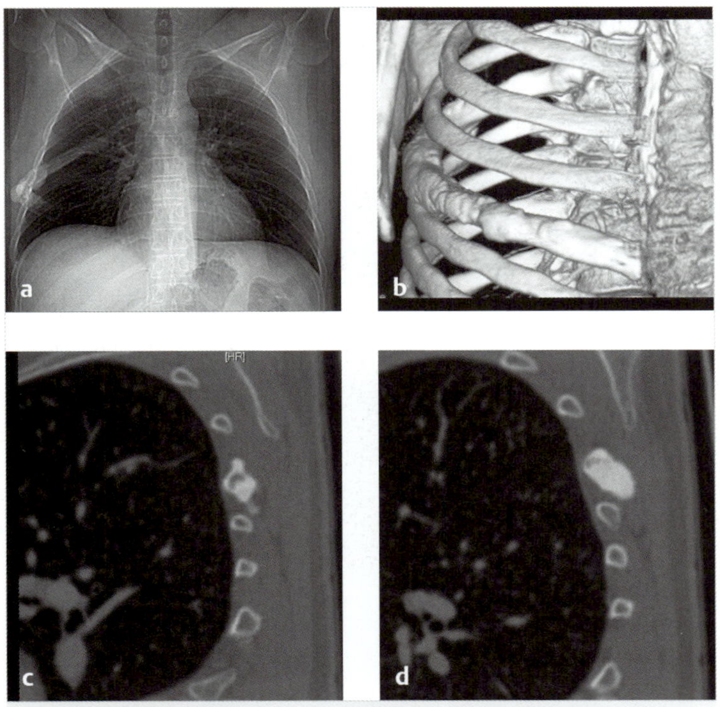

Fig. 5.20 a–d Congenital hyperostosis?

▶ **Trauma?** No trauma history.

▶ **Inflammation?** No, the negative history and incidental finding do not suggest an inflammatory process.

▶ **Tumor?** No, the very fact that the hyperostosis involves the entire rib, and thus follows an ontogenetically defined structure, does not suggest a tumor.

Synopsis and Discussion

Based on the data described above, it is not difficult to interpret the finding as melorheostosis, a congenital postzygotic skeletal disorder characterized by a radial pattern of ivorylike hyperostosis involving one or multiple bones, usually on one side. The changes in the classic form are located both inside and outside the affected bone. Further details on melorheostosis are presented in Case 17 and Case 99.

▶ Fig. 5.21 illustrates another case of melorheostosis involving the ribs. The 31-year-old man had a 5-year history of increasing swelling from the subscapular to cervical region accompanied by slight livid discoloration of the skin. The radiographs in ▶ Fig. 5.21 **a, b** show ivorylike hyperostosis on and in the 1st rib and the 4th through 10th ribs on the right side. Additional sclerotic areas are visible in the right portions of the T5 through T10 vertebrae, increasing in width from above downward. The radial and segmental arrangement of the dense sclerotic areas is consistent with melorheostosis, which is the only realistic diagnosis. The soft-tissue changes that prompted the imaging work-up represent additional cutaneous and subcutaneous lesions, which are found in approximately 60% of patients with melorheostosis. Unfortunately, we were unable to obtain MR images of the soft-tissue changes in this patient.

Final Diagnosis

Melorheostosis on and in the fifth rib.

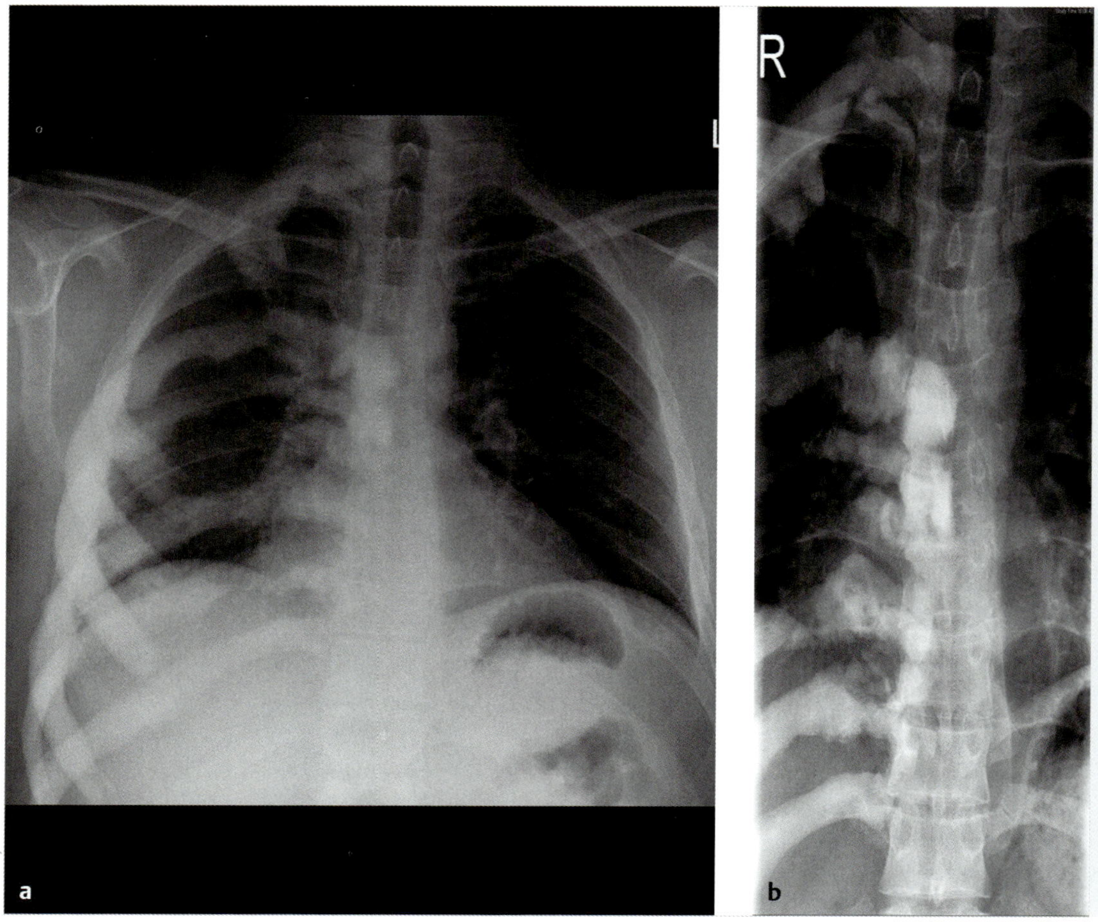

Fig. 5.21 a, b Melorheostosis of the ribs in a 31-year-old man.

Comments

Extremely dense, ivorylike hyperostosis on and in a bone with a segmental and radial distribution always indicates melorheostosis. The clinical hallmark may be cutaneous and subcutaneous soft-tissue changes. Imaging then reveals the osseous changes that are specific for melorheostosis. The cutaneous and soft-tissue changes in these cases represent the tip of the iceberg in the truest sense of the metaphor.

Case 89 (▶ Fig. 5.22)

Case description

- *Referral:* self-referral by the patient.
- *Prior history and clinical question:* A 31-year-old woman had a long history of known hereditary multiple exostosis disease. Before embarking on a prolonged stay abroad, she wanted to know whether the very prominent exostosis on her left upper anterior chest wall was malignant and should be removed. She claimed that the size of the mass had not changed in recent years. Physical examination revealed a bony-hard mass in the region of the left clavicular head (sternal end of the clavicle; see ▶ Fig. 5.22 **a**).

Radiologic Findings

The series of CT scans in ▶ Fig. 5.22 **b–e** show an unusually large cartilaginous exostosis (osteochondroma) with mature trabecular structures. The exostosis does not originate from the clavicle but from the left first rib. This is most clearly depicted in ▶ Fig. 5.22 **d**. The clavicle is displaced anteriorly and is eroded. MRI (▶ Fig. 5.22 **f**) shows a thin cartilage cap (arrows) just 2 to 3 mm thick over the head of the exostosis. Note the additional large exostoses on both scapulae.

Assignment to a Possible Basic Entity

The patient had a known multiple exostosis disease, so there is no difficulty in defining a basic entity. As for the question of whether the prominent exostosis on the first rib is malignant, see Synopsis and Discussion and Comments sections below.

Synopsis and Discussion

The clinically impressive exostosis is composed of mature cancellous bone based on enchondral ossification. The cartilage cap over the exostosis, which represents its growth zone, is thin, indicating that the lesion is unlikely to undergo significant further growth. A look at the list of criteria for secondary chondrosarcoma in Case 85 shows that the lesion meets none of the listed criteria except for the first two (size and location near the trunk). This is sufficient to exclude a secondary or eccentric chondrosarcoma and preclude its future occurrence. It is safe for the patient to proceed with her plans for a lengthy trip abroad. The same considerations apply to the other exostoses on the scapula, which require no further discussion. Aside from oncologic aspects, a "prophylactic" removal of the exostosis would carry significant risks ranging from a pneumothorax to instability of the clavicle and its articulations.

▶ Fig. 5.23 illustrates a solitary costal osteochondroma that arises close to the head of the rib and is very mature. The space between the peripheral outline of the exostoses and the adjacent vertebral arch and spinous process may be occupied by a cartilage cap measuring several millimeters to a maximum of 1 cm in thickness. This can be proven only by MRI. But the estimated thickness of the hypothetical cartilage cap is not worrisome in the 27-year-old asymptomatic man, and there is no oncologic indication for prophylactic removal of the tumor.

For comparison, ▶ Fig. 5.24 shows an *enchondroma* in posterior portion of the right second rib in an asymptomatic 29-year-old man. The finding was noted on a chest radiograph. The tumor has grown posteriorly from the rib by expansion, raising a "bulge" in the cortical bone. The ossification pattern is very typical of a cartilage-forming lesion. The differential diagnosis would include enchondroma protuberans (see also ▶ Fig. 5.15 in Case 85), but the intact solid bony shell over the lesion does not support that diagnosis in the present case.

Final Diagnosis

Very large exostosis or osteochondroma on the anterior side of the left first rib with no evidence of secondary chondrosarcoma in a patient with multiple cartilaginous exostosis disease.

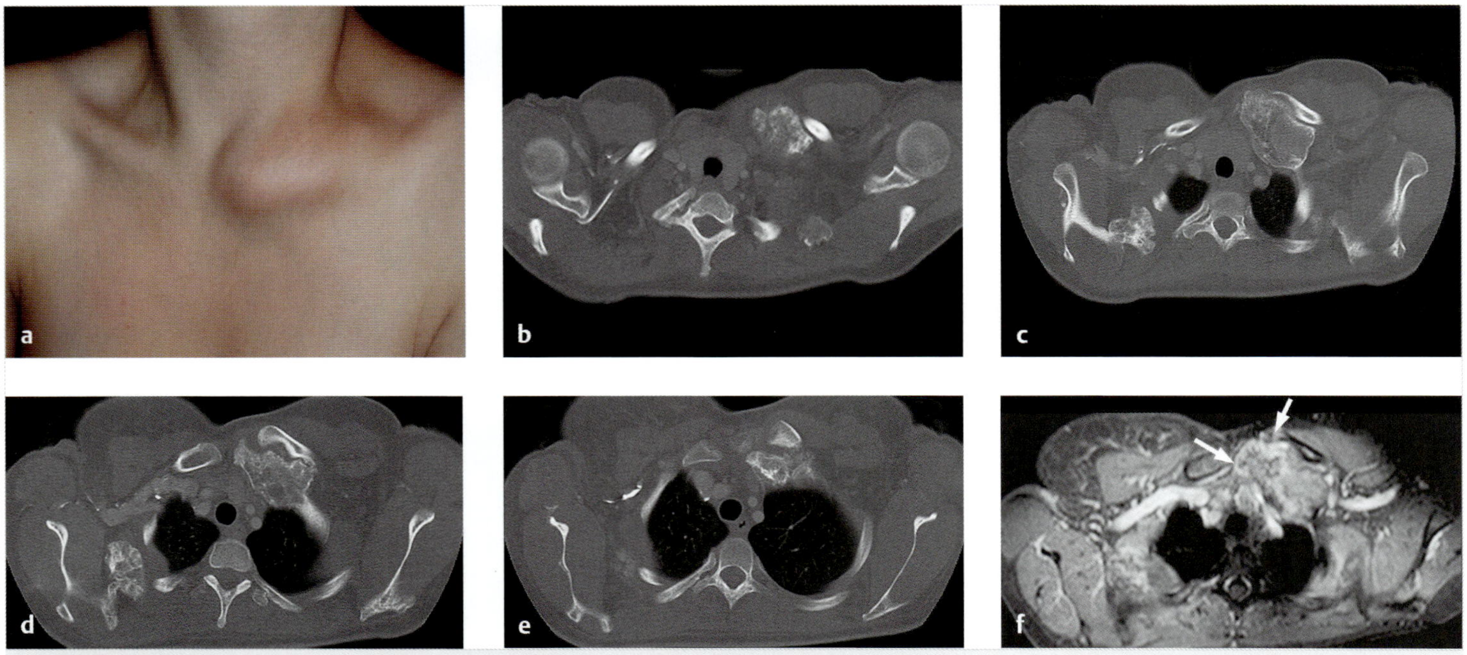

Fig. 5.22 a–f Known multiple exostosis disease: chondrosarcoma?

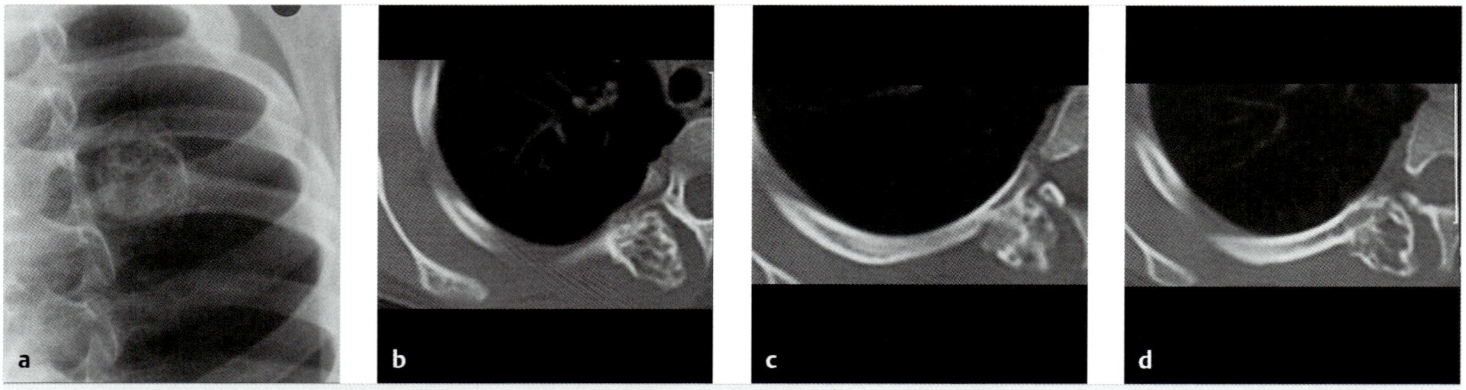

Fig. 5.23 a–d Solitary osteochondroma near the head of a rib.

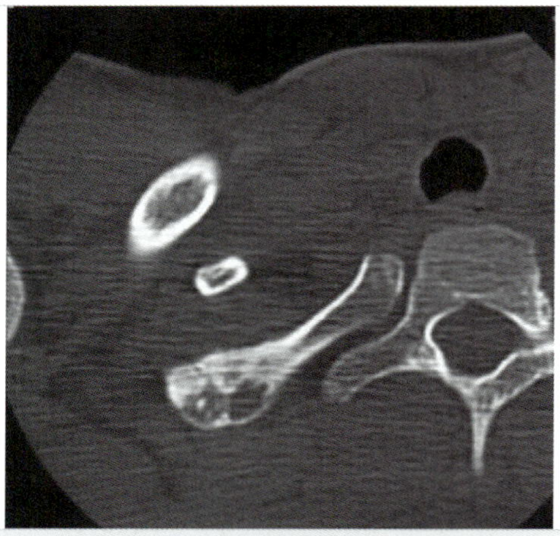

Fig. 5.24 Enchondroma in the second rib.

Comments

In themselves, size and location near the trunk are not radiologic proof of a secondary chondrosarcoma in a patient with exostosis disease. The only compelling criteria for a malignant process are the presence of a thick cartilage mass, size progression, pain, and ossifications separate from the body of the exostosis (see Case 85).

Case 90 (▶ Fig. 5.25)

Case description

- Referring physician: radiologist.
- Prior history and clinical question: A 23-year-old woman complained of occasional pain in her left lateral chest wall while riding on horseback. The radiologist sought confirmation of apparent fibrous dysplasia.

Radiologic Findings

The radiograph (▶ Fig. 5.25) shows an elongated osteolytic area in the left sixth rib associated with moderate expansion of the bone. The lesion has smooth margins, and its interior shows ground-glass density.

Pathoanatomic Background of the Findings

An expansile lesion with smooth margins, no destruction of the (often newly formed) cortical bone, and an interior ground-glass appearance always suggest a benign connective-tissue process associated with the formation of woven bone.

Assignment to a Possible Basic Entity

▸ **Normal variant or malformation?** No, there is no known precedent in a rib.

▸ **Trauma?** No trauma history. Horse riding in itself, without a fall, does not lead to expansive rib changes.

▸ **Inflammation?** No clinical manifestations. The complaint of pain in the left chest wall while riding on horseback is not necessarily referable to the radiologic lesion.

▸ **Tumor or tumorlike lesion?** Yes. The expansive component of the lesion immediately suggests a tumor or tumorlike lesion.

Synopsis and Discussion

Interpreting the pathoanatomic background of the lesion as a benign, fibrous (woven) bone-forming process, plus the mild clinical complaints, which may not even relate to the lesion itself, are suggestive of *fibrous dysplasia*. This diagnosis is also supported by the fact that the ribs are the second most common site of occurrence of fibrous dysplasia in a flat bone. The main clinical and radiologic features of fibrous dysplasia are illustrated in Case 7. An expansile lesion with a ground-glass pattern is the hallmark of fibrous dysplasia.

The tumorlike growth of fibrous dysplasia never transcends compartment boundaries, even in the aggressive polyostotic form, and the lesion never infiltrates adjacent soft tissues. This is clearly illustrated by the sectional images in ▸ Fig. 5.26: a 45-year-old asymptomatic woman (a, b); a 50-year-old man, another incidental finding (c–e); and a 40-year-old woman with occasional pain in the right upper anterior chest wall, especially in the second half of her menstrual cycle (f–i). Despite the often significant degree of bone expansion, the lesions always respect compartment boundaries. Many lesions in their active phase may undergo regressive changes such as intralesional hemorrhage and liquefaction (see also Case 7, Case 112, and Case 110), with an associated loss of the classic ground-glass appearance on radiographs and CT scans. This may also lead to problems of differential diagnosis. "Older" lesions may show heavy ossification and regressive fatty infiltration, resulting in fibro-osseous lesions that can no longer be identified even by histologic examination (see ▸ Fig. 4.42 in Case 73 and Case 133).

To aid in the differential diagnosis of an expansile rib lesion, ▸ Fig. 5.27 illustrates a brown tumor in an anterior rib (arrow in ▸ Fig. 5.27 **a**). A brown tumor can be diagnosed by noting the rarefied and indistinct structures of the affected rib and all other ribs appearing in the image. An incipient brown tumor is found at the chondro-osseous junction of the next higher rib. A radiograph of the hand (▸ Fig. 5.27 **b**) can confirm this diagnosis without the need for laboratory tests. The radiograph shows highly specific changes: rarefied and ill-defined cancellous trabeculae due to osteoclastic resorption and fibrous tissue replacement along with cortical thinning and striations, especially in the middle phalanges, caused by endosteal, periosteal and subperiosteal resorption and osteoclastic widening of the haversian canals. Whole-body scintigraphy would show a superscan in which the areas of intense bone turnover and the brown tumors "suck up" all the tracer activity (see also Case 15 and Case 111).

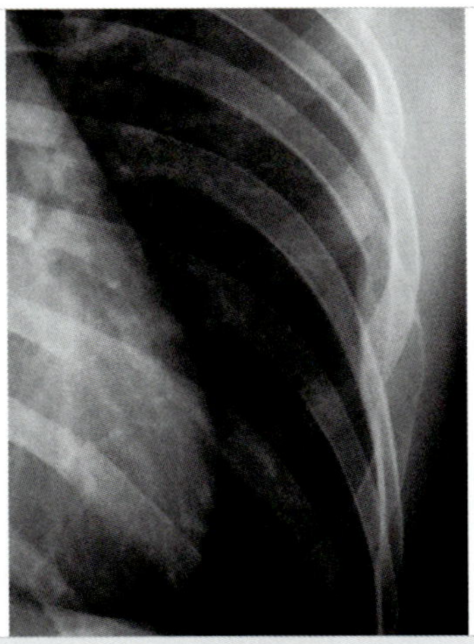

Fig. 5.25 Incidental finding in the left sixth rib.

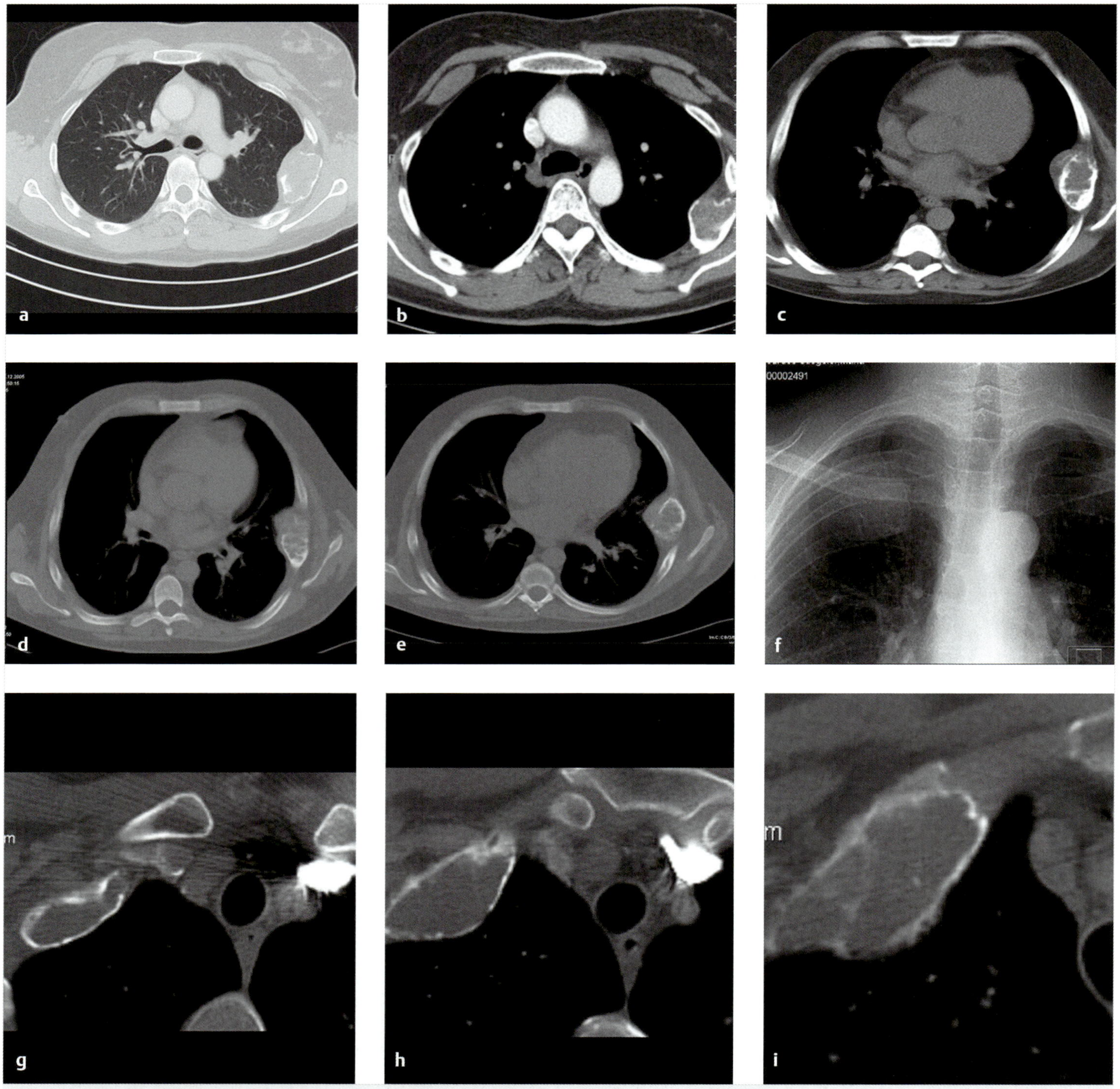

Fig. 5.26 a–i CT images and plain radiograph of fibrous dysplasia in three different patients.

Final Diagnosis

Typical fibrous dysplasia in the left sixth rib.

Comments

An expansile osteolytic lesion with an internal ground-glass pattern in the rib of a more or less asymptomatic patient is highly specific for fibrous dysplasia.

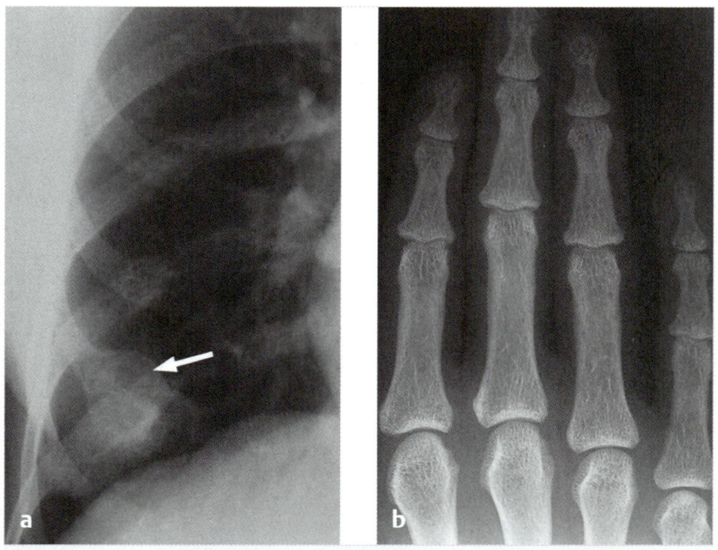

Fig. 5.27 a, b Brown tumor of hyperparathyroidism in an anterior rib and corresponding hand radiograph.

Case 91 (▶ Fig. 5.28)

Case description

- Referring physician: radiologist.
- Prior history and clinical question: A 40-year-old man, otherwise healthy, complained of occasional retrosternal pain. A structural alteration in the right ninth rib was noted incidentally on a chest radiograph. MRI (not pictured here) showed a nonspecific finding with inhomogeneous T1w and T2w signal intensity. Since we were apparently dealing with a primary osseous process, we recommended a CT examination.

Radiologic Findings

The CT scans in ▶ Fig. 5.28 show a slightly expansile lesion with sharply defined margins in the posterolateral portion of the right ninth rib. At the center of the lesion is an elliptical ossification that has an ossified capsule in its upper portion and a more fibrous structure inferiorly. The interior of the ossified figure is inhomogeneous, with an attenuation similar to that of the cancellous bone in the adjacent uninvolved rib. Between the expanded cortex and central ossified figure is an intermediate layer that includes fat attenuation values.

Pathoanatomic Background of the Findings

The lesion definitely consists of at least three different tissue components (fat, bone, and connective tissue). The harmonious expansion of the fully intact and minimally thinned cortex, the smooth borders of the lesion relative to healthy bone, and the detection of fat attenuation in the intermediate zone between the cortex and central ossification suggest an apparently older lesion. The fat component suggests something benign. The encapsulated central figure in the lesion does not conform to a cartilaginous ossification pattern but is more consistent with dystrophic connective-tissue ossification.

Assignment to a Possible Basic Entity

▶ **Normal variant or malformation?** Not known to occur in this form, although it would fit the incidental nature of the finding.

▶ **Trauma?** Not recalled. An old, consolidated rib fracture is usually solid and the cortex would not be thinned and expanded.

▶ **Inflammation?** No clinical manifestations.

▶ **Tumor or tumorlike lesion?** Very likely, but apparently benign as indicated by the mass effect of the lesion and its smooth margins.

Synopsis and Discussion

When we consider that the lesion was detected incidentally, and if we assume that it is a *benign tumor or tumorlike lesion,* the following entities may qualify:

- Old focus of fibrous dysplasia that has undergone regressive changes with partial fatty infiltration and central ossification, probably dystrophic
- Old infarcted intraosseous lipoma (the central ossified figure would be the "nidus," indicating central ossified necrosis)
- Old infarcted hematopoietic hyperplasia with central ossification (rare; the central ossified figure would then be interpreted as the dystrophic ossification of a central infarction in hematopoietic hyperplasia)

Since we are dealing with a benign incidental finding, there is no need for further investigation (e.g., by biopsy), especially from an oncologic standpoint. We know from experience that such lesions have a nonspecific histology ("fibro-osseous lesion"), and we simply advised the patient to "forget the lesion."

For comparison, ▶ Fig. 5.29 illustrates a grade III *chondrosarcoma* in a rib. The elderly patient had noticed an increasingly painful, firm swelling at that location for some time, which he initially attributed to a direct impact. A long segment of the rib has been completely destroyed and replaced by a soft-tissue mass with flocculent calcifications. These findings, together with the advanced age of the patient and the location on the trunk and in a rib (10% of all chondrosarcomas occur in the ribs!), are consistent with a malignant cartilage-forming tumor.

▶ Fig. 5.30 illustrates another chondrosarcoma, occurring this time in a 44-year-old woman who complained of a painful lump in the right anterior chest wall. Her family doctor diagnosed the lesion as "Tietze syndrome." We do not believe that this condition actually exists as a separate entity, but unfortunately it is still occasionally evoked for purposes of convenience (see also Case 98).

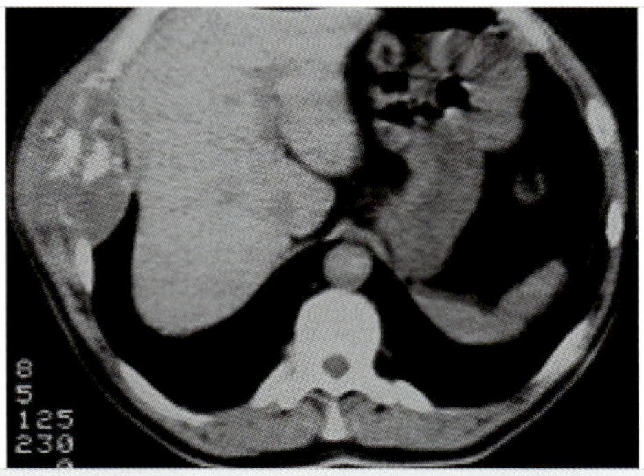

Fig. 5.29 Chondrosarcoma in the rib of an elderly man.

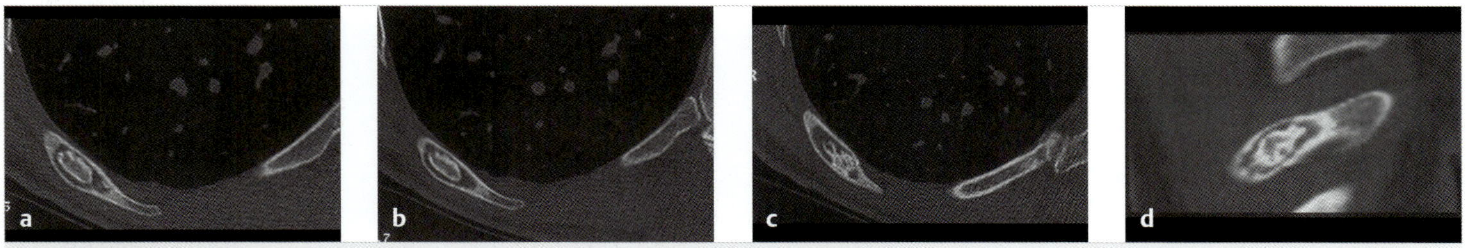

Fig. 5.28 a–d Sequestra?

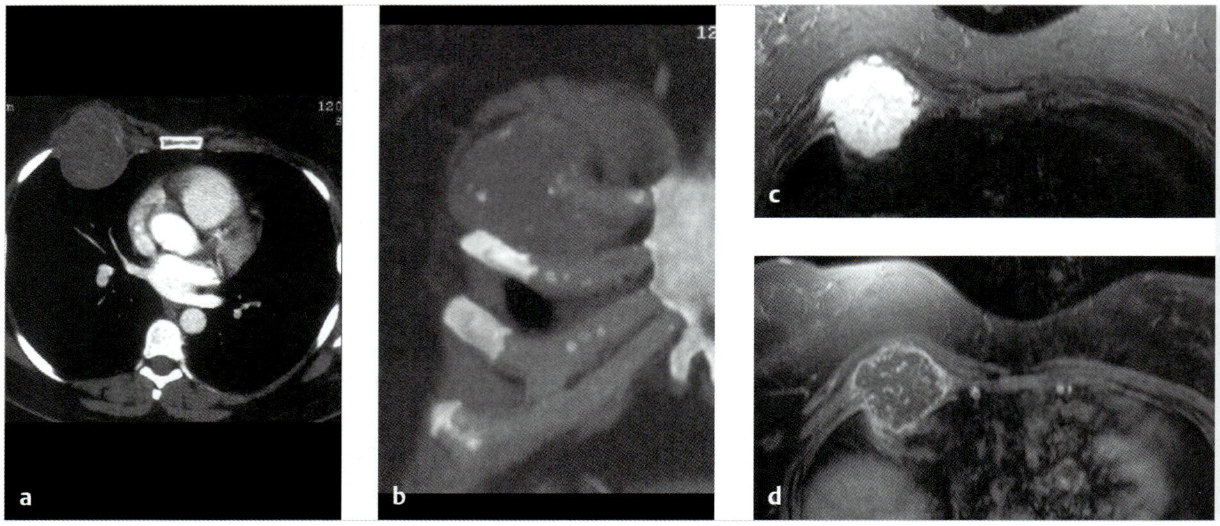

Fig. 5.30 a–d Chondrosarcoma in the chest wall of a 44-year-old woman.

This caused the true diagnosis to be delayed for several months. The cartilaginous nature of the tumor is evidenced by the fine calcifications within the tumor mass (▶ Fig. 5.30 **a, b**), its lobular architecture on unenhanced MRI (STIR sequence in ▶ Fig. 5.30 **c**), and the intense septal and peripheral enhancement following IV contrast administration (▶ Fig. 5.30 **d**).

Final Diagnosis

Old benign, fibro-osseous lesion that cannot be assigned to a specific entity.

Comments

Mass lesions detected incidentally in a rib that have multiple components and show fat attenuation should be left alone ("don't touch me" lesion).

Case 92 (▶ Fig. 5.31)

Case description

- Referring physician: radiologist.
- Prior history and clinical question: This is a "historical" case intended to illustrate how a correct radiologic diagnosis can be made quickly and directly with a minimum of radiologic investigations. The patient was a 69-year-old colleague, otherwise healthy, who had experienced a dull, focal rib pain in his right lower posterolateral chest wall for several weeks. He noticed a stabbing pain after a severe cough, and this finally prompted a radiologic evaluation. Fluoroscopically guided radiographs (▶ Fig. 5.31 **a, b**) showed a destructive osteolytic process with a spontaneous fracture in the posterolateral portion of the eighth rib (arrows). Whole-body bone scans (▶ Fig. 5.31 **c**) revealed no additional lesions. What should be the further course of action?

Radiologic Findings

As noted above, the spot films showed a complete osteolytic lesion without significant matrix ossification with a spontaneous fracture in the posterolateral eighth rib. The bone scan showed no additional lesions. The chest radiograph was normal.

Pathoanatomic Background of the Findings

The spontaneous fracture has a potentially broad pathoanatomic background ranging from a solitary metastasis from an unknown primary tumor or a solitary plasmacytoma, to a primary bone tumor with no appreciable matrix formation on plain radiographs.

Assignment to a Possible Basic Entity

▶ **Normal variant or malformation?** Not known to occur in this form, and not consistent with the marked clinical manifestations.

▶ **Trauma?** No, the patient has a spontaneous fracture with no known trauma history (see also Case 93).

▶ **Inflammation?** No. Osteomyelitis (e.g., due to a staphylococcal infection) would not be a realistic cause of osteolysis and spontaneous fracture in an otherwise healthy older man. Since our colleague had never been in the tropics, we must also exclude a rare infection associated with large granuloma formation. A solitary focus of Paget disease in the lytic stage generally does produce a spontaneous fracture.

▶ **Tumor or tumorlike lesion?** Yes. Osteolysis with a spontaneous fracture always suggests an underlying tumor, see details below in Synopsis and Discussion.

Synopsis and Discussion

As noted under Pathoanatomic Background of the Findings, the differential diagnosis of this case includes a broad range of possibilities. The patient asked about possible further actions:

- Extensive search for a primary tumor
- CT
- Rapid percutaneous biopsy

We chose the third option, since the first two options would have required histologic confirmation anyway. The detection of prostate cancer, for example, would not necessarily have meant that the rib lesion was metastatic to that disease. The detection of paraproteins would have suggested plasmacytoma, but that would not necessarily have established the etiology of the rib lesion. To our surprise, histology revealed an eosinophilic granuloma (focus of Langerhans-cell histiocytosis), which is extremely unusual for a patient of this age. Given the harmless nature of the diagnosis, it was appropriate to take the shortest path to a useful diagnosis. Because histologic confirmation is still the gold standard for a nonspecific osteolytic lesion, we recommend early histologic investigation as a routine action, especially since modern techniques of percutaneous biopsy are well tolerated by patients. As expected, the lesion resolved completely within 1 year; no additional lesions occurred.

▶ Fig. 5.32 illustrates another case of Langerhans-cell histiocytosis in an older patient. The 56-year-old man complained of increasing respiratory difficulty and skeletal pain, especially in the upper legs. He had had significant tooth loss in the previous year, and he was a chain smoker. A whole-body bone scan (▶ Fig. 5.32 **d**) showed three hot spots in the calvarium along with foci in the maxilla and mandible, in both proximal humeri, in both proximal femurs, in the left distal femur, and in the left fifth and eighth ribs. Radiographs showed multiple osteolytic skeletal lesions that

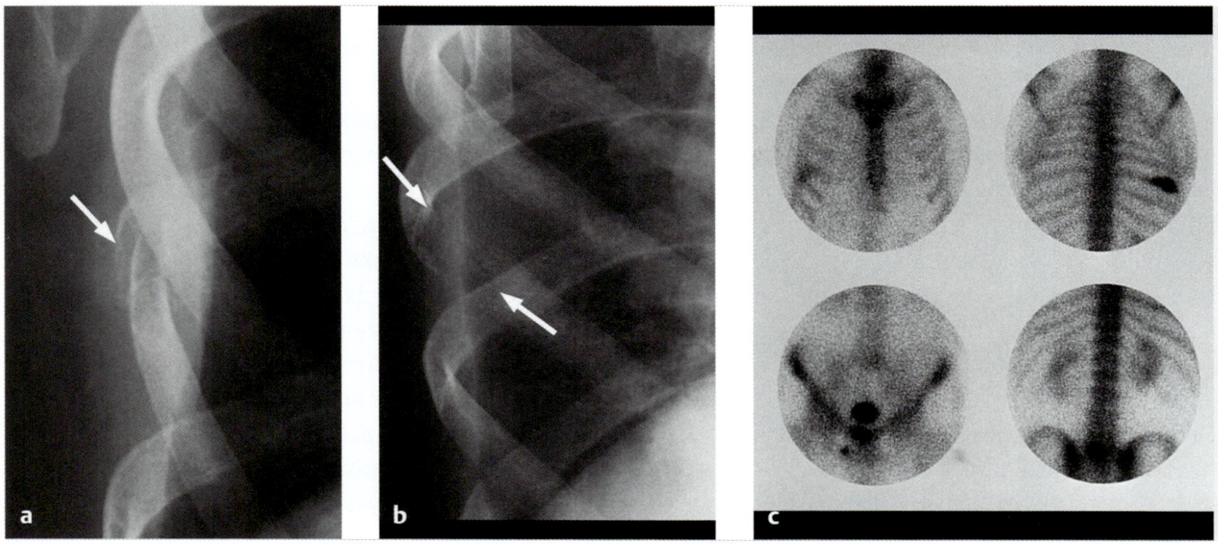

Fig. 5.31 a–c Unexplained osteolytic lesion in the eighth rib. Further course of action?

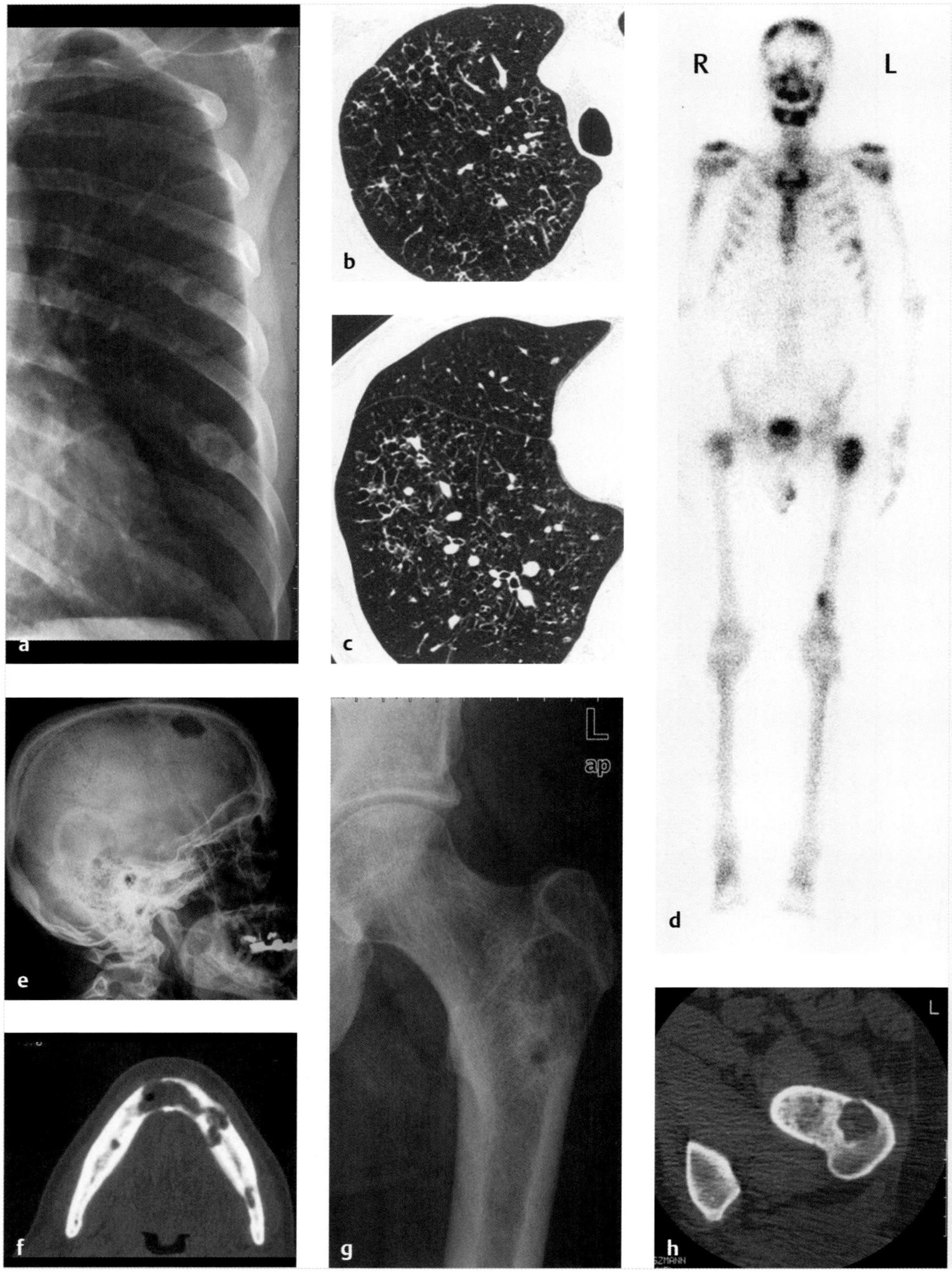

Fig. 5.32 a–h Multisystemic Langerhans-cell histiocytosis in a 56-year-old man.

could not be further classified—although the smoking history suggested metastatic lung cancer, which was also supported by the presence of unusual lung findings.

We were asked for further clarification of the multiple findings. The chest radiograph showed osteolytic areas in the posterolateral portions of the left fifth and seventh ribs with dense sclerotic margins (▶ Fig. 5.32 **a**) that were probably reparative in nature. The lesion in the left proximal femur also had sclerotic margins, suggesting a benign process. The disordered appearance of the lung parenchyma on the chest radiograph may have indicated bronchoalveolar carcinoma or lymphangiomatosis, for example, which prompted us to order CT scans (▶ Fig. 5.32 **b, c**). In addition to fibrosis, CT showed innumerable small lesions with central cavitation—a pattern that is very typical of Langerhans-cell histiocytosis (see also Case 24), especially in smokers. The skeletal foci in the ribs (▶ Fig. 5.32 **a**), skull (▶ Fig. 5.32 **e**), mandible (▶ Fig. 5.32 **f**), and proximal femoral metaphyses (left side shown in ▶ Fig. 5.32 **g, h**) are consistent with multisystemic Langerhans-cell histiocytosis. Histologic confirmation was still indicated, however. Since percutaneous lung biopsy posed a relatively high risk of pneumothorax, we biopsied the lesion in the left femur, which was initially negative. Additional unproductive biopsies were taken over the next 3 weeks, yielding only necrotic tissue or connective tissue. Finally the sixth biopsy was diagnostic and confirmed our presumptive diagnosis of Langerhans-cell histiocytosis. The problem of unproductive biopsies in Langerhans-cell histiocytosis is explored further in Case 24. Viewed in its entirety, the present case is virtually pathognomonic for a protracted course of multisystemic Langerhans-cell histiocytosis in which the skeletal lesions have already undergone reparative processes.

Final Diagnosis

Symptomatic focus of Langerhans-cell histiocytosis (eosinophilic granuloma) in the right eighth rib with an associated spontaneous fracture.

Comments

An osteolytic rib lesion with a spontaneous fracture in an elderly patient may occasionally signify Langerhans-cell histiocytosis. Multisystemic Langerhans-cell histiocytosis is the diagnosis of first choice in patients with a history of smoking, multiple skeletal foci, and disseminated pulmonary lesions with central cavitation.

Case 93 (▶ Fig. 5.33)

Case description

- Referring physician: radiologist.
- Prior history and clinical question: A 64-year-old man suffered from posttraumatic fractures of the right sixth through eighth ribs and a bloody pleural effusion. The effusion was managed by percutaneous drainage. The possibility of a bacterial infection (pleural empyema) was noted. The fractures did not heal over time, and the case was referred to us for determination of the cause.

Radiologic Findings

Spot radiographs taken 3 weeks after the fractures occurred (▶ Fig. 5.33 **a**) demonstrated fractures of the right sixth through eighth ribs with marked diastasis of the bone ends. Spot films taken approximately 8 weeks later (▶ Fig. 5.33 **b**) still showed no evidence of fracture healing (consolidation of the fracture site, callus formation, etc.). The anterior ends of the fractured seventh and eighth ribs had a "licked candy stick" appearance and were widely separated from the posterior fracture ends. This appearance did not change in subsequent months. A chest radiograph obtained 6 months later (▶ Fig. 5.33 **c**) showed that the portion of the clavicle adjacent to the acromioclavicular joint was absent on both sides. The finding is especially pronounced on the left side, as shown by the spot film in ▶ Fig. 5.33 **d**.

Location

The osteolytic changes affect only the distal portions of the fractured ribs and the peripheral portions of both clavicles.

Pathoanatomic Background of the Findings

The resorption of distal (acral) bone segments or of fractured bone ends indicates a trophic process known as acro-osteolysis.

Assignment to a Possible Basic Entity

▶ **Normal variant or malformation?** No. The follow-up radiographs, especially of the osteolytic rib changes, exclude a normal variant.

▶ **Trauma?** The follow-up proves that trauma was certainly a precipitating cause of the acro-osteolytic changes in the ribs and clavicles. On a chest radiograph taken the day of the injury (not pictured here), the clavicles were still intact.

▶ **Inflammation?** No, follow-up showed no signs of osteitis or osteomyelitis such as reactive or reparative sclerosis. Although little was known about the history of osteolytic rib changes and possible pleural empyema, the patient definitely did not have a history of clavicular changes.

▶ **Tumor or tumorlike lesion?** No, there was no evidence of a mass lesion.

▶ **Perfusion disorder?** Yes, see in Synopsis and Discussion.

Synopsis and Discussion

The vanishing or "melting away" of peripheral bone segments with no associated sclerosis or periosteal reaction is known as acro-osteolysis. As a rule, distal (acral) bone segments do not have a collateral blood supply, and so any disruption of blood flow due to trauma or a trophic disturbance of neurovascular regulation, for example, will lead to necrosis. If the necrosis of peripheral bone segments occurs gradually, especially in the distal phalanges or clavicles, radiographs will not show fragmentation or other phenomena that are otherwise typical of osteonecrosis. The "licked candy stick" appearance is the radiographic hallmark of acro-osteolysis (see also Case 79).

But there is another theory, based partly on histologic studies, that relates particularly to acro-osteolysis in the ribs and clavicle:

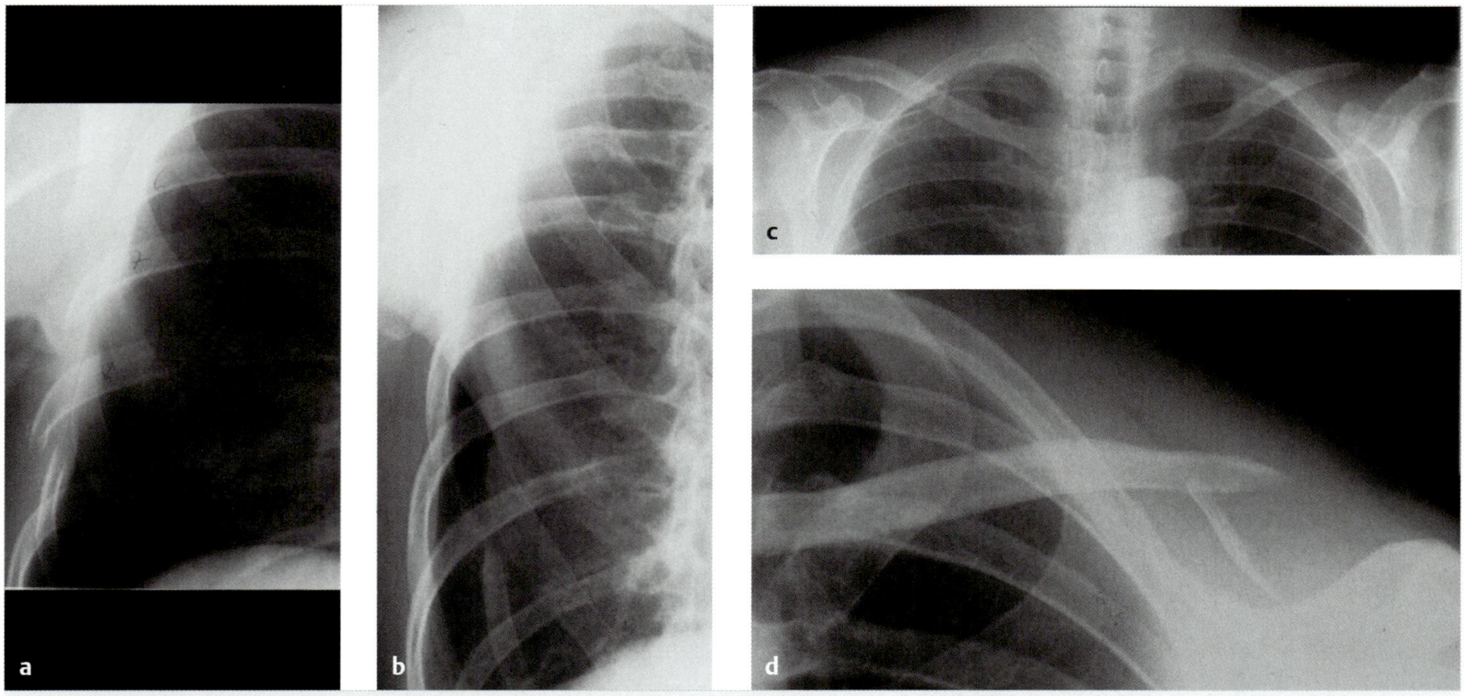

Fig. 5.33 a–d Multiple nonhealing rib fractures: cause? Radiographs were taken in November 2000 (a), January 2001 (b), and July 2001 (c, d).

When the neural vascular supply is disturbed due to trauma or some other cause, this may lead to increased vascularization and hyperperfusion of bone areas distal to the site of the disturbance. This incites an excessive, uncontrolled osteoclast stimulation that culminates in resorption of the acral bone segments. This increased vascularization is indistinguishable from angiomatosis by conventional histologic methods, so it would be appropriate to discuss vanishing bone disease (phantom bone disease, massive osteolysis, Gorham–Stout disease) as a diagnosis for the present case (see also Case 11 and Case 54). Trauma has also been cited as a possible precipitating cause in vanishing bone disease. It is generally accepted that angiomatous changes in the skin and synovium, for example, can be induced by trauma.

Final Diagnosis

Trauma-induced acro-osteolysis of three ribs and both clavicles.

Comments

The tapered "candy stick" appearance on radiographs (distal bone resorption with no associated sclerosis or periosteal reaction) indicates a perfusion disorder in the affected bone. Histologic examination generally does not add useful information.

Case 94 (▶ Fig. 5.34)

Case description

- Referring physician: orthopedist.
- Prior history and clinical question: A 39-year-old man had suffered rib pains of variable location and intensity for many years. It was felt that the rib changes shown in ▶ Fig. 5.34 **a, b** were due to enchondromatosis. The orthopedist requested a second opinion. When asked, he stated that the patient had an unusual number of café-au-lait spots, especially on the trunk.

Radiologic Findings

The chest wall radiographs (▶ Fig. 5.34 **a, b**) demonstrate expansile lesions with a "soap-bubble" appearance in almost all the ribs, with sparing of the central rib segments on the left side. Some of the lesions have a ground-glass appearance. The CT scans in ▶ Fig. 5.34 **c** show that the masses respect the bone boundaries but that some are outlined by a very thin shell of periosteal calcification. Fluid levels (arrows) are visible in the middle and lower panels of ▶ Fig. 5.34 **c**. The scapulae are also affected. Other changes were noted elsewhere in the skeleton but are not described here.

Location

The epicenters of the expansile lesions are located in the ribs.

Pathoanatomic Background of the Findings

The terms "soap-bubble appearance" and "ground-glass appearance" form a pattern that immediately suggests fibrous dysplasia with marked regressive changes. This interpretation is also supported by the fluid levels on representative CT scans. They are formed by the interface of two fluid media that have different densities—analogous to the fluid–fluid levels on MRI, which have a different physical explanation (see Case 45).

Assignment to a Possible Basic Entity

Since the pathoanatomic background already implies a diagnosis of fibrous dysplasia, we may shorten the interpretation process and proceed directly to the synopsis and discussion.

Synopsis and Discussion

The patient has a polyostotic form of regional (confined to the thorax) fibrous dysplasia, whose key features are:

- a long history,
- café-au-lait spots (indicating a systemic disease process),
- soap-bubble expansion of the affected rib areas,
- ground-glass pattern within the lesions, reflecting the presence of poorly calcified woven bone,
- respects bone boundaries, and
- fluid levels.

The lesions are always more active and aggressive in the polyostotic form; that is, the expansile lesions are larger and exhibit more dynamic changes. These changes include necrosis with liquefaction and intralesional hemorrhage (fluid levels on sectional imaging), followed later by regional fatty infiltration and bizarre ossification. Secondary aneurysmal bone cysts are also observed in larger lesions. Polyostotic forms of fibrous dysplasia have a high association with skin changes such as café-au-lait spots. Fibrous dysplasia is associated with hormonal disorders in McCune–Albright syndrome, in which the radiographic bone changes may assume even more grotesque forms.

The initial suspicion of enchondromatosis was not entirely unfounded, as that condition is likewise associated with bone expansion and deformity that begin in early childhood. The changes are generally unilateral, however. Lesions in the Ollier type of enchondromatosis, for example, usually display a lobular or column-shaped morphology, and the lesions often have an unmistakable cartilaginous ossification pattern (see Case 115 and Case

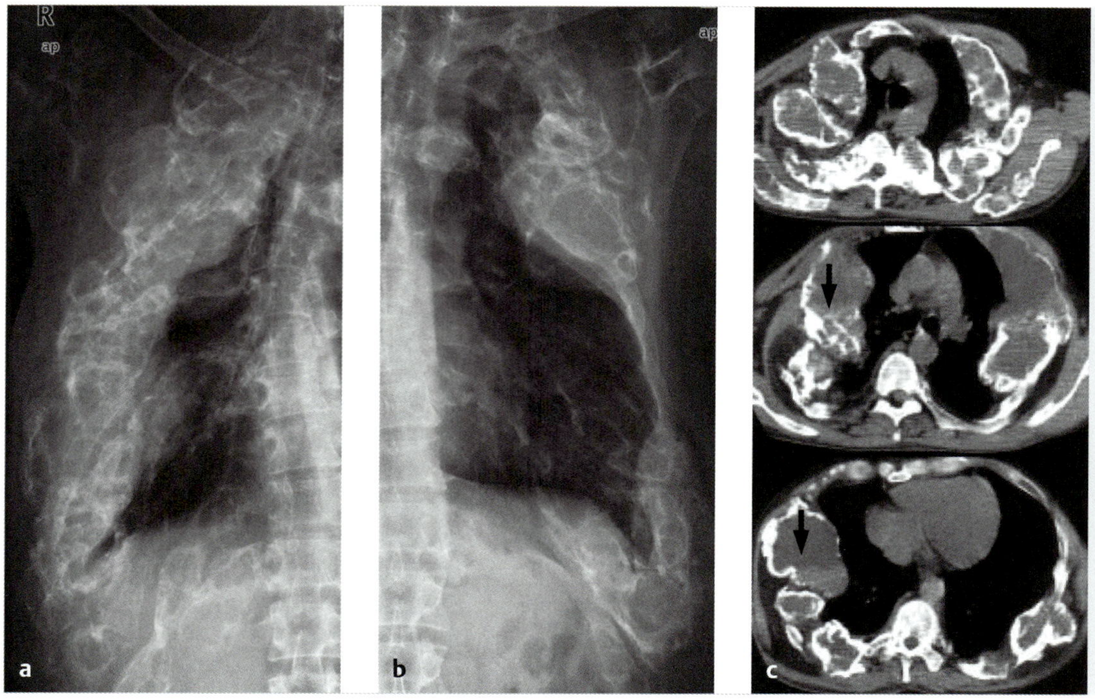

Fig. 5.34 a–c Enchondromatosis?

120). One should be careful, however, since the lesions in fibrous dysplasia may also have a cartilaginous component, especially with involvement of the lower limbs. The origin of these cartilaginous components is not fully understood.[18]

The differentiation between polyostotic fibrous dysplasia and enchondromatosis is important because fibrous dysplasia has only about a 0.5% rate of secondary malignant transformation, compared with almost 60% for enchondromatosis. Thus, patients with enchondromatosis require constant, close-interval clinical and radiologic follow-ups, which are unnecessary in fibrous dysplasia patients from an oncologic standpoint. In the rare cases of osteosarcoma, fibrosarcoma, or chondrosarcoma occurring within a focus of polyostotic fibrous dysplasia, the tumor is manifested by unusually severe pain, swelling, or other signs. Imaging will document a transformation from the classic signs of fibrous dysplasia to the corresponding signs of sarcoma, most notably the infiltration of surrounding structures.

Further details on fibrous dysplasia may be found in Case 4, Case 7, Case 8, Case 20, Case 36, Case 58, Case 90, and Case 112.

Final Diagnosis

Polyostotic fibrous dysplasia of the ribs and scapulae.

Comments

Expansile “soap-bubble” lesions of the ribs or other flat bones combined with a ground-glass pattern suggest an aggressive, polyostotic form of fibrous dysplasia.

5.4 Sternum

Case 95 (▶ Fig. 5.35)

Case description

- *Referring physician:* This case was kindly furnished to us by Prof. Dr. J. Schäfer, University of Tübingen.
- *Prior history and clinical question:* A 14-year-old boy presented with pain in the lower sternum.

Radiologic Findings

The CT images in ▶ Fig. 5.35 **a–d** demonstrate a punched-out defect in the left upper portions of the third segment of the body of the sternum. The attenuation values in the lesion range from 92 to 163 HU. The cortex is partially destroyed. MRI after IV contrast administration shows only moderate enhancement (▶ Fig. 5.35 **e**). Diffuse hyperintensity is noted throughout the third sternal segment and in the lower portions of the second segment. Definite matrix calcification is not demonstrable by CT.

Pathoanatomic Background of the Findings

Findings indicate a solid destructive process that is moderately perfused but has incited a significant proton-rich perifocal reaction.

Assignment to a Possible Basic Entity

▶ **Normal variant or malformation?** No known precedents. Clinical manifestations and MRI findings are also inconsistent with a normal variant or malformation.

▶ **Trauma?** No trauma history.

▶ **Inflammation?** No clinical manifestations, and imaging shows no evidence of an abscess or paraosseous edema.

▶ **Tumor?** Yes, but what kind? Primary bone tumors are extremely rare in the sternum. The present case shows no matrix mineralization that might indicate a bone-forming or cartilage-forming tumor. The marked edema-like signal surrounding the destructive process could signify an osteoid osteoma, osteoblastoma, or perhaps even a chondroblastoma. The marked perifocal reaction is not characteristic of eosinophilic granuloma (Langerhans-cell histiocytosis), though apparently it may occur (see ▶ Fig. 4.12 in Case 55) due to local bone weakening or destruction. All in all, a benign tumor appears more likely than a malignancy owing to the apparent absence of spread to surrounding structures. The etiology in this case can be established only by histology; afterward the radiologist may consider the histologic diagnosis to be plausible or implausible, and the latter conclusion should prompt further evaluation of the case.

Synopsis and Discussion

The tumor was excised, and histology identified it as osteoblastoma. This diagnosis was confirmed by a reference pathologist. From a radiologic standpoint, the lesion did not exhibit the characteristic features of an osteoblastoma:

- very good to extreme vascularization or perfusion
- matrix mineralization

The location is also unusual for osteoblastoma, although the tumor may occur in any bone. Sites of predilection in descending

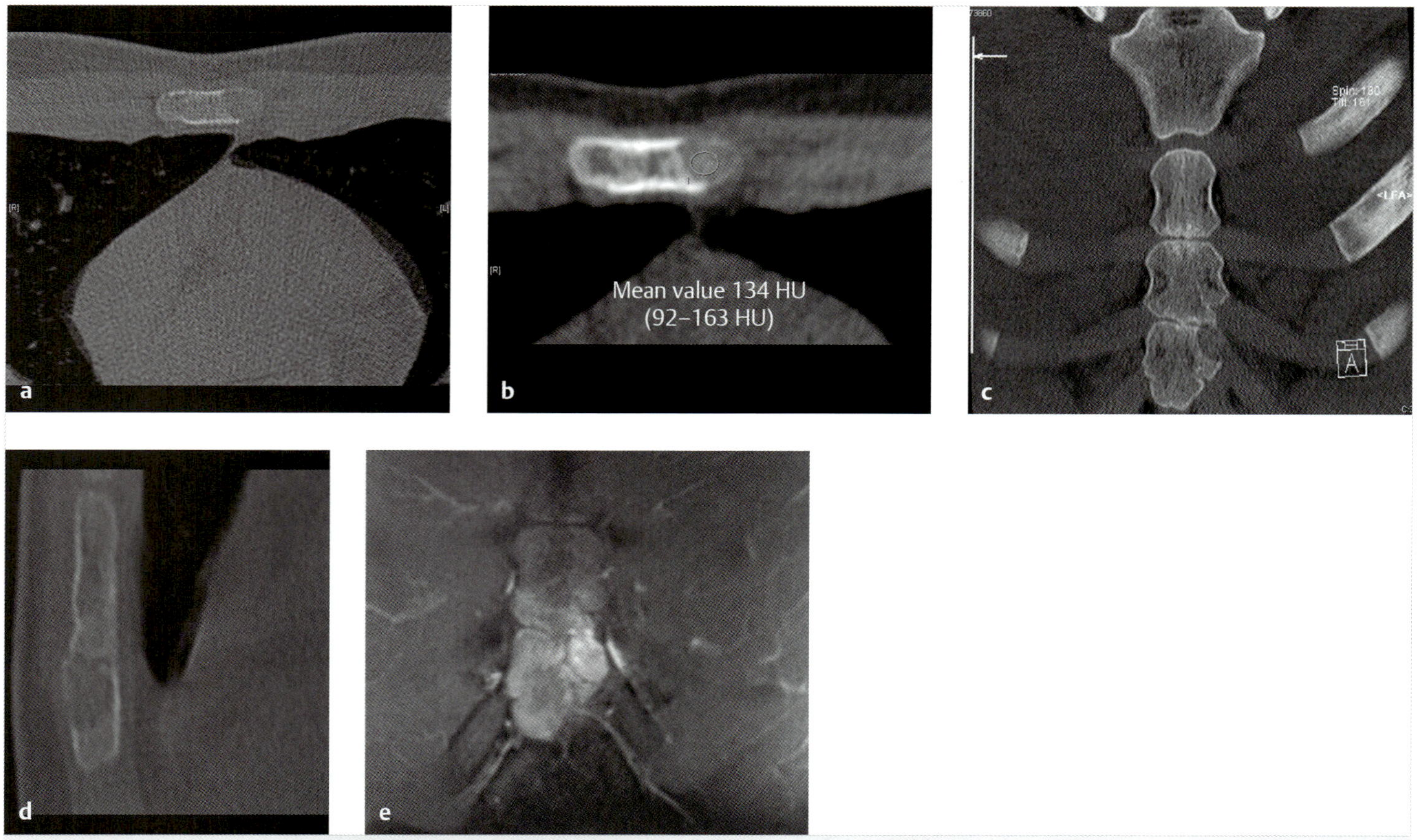

Fig. 5.35 a–e Can this case be solved by biopsy or radiology?

order of frequency are the spine, skull, pelvis, hand/foot, and large tubular bones. We have not previously encountered an osteoblastoma in the sternum, but this does not mean that it cannot occur there. With such an unusual location, however, it is not surprising that the lesion would have an unusual radiologic presentation. To date there have been no publications on the specific features of an osteoblastoma located in the sternum of a still-growing skeleton, so there are no solid counterarguments to a histologic diagnosis. Because osteoblastomas have a propensity for recurrence, the boy should be followed clinically and radiologically for the next 2 years.

Final Diagnosis

Osteoblastoma in the third segment of the body of the sternum.

Comments

It is not uncommon for tumors at unusual sites to have a surprising histologic diagnosis, especially since it appears that lesions at unusual sites tend to have atypical radiologic features.

Case 96 (▶ Fig. 5.36)

Case description

- Referring physician: radiologist.
- Prior history and clinical question: A 61-year-old woman had a 7-month history of increasing pain and swelling in the sternum. On touching her sternum, the patient felt a vibrating sensation that was confirmed by the attending colleague. CT and MR images were obtained. We were consulted to identify the tumor entity.

Radiologic Findings

The manubrium sterni is expanded by a space-occupying lesion that contains soft tissue and bizarre septum-like ossifications with a honeycomb appearance (▶ Fig. 5.36 **a, b**). The soft-tissue structures also show some evidence of extension into the retrosternal space. Gaps present in the anterior and posterior bony walls of the lesion are appreciated most clearly in the coronal reformatted image (▶ Fig. 5.36 **c**). MRI after contrast administration (▶ Fig. 5.36 **d**) shows intense enhancement with contrast pools, small rounded spots, and serpiginous figures.

Pathoanatomic Background of the Findings

Contrast-enhanced MRI clearly demonstrates the presence of vascular structures that have partially replaced the bone. The honeycomb structure on CT also indicates a predominantly vascular process (see also Case 3, Case 22 and Case 154). The gaps in the anterior and posterior walls of the lesion represent passageways for vessels.

Assignment to a Possible Basic Entity

▶ **Normal variant or malformation?** No. The clinical and radiologic manifestations appear to have developed only in recent years.

▶ **Trauma?** The patient could not recall any previous trauma.

▶ **Inflammation?** No clinical manifestations (e.g., local warmth).

▶ **Tumor or tumorlike lesion?** Yes. There is definitely a space-occupying lesion with a predominantly vascular structure.

Synopsis and Discussion

Only a hypervascular tumor fits all of the above data. The following entities should be considered:

- Primary vascular tumor or vascular malformation
- Hypervascular metastasis (e.g., from renal cell carcinoma)
- Hypervascular primary bone tumor (e.g., osteoblastoma)

Although the clinical findings (palpable thrill over the sternum, no known primary tumor, negative abdominal ultrasound) suggest a primary vascular process, most likely a vascular malformation, radiology could not exclude a hypervascular primary bone tumor or bone metastasis, so biopsy was indicated. Histology revealed "portions of a cavernous hemangioma of bone." The lesion was treated surgically, and most of it was excised. Seven years after surgery the patient was free of complaints and there is no radiologic evidence of recurrence.

We might question the diagnosis of cavernous hemangioma by noting that most hemangiomas are congenital tumors that resolve spontaneously as the patient grows. This particularly applies to hemangiomas of the skin. But even vertebral hemangiomas, a common incidental finding in the spine, generally represent "war memorials," that is, hemangiomas that have regressed and appear on sectional images as a rarefied, honeycomblike bone area occupied by fatty tissue while showing no signs of an active vascular tumor process. When a symptomatic, active vascular process is diagnosed in an adult, it is generally a vascular malformation (e.g., venous or arteriovenous malformation, (see Case 154). These processes are usually progressive and therefore require treatment (e.g., vascular occlusion by catheter, sclerotherapy, etc.). In the present case, finding a palpable thrill over the lesion was sufficient to suggest a vascular malformation, and this was supported by intraoperative findings (enlarged vessels, heavy bleeding).

Final Diagnosis

Vascular malformation in the manubrium sterni.

Comments

An expansile bone lesion with a honeycomb structure that shows intense enhancement on MRI with vascular lakes and obvious vascular structures in adults is usually a vascular malformation, which pathologists generally describe morphologically as a hemangioma.

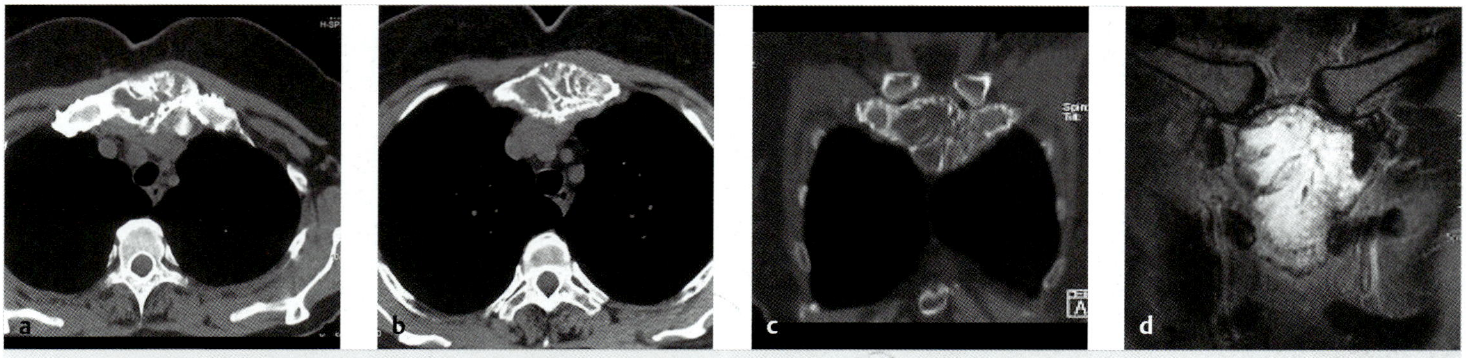

Fig. 5.36 a–d Palpable thrill over the sternum. Can this case be solved by radiology?

5.5 Anterior Chest Wall as a Whole

Case 97 (▶ Fig. 5.37)

Case description

- Referring physician: radiologist.
- Prior history and clinical question: A 35-year-old woman complained of intolerable pain in the right parasternal area and posterior lower chest. She claimed that her pains had worsened after pregnancy and during lactation. The referring radiologist requested confirmation of his diagnosis.

Radiologic Findings

The MR images in ▶ Fig. 5.37 **b, c** show areas of increased edema-like signal intensity in the upper right quadrant of the manubrium sterni and adjacent soft tissues, also in the upper body of the sternum and adjacent structures on the right side. The CT image (▶ Fig. 5.37 **a**) reveals sclerotic changes around the manubriosternal synchondrosis, mixed destructive and sclerotic changes in the first manubriocostal synchondrosis, and—just visible in the section—sclerosis in the second sternocostal synchondrosis (only the most representative images are shown in the figure). Spinal MRI in ▶ Fig. 5.37 **f** shows increased signal intensity at the anterior inferior corner of the T11 vertebral body; a similar finding was noted at the upper left corner of T12 (not pictured here). Correlative CT shows a mixed pattern of bone destruction and proliferation at the diskoligamentous attachment of T11 and T12 (▶ Fig. 5.37 **d, e**).

Location

All of the above changes are located at the following entheses in the anterior chest wall, see the anatomic diagram in ▶ Fig. 5.38:

- Manubriosternal synchondrosis
- Costomanubrial synchondrosis and ligament
- Costosternal synchondrosis and ligament

The changes in the two lower thoracic vertebrae are also located at an enthesis: the discovertebral junction.

Pathoanatomic Background of the Findings

The mixed radiologic pattern of bone destruction and proliferation at entheses is typical of a chronic, nonbacterial inflammation, that is, an enthesitis with associated osteitis, which explains the edema-like signal on MRI. The findings are based on a generalized enthesitis in the anterior chest wall and lower thoracic spine.

Assignment to a Possible Basic Entity

The pathoanatomic substrate for the radiologic changes is identified by name in the previous paragraph, so we may proceed to the discussion.

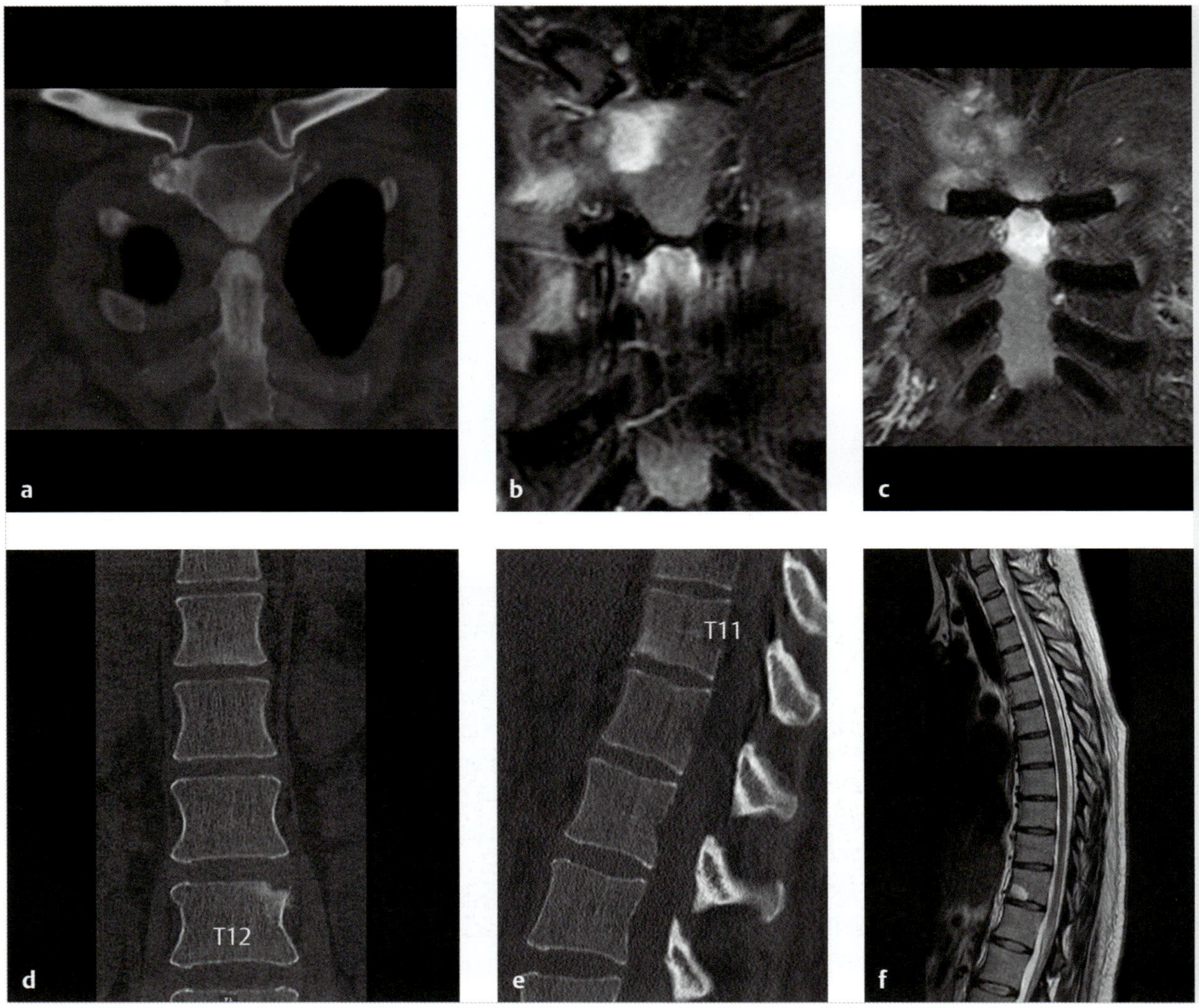

Fig. 5.37 a–f Severe pain in radiologically abnormal regions. Indication for biopsy?

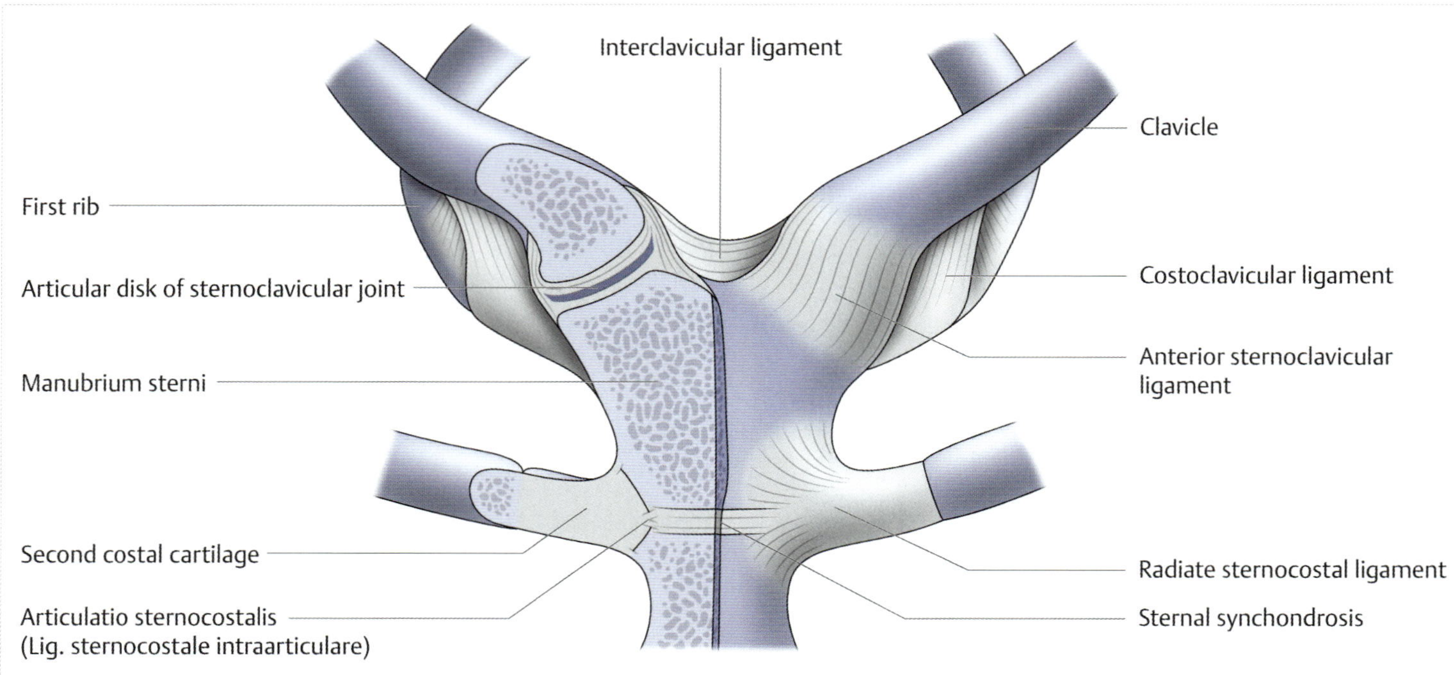

Fig. 5.38 Anatomy of the anterior chest wall. Note the countless ligament attachments and chondro-osseous junctions, all of which function as entheses.

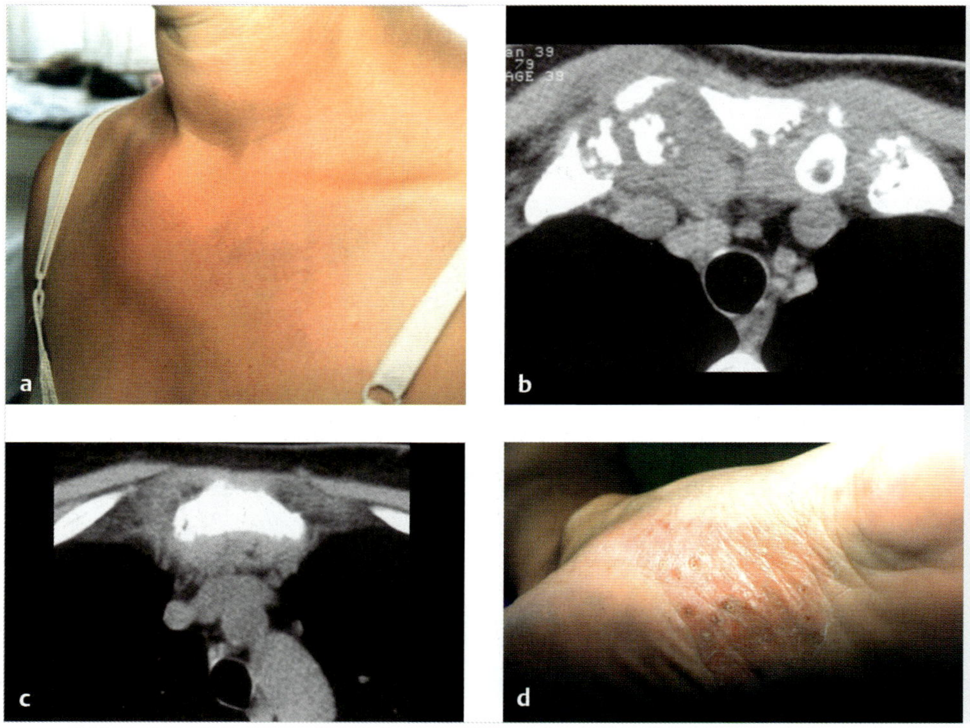

Fig. 5.39 a–d Clinical and CT findings in pustulosis palmoplantaris.

Synopsis and Discussion

The patient suffers from a generalized enthesitis that may be classified as belonging to the group of (seronegative) spondyloarthritis. The distribution pattern of the changes is consistent with psoriatic arthritis, although no visible signs of psoriasis or pustulosis palmoplantaris were noted when the images were obtained. The family history was also negative for psoriasis, and the personal history and clinical presentation showed no evidence of Reiter symptoms or bowel disease. Since the patient may eventually develop psoriasis or pustulosis palmoplantaris—though we do not believe the hypothesis of psoriatic arthritis or spondyloarthritis without psoriasis—it appears reasonable to offer a preliminary diagnosis of "undifferentiated spondyloarthritis." Also, we cannot justify a classification of ankylosing spondylitis or spondyloarthritis because the case does not meet the necessary diagnostic criteria (e.g., the Ankylosing Spondylitis Assessment Study [ASAS] criteria). The disease in the present case is still in an initial phase, and it is hoped that antirheumatic drug therapy, especially with tumor necrosis factor α blockers or antagonists, can prevent progression of the disease.

The initial changes in the anterior chest wall may progress to sternocostoclavicular hyperostosis (SCCH; synonyms: sternocostal arthro-osteitis, intersternocostoclavicular ossification), which is often associated initially with significant complaints, painful swelling, and soft-tissue inflammation that is detectable by imaging. This occurred in one patient with a variant of psoriasis, namely pustulosis palmoplantaris (PPP) (▶ Fig. 5.39). The "bull's head sign" on bone scans is a typical finding (▶ Fig. 5.40 and ▶ Fig. 5.43 **d**).

SCCH may also have an asymmetric onset, as in the case of a 44-year-old woman with classic psoriasis (▶ Fig. 5.41 **a–f**). The mixed pattern of bone destruction and proliferation in this and another case (43-year-old woman, ▶ Fig. 5.42 **a–d**) is clearly demonstrated by CT and can be documented but not proven by MRI, as demonstrated in ▶ Fig. 5.42 **a**.

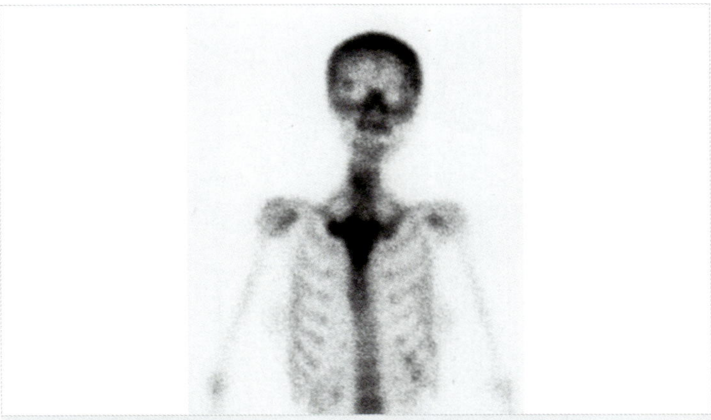

Fig. 5.40 "Bull's head" sign.

The late stage is marked by plaque-like ossification in the sternocostoclavicular region (▶ Fig. 5.43 **a–c, e**).

The dominant feature in some cases is manubriosternal synchondritis, as illustrated by the case of a woman with PPP and spondyloarthritis in a lower thoracic vertebra (▶ Fig. 5.44). As in other forms of spondyloarthritis, concomitant involvement of the costotransverse joints is a typical finding (▶ Fig. 5.43 **b**).

Diseases from the group of seronegative spondyloarthropathies that are associated with pustular skin lesions are also called SAPHO syndrome or, more specifically, pustular arthro-osteitis (PAO) or enthesio-osteitis (PEO), as illustrated in Case 39 and Case 40. Based on information from dermatologists and our own observations, PPP is more prevalent among smokers. We even had a case in which PPP plus extensive destructive-proliferative changes in the scapula and SCCH (see ▶ Fig. 5.13 in Case 84) regressed over a period of 10 years after the patient quit smoking. Clinical experience indicates that otherwise a spontaneous remission over a long period is unlikely to occur.

Preliminary Diagnosis

Undifferentiated spondyloarthritis with involvement of the sternocostoclavicular region; possible incomplete form of psoriatic spondyloarthritis.

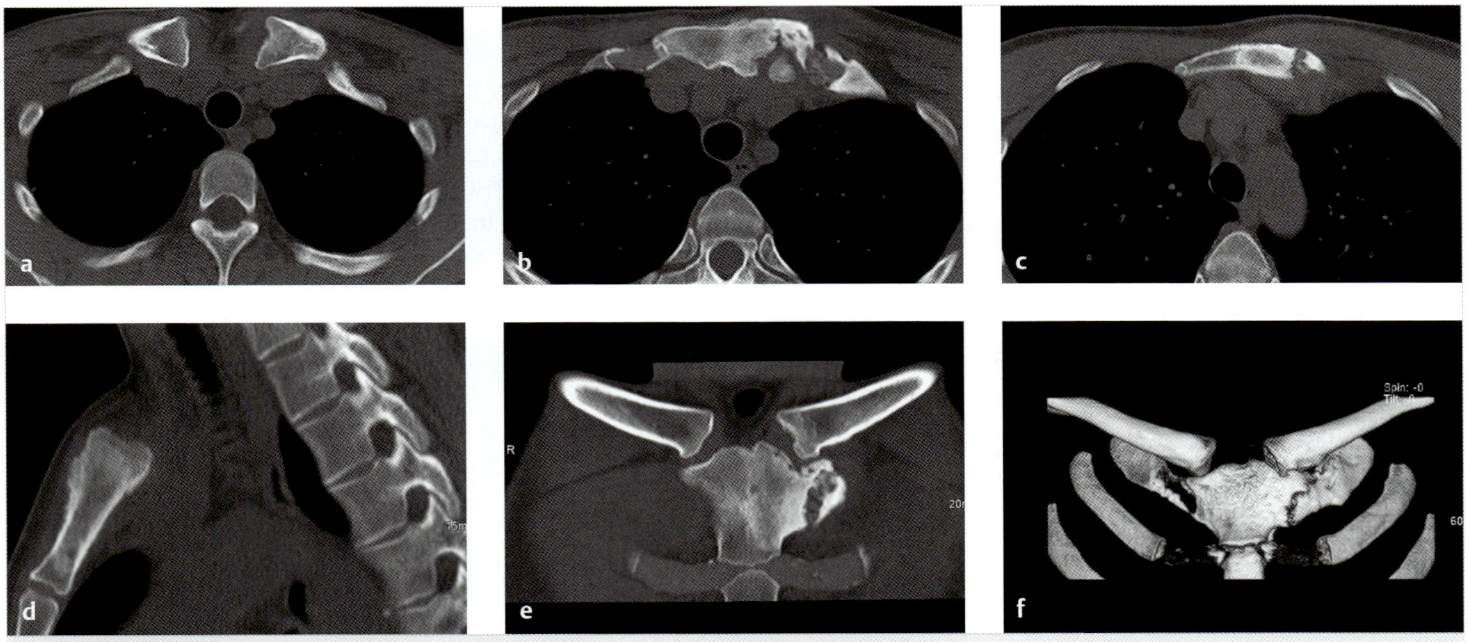

Fig. 5.41 a–f Asymmetric onset of SCCH in a 44-year-old woman.

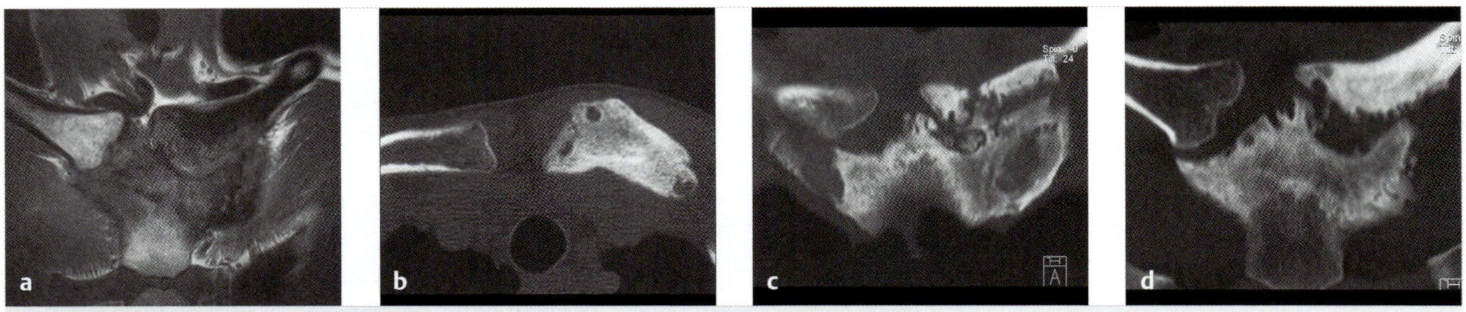

Fig. 5.42 a–d Mixed bone destruction and proliferation in SCCH.

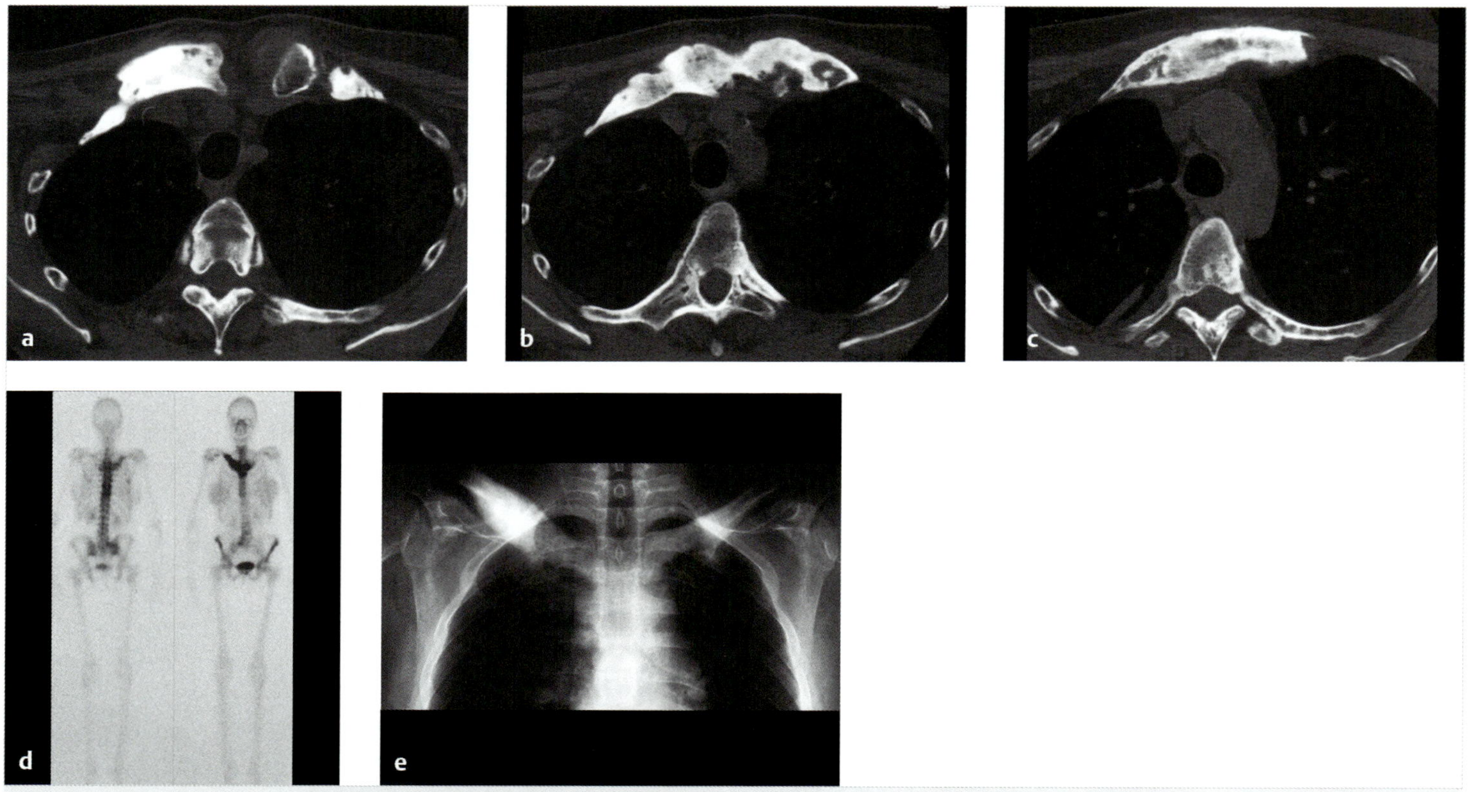

Fig. 5.43 a–e Plaque-like ossification in a late stage of SCCH.

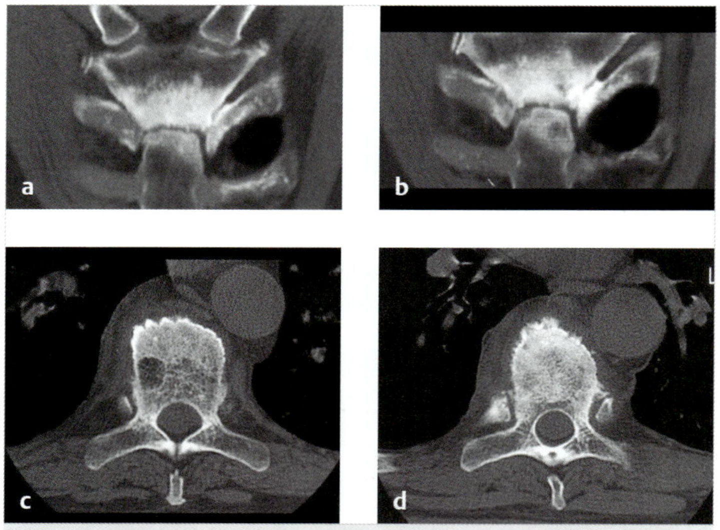

Fig. 5.44 a–d Manubriosternal synchondritis in a patient with pustulosis palmoplantaris and spondyloarthritis.

Comments

Destructive-proliferative changes in the entheses of the anterior chest wall and diskovertebral attachments are highly specific for psoriatic spondyloarthritis and, when pustulosis palmoplantaris (PPP) is present, for pustular arthro-osteitis (PAO) or enthesio-osteitis (PEO) or a SAPHO syndrome. But if neither psoriasis nor PPP is present clinically, these changes should be interpreted initially as an undifferentiated spondyloarthritis.

Case 98 (▸ Fig. 5.45)

Case description

- Referring physician: orthopedist.
- Prior history and clinical question: A 61-year-old patient had been aware of an indolent swelling on her right upper anterior chest wall for 6 weeks. Serum testing was negative for an inflammatory process, and rheumatoid factors were also negative. The sternal end (head) of the clavicle was prominent and springy on palpation. The referring orthopedist asked about a possible Tietze syndrome.

Radiologic Findings

The head of the right clavicle (sternal end) is subluxated anterosuperiorly. It is sclerotic and partially fragmented in its lower portion. The clavicular notch of the manubrium has irregular margins and is sclerotic. The soft tissues around the joint show significant thickening. Small, rounded lucencies are visible in the clavicular head on CT (▸ Fig. 5.45 **a–d**).

Location

The epicenter of the changes is located in the manubrioclavicular joint.

Pathoanatomic Background of the Findings

This case definitely involves a process originating from the manubrioclavicular joint. The (reactive) sclerosis indicates a longstanding arthropathy.

Assignment to a Possible Basic Entity

▸ **Normal variant or malformation?** No known precedents. Also, the process in the right manubrioclavicular joint has been symptomatic for only 6 weeks; this is inconsistent with a congenital condition.

▸ **Trauma?** The patient has no history of acute or chronic trauma.

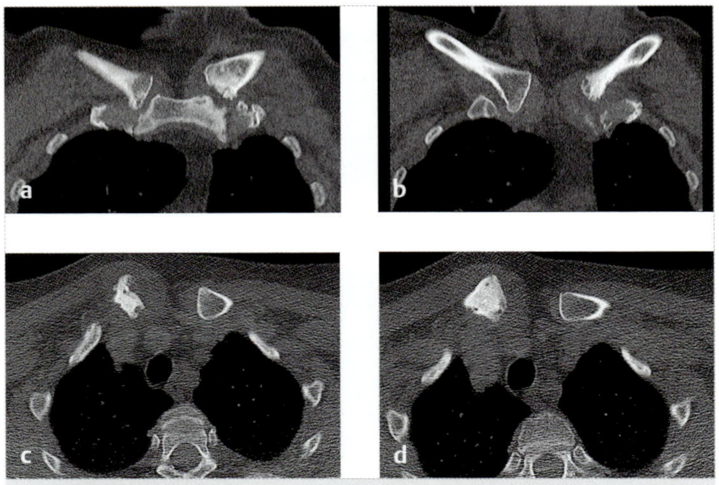

Fig. 5.45 a–d Tumor or chronic inflammation (a, b rendered with the sides reversed)?

▸ **Inflammation?** Certainly not a bacterial arthritis, but more likely a secondary, abacterial inflammation as in activated osteoarthritis. There is no clinical or laboratory evidence of rheumatic inflammation.

▸ **Tumor or tumorlike lesion?** No, the concentric thickening of the surrounding soft tissues signifies a primary articular process. With a tumor arising from the synovial membrane (e.g., synovial chondromatosis), we would expect to see eccentric thickening probably accompanied by erosive changes.

▸ **Perfusion disorder?** This is conceivable since the changes involve the end of the clavicle, but involvement of the clavicular notch and articular soft tissues is more suggestive of a primary articular process.

▸ **Regressive change?** Yes, see details in Synopsis and Discussion below.

Synopsis and Discussion

As we have seen, the mild clinical signs suggest a degenerative articular process. The following radiologic findings point to a primary degenerative process:
- Sclerosis of both articulating members
- Anterosuperior subluxation of the clavicular head
- Small lucencies in the clavicular head, which may be interpreted as subchondral cysts

The manubrio- or sternoclavicular joint is inherently incongruent and lacks stability owing to the very shallow clavicular notch of the manubrium and the slightly convex or sometimes concave end of the clavicle—especially when we consider that the joint capsule is relatively large and the articular disk, which should produce a buffering effect, is subject to early regressive changes that may begin by 20 to 30 years of age. When osteoarthritis is present, therefore, the clavicular head may easily follow the path of least resistance and subluxate anterosuperiorly. When combined with sclerosis of the articulating surfaces and subchondral cysts, this subluxation is highly specific for a diagnosis of *osteoarthritis of the manubrio- or sternoclavicular joint.*

The small bone fragment visible at the posteroinferior and medial end of the clavicle (▸ Fig. 5.45 **a**) is located in a defect in the joint contour and thus originates from the clavicular head. It very likely results from circumscribed bone necrosis in a setting of osteoarthritis, which is not at all unusual in other osteoarthritic joints. We do not believe that the bone fragment warrants a diagnosis of primary *aseptic necrosis* ("Friedrich disease"), in as much as we doubt that this condition, first described by Friedrich in 1924 (!), really exists as a separate entity.[13]

While the referring orthopedist suggested a diagnosis of *Tietze syndrome*, we again doubt that this is a separate disease entity. In 1921 Tietze described a painful and tender swelling of unknown cause, usually self-limiting and most commonly affecting the region of the second and third sternocostal junction. Since sectional imaging studies were unavailable at that time, there was no way to define the precise anatomic location of this obscure condition. Did it originate in the cartilage, entheses, or bone? Swellings of this kind can have many potential causes including a degenerative or inflammatory rheumatic enthesitis, chondritis, or chondronecrosis. With modern diagnostic modalities (including percutaneous biopsy) and criteria, we can differentiate among these entities and there is no longer any justification for making a catch-all diagnosis of "Tietze syndrome."

Final Diagnosis

Osteoarthritis of the right manubrio- or sternoclavicular joint with anterosuperior subluxation of the clavicular head.

Comments

When a woman in her 50s or 60s looks in the mirror and notices that the medial end of the clavicle appears prominent, and that site is noted clinically to be slightly tender and springy on palpation, this most likely indicates simple osteoarthritis of the manubrio- or sternoclavicular joint. Syndromes described almost a century ago, such as Friedrich disease and Tietze syndrome, no longer have a place in modern diagnostic radiology.

6 Upper Limb

6.1 Upper Arm

Case 99 (▶ Fig. 6.1)

Case description

- Referring physician: radiologist.
- Prior history and clinical question: When examined during a regular checkup 1 year earlier, a 7-year-old boy had been diagnosed with a "functional abnormality" of the right thumb that was not further specified. In a subsequent preschool examination, the boy had difficulty in fully extending his right knee. His mental and physical development was normal, and he had a negative family history. Radiographs were obtained and the radiologist offered a tentative diagnosis of melorheostosis.

Radiologic Findings

The radiograph of the right hand (▶ Fig. 6.1 **c**) shows dense linear and columnar ossifications in the first, second, fourth and fifth metacarpals, also in the proximal phalanges of those fingers, the distal phalanges of the first and fifth fingers, and the middle phalanx of the fifth finger. Incipient sclerosis is noted in the middle phalanges of the third and fourth fingers. Focal opacities are visible in all the carpal bones and in the radial epiphysis. The thumb

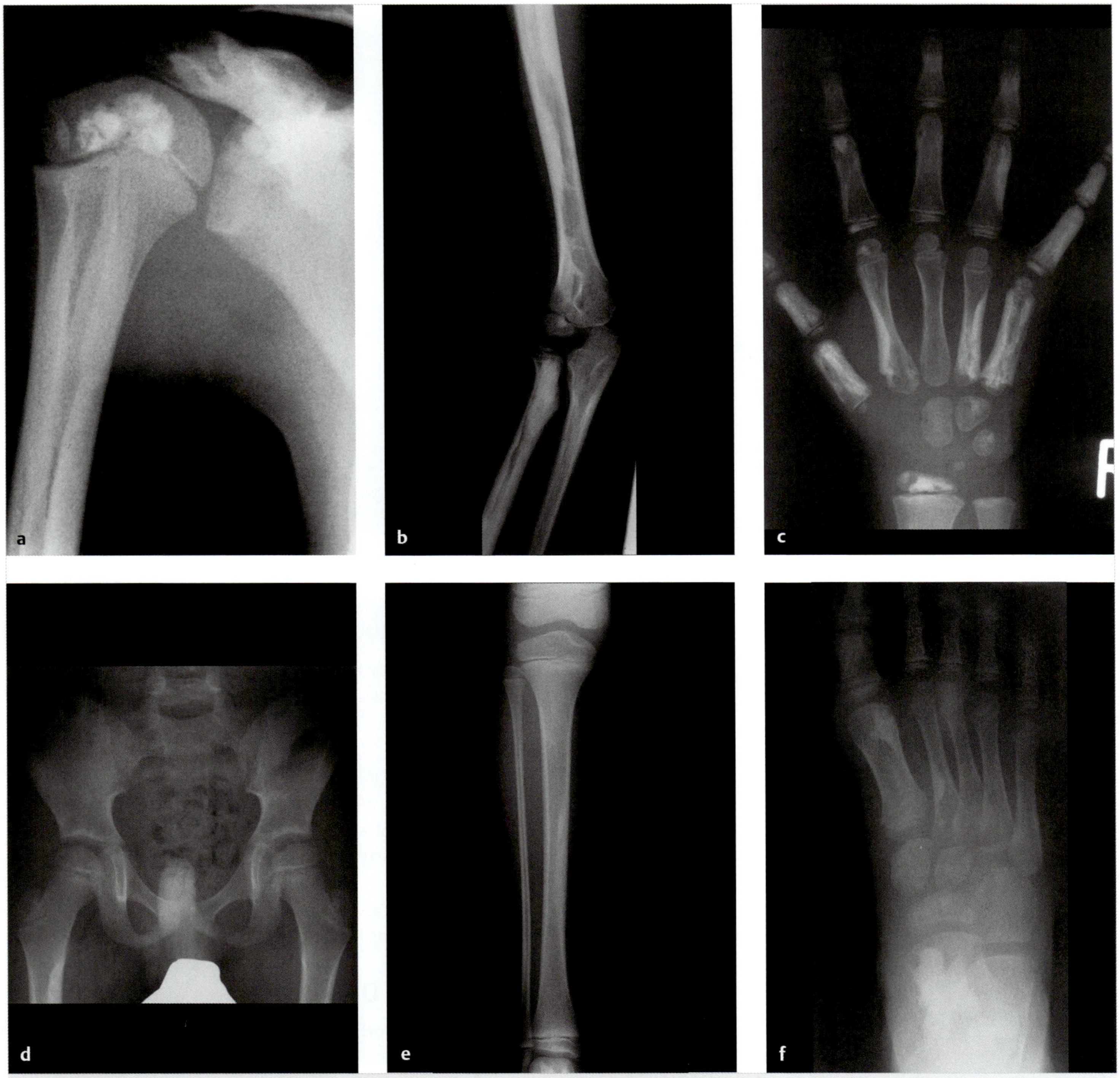

Fig. 6.1 a–f Functional abnormality of the right thumb and an extension deficit in the right knee. Congenital or acquired hyperostosis?

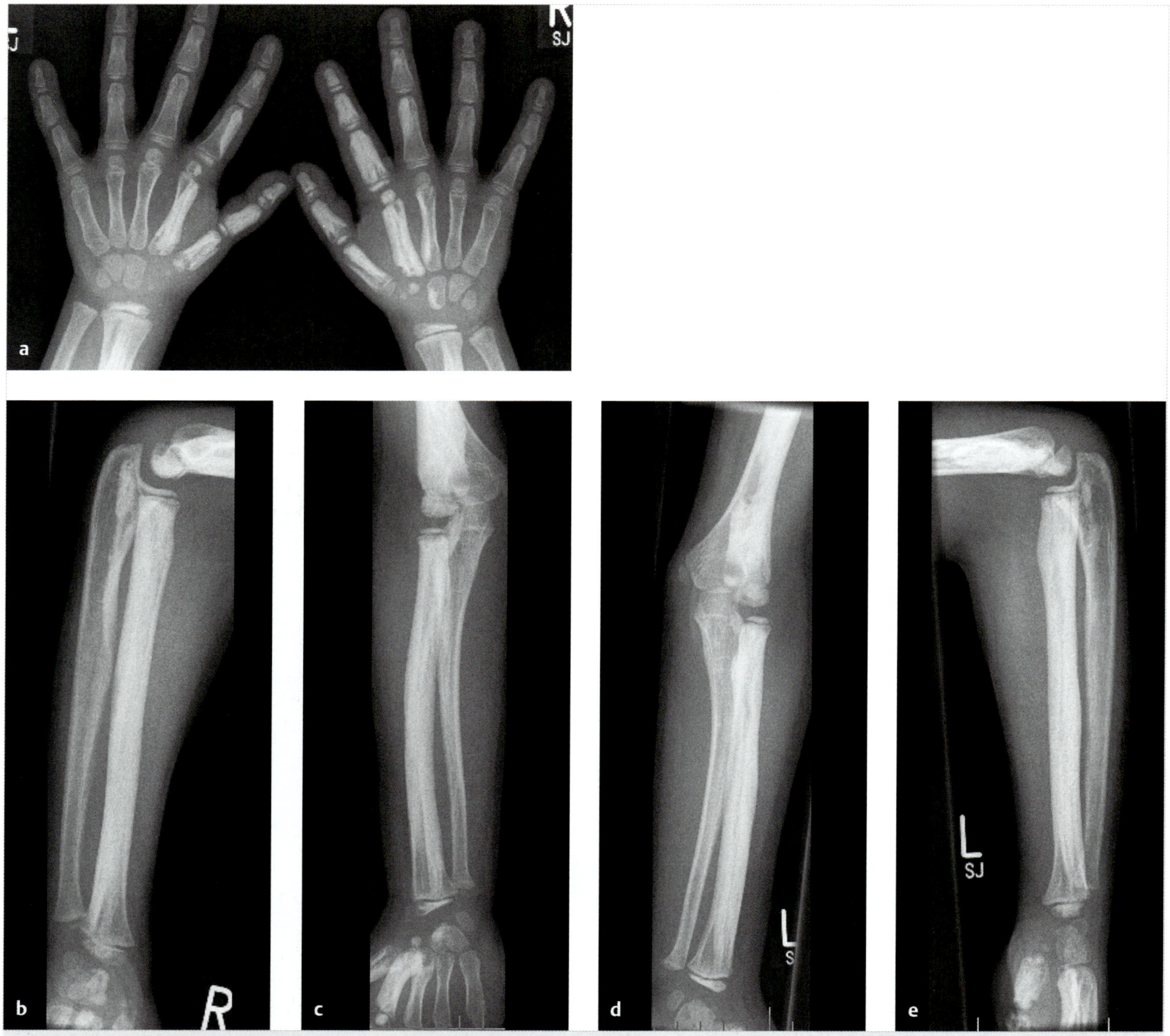

Fig. 6.2 a–e Bilateral melorheostosis in a 10-year-old boy.

appears slightly too short. Very dense bands and foci of sclerosis are also noted in the right scapula, throughout the humerus, and in the radius and ulna (▶ Fig. 6.1 **a, b**). Other areas of abnormal endosteal sclerosis are present in the epiphysis of the right femoral head, on the medial side of the right proximal femoral diaphysis (▶ Fig. 6.1 **d**), in the right tibial shaft (▶ Fig. 6.1 **e**), and in the talus of the right foot, which shows a more clumplike pattern of sclerosis (▶ Fig. 6.1 **f**).

Location

The areas of abnormal sclerosis are endosteal and occur only on the right side (images of the contralateral side are not pictured here). Their distribution, therefore, is unilateral and segmental.

Pathoanatomic Background of the Findings

The unilateral segmental distribution of the sclerotic areas, some showing an ivory density, and the age of the patient are suggestive of bone dysplasia with too much bone.

Assignment to a Possible Basic Entity

▶ **Normal variant or malformation?** Yes. The findings are typical of melorheostosis affecting the limb bones on the right side of the body.

▶ **Inflammation?** No history. Reactive inflammatory bone formation is rarely as solid and well circumscribed as in this case. We do not know of an inflammatory bone process that would have a segmental distribution limited to one side of the body.

▶ **Tumor?** Multifocal osteosarcomas do occur, but not in a unilateral distribution as in this case.

Synopsis and Discussion

The endosteal, melorheostotic new bone formation can be described morphologically as showing a mixed striate, osteoma-like (osteopathia striata–like) pattern combined with a "flowing candle wax" appearance. There is no other reasonable differential

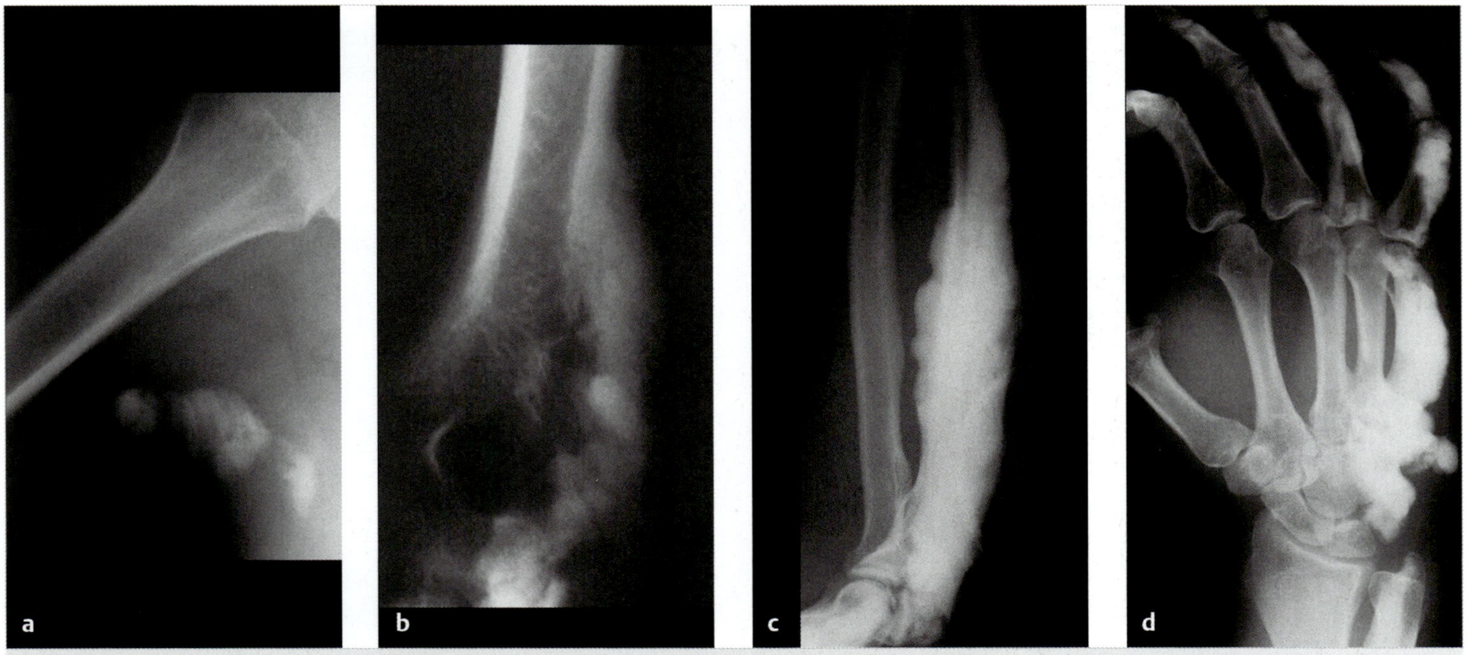

Fig. 6.3 a–d Melorheostosis of the right upper limb in a 36-year-old man.

diagnosis. Further information on melorheostosis can be found in Case 17 and Case 88. We attribute the child's clinical complaints to fibrotic soft-tissue changes in the thumb and about the knee, which occur in approximately 60% of patients with melorheostosis (see also Case 88). These fibrotic changes may eventually ossify (see ▶ Fig. 6.3 **below**) and, when viewed in isolation, can mimic myositis ossificans (▶ Fig. 6.3 **a**).

▶ Fig. 6.2 shows an unusual case of bilateral involvement by melorheostosis with clear-cut radiographic features in a 10-year-old boy with brachydactyly of the thumbs and index fingers. The ossifications are more pronounced on the radial side as they follow the distribution of "sclerotomes," or skeletal zones supplied by individual sensory spinal fibers. We attribute the brachydactyly to associated soft-tissue changes in the affected phalanges leading to growth disturbance.

▶ Fig. 6.3 illustrates the case of a 36-year-old man with pronounced melorheostosis of the right upper limb, again presenting unmistakable radiomorphologic features ("candle wax" pattern on the distal humerus, radius, and bones of the hand). Note the ossification in the right axilla. Marked subcutaneous fibrotic changes, associated with considerable pain, were found on the right forearm and the ulnar side of the hand. The symptoms had begun in puberty, and the patient eventually lost the use of his right arm. Note the segmental distribution of the changes on the ulnar side, again following the sclerotomes as in the previous case (▶ Fig. 6.2).

Final Diagnosis

Melorheostosis.

Comments

A segmental arrangement of solid ossifications in the upper and/or lower limb distributed along sclerotomes always indicates melorheostosis. Since the disease may be complicated by soft-tissue changes, it should not be dismissed as a harmless normal variant.

Case 100 (▶ Fig. 6.4)

Case description

- Referring physician: pediatrician.
- Prior history and clinical question: An 18-year-old male had a complex condition that included epilepsy, dementia, muscular dystrophy, nephrocalcinosis type 1, etc. He had been on anticonvulsant medication (sodium valproate) for a number of years. Because the patient developed severe osteoporosis with an osteomalacic component (resulting from the muscular dystrophy and anticonvulsant therapy) with repeated bone fractures, treatment with cholecalciferol was tried but was unsuccessful. Bisphosphonates were started 2 years previously in an effort to treat the osseous changes. Follow-up radiographs of the upper and lower limbs showed a surprising finding, which was referred to us for investigation.

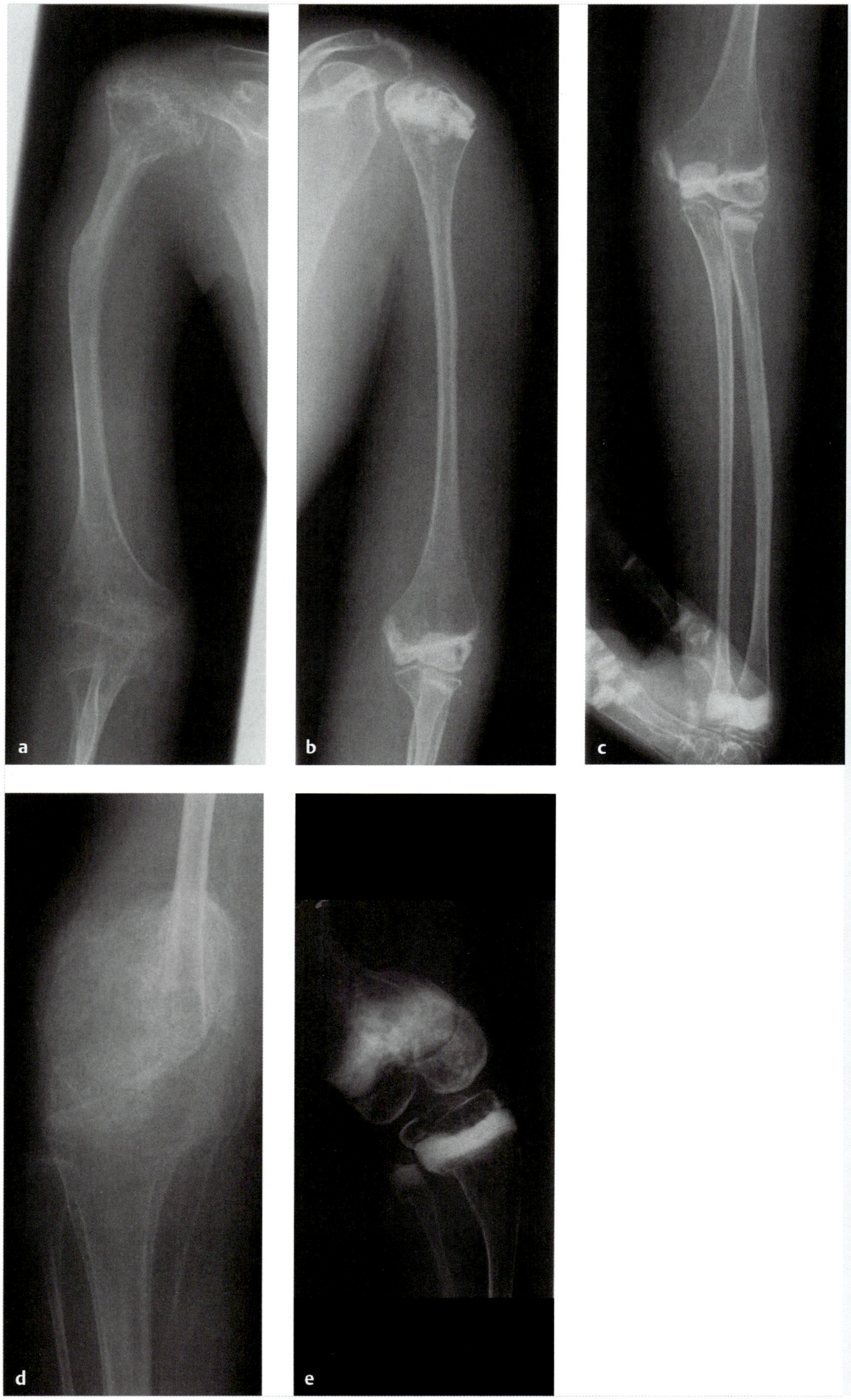

Fig. 6.4 Congenital or acquired hyperostosis? Two radiographs were taken in 2002 (a, d), the other radiographs in 2004 (b,c,e).

Radiologic Findings

Current radiographs of the upper and lower limbs taken in 2004 (▶ Fig. 6.4 **b, c, e**) initially show a very severe narrowing and developmental disturbance of the imaged long bones (epiphyseal plates still open in an 18-year-old!) with severe bowing of the bones about the right knee joint. Dense sclerotic changes are visible in the metaphyses. A radiograph of the right arm in 2002 (▶ Fig. 6.4 **a**; a prior radiograph of the left side does not exist) shows varus bowing caused by an old malunited fracture at the junction of the middle and upper thirds of the diaphysis; there is no metaphyseal sclerosis. A radiograph of the right knee in 2002 (▶ Fig. 6.4 **d**) shows a fracture of the femoral metaphysis that healed with gross deformity and excessive callus formation, but without sclerotic changes.

Location

The unusual opacities on the 2004 radiographs are confined to the metaphyses.

Pathoanatomic Background of the Findings

The unusual zones of metaphyseal sclerosis are acquired, as they did not exist 2 years earlier. They represent new bone.

Assignment to a Possible Basic Entity

The metaphyseal opacities apparently result from the bisphosphonate therapy initiated 2 years earlier. The patient's overall condition and medication did not change during that period. Given this plausible chain of causality, we do not need to consider the usual range of basic entities.

Synopsis and Discussion

This young man has a complex skeletal disorder that may be described as a severe developmental abnormality characterized by significant osteoporosis with an osteomalacic component. It results from a lifetime of muscular dystrophy and chronic anticonvulsant drug therapy, which is known to cause osteomalacia in some patients.

Bisphosphonates inhibit the osteoclastic breakdown of bone, leading to decreased bone resorption. This effect appears first in the metaphyses because they directly adjoin the growth plate, whose metaphyseal side consists of the "zone of provisional (or preparatory) calcification." When resorption in this zone is absent or greatly diminished, the result is dense bone formation similar to that in marble bone disease. Intermittent bisphosphonate therapy in a growing skeleton may give rise to thin, sclerotic metaphyseal bands in the long tubular bones. The bands are directed parallel to the growth plates, with each line representing one treatment cycle. Only their extreme radiographic density distinguishes these bands from metaphyseal growth lines (Harris lines), which result from episodic growth (as a normal variant or growth disturbance) and resemble the growth rings of a tree.

Long-term bisphosphonate therapy, as in the present case, may induce the development of broader and denser bands. Dense bands (▶ Fig. 6.4 **c**) may also appear around the apophyses and around small round and irregular bones (carpals, tarsals), whose actual growth zone is located between the ossification center and articular cartilage (synonyms: acrophysis, spherical growth plate). "Growth rings" may also develop in the vertebral bodies due to bisphosphonate therapy and create a "bone in bone" pattern like that seen in marble bone disease.

Final Diagnosis

Dense metaphyseal bands induced by bisphosphonate therapy.

Comments

Bisphosphonate therapy in the growing skeleton may induce unusual zones of metaphyseal sclerosis that result from the inhibition of osteoclastic and osteocytic bone resorption.

Case 101 (▶ Fig. 6.5)

Case description

- Referring physician: orthopedist.
- Prior history and clinical question: A 57-year-old woman presented with a long history of left shoulder pain. She stated that the pain would worsen from time to time, becoming intolerable. She claimed good response to nonsteroidal anti-inflammatory drugs. MRI raised suspicion of a neoplastic process. Otherwise the patient was in good health.

Radiologic Findings

The coronal STIR image in ▶ Fig. 6.5 **a** shows a large area of edema-like signal occupying the left humeral head and proximal metaphysis. The axial T1-weighted (T1w) image in ▶ Fig. 6.5 **b** shows an elliptical signal void bordering the posterior circumference of the humeral head, just behind the greater tuberosity. The lesion has a peripheral rim of intermediate signal intensity, creating a target pattern.

Location

The possible cause of the edema-like signal is located in the bone (▶ Fig. 6.5 **b**) but lies directly beneath the infraspinatus tendon and a possible bursa.

Pathoanatomic Background of the Findings

The two principal findings on MRI are a large area of edema-like signal and a signal void located behind the greater tuberosity. It is logical to assume that both findings are related. The low signal intensity of the focal lesion suggests that it is osseous or has a low proton density. We ordered CT scans as a simple, straightforward way to resolve these questions. CT definitely shows a calcific process within a bone defect (▶ Fig. 6.5 **c, d**). Between the rim of the osteolytic defect and the calcific lesion is a transitional zone whose intermediate signal intensity suggests synovial tissue or a kind of capsule, but may also represent uncalcified osteoid, for example. Thus, the findings may indicate a tumor with pronounced perifocal edema such as osteoid osteoma, an enthesitic process that has eroded into the bone, or even a primary inflammatory process.

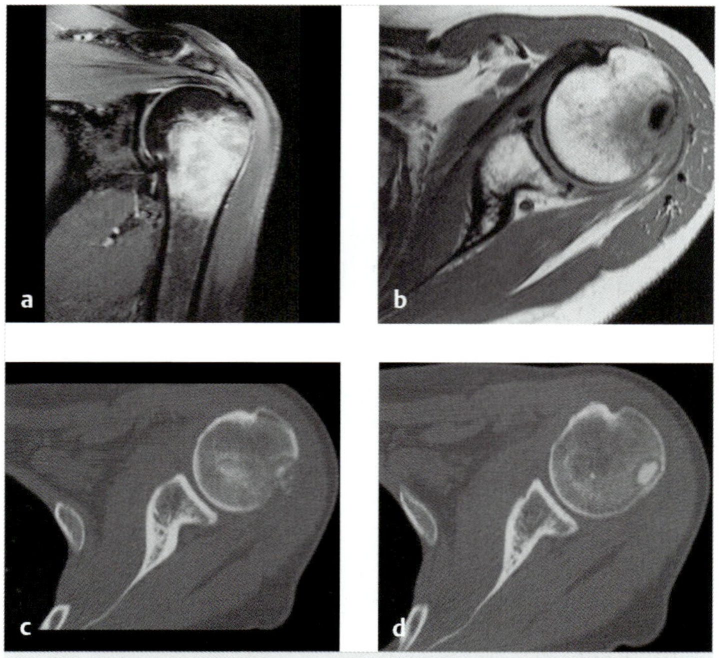

Fig. 6.5 a–d Tumor in the humeral head?

Assignment to a Possible Basic Entity

▶ **Normal variant or malformation?** No, the clinical presentation alone indicates a significant disease process.

▶ **Trauma?** The patient did not give a history of acute trauma. On the other hand, the principal finding is located below a region that is subject to constant, significant stress, namely an enthesis.

▶ **Inflammation?** The edema-like signal may be interpreted as a reactive inflammatory process or osteitis. The lesion just behind the humeral head could be a sequestrum.

▶ **Tumor?** Quite possibly, an osteoid osteoma with a calcified nidus and marked perifocal edema.

Synopsis and Discussion

The above considerations give us the following differential diagnosis:

1. Osteomyelitis with a sequestrum
2. Osteoid osteoma
3. Calcified tendinitis and/or bursitis that has eroded into the bone

▶ **On differential diagnosis 1** This diagnosis is not consistent with the history. With bacterial osteomyelitis, the patient would have had a shorter history, fever, and other signs. She had no risk factors for osteomyelitis such as diabetes mellitus.

▶ **On differential diagnosis 2** This diagnosis is not supported by the patient's age or history. Osteoid osteoma would most likely be characterized by constant pain and a shorter history.

▶ **On differential diagnosis 3** This diagnosis is supported by the following findings:

- *Location:* The location is typical of a calcifying tendinitis or bursitis periodically eroding into the bone. The calcified material in the bone is resorbed after these acute episodes, and any extraosseous calcification at the perforation site has disappeared. The shoulder with its numerous entheses (tendons and capsular attachments) is a musculoskeletal weak point that is subjected to constant heavy loads.
- *Age of the patient:* Calcifying tendinitis or bursitis typically occurs in older individuals.
- *History:* The history consists of several years of intermittent shoulder pain with periodic exacerbations. During the exacerbations, a nonspecific, highly inflammatory process develops in the tendon attachment or bursa leading to resorption of the adjacent bone and eventual breakthrough (of the calcifications) into the bone.

▶ Fig. 6.6 shows an almost identical case in a 67-year-old man with calcifying tendinitis or bursitis eroding into the bone. He

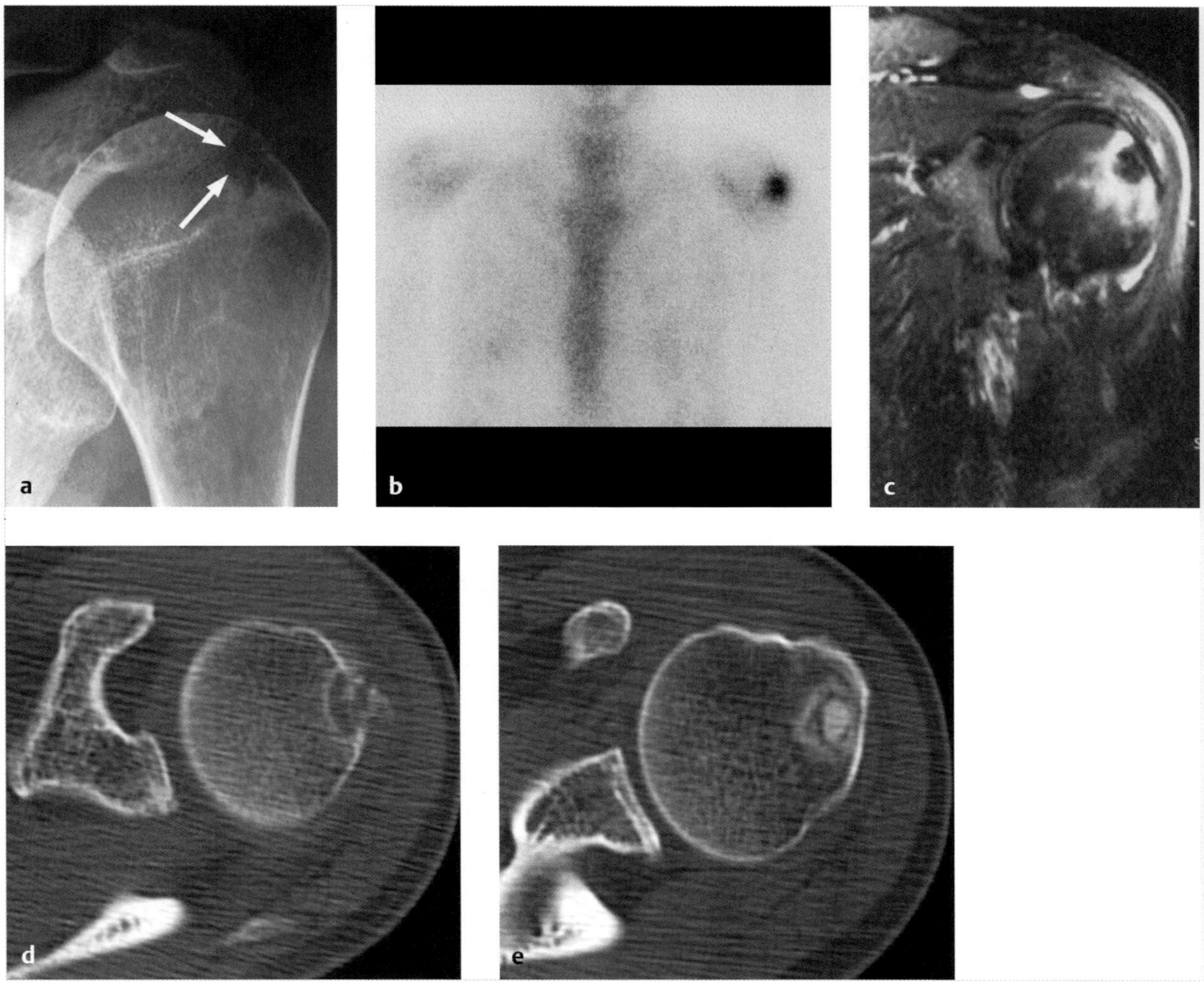

Fig. 6.6 a–e Calcifying tendinitis or bursitis with bone erosion and perforation in a 67-year-old man.

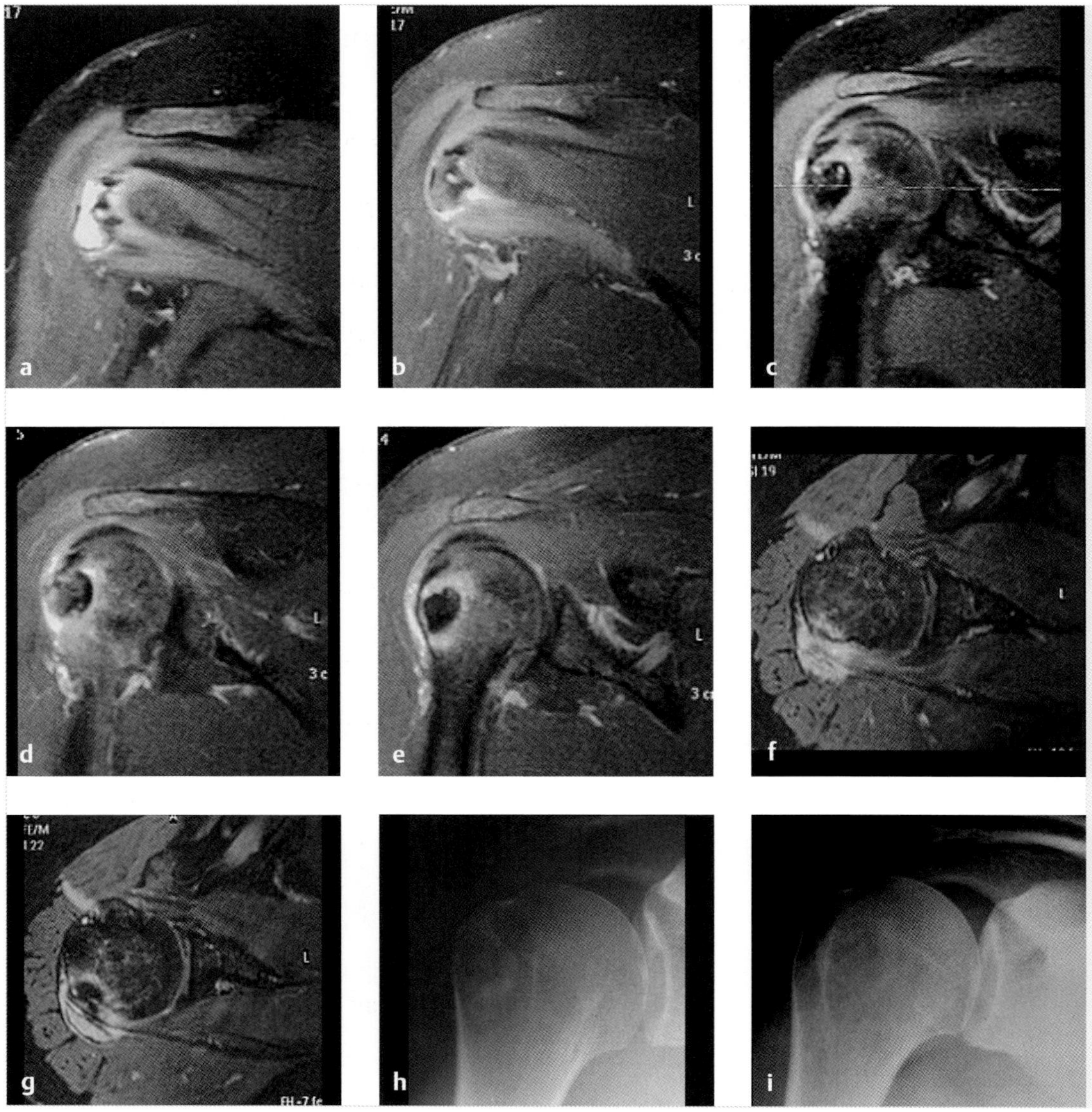

Fig. 6.7 a–i Calcifying tendinitis or bursitis with bone erosion in a 57-year-old woman. The last shown radiograph (i) was taken at 3-month follow-up.

was seen 2 weeks after experiencing an acute, stabbing pain in his left shoulder lasting approximately 48 hours. The radiograph (arrows in ▶ Fig. 6.6 **a**) showed an osteolytic area in the region of the greater tuberosity. The bone scan (▶ Fig. 6.6 **b**) showed focal increased uptake, and MRI (▶ Fig. 6.6 **c**) showed marked edema-like signal intensity around a hypointense focus, which CT (▶ Fig. 6.6 **d, e**) identified as a calcified mass. The scan in ▶ Fig. 6.6 **d** clearly documents the pathogenesis of the process: An extraosseous calcified mass relating to the calcified tendon or bursa is continuous with an intraosseous calcified mass through a defect in the cortex.

Another case of cortical erosion by calcifying tendinitis or bursitis is illustrated in ▶ Fig. 6.7. The patient, a 57-year-old woman, had hyperacute pain symptoms several days before MRI. Her right shoulder was swollen and warm to the touch, mimicking arthritis. The MR images (▶ Fig. 6.7 **a–g**) are self-explanatory. A radiograph (▶ Fig. 6.7 **h**) at the time of MRI showed an osteolytic area in the greater tuberosity, in which ground-glass opacities could be seen. After 3 months of intensive therapy with nonsteroidal anti-inflammatory drugs, her clinical symptoms resolved completely and a radiograph (▶ Fig. 6.7 **i**) showed increasing bony consolidation of the osteolytic area. It should be added that the osteolytic area displayed by radiographs should not be confused with the normal sparseness of trabecular structures in that region.[17]

Final Diagnosis

Calcifying tendinitis or bursitis that eroded into the bone.

Comments

When interpreted by themselves, MR images of calcifying tendinitis or bursitis with cortical erosion may lead to misinterpretation. CT scans should be added to enable detection of the calcified structures.

Case 102 (▶ Fig. 6.8)

Case description

- Referring physician: orthopedist.
- Prior history and clinical question: A 7-year-old boy was noted incidentally to have a posterolateral bony prominence at the junction of the proximal and middle thirds of the humeral diaphysis. Tumor?

Radiologic Findings

Radiographs of the humerus (▶ Fig. 6.8 **a, b**) demonstrate a prominence in the area of the deltoid tuberosity. On CT scans (▶ Fig. 6.8 **c, d**) the cortex of the adjacent humerus appears to be continuous with the prominence. The area within the prominence shows ground-glass opacity adjoining the fat-containing medullary cavity. Bone scans (▶ Fig. 6.8 **e**) show no abnormalities in either humerus.

Location

The prominence is located in the anatomic region of the deltoid tuberosity.

Pathoanatomic Background of the Findings

The harmonious structure of the prominence in the region of a physiologic "roughness" or bony protrusion with a rough surface (tuberosity) at the attachment of the deltoid muscle, plus the incidental detection and negative bone scan, are not consistent with a true pathologic finding. The prominence appears to contain cancellous bone, which would explain the ground-glass attenuation on CT. This makes the diagnosis clear, and there is no need to consider a range of basic entities.

Synopsis and Discussion

If the child had pain in the affected region and a positive bone scan, the differential diagnosis would still include a stress-induced enthesiopathy (see Case 75, Case 77, Case 103, Case 104, and Case 151). Other possibilities such as a flat osteochondroma or osteoblastoma lack any real basis, as we are dealing with a physiologic finding that varies in different individuals depending on body habitus and stress levels.

▶ Fig. 6.9 shows the case of a 53-year-old man with nonspecific complaints in his left upper arm 3 years after receiving an early-summer meningoencephalitis vaccination at that site. Even at the time of imaging, the symptoms subsided in response to local massage. The imaging studies had been ordered for investigation of a shoulder contusion, but the patient asked that imaging be extended to cover his left upper arm. The deltoid tuberosity appears prominent on MRI (▶ Fig. 6.9 **a, b**) and contains cancellous bone and fatty tissue. The adjacent medullary cavity contains normal fat plus a linear, medially angled structure that is hyperintense in the water-sensitive sequence (▶ Fig. 6.9 **a**) and is devoid of signal on the T1w image (▶ Fig. 6.9 **b**). This may represent a vascular structure. CT images in various projections (▶ Fig. 6.9 **e–h**) show disorganized intraosseous bone tissue in which fatty marrow spaces can be seen. Anatomic diagrams of the humerus (▶ Fig. 6.9 **c, d**) illustrate the complex anatomy in the region of the deltoid tuberosity, especially in the posterior view (▶ Fig. 6.9 **c**), with a vascular foramen and the groove for the ulnar nerve. It is easy to see how regressive changes might develop in and on this enthesis in response to repetitive stresses, including focal inflammation with intramedullary involvement, fat necrosis leading to metaplastic bone formation, and other changes. Any suspicion of a tumor process ("A tumor cannot be excluded.") is untenable, and further follow-ups are unnecessary. The clinical complaints cannot be attributed to the finding, which we therefore classify as incidental.

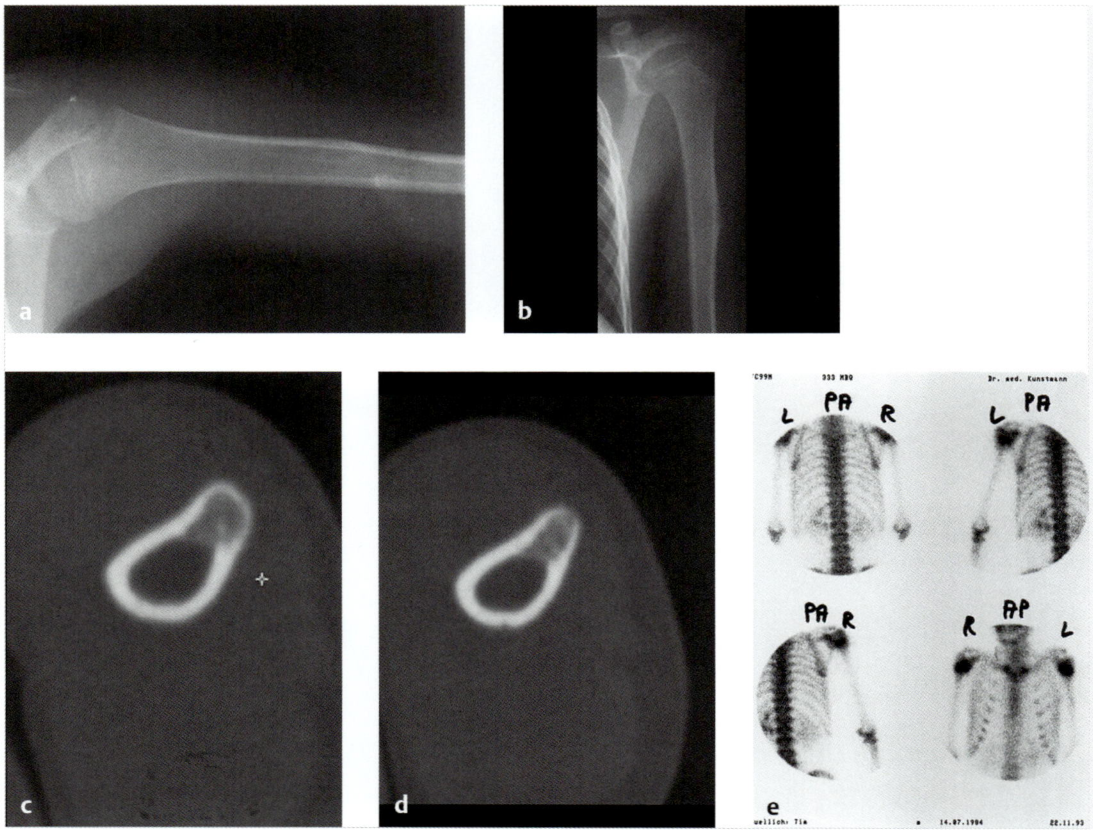

Fig. 6.8 a–e Exostotic tumor?
AP = anteroposterior
PA = posteroanterior

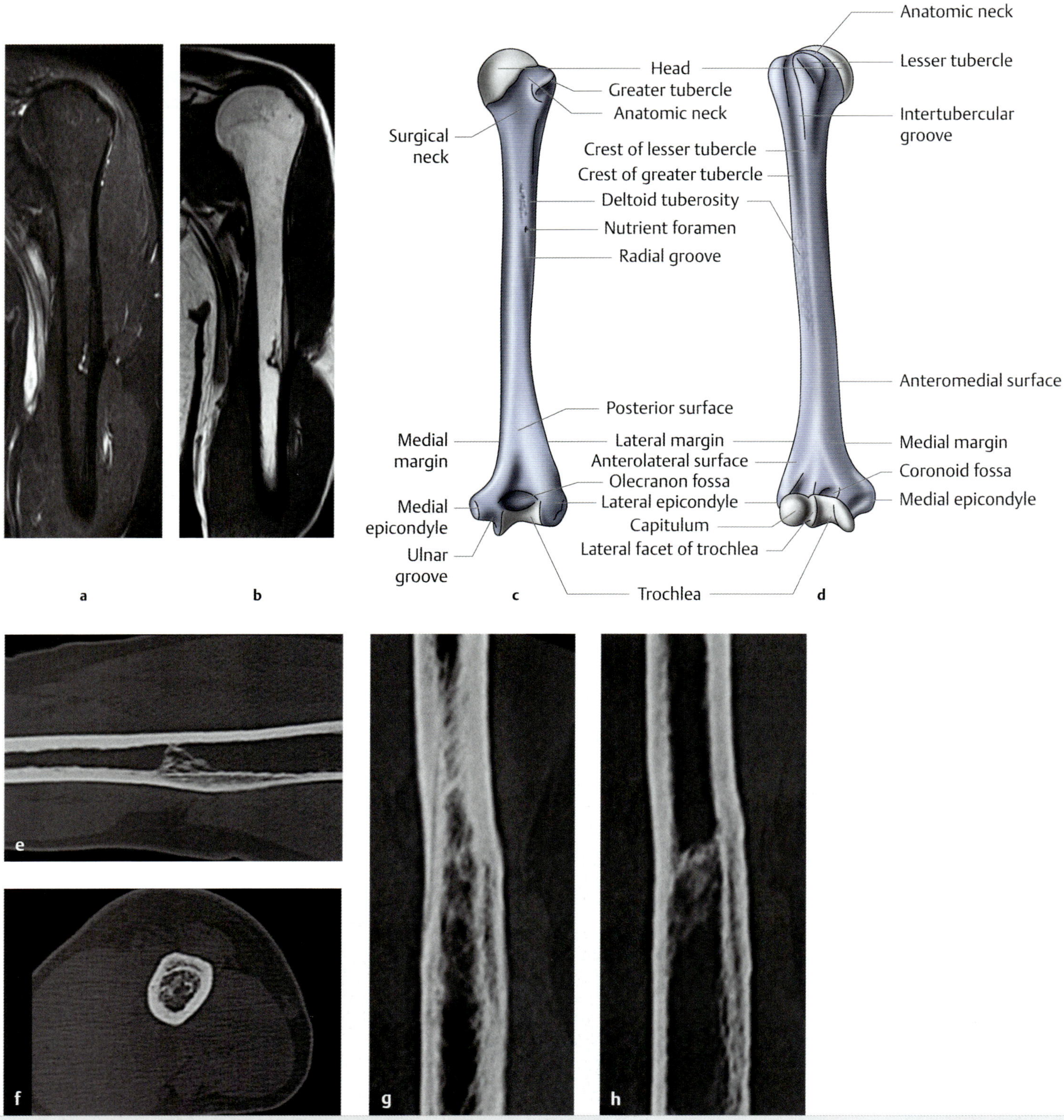

Fig. 6.9 a–h Incidental finding on the deltoid tuberosity of a 53-year-old man.

Final Diagnosis

Slightly prominent but normal deltoid tuberosity.

Comments

Incidental findings, especially at an enthesis, most likely represent normal findings or variants. Cases of this kind do not require follow-up, which would cause needless concern for the patients and their families.

Case 103 (▶ Fig. 6.10)

Case description

- Referring physician: pathologist.
- Prior history and clinical question: A 51-year-old woman with a history of breast cancer underwent a bone scan for investigation of mild back pain. The scan showed slight focal uptake in the proximal left humerus. The patient had no complaints in that area; she was otherwise healthy with no evidence of metastasis. She was an avid golfer.

Radiologic Findings

The whole-body bone scan (▶ Fig. 6.10 **b**) was normal except for a focal area of slightly increased uptake in the left proximal humeral diaphysis. The radiograph (▶ Fig. 6.10 **a**) showed a circumscribed lucency in the slightly prominent deltoid tuberosity, corresponding to the site of increased uptake. MRI (▶ Fig. 6.10 **c–e**) showed no significant pathology at the site of increased uptake.

Location

As described above, the osteolytic focus showing moderate tracer uptake is located in the deltoid tuberosity, and thus in an enthesis.

Pathoanatomic Background of the Findings

The location of the radiologic findings is suspicious for an enthesiopathy. A solitary cortical metastasis or primary bone tumor (e.g., osteoid osteoma) is unlikely due to the incidental nature of the finding (see Normal variant or malformation? and Synopsis and Discussion below).

Assignment to a Possible Basic Entity

▶ **Normal variant or malformation?** There is no consensus as to whether an incidental imaging finding (increased uptake, lucency) at an enthesis should still be considered a normal variant if the patient has no complaints. This view is supported by the observation that entheses, where soft-tissue structures are attached to bone, are generally exposed to greater stresses than other skeletal regions. This makes them areas of least resistance that are considerably more susceptible to any and all stimuli than other regions. Based on this concept, even mild stress reactions may produce clinically silent effects that can now be visualized by sensitive modalities such as bone scintigraphy and MRI. Also, there are undoubtedly significant interindividual differences in the sensitivity of entheses to stress depending on factors such as body habitus and stress levels. We tend to classify these findings as normal variants. Note that this does not apply to enthesiopathies from the rheumatoid group (enthesitis) or severe stress-

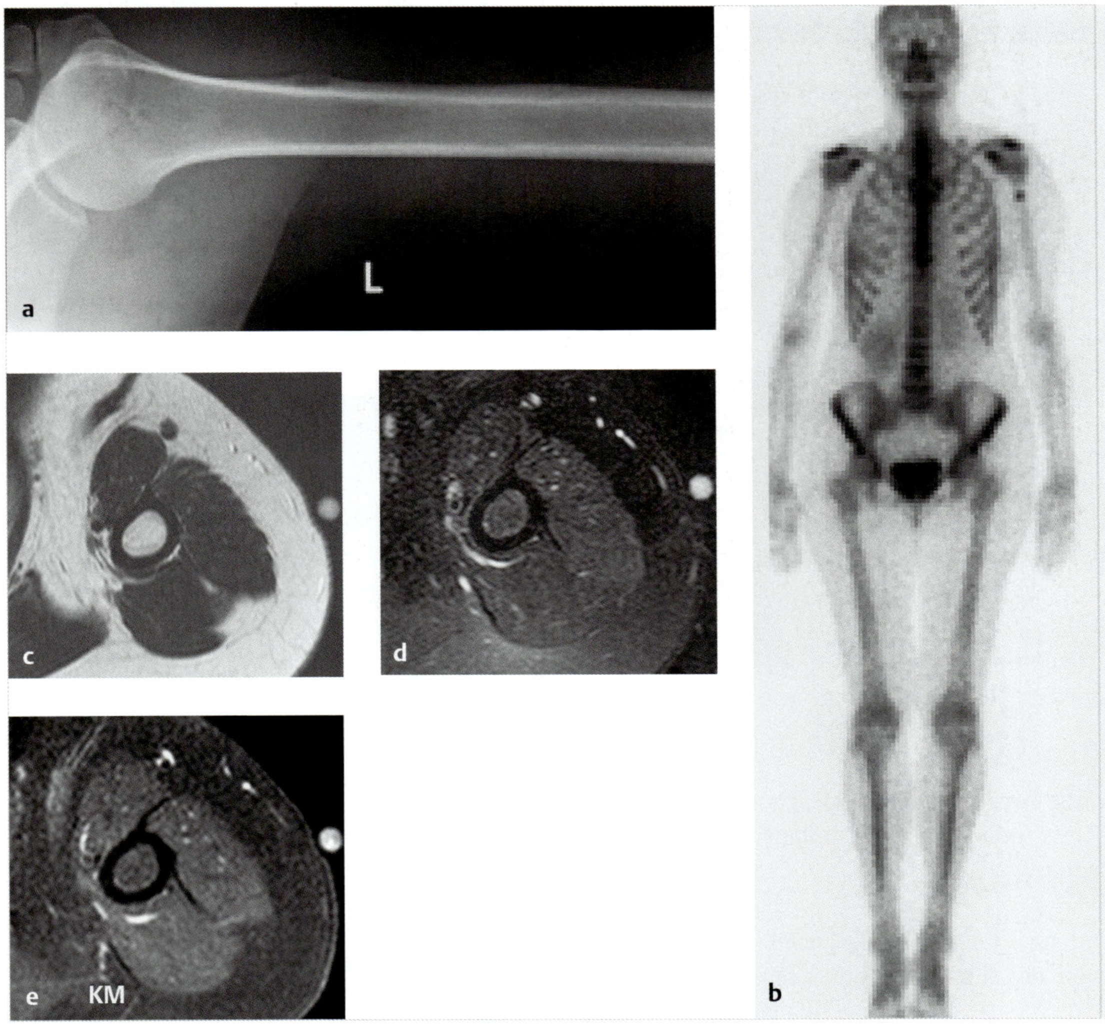

Fig. 6.10 a–e Patient with a history of breast cancer. Metastasis?

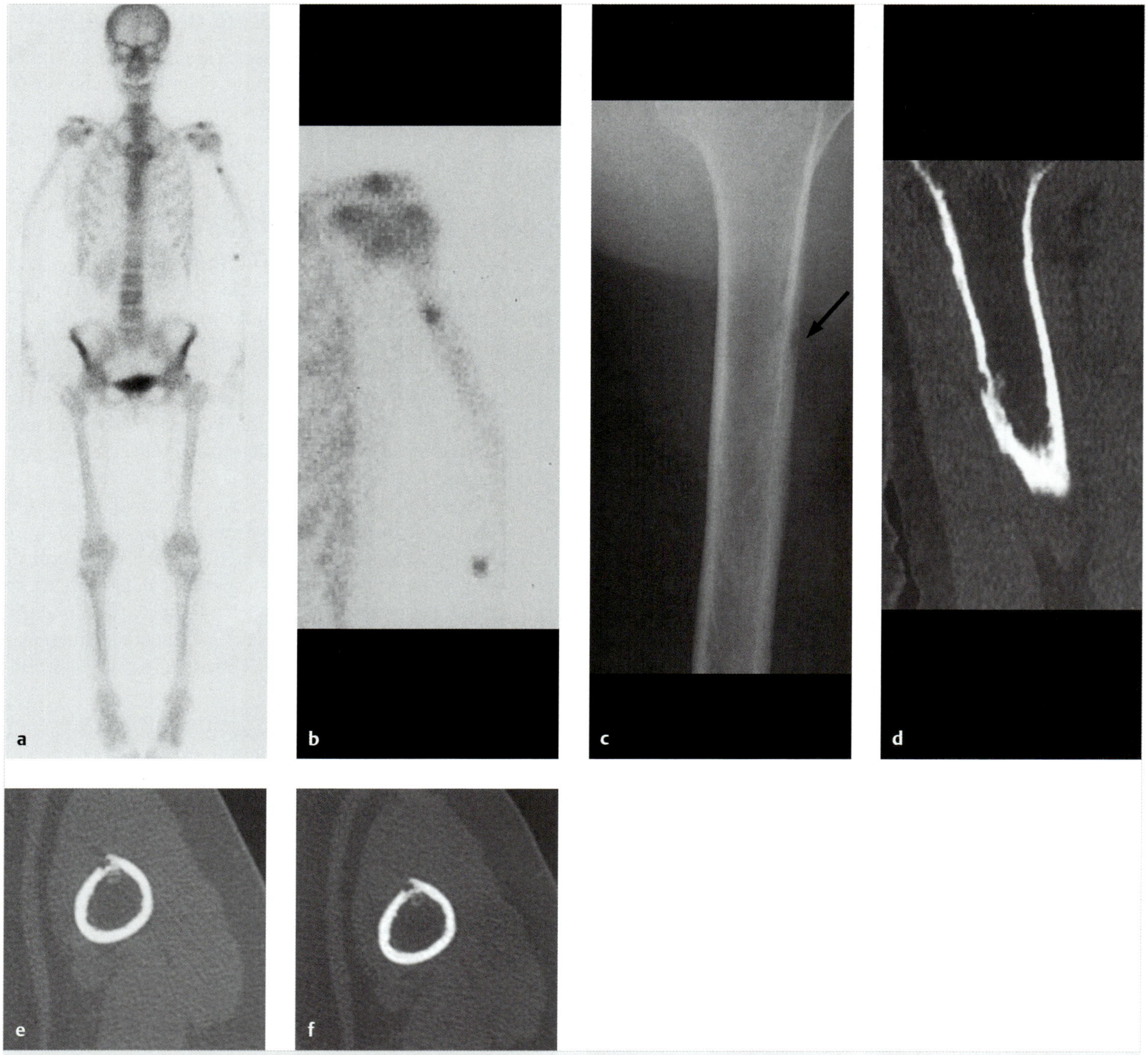

Fig. 6.11 a–f Calcifying tendinitis with cortical erosion and perforation in a 62-year-old woman.

induced changes, which generally are associated with clinical symptoms.

▶ **Trauma?** Yes, in the form of chronic traction injury (see section Normal variant or malformation?). The patient is an avid golfer.

▶ **Inflammation?** Certainly not in the form of osteomyelitis, given the absence of clinical signs. Stress-induced reactive inflammatory changes are discussed above.

▶ **Tumor?** No. An osteoid osteoma, for example, would generally be associated with pain. It would also show more tracer uptake on the bone scan (the "double density sign," see Case 74 and Case 144). A cortical metastasis would also produce greater uptake in addition to clinical complaints and positive MRI. In any case, a solitary metastasis in an enthesis would be an extremely rare occurrence that should be considered only after all other possibilities have been excluded. It would require an excisional biopsy.

Synopsis and Discussion

Based on the above considerations, the finding in the left proximal humerus appears to be a clinically silent stress reaction at the deltoid muscle attachment. It may be classified as a harmless associated finding or, as we prefer, a normal variant. There is no need for excisional biopsy or imaging follow-ups.

By contrast, ▶ Fig. 6.11 illustrates the case of a 62-year-old woman with a history of breast cancer. She complained of pain in her left upper arm which occurred approximately 3 weeks before imaging and responded well to nonsteroidal anti-inflammatory drugs. A spot radiograph of the humerus showed an osteolytic lesion or lucency at the crest of the greater tubercle (arrow in

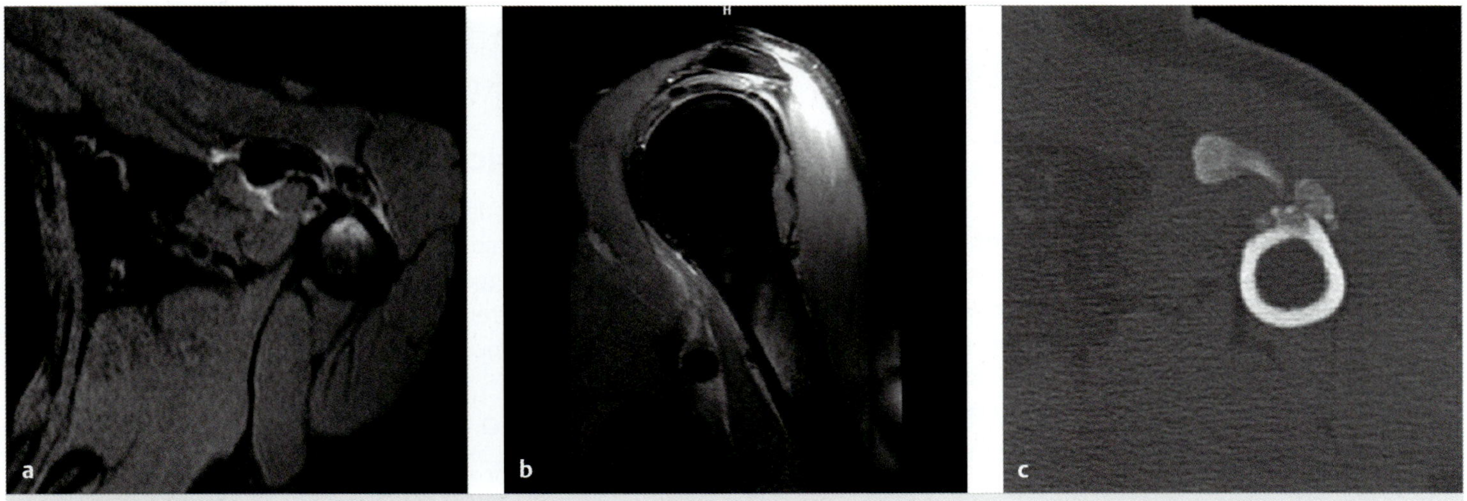

Fig. 6.12 a–c Osseous involvement by calcifying tendinitis in a 47-year-old woman.

▶ Fig. 6.11 **c**). The bone scan showed slightly increased uptake at that location (▶ Fig. 6.11 **a, b**). CT (▶ Fig. 6.11 **d–f**) showed a defect in the anterior cortex or in the crest of the greater tubercle (see ▶ Fig. 6.9 **d** in Case 102). Below the defect was a small intramedullary calcification that has the same diameter as the defect. This made the diagnosis clear: cortical erosion and perforation by a somewhat longstanding calcifying tendinitis of the pectoralis major, which inserts on the crest. This refuted the earlier suspicion of a metastasis and eliminated the need for excisional biopsy.

Another case of calcifying tendinitis of the pectoralis major tendon is illustrated in ▶ Fig. 6.12. The 47-year-old woman had experienced acute pain in the proximal anterior upper arm several weeks earlier. At the time of imaging (MRI, CT), there were still marked signs of inflammation at the tendon attachment as indicated by edema-like signal with involvement of the medullary cavity. The latissimus dorsi tendon was also involved at its adjacent attachment on the crest of the lesser tubercle. The patient was a dental assistant, and we believe that constant arm use in an externally rotated position was the decisive chronic stress factor.

Final Diagnosis

Clinically silent stress reaction at the deltoid muscle attachment.

Comments

An asymptomatic focus of increased tracer uptake at the deltoid muscle attachment may reasonably be interpreted as a normal variant.

Case 104 (▶ Fig. 6.13)

Case description

- *Referring physicians:* oncologist, orthopedist.
- *Prior history and clinical question:* The patient was a 34-year-old man with non-Hodgkin lymphoma in remission. For several weeks he experienced increasing pain in the left shoulder region, most pronounced after exercise. Clinical examination largely excluded a primary shoulder process due to absence of a capsular pattern. MRI yielded a confusing finding in the proximal medial humeral metadiaphysis that was considered suspicious for a tumor. But the absence of any other clinical or laboratory signs of a recurrence cast doubt on that suspicion.

Radiologic Findings

Water-sensitive MR images (▶ Fig. 6.13 **a, b**) showed an edema-like signal in the proximal medial humeral metadiaphysis with both an extra- and intraosseous component. A contrast series (not pictured here) showed moderate enhancement. Since these findings yielded little information, we ordered a simple radiograph and CT scans. The radiograph (▶ Fig. 6.13 **f**) shows a circumscribed, broad-based area of new bone formation on the medial humeral cortex. The latter is somewhat gray in appearance ("gray cortex") and shows circumscribed resorption under the distal portion of the new bone. This is displayed more clearly on CT scans (▶ Fig. 6.13 **c–e**), which show fine ossification within the circumscribed area of resorption (arrow in ▶ Fig. 6.13 **e**).

Location

The edema-like signal has both an intra- and extraosseous component, so its epicenter may be located in the cortex and its fibro-osseous junctions, the entheses. This would correspond anatomically to the area where the pectoralis major, latissimus dorsi, and teres major muscles attach to the crests of the lesser and greater tubercles of the humerus.

Pathoanatomic Background of the Findings

Based on the location of the circumscribed new bone, it may result from a stress-induced reactive process. But the finding in ▶ Fig. 6.13 **e** also suggests an osteoid osteoma with a central calcified nidus and surrounding reactive hyperostosis. A final possibility is an osseous focus of non-Hodgkin lymphoma.

Assignment to a Possible Basic Entity

▶ **Normal variant or malformation?** Unlikely, since the finding is apparently symptomatic, although we should consider the statements made in Case 103 under Normal variant or malformation?

▶ **Trauma?** The hyperostotic and resorptive changes are located at entheses, which immediately suggests a stress-induced change.

▶ **Inflammation?** Not in the form of bacterial osteomyelitis, but quite possibly in the form of stress-induced reactive osteitis.

▶ **Tumor?** If we interpret the finding marked by an arrow in ▶ Fig. 6.13 **e** as one feature of osteoid osteoma (nidus with central calcification), this possibility is worth considering.

Synopsis and Discussion

As in most complex cases, the key to a correct diagnosis lies in the history. Our differential diagnosis led us to elicit more detailed information about the patient's history. He said that he had started an intensive physical training program in recent months

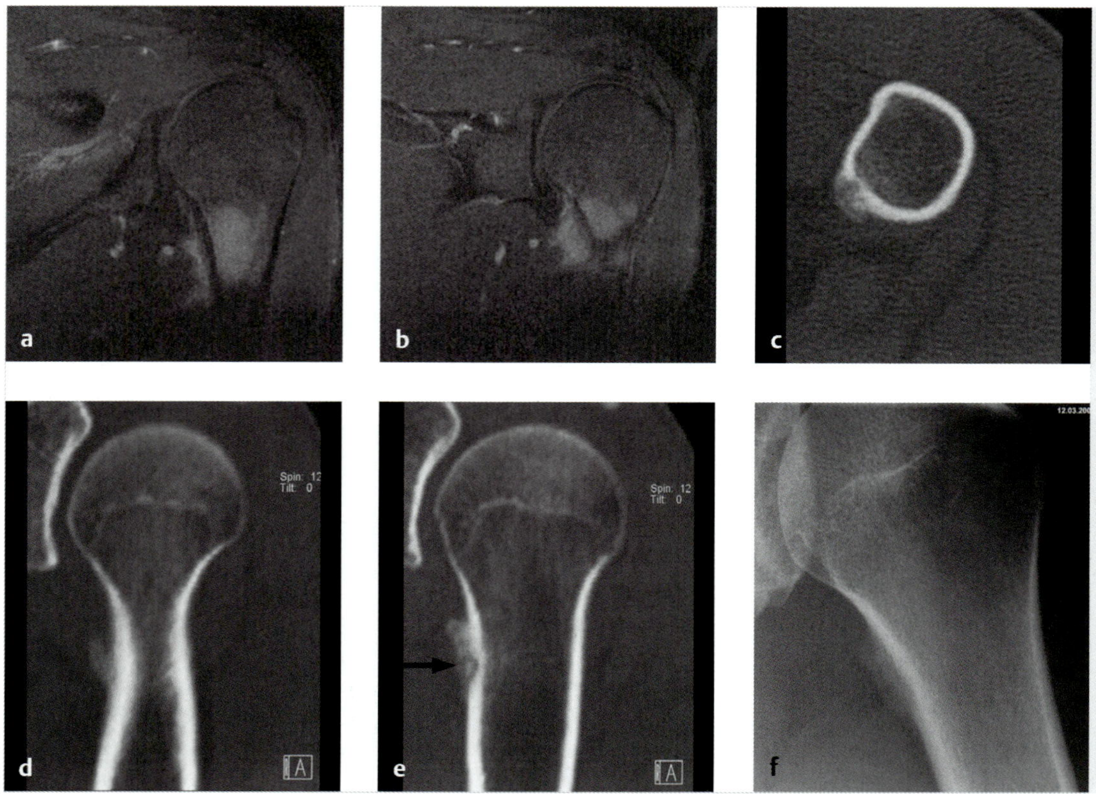

Fig. 6.13 a–f Osteoid osteoma?

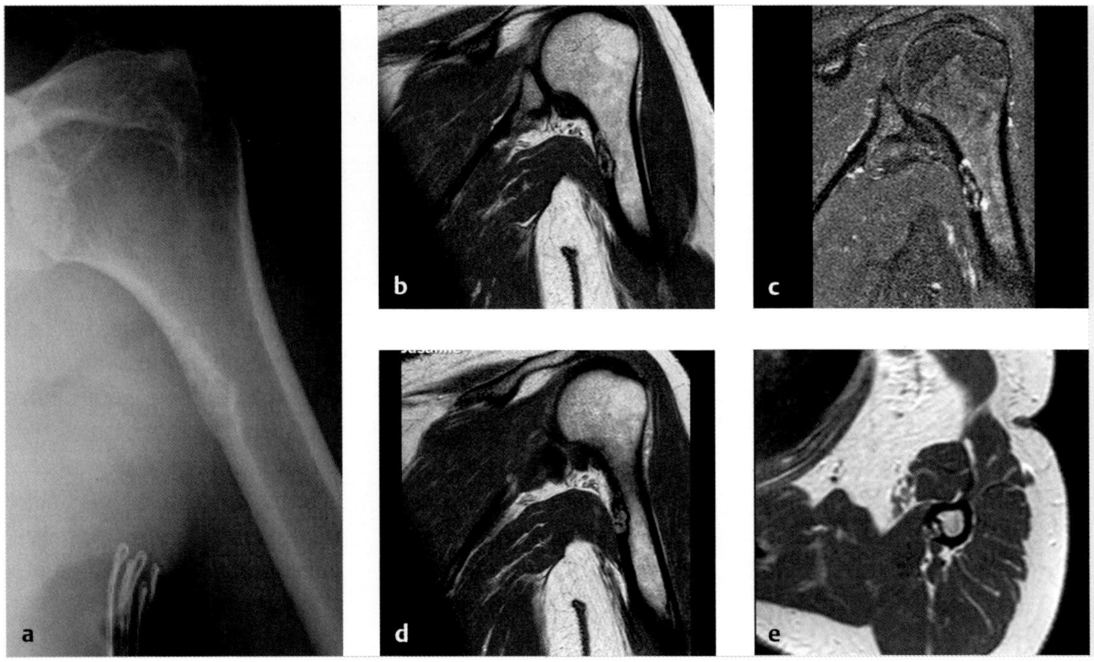

Fig. 6.14 a–e Stress-induced enthesiopathy of the humerus, simulating a tumor.

that included chest expander workouts, swimming, a rowing machine, and other exercises intended to "restore him to complete health." His symptoms began after he started the training program. He claimed to have little or no pain at rest.

This information excluded neoplasia from the differential diagnosis, as both a cortical osteoid osteoma and a focus of non-Hodgkin lymphoma would also have caused pain at rest. In summary, the following findings confirm the diagnosis of stress-induced enthesiopathy at the attachments of the muscles listed above:

- There is a direct link between the start of a rigorous exercise program and the onset of shoulder pain.
- The epicenter of the changes is located in the fibro-osseous junction region, specifically at the entheses of the aforementioned muscles. These muscles are the principal actors in the physical exercises listed above.
- CT scans showed that the configuration of the new bone formation was sharply tapered superomedially, following the course of the tendons.
- The stress on the entheses of the left humerus began from a "cold start," that is, an abrupt onset of rigorous physical training after more than 6 months of inactivity.

Because the oncologist did not believe us and continued to suspect recurrent lymphoma, he ordered a biopsy, which confirmed our diagnosis. The ossifications were scraped off during the biopsy and the tendons reattached, resulting in a relief of complaints.

▶ Fig. 6.14 shows a similar case of stress-induced enthesiopathy of the left humerus simulating a tumor in a 56-year-old woman.

For comparison, ▶ Fig. 6.15 shows the case of a 24-year-old man with an osteoid osteoma in the proximal medial humeral metaphysis. The central ossified nidus creates a target pattern on MRI (central signal void surrounded by a hyperintense ring) with significant reactive perifocal edema (▶ Fig. 6.15 **a–c**). The radiograph (▶ Fig. 6.15 **d**) is typical, showing a osteolytic nidus with central ossification (tumor-produced osteoid) and marginal sclerosis, which also involves the adjacent periosteum on the medial side. The patient had extreme pain that was non–exercise-related

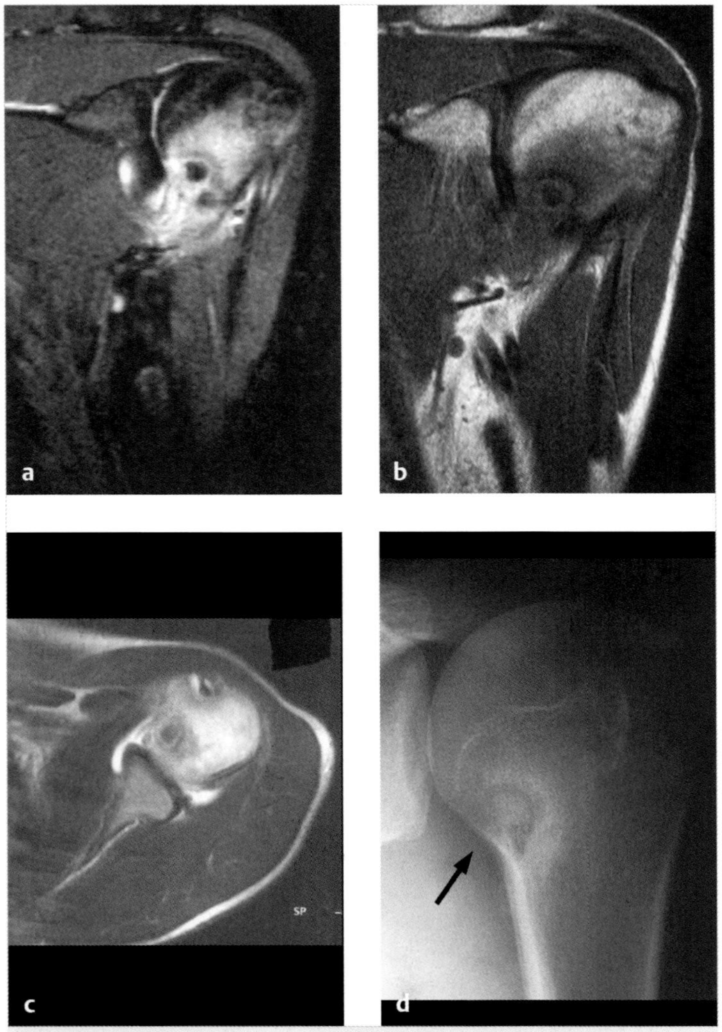

Fig. 6.15 a–d Osteoid osteoma in the proximal humerus of a 24-year-old man.

and worse at night. Unlike the cases in ▶ Fig. 6.13 and ▶ Fig. 6.14, the lesion is intracapsular. The humeral head shows marked demineralization resulting from edema with osteoclastic stimulation.

Final Diagnosis

Stress-induced enthesiopathy at the attachments of the pectoralis major, latissimus dorsi, and teres major tendons.

Comments

Besides the location and morphology of a finding, the history may provide an essential clue in solving the diagnostic puzzle.

Case 105 (▶ Fig. 6.16)

Case description

- Referring physician: radiologist.
- Prior history and clinical question: A 14-year-old boy complained of aching pains in his right upper arm, initially mild but recently increasing, and unrelated to exercise. The radiograph showed a "roughness" on the proximal medial cortex of the humeral diaphysis, which could not be definitely classified even when imaged by MRI.

Radiologic Findings

The medial humeral circumference has been replaced by a patchy destructive process that is associated with some degree of new bone formation (▶ Fig. 6.16 **a, b**). Water-sensitive MRI sequences (▶ Fig. 6.16 **c, d**) show a hyperintense band that is undulating at its interface with the bone. The underlying cortex appears slightly thickened (▶ Fig. 6.16 **d**). It has conformed to the wavy shape of the hyperintense structure, the "waves" indicating the variable thickness of the hyperintensity. The representative CT scan in ▶ Fig. 6.16 **e** demonstrates the eroded cortical bone, which is thickened posteromedially.

Location

The radiologic changes are located in and on the humeral cortex. They are probably subperiosteal.

Pathoanatomic Background of the Findings

Based on its signal intensity, the bandlike structure may be composed of cartilage. In this case the underlying cortical changes would be interpreted as erosions combined with reactive-reparative new bone formation. Ultimately, however, the hyperintense structure could be any proton-rich process (e.g., nonmineralized osteoid).

Assignment to a Possible Basic Entity

▶ **Normal variant or malformation?** No, this is not consistent with a hyperintense layer overlying the eroded cortex. This pattern is not known to occur with a normal variant or malformation.

▶ **Trauma?** No trauma history.

▶ **Inflammation?** No, an inflammatory process of this extent would produce systemic signs. An inflammation in the form of periosteal osteitis or periostitis, for example, would also be associated with perifocal edema, which is absent on MR images (▶ Fig. 6.16 **c, d**).

▶ **Tumor?** If the proton-rich structure is cartilaginous, it could be a periosteal chondroma. If it is nonmineralized osteoid, the lesion could be a periosteal osteosarcoma. The latter would be consistent with the cortical thickening on the posteromedial circumference, which could be interpreted as ossified tumor osteoid. Other possibilities are reactive-reparative new bone formation or solid ossified cartilage.

Synopsis and Discussion

Since the identity of the hyperintense structure on the eroded cortex could not be positively established by imaging, biopsy was necessary. When interpreted in the light of radiologic findings, the lesion was identified histologically as *periosteal chondroma*. These entities are benign and extremely rare. They develop on the bone surface, are covered by periosteum, may erode the underlying cortex and, as in our case, may also lead to reactive-reparative new bone formation. Its base, or the layer applied to the cortex, may also undergo enchondral ossification over time. Unlike enchondromas, periosteal chondromas are painful due to their contact with the periosteum. Sites of predilection are the humerus, tibia, femur, and small tubular bones, especially in the hand. This periosteal chondroma may be the initial manifestation

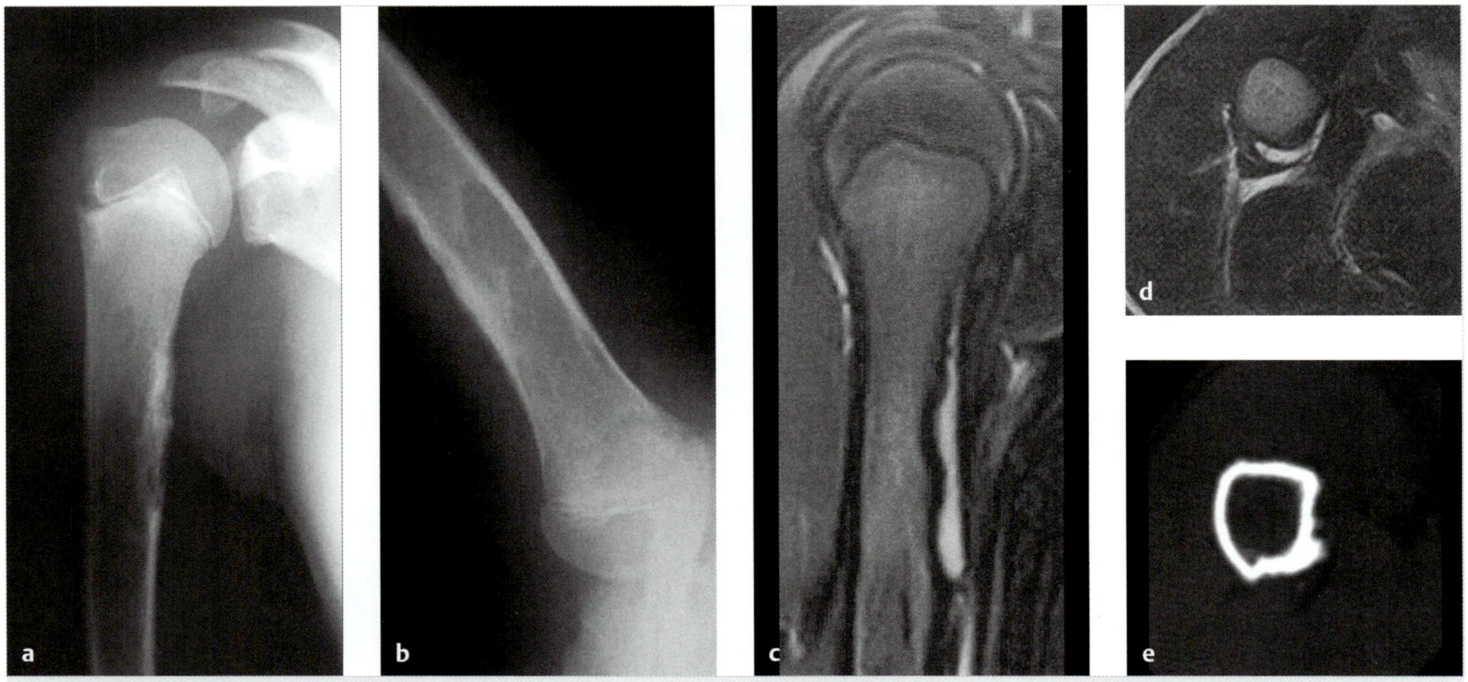

Fig. 6.16 a–e Insertional tendinopathy?

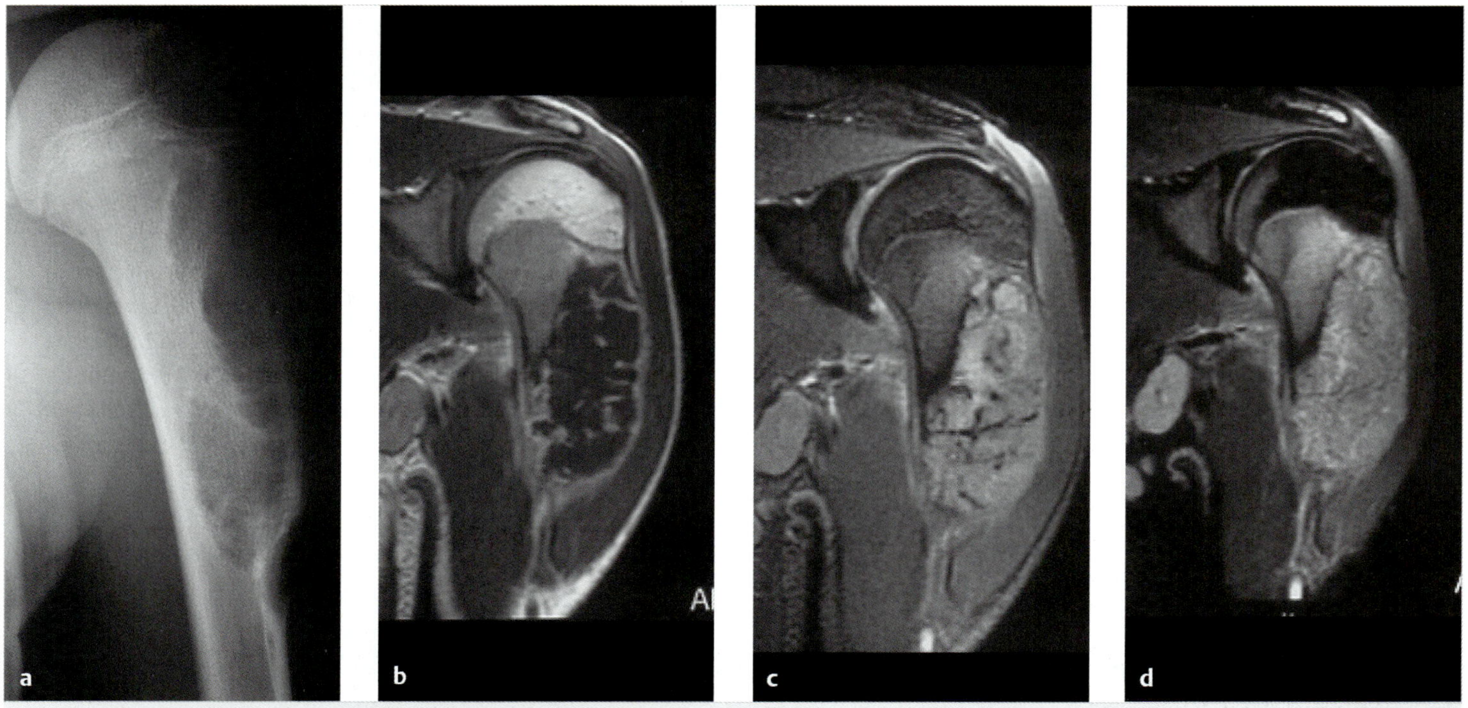

Fig. 6.17 a–d Periosteal chondroma in a 15-year-old boy.

of enchondromatosis, which is why—as in the case in ► Fig. 6.17—the patient should be followed for 2 years by whole-body MRI (see also Case 115, Case 116, and Case 120).

Differentiation is mainly required from *periosteal osteosarcoma* (see ► Fig. 7.27 in Case 144), which normally has a larger paraosseous tumor component with dense matrix ossification and spicules. Periosteal chondrosarcoma is another extremely rare entity that can only be diagnosed histologically.[18]

Another possibility is *periosteal desmoid*, better known as a cortical irregularity. This is a tumorlike lesion that we interpret as a local desmoid reaction to trauma that arises from the periosteum and spreads to the cortex.[18] It most commonly occurs at muscular insertions, similar to a fibrous metaphyseal defect (adductor or gastrocnemius insertions, etc.).

► Fig. 6.17 illustrates another case of periosteal chondroma in a 15-year-old boy. The tumor has caused a saucer-shaped area of bone resorption. The diagnosis is suggested by the lobular structure of the lesion, which is clearly depicted by MRI.

Final Diagnosis

Periosteal chondroma.

Comments

By following a systematic approach that takes into account all imaging details, we can formulate a correct differential diagnosis even for rare lesions such as periosteal tumors and direct the histologist in making an interpretation.

Case 106 (▶ Fig. 6.18)

Case description

- Referring physician: radiologist.
- Prior history and clinical question: A 16-year-old youth presented with a firm, painless mass in his left upper arm. The radiologist accurately diagnosed an osteochondroma (cartilaginous exostosis). He asked us to explain the unusual configuration of the tumor and suggest further actions. On physical examination, no additional exostoses were palpable at sites of predilection (metaphyses of long tubular bones).

Radiologic Findings

While the anteroposterior (AP) radiograph (▶ Fig. 6.18 **a**) shows a very typical sign of osteochondroma (round or elliptical sclerotic rim from which the body of the exostosis arises), the axillary view (▶ Fig. 6.18 **b**) shows a slight cortical elevation with a central saucer-shaped depression. A mushroom-shaped mass with a stalk and head projects distally from the central depression. The CT scans in ▶ Fig. 6.18 **c, d** show an open communication between the medullary cavity of the affected humerus and exostosis. ▶ Fig. 6.18 **c** shows a discontinuity in the exostosis, while two further images show small adjacent bone fragments (▶ Fig. 6.18 **d, e**). The last CT scan in this series (▶ Fig. 6.18 **f**) shows a rounded shaped figure that contains cancellous bone bounded by a thin cortex. The 3D reconstruction in ▶ Fig. 6.18 **g** clearly shows that the pedicle of the exostotic structure has broken free of its base.

Location

The exostotic structure developed from the proximal humeral metaphysis.

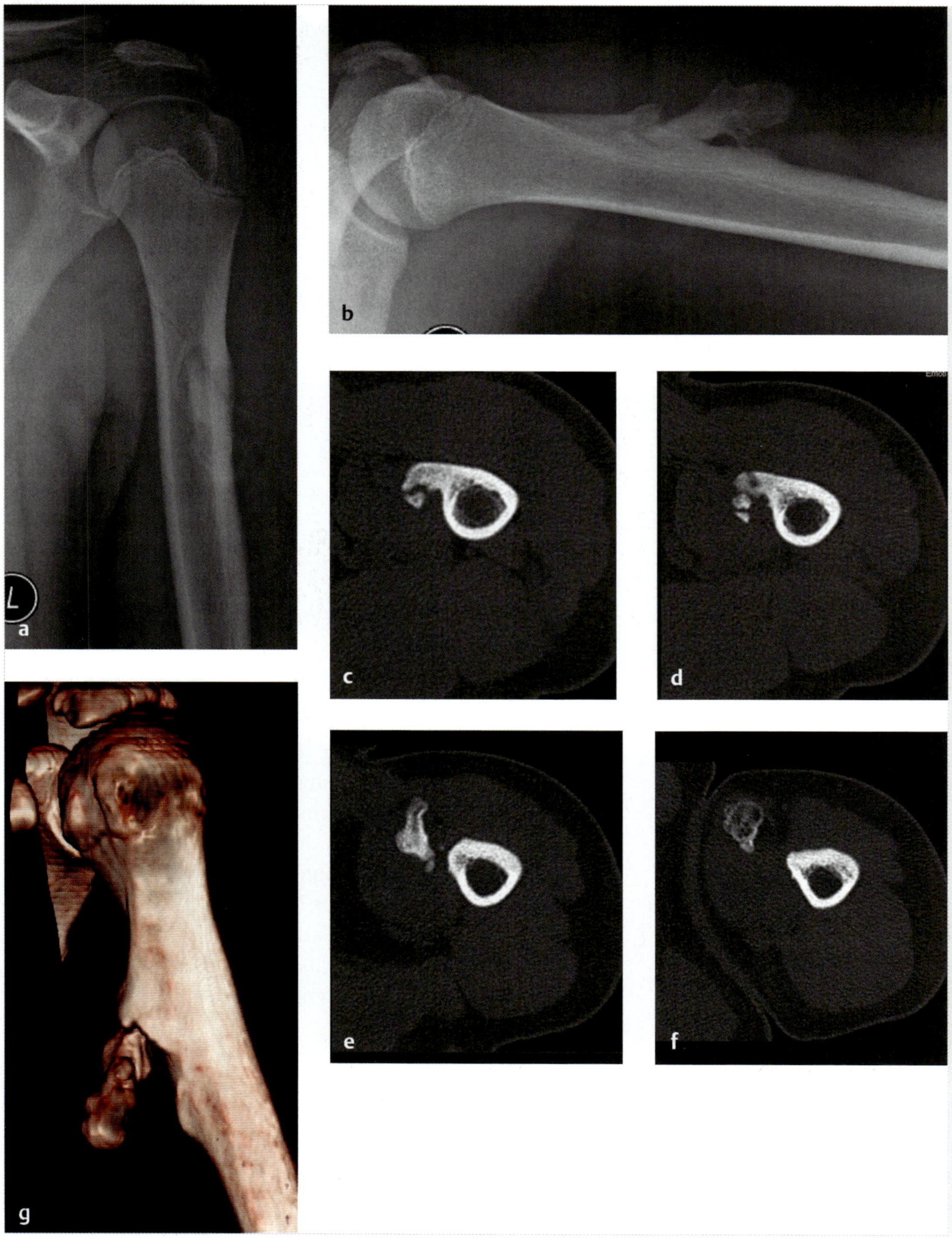

Fig. 6.18 a–g Cartilaginous exostosis?

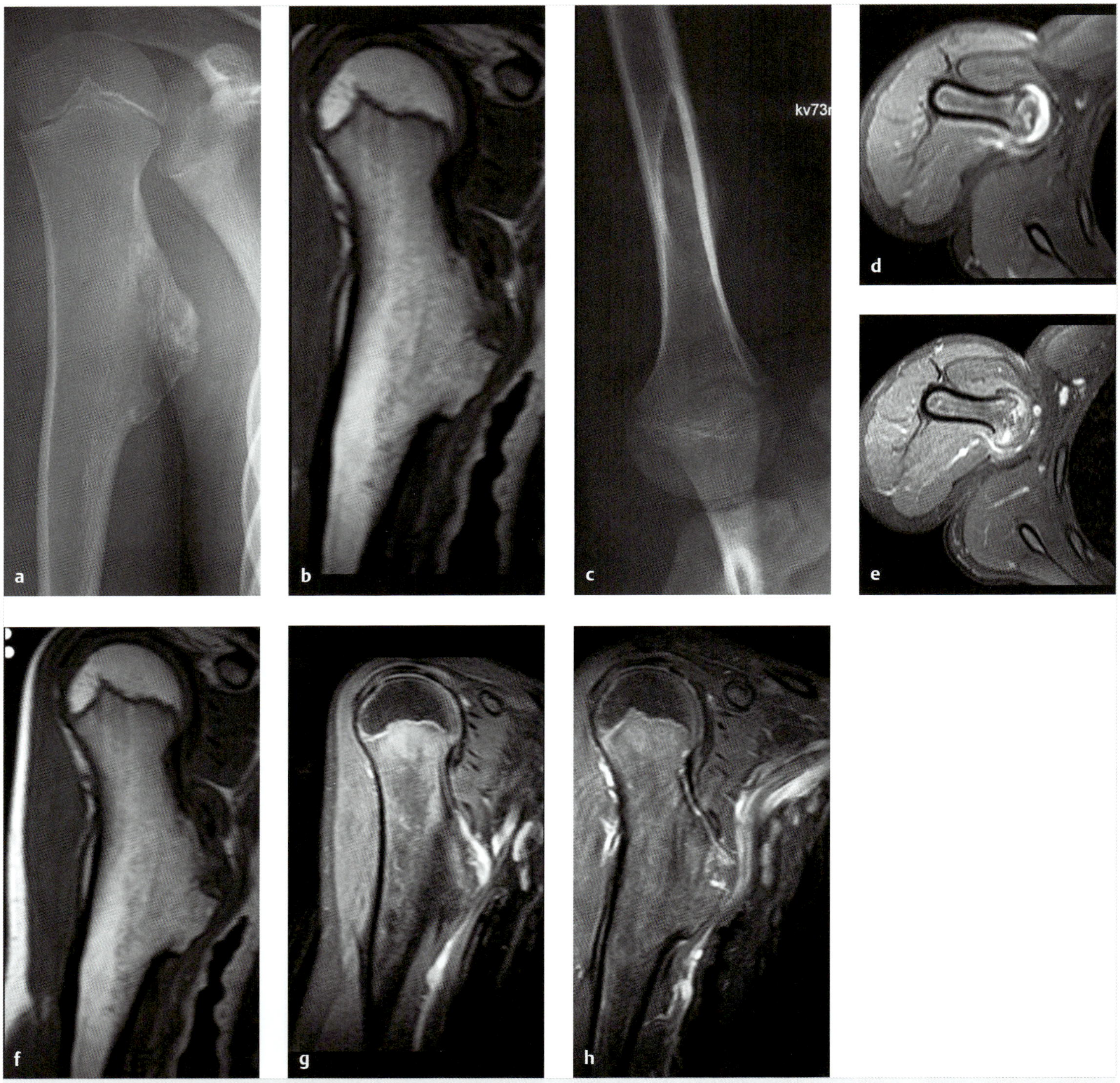

Fig. 6.19 a–h Classic broad-based cartilaginous exostosis in an 11-year-old boy.

Pathoanatomic Background of the Findings

The lesion is definitely an osteochondroma with an atypical pedicle.

Assignment to a Possible Basic Entity

The pathoanatomy of the lesion is sufficient to assign it to a basic entity.

Synopsis and Discussion

The main criteria for diagnosing a pedunculated osteochondroma or pedunculated cartilaginous exostosis are met: There is an open connection between the stalk of the exostotic paraosseous structure and the medullary cavity of the humerus. A stalk is present, surmounted by a head containing demonstrable cancellous bone with fat marrow spaces. The growth of the exostosis is directed away from the joint, following the direction of muscle pull, and the lesion has a typical metaphyseal location. Apparently the stalk broke off at some time or other, which is not uncommon with pedunculated exostoses. Cases are known in which the exostosis patient could not recall a specific injury that caused the break, especially if the patient engaged in contact sports such as soccer or handball.

The MR images for this case (not pictured here) showed that the head of the exostosis did not have a significant cartilaginous cap, meaning that this osteochondroma will not undergo additional growth. Since the unfortunately exposed location of the osteochondroma would predispose to further trauma, we recommended surgical removal. Accessory bursae may also form over exposed lesions of this kind; they may become inflamed and cause distressing pain (malignant transformation?). It should be added that prophylactic removal of a solitary osteochondroma is not indicated on oncologic grounds.

▶ Fig. 6.19 illustrates a classic broad-based (sessile) cartilaginous exostosis or broad-based osteochondroma in an 11-year-old boy. This lesion has a cartilaginous cap 3 to 5 mm thick, indicating a propensity for additional growth. As the MR images clearly demonstrate, the head of the exostosis directly abuts the neurovascular bundle, so it would be advisable to consider surgical removal. We have seen several cases in which trauma led to vascular contusions with pseudoaneurysm formation or nerve contusions with associated palsies.

Final Diagnosis

Solitary pedunculated osteochondroma (cartilaginous exostosis) that has broken off from the humerus.

Comments

Otherwise harmless, solitary, pedunculated osteochondromas may occasionally fracture. Surgical removal should be considered for both pedunculated and sessile osteochondromas that are in close proximity to neurovascular structures.

Case 107 (▶ Fig. 6.20)

Case description

- Referring physician: radiologist.
- Prior history and clinical question: A 50-year-old man was referred to another institution for the MRI investigation of shoulder pain. Images showed an incidental finding in the humerus that was difficult to classify.

Radiologic Findings

The MR images in ▶ Fig. 6.20 **a, b** show expansion of the humeral shaft associated with inhomogeneous signal intensity in the bone. The medullary cavity appears intact based on its high signal intensity in the T1w image (▶ Fig. 6.20 **b**). The radiograph that we ordered (▶ Fig. 6.20 **c**) shows thickening of the humerus cortex, which appears split open in the proximal third of the diaphysis and proximal portions of the middle third. This is particularly clear when compared with the cortex at more distal levels. The distal extension of the changes has a V-shaped configuration that projects distally (arrow in ▶ Fig. 6.20 **c**) and is best displayed by the reformatted CT images in ▶ Fig. 6.20 **d–f** (see arrow in ▶ Fig. 6.20 **d**). The medullary cavity is intact, as shown in the axial scans (▶ Fig. 6.20 **h, i**). The humeral head shows a coarse, rarefied trabecular pattern (▶ Fig. 6.20 **c, g**).

Location

The changes described above begin in the epiphysis and extend into the proximal part of the middle third of the diaphysis, thus affecting the cancellous bone of the humeral head and the cortical bone of the shaft.

Pathoanatomic Background of the Findings

The bone shows structural alterations and volume expansion that apparently began in the proximal epiphysis (coarse trabecular pattern) and spread into the mid-shaft. At that level the process still appears to be very active, which could account for the V-shaped configuration (see details in Synopsis and Discussion below).

Assignment to a Possible Basic Entity

▶ **Normal variant or malformation?** No, because the bone shows active structural transformation.

▶ **Trauma?** No, there is no history of acute or chronic trauma.

▶ **Inflammation?** No, not in the form of bacterial osteomyelitis (see Case 109) owing to a lack of clinical manifestations. Yes, in the form of a chronic, nonbacterial inflammatory process, which can be classified as primary rather than reactive. This occurs only in Paget disease.

▶ **Tumor?** No, there are no signs of a mass lesion or destructive changes, only signs of chronic structural transformation.

Synopsis and Discussion

The findings in the proximal right humerus are typical of Paget disease. The proofs are as follows:

- *Continuous involvement of a long segment:* starting in the epiphysis and extending to the shaft. The bone always shows sclerotic changes where the process began. Where it is still active, bone resorption around the haversian canals has caused splitting of the cortex. The front of the process resembles a drill bit ("cutting cone" of bone resorption), which appears V-shaped on radiographs and especially on bone scans (see ▶ Fig. 6.21 **i** in a similar case and ▶ Fig. 7.20 **b** in Case 140). It is believed to advance at a rate of approximately 1 cm/year.
- *Widening of the affected bone with a coarse trabecular pattern and splitting of the cortex.*
- *Preservation of medullary fat:* useful differentiating feature from a neoplastic or bacterial inflammatory process.
- *Age of the patient:* Current thinking is that the disease begins in youth or middle age. Because it is asymptomatic in the great majority of cases, it is usually detected incidentally at a later age. More than 90% of patients are over age 40 years when the disease is discovered. It is estimated that 3 to 4% of persons over age 40 in Central Europe have Paget disease. Based on this figure and the fact that the prevalence doubles in each successive decade after age 50, the structural changes in the humerus of our patient very likely represent Paget disease from a statistical standpoint alone.
- *Absence of complaints:* On further inquiry, the patient was found to have a typical capsular pattern, meaning that his complaints were referable to an ordinary degenerative process.

▶ Fig. 6.21 **a–i** illustrates a case of Paget disease of the humerus (67-year-old man with shoulder pain) that has very similar radiologic features. Note the coarse trabecular pattern in the humeral head on the CT scout view and coronal reformatted images in ▶ Fig. 6.21 **f–h**. The fatty marrow spaces among the structurally altered trabeculae are fully intact (▶ Fig. 6.21 **h**; measured attenuation values as low as –70 HU). A whole-body bone scan (▶ Fig. 6.21 **i**) shows additional sites of involvement in the left leg (less active in the femur than in the tibia, but involving a longer segment and therefore older), in the mid-thoracic spine, upper lumbar spine, and left pubis and acetabulum. This is a polyostotic form of Paget disease, therefore. Serum alkaline phosphatase was only moderately elevated at 278 U (normal range = 40–129 U) because the disease, aside from the humerus and tibia, had apparently entered a more chronic stage.

For comparison, ▶ Fig. 6.22 shows a case of osseous involvement by non-Hodgkin lymphoma. Clinically the patient had massive swelling and severe pain in the left shoulder. Soft-tissue infiltration about the humeral head, which shows patchy opacities, is clearly documented by obliterated fat planes on a conventional radiograph (▶ Fig. 6.22 **a**) and especially on MRI (▶ Fig. 6.22 **b, c**). The fatty marrow spaces are infiltrated; the epicenter of the process is located in the medullary cavity. The structural transformation of the bone is explained by a mixed pattern of bone destruction, necrosis, and reparative and metaplastic woven bone formation.

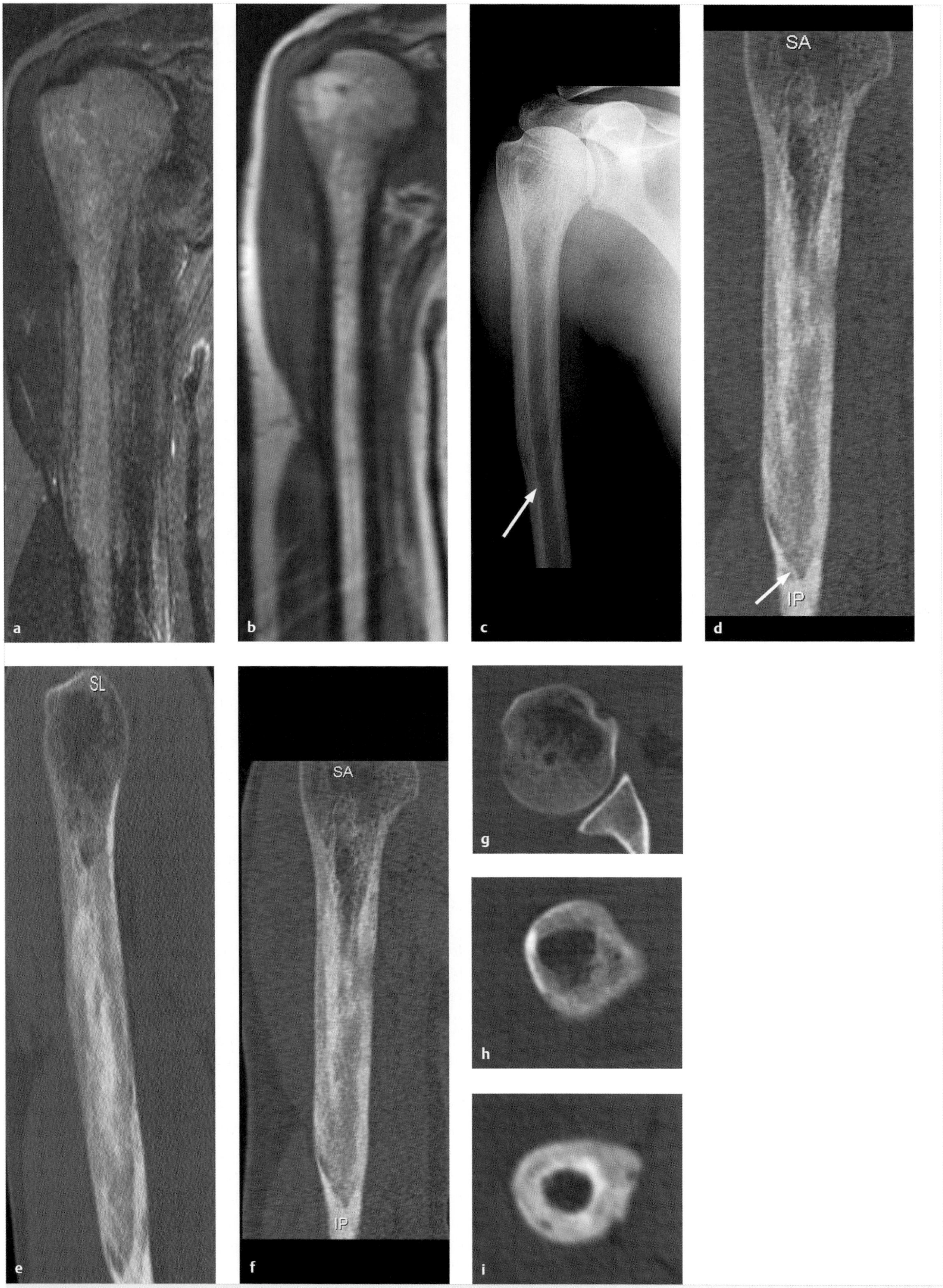

Fig. 6.20 a–i Congenital hyperostosis, fibrous dysplasia, or chronic osteomyelitis?

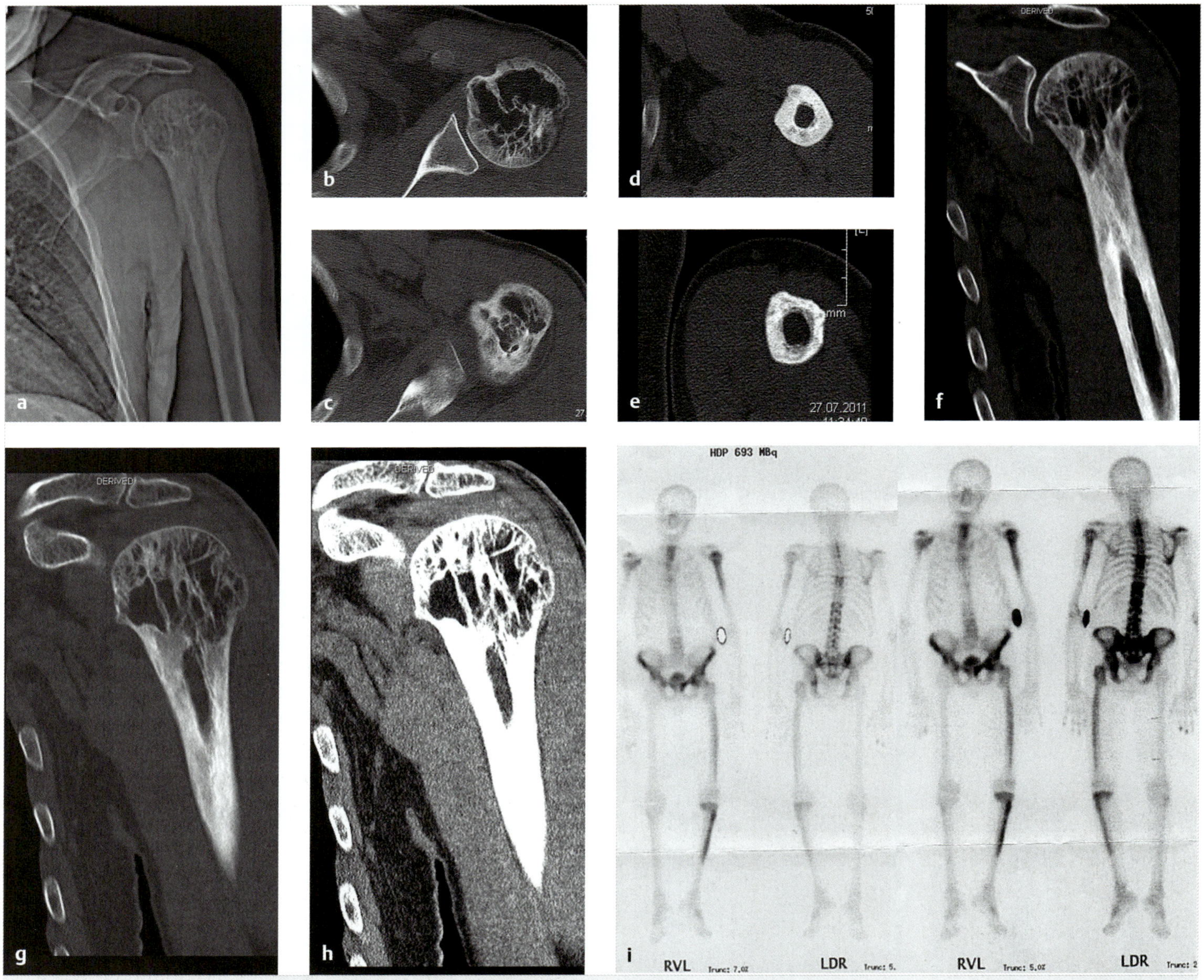

Fig. 6.21 a–i Polyostotic Paget disease in a 67-year-old man.

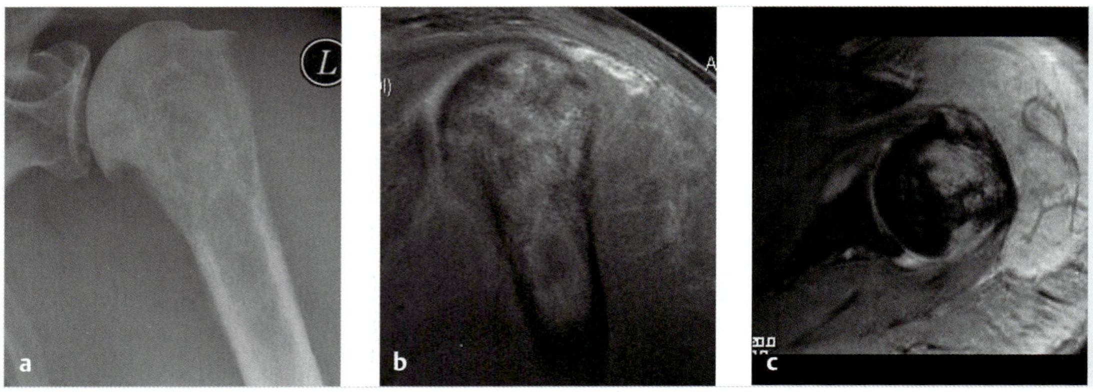

Fig. 6.22 a–c For comparison: osseous involvement by non-Hodgkin lymphoma.

Final Diagnosis

Paget disease of the humerus.

Comments

Asymptomatic structural changes involving a long bone segment and associated enlargement and a V-shaped interface with uninvolved bone are diagnostic of Paget disease. This disease can be confidently diagnosed from radiologic findings; excisional biopsy is unnecessary.

Case 108 (▶ Fig. 6.23)

Case description

- *Referral:* self-referral by the patient.
- *Prior history and clinical question:* A pathologic process in the medullary cavity of the left proximal humerus was detected incidentally in a 45-year-old man after a skiing accident. But this process had already been correctly diagnosed as a typical calcifying enchondroma 2 years earlier. The patient came to us, wanting to know about the prognosis and possible further course of action.

Radiologic Findings

The radiographs taken in 2010 (▶ Fig. 6.23 **a, b**) show fine, popcornlike calcifications in the right proximal humeral diaphysis; the cortex is intact. The MR images in ▶ Fig. 6.23 **c–f** show that the lesion has a lobular structure. The lobules have low signal intensity on the T1w image (isointense to muscle, ▶ Fig. 6.23 c) and high signal intensity on the T2w images (▶ Fig. 6.23 **d, f**). The postcontrast image (▶ Fig. 6.23 **e**) demonstrates septal enhancement among the lobules. MR images obtained after a prior accident in 2008 (▶ Fig. 6.23 **g–j**) ultimately showed identical findings using a slightly different technique.

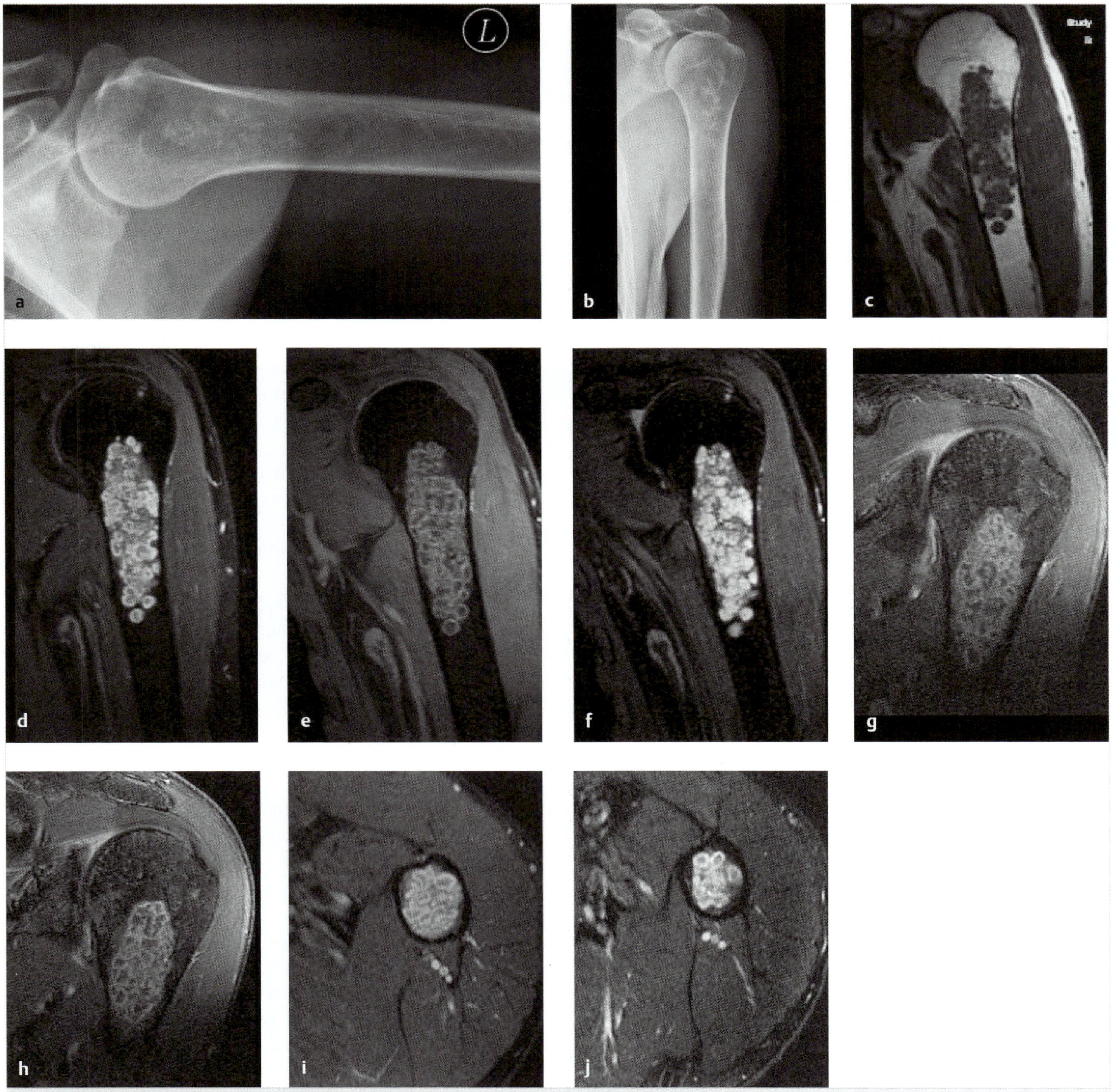

Fig. 6.23 a–j Calcifying enchondroma. Signs of malignant transformation? The images in a–f were obtained in 2010. Those in g–j date from an earlier injury in 2008.

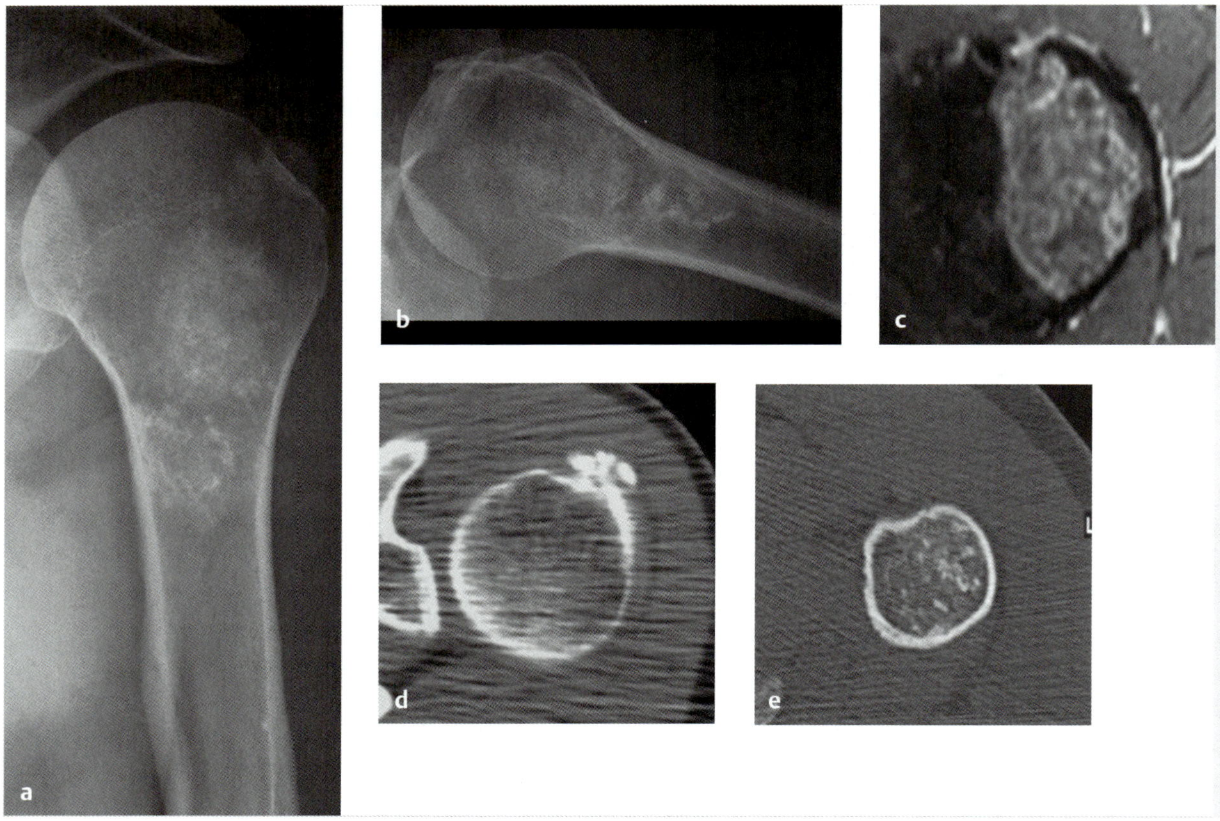

Fig. 6.24 a–e Calcifications at the tendon insertion on the greater tubercle and/or calcifying bursitis as the cause of acute shoulder pain in a 54-year-old man with enchondroma in the proximal humerus.

Location

The changes are intraosseous, located in a diametaphyseal segment of the humerus.

Pathoanatomic Background of the Findings

Intraosseous calcifications with a popcornlike pattern are proof of a cartilage-forming tumor. The popcorn pattern is a summation effect produced by ossified shells on the individual cartilage lobules and/or their stroma. The MRI findings of small, round foci with little or no T1w signal intensity and high T2w signal intensity are also typical of a cartilage-forming tumor. The septal enhancement described above is explained by contrast uptake in the interlobular stroma, which generally has a rich blood supply with an active tumor. A pathoanatomic interpretation of the radiologic findings, including their location, definitely indicates a cartilage-forming tumor. The lesion is probably benign due to the absence of clinical complaints.

Assignment to a Possible Basic Entity

Because the engrammatic link between the imaging signs and a pathoanatomic background (popcorn pattern = calcified cartilage lobules, lobular structure with low T1w signal intensity and high T2w signal intensity, septal enhancement) has already assigned the lesion to a basic entity, there is no need to consider other possible candidates in the differential diagnosis.

Synopsis and Discussion

Calcifying enchondromas occurring at a typical location in the diametaphyses of long tubular bones (humerus, femur, tibia) are purely incidental findings in most cases. They are detected after accidents or fortuitously in the humerus, for example, in patients with clinically symptomatic periarthropathia calcificans.

Grade I chondrosarcoma (more commonly known as an atypical cartilaginous tumor), which may have identical radiologic features, is generally distinguished from calcifying enchondroma by the cardinal symptom of pain. The pain associated with chondrosarcoma is non–exercise-related and is described as boring and also present at night. The radiologic signs of grade I chondrosarcoma are as follows:

- Significant cortical bone destruction (more than two-thirds of the cortical thickness over a long segment), also called scalloping
- Significant bone expansion, cortical thickening, and periosteal reaction
- Large lesion more than 10 cm in its longitudinal dimension
- Intense, inhomogeneous and/or septal enhancement on post-contrast MRI
- Very intense tracer uptake on radionuclide bone scan

Besides pain, at least two of the above criteria must be met for a diagnosis of grade I chondrosarcoma. The present case meets none of these criteria.

Because a benign calcifying enchondroma more than 10 cm in its longitudinal dimension located near the trunk may develop into a low-grade chondrosarcoma over an approximately 20-year period, if only in about 5% of cases, it is reasonable to ask whether prophylactic curettage would be appropriate for a calcifying enchondroma detected in patients under 40 to 50 years of age. We generally favor this procedure because removal of the tumor can spare the patient years of follow-up examinations. In patients over 55 to 60 years of age, there is no oncologic rationale for surgical intervention. In any case we consider biopsy to be obsolete, as the known inhomogeneity of solid tumors creates a high risk of an unrepresentative sample (see ▶ Fig. 6.26). A detailed discussion of this problem can be found in Freyschmidt et al (2010).[18] In the present case, we explained the risks and options to the

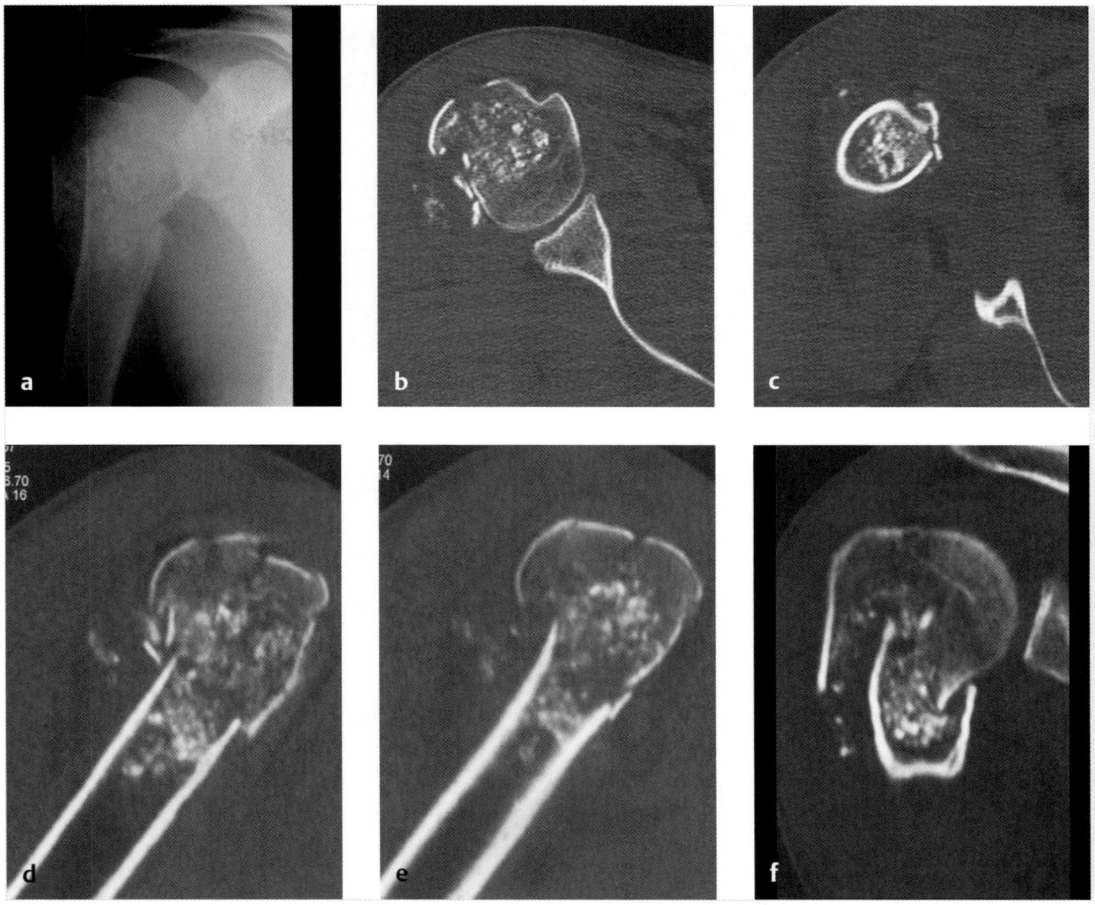

Fig. 6.25 a–f Grade I chondrosarcoma in a 48-year-old woman with a spontaneous fracture of the proximal humerus.

unworried patient, who accepted our recommendation for a follow-up examination at 2 to 3 years.

▶ Fig. 6.24 shows a radiologically similar case in which a 54-year-old man was found to have a tumor during the MRI investigation of highly acute left shoulder pain after a tennis injury. Based on the MR images alone, the tumor was initially blamed for the shoulder pain and was interpreted as malignant. But subsequent radiographs and CT detected calcifications at the tendon insertion on the greater tubercle and/or calcifying bursitis, which was considered the cause of the acute pain. More than 10 years' follow-up showed no clinical or radiologic changes.

▶ Fig. 6.25 presents the case of a 48-year-old woman who suffered a spontaneous fracture of the right proximal humerus after a trivial injury. She claimed to have had right shoulder pain long before the trauma, which her family doctor treated as osteoarthritis. The humeral head and subcapital region were comminuted, as shown by the CT images in ▶ Fig. 6.25 **b–f**, which were acquired several days after the radiograph (▶ Fig. 6.25 **a**). Tumor tissue has been pressed into the soft tissues as indicated by fine, paraosseous matrix calcifications. As much of the tumor as possible was removed by curettage and the cavity filled with methylmethacrylate cement. The lesion was identified histologically as grade I chondrosarcoma, not a poorly differentiated chondrosarcoma as was initially assumed based on the spontaneous fracture. The decisive criteria for diagnosing chondrosarcoma in this case were the pain history and spontaneous fracture.

The case shown in ▶ Fig. 6.26 involves a 70-year-old woman with a focal grade I chondrosarcoma (criterion: invasive growth) diagnosed in a biopsy specimen 1 to 2 mm in diameter. The patient had fallen 3 months earlier, sustaining a subcapital humeral fracture. The biopsy was motivated by persistent pain after the trauma. The patient had no complaints prior to the fall. Based on

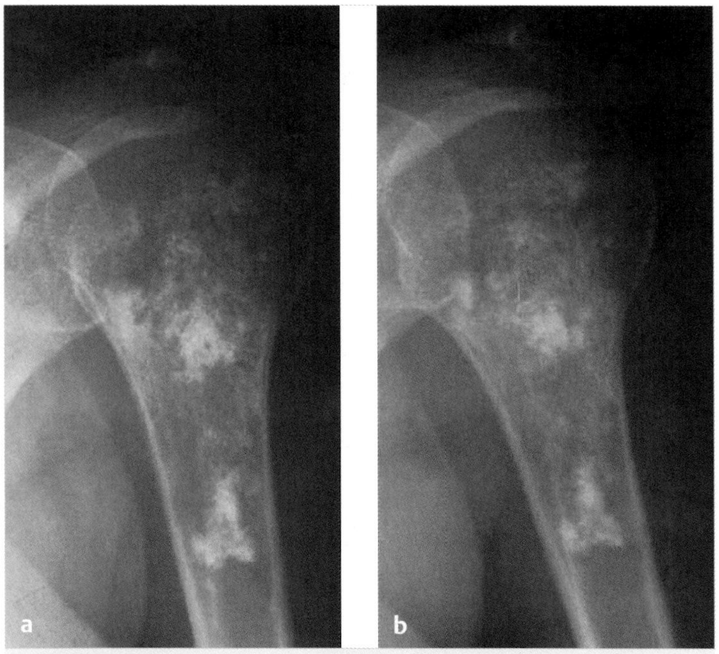

Fig. 6.26 a, b Focal grade I chondrosarcoma of the proximal humerus in a 70-year-old woman.

this diagnosis, curettage was performed and histology yielded the surprising diagnosis of a pure enchondroma. This case not only illustrates the problems involved in the biopsy of large, purely intraosseous enchondromas, but also proves that chondrosarcomas may develop from enchondromas. Apparently the very small sarcomatous component of the lesion was insufficient to cause the hallmark pain that usually distinguishes chondrosarcoma from enchondroma. Based on a tumor doubling time of approximately 200 days for a well-differentiated chondrosarcoma,[44] it would take an estimated 6 years for the sarcomatous component of the lesion to reach a volume of 10 cm^3 (approximately 2.2 cm × 2.2 cm × 2.2 cm), at which time the patient may become symptomatic.

Final Diagnosis

Calcifying enchondroma of the proximal humerus, detected as an incidental finding.

Comments

Calcifying enchondromas in long tubular bones are common incidental findings. There are well-established differentiating criteria from intraosseous grade I (low-grade) chondrosarcoma (atypical cartilaginous tumor). Excisional biopsy is not required for this differential diagnosis except in a few highly selected cases.

Case 109 (► Fig. 6.27)

Case description

- Referring physician: surgeon.
- Prior history and clinical question: A 56-year-old man had experienced pain in the right upper arm for many months. The patient was an alcoholic with decompensated hepatic cirrhosis.

Radiologic Findings

The cortex of the right proximal and middle humeral shaft shows significant structural alterations: It is "gray" and undulating on the endosteal side with an alternation between focal thickening and thinning. Compare the altered cortex with the normal cortex on the distal third of the shaft (► Fig. 6.27 **a**). A representative axial CT scan in ► Fig. 6.27 **c** also demonstrates cortical resorption on the periosteal side (arrow). The attenuation values in the medullary cavity range from 30 to 60 HU. The coronal reformatted image in ► Fig. 6.27 **b** shows a small element of very high density. Other slices (not pictured here) showed additional small densities. The bone scans in ► Fig. 6.27 **d** show very intense uptake in the proximal two-thirds of the right humerus.

Location

The changes are reflected mainly in the cortex, medullary cavity, and periosteal side of the bone. Involvement of the diaphysis is apparent on radiography and CT. The bone scan shows involvement of the proximal epimetaphysis.

Pathoanatomic Background of the Findings

Based on the criterion of the "hot" bone scan, we are dealing with an active process. "Gray" cortex always indicates structural transformation, which is usually inflammatory or stress-related but may also have a neoplastic cause. The transformation process occurs on the endosteal *and* periosteal sides. This would be unusual for an intramedullary tumor, which would be more likely to cause pure scalloping (erosion of the inner cortical surface) and a periosteal reaction (solid, interrupted, or lamellated) rather than external destruction. This finding would be consistent with an inflammatory process, however. The overall picture favors the interpretation of an inflammatory process.

Assignment to a Possible Basic Entity

► **Trauma?** The patient did not give a history of acute trauma, although chronic or repetitive trauma would be possible in an alcoholic. A stress fracture is known to alter cortical structure, but not over such a long segment. In any case the absence of a visible fracture line excludes this possibility.

► **Inflammation?** Yes, specifically bacterial osteomyelitis, which typically arises from the medullary cavity and spreads beneath the periosteum through vascular channels. This interpretation is also supported by the small sequestra detected by CT. Paget disease (see Case 107) is inconsistent with the relatively high density in the medullary cavity, which suggests an inflammatory secretion along with granulation tissue and necrosis.

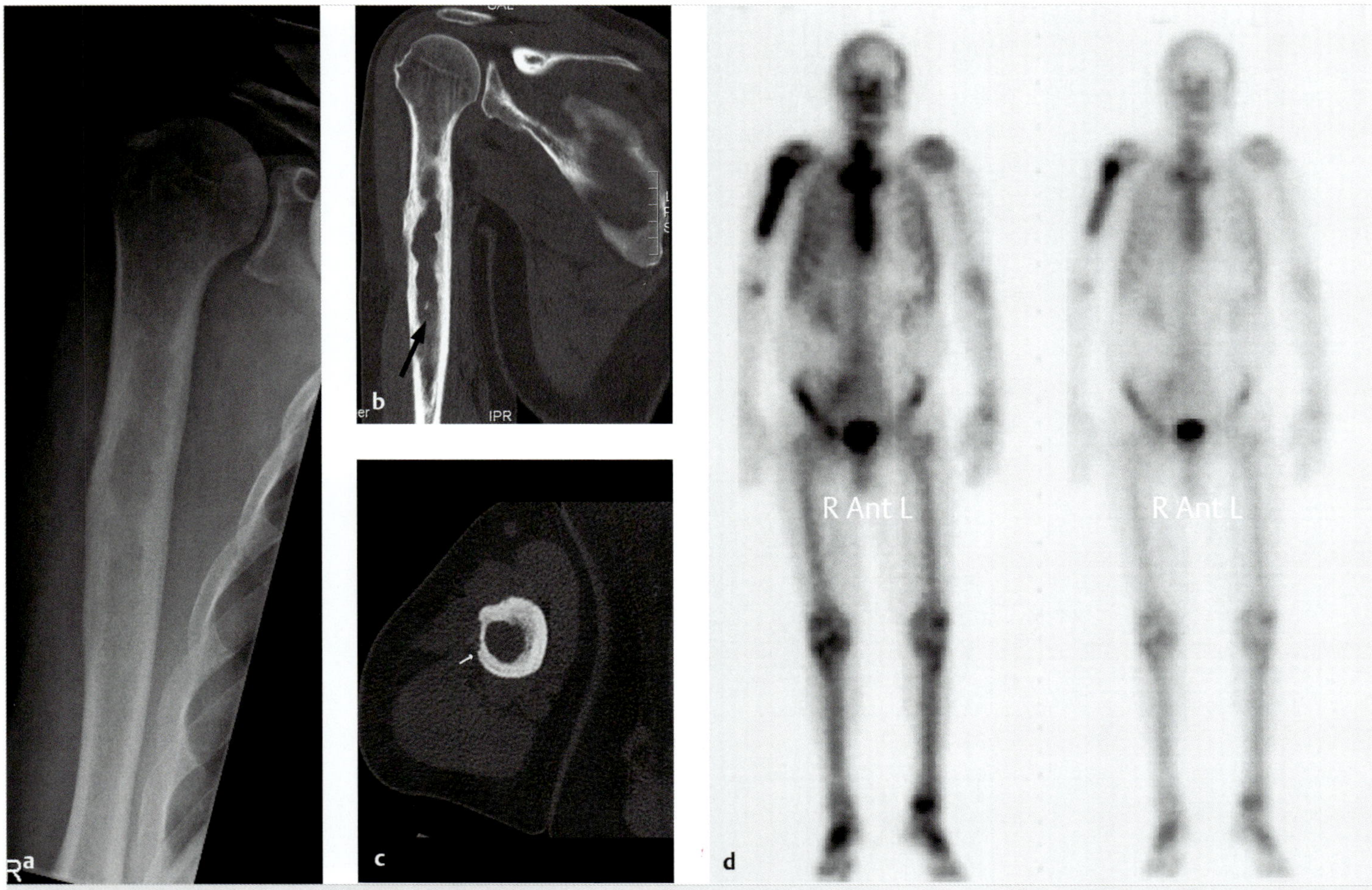

Fig. 6.27 a–d Chondrosarcoma?

▸ **Tumor?** No, the key arguments against a neoplastic process were discussed under Pathoanatomic Background of the Findings. A heavily necrotic tumor such as lymphoma would be a possibility, however (see also Case 86).

▸ **Perfusion disorder or necrosis?** Definitely not a primary cause, as we do not see fragmentation, and the bone scan would show cold spots or a generally inhomogeneous pattern. We may assume, however, that perfusion defects and necrotic processes have taken place within the extensive process.

Synopsis and Discussion

Based on the differential considerations above, there is an urgent need for an excisional biopsy from the medullary cavity, cortex, and paraosseous compartment. We reported to the pathologist that the most likely radiologic diagnosis was chronic osteomyelitis, and that was confirmed histologically. As in many cases of chronic osteomyelitis, a causative organism could not be identified.

Now osteomyelitis in the diaphysis of a long tubular bone is very unusual. We assume that the scintigraphic involvement of the proximal epimetaphysis was a purely trophic, sympathetic process. Hematogenous osteomyelitis in adults most commonly occurs in the spine (in the form of spondylitis or spondylodiskitis). The primary focus in children is generally located in the metaphysis of a tubular bone. The key to understanding the unusual location lies in the patient's history: As a chronic alcoholic with decompensated hepatic cirrhosis, he is immunocompromised. Since the patient comes from Eastern Europe, there could be other immunocompromising factors that were not identified.

The chronic nature of the process probably explains the absence of periosteal new bone formation. The hepatic cirrhosis may also be a factor: the proteins produced or metabolized at that site were insufficient for periosteal bone formation to occur.

Final Diagnosis

Unusual chronic hematogenous osteomyelitis in an immunocompromised patient.

Comments

In an adult whose radiologic findings are consistent with osteomyelitis but occur at an atypical location, a diagnosis of osteomyelitis should be considered if there are factors in the patient's history (e.g., diabetes mellitus, alcoholic liver disease, AIDS, etc.) that could compromise the immune system.

Case 110 (▶ Fig. 6.28)

Case description

- Referring physician: orthopedist.
- Prior history and clinical question: A 39-year-old man presented with a long history of pain, predominantly in the chest wall. This case was previously described in detail as Case 94, focusing on the chest wall changes caused by polyostotic fibrous dysplasia and their differentiation from enchondromatosis.

This section reviews additional fibrous dysplastic changes in the upper limbs of the same patient (▶ Fig. 6.28 **a–e**). Because the diagnosis is clear-cut, we will depart from our customary systematic approach to making a diagnosis.

There is virtually no other diagnosis than enchondromatosis that would explain the extensive osteolytic and expansile changes, aside from extremely rare hereditary conditions (e.g., osteoectasia with hyperphosphatasia, also called juvenile Paget disease). Fibrous dysplasia tissue has almost completely replaced normal bone in both upper limbs. The diaphyses exhibit lytic changes with paper-thin residual cortex plus expansile soap-bubble lesions. In contrast to pure osteolysis caused by noncalcifying tumor tissue, for example, the right radial diaphysis and left humeral diaphysis have a ground-glass appearance typical of fibrous dysplasia (see also Case 4, Case 7, Case 8, Case 20, Case 36, Case 58, and Case 139). This is explained by calcifying connective tissue. The marked expansile areas in the right proximal radial metaepiphysis (▶ Fig. 6.28 **a, b**) and distal right humerus (▶ Fig. 6.28 **c**—this radiograph was taken later than the views in ▶ Fig. 6.28 **a, b**) are a result of regressive processes with necrosis, intraosseous hemorrhage with liquefaction, and fatty infiltration.

Several findings are not characteristic of enchondromatosis: absence of a lobular lesion structure, absence of at least partial enchondromatous bone formation, and the bilateral pattern of spread. Moreover, the marked aggressiveness of the changes, also displayed by the case of another patient, shown in ▶ Fig. 6.29, is typical of polyostotic fibrous dysplasia.

The latter patient, 10 years old when first examined (▶ Fig. 6.29 **a**), had extensive osteolytic changes in the right humerus that were correctly interpreted as fibrous dysplasia. The pronounced eccentric expansion at the junction of the proximal and middle thirds of the humeral shaft, with small flecks of calcifications, represented a cartilaginous component of the fibrous dysplasia (fibrous dysplasia with cartilaginous differentiation); this is not unusual in larger lesions. At the time the boy had no complaints at all, despite his intensive tennis training. The osteolytic changes had increased by 14 years of age (▶ Fig. 6.29 **b**). Because the boy was experiencing a growth spurt with a predicted final height of 2 m, testosterone therapy was started at a different institution 3 months before the radiograph in ▶ Fig. 6.29 **c**, also in the hope of stopping the progression of fibrous dysplasia—even though it was known that fibrous dysplasia may undergo clinical and morphologic changes in response to hormonal stimuli. The therapy triggered an explosive activation of the fibrous dysplasia with grotesque volume expansion (▶ Fig. 6.29 **c, d**). The surrounding soft tissues were atrophic. Sectional images (not pictured here) documented liquefaction of the fibrous dysplasia. The condition was managed by surgical resection and reconstruction with a humeral shaft allograft, which healed without complications. Six years later there was a recurrence at the proximal end of the graft, which was also successfully treated surgically. At that time radiographs of the right shoulder, forearm, and right hand (▶ Fig. 6.29 **e, f**) revealed additional foci of fibrous dysplasia, which showed cartilaginous differentiation in the second and third fingers. A detailed account of this case is presented in Freyschmidt et al. (2010).[18] The ground-glass appearance in the proximal radius (▶ Fig. 6.29 **e**), which is typical of fibrous dysplasia, would be helpful for anyone seeing the case at the time of the second roentgen series without knowing the prior history.

Final Diagnosis

Polyostotic fibrous dysplasia.

Comments

The cardinal features of fibrous dysplasia are osteolytic changes combined with a ground-glass appearance. Regressive changes may lead to soap-bubble expansion of the lesions. The changes in polyostotic fibrous dysplasia are more aggressive.

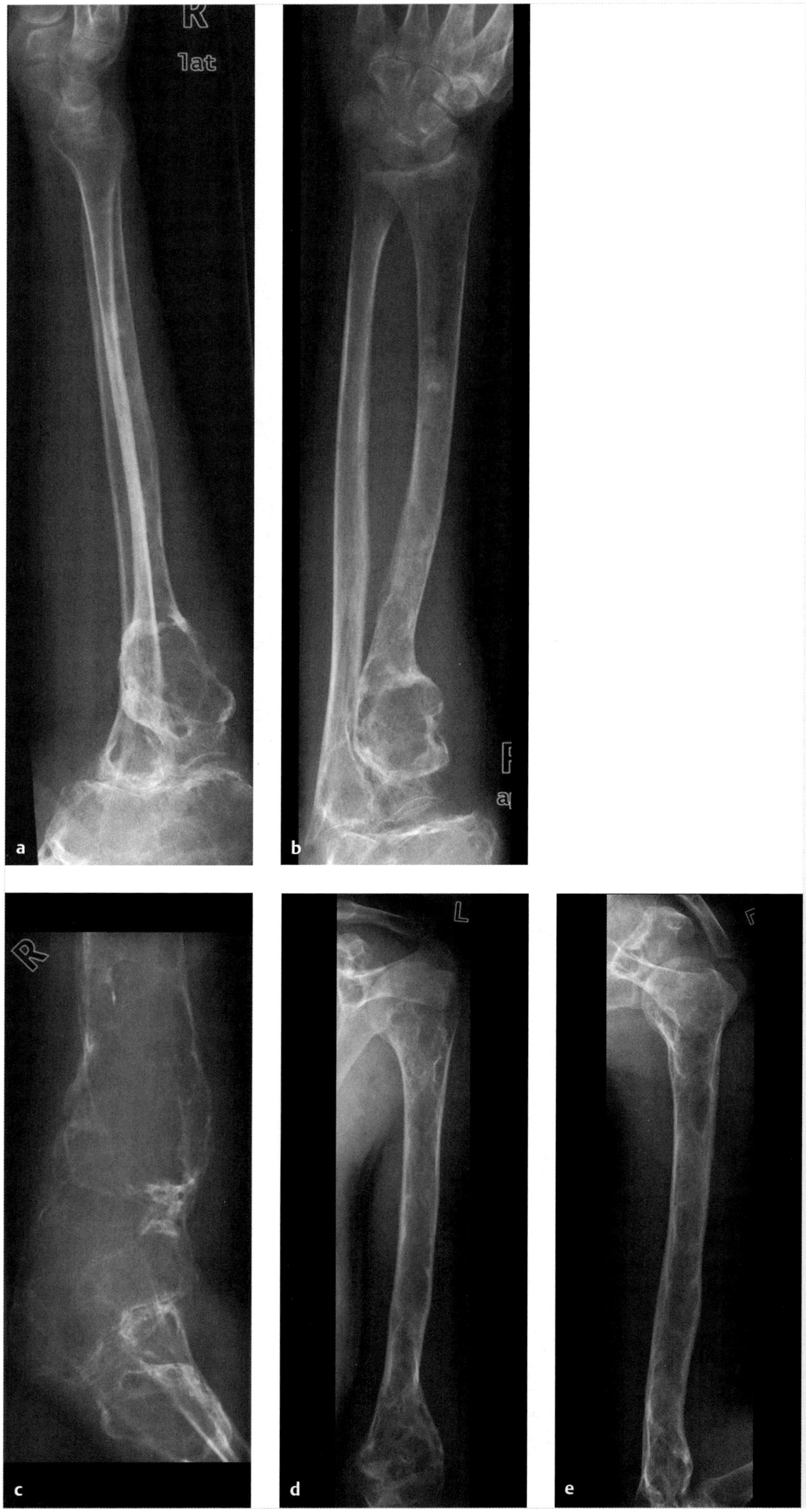

Fig. 6.28 a–e Enchondromatosis?

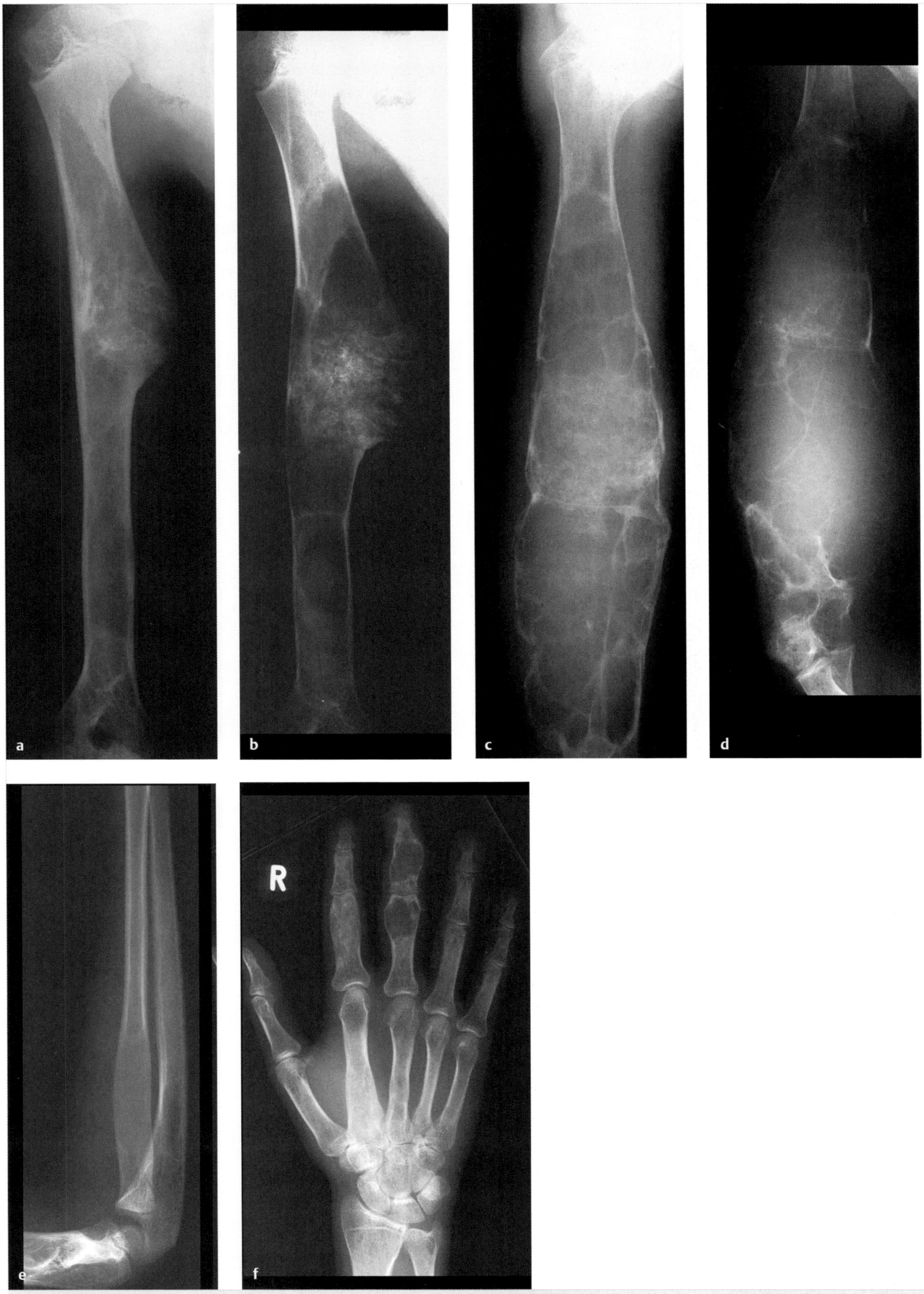

Fig. 6.29 Fibrous dysplasia at age 10 years (a), 14 years (b), 16 years (c), 18 years (d), and 24 years (e, f).

6.2 Forearm

Case 111 (▶ Fig. 6.30)

Case description

- Referring physician: orthopedist.
- Prior history and clinical question: A 50-year-old woman had pain in her right elbow joint radiating to the forearm. She had not been feeling well, was depressed, and also had cardiac complaints. A destructive process in the right proximal ulna was biopsied, and histology gave the impression of a somewhat atypical giant cell tumor. Question: Are the radiologic findings consistent with a giant cell tumor?

Radiologic Findings

The normal trabecular pattern is absent in the right proximal ulnar epiphysis, metaphysis, and diaphysis, and the cortex is greatly thinned and partially disrupted (▶ Fig. 6.30 **a, b**). T2w MRI (▶ Fig. 6.30 **c**) shows focal, water-equivalent hyperintensities in the area of radiologic osteolysis, which exhibits fluid–fluid levels on the axial image in ▶ Fig. 6.30 **e**. Images after intravenous (IV) contrast administration (▶ Fig. 6.30 **d, f**) show marked inhomogeneous enhancement, with a number of enhancing septa around hypointense areas. Paraosseous hyperintensities are visible on all MR images. The whole-body bone scan (▶ Fig. 6.30 **g**), besides showing intense cranial uptake, is remarkable by the nonvisualization of soft tissues, particularly the kidneys, bladder, and

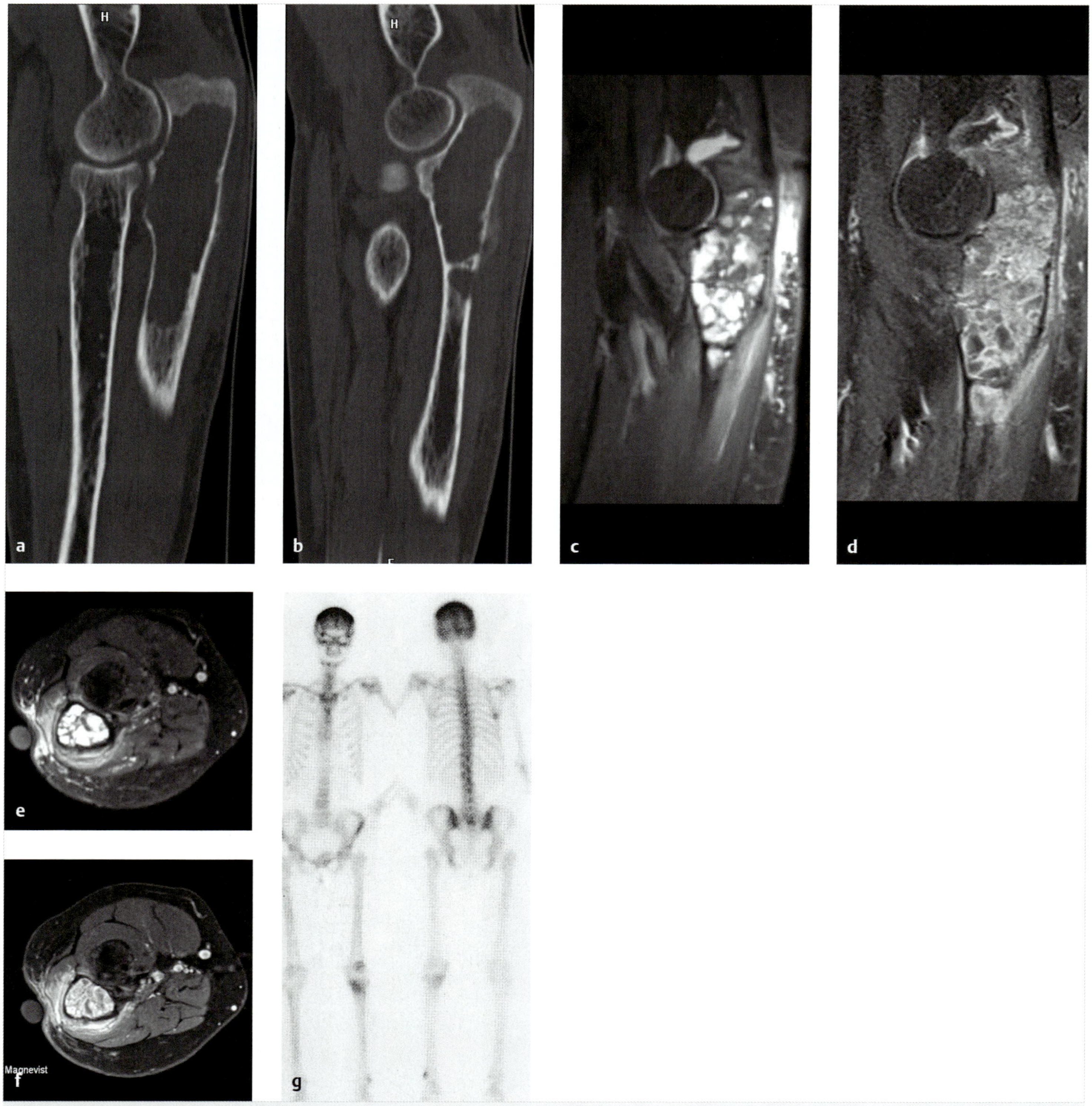

Fig. 6.30 a–g Giant cell tumor?

muscles (e.g., in the legs). Slightly increased uptake is noted in the right upper tibia and patella. Sectional images of the right arm (not pictured here) showed intense enhancement about the right elbow joint.

Location

The pathologic changes are located in the proximal ulnar epiphysis, metaphysis, and diaphysis and have a paraosseous component.

Pathoanatomic Background of the Findings

The lesion in the proximal ulna contains solid and liquid areas, as indicated by the fluid–fluid levels.

Assignment to a Possible Basic Entity

► **Inflammation?** No clinical manifestations. The region around the right elbow joint is only slightly warm to the touch.

► **Trauma?** No trauma history.

► **Tumor?** Very likely, since normal bone structures have been replaced by other tissues. Considering the fluid–fluid levels, we may be dealing with a primary or secondary aneurysmal bone cyst. With a primary aneurysmal bone cyst, at least 70% of the lesion should exhibit fluid–fluid levels; this is not true in the present case. This leaves only secondary aneurysmal bone cysts. But when we note the preliminary histologic finding, we might also consider a giant cell tumor with regressive changes. This would fit the location of the lesion, although the proximal ulna would be a rare site of occurrence for a giant cell tumor. But lesions that contain giant cells and cavities with hemorrhagic fluid levels may also occur in a solid aneurysmal bone cyst (reparative giant cell granuloma) or within a brown tumor of hyperparathyroidism.

Synopsis and Discussion

Based on the above considerations, our differential diagnosis consists of a giant cell tumor, solid aneurysmal bone cyst, and brown tumor. This led us to revisit the staging whole-body bone scan, which is actually a *superscan* in which all activity is "sucked" into the bone leaving no uptake for the soft tissues. Superscans are often interpreted as normal because when the gamma camera reaches a certain count (here, in the skull), it automatically turns off and does not register the true magnitude of the tracer uptake. This may occur with a diffuse metastasizing bone disease, for example, but it is very characteristic of hyperparathyroidism. This is further supported by the very intense uptake in the skull. In summary, we may attribute the destructive process to a brown tumor of hyperparathyroidism. Because the patient had no signs of renal failure, the hyperparathyroidism is primary. This diagnosis is consistent with the general clinical complaints reported by the patient. Serum parathormone was finally determined and showed a very abnormal elevation.

Final Diagnosis

Brown tumor of primary hyperparathyroidism.

Comments

The histologic diagnosis of an atypical giant cell tumor should always prompt further testing for a possible brown tumor in hyperparathyroidism.

Case 112 (▶ Fig. 6.31)

Case description

- Referring physician: surgeon.
- Prior history and clinical question: A 26-year-old woman complained of pain in her right elbow following an impact trauma during soccer. The pain was attributed to a small cortical fracture in the radial tuberosity seen on an AP radiograph (not pictured here). This was consistent with clinical findings (pain exacerbated by flexion and supination). An expansile process (Lodwick grade IA) was also noted incidentally at the level of the fracture site (▶ Fig. 6.31**a**); it had ground-glass opacity and was therefore interpreted as fibrous dysplasia. The arm was immobilized at the elbow joint for 3 weeks. Approximately 3 months later the patient returned with new complaints of pain in her right elbow joint. The ground-glass opacity was no longer present on radiographs (▶ Fig. 6.31 **b, c**), which now showed increased expansion of the bone with marked thinning of the surrounding cortex. The surgeon suspected a malignant process and recommended biopsy.

Radiologic Findings

The confusing images in ▶ Fig. 6.31 **b, c** show a Lodwick grade IB lesion. The cortex is greatly thinned but not destroyed. Soap-bubble areas of very low density are visible within the osteolytic process.

Pathoanatomic Background of the Findings

The radiographic signs of increasing destruction of the woven bone and progressive thinning of the cortex over a 3-month period can actually be explained only by regressive processes within the lesion (cystic transformation due to intralesional hemorrhage, etc.), raising suspicion of a secondary aneurysmal bone cyst. Malignant "transformation" in 3 months is not realistic; at most we might consider the activation of a tumor that is already malignant, but this would not be consistent with the absence of complaints before the trauma or the Lodwick IB grade lesion.

Assignment to a Possible Basic Entity

Because the lesion in the proximal radius is obviously a tumor or tumorlike lesion, any attempt to assign the lesion to a different basic entity would be purely academic and may be omitted here.

Synopsis and Discussion

Given the risk of spontaneous fracture, the lesion was curetted and the defect was filled with cancellous bone. Gross examination showed a slightly blood-tinged fluid in a "pulpy" tissue, reflecting a trauma-induced (and histologically verifiable) regressive cystic transformation of fibrous dysplasia tissue. A secondary aneurysmal bone cyst was not confirmed.

This case clearly illustrates that trauma to a tumor or tumorlike lesion may lead to very rapid changes in its morphology.

Final Diagnosis

Regressive cystic transformation of fibrous dysplasia due to trauma.

Comments

Trauma can transform the typical, benign-appearing morphology of fibrous dysplasia into an aggressive morphology.

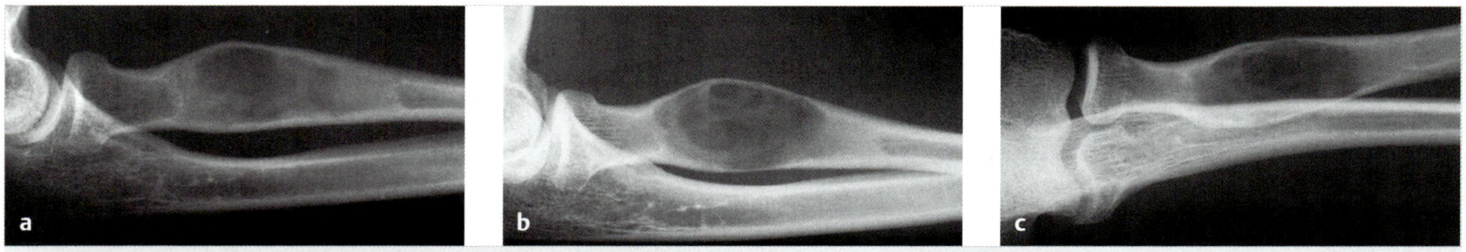

Fig. 6.31 a–c Unexplained morphologic change (from a to b) of an expansile lesion in the proximal radius.

Case 113 (▶ Fig. 6.32)

Case description

- Referring physician: radiologist.
- Prior history and clinical question: A 47-year-old woman had a 2-year history of pain in her right proximal forearm, which was most pronounced during forearm rotation. The patient worked in a carpentry shop. Tenderness was noted over the proximal radius on physical examination, and pronation/supination was limited to 30–40°.

Radiologic Findings

Unfortunately, conventional radiographs were not available. The CT images in ▶ Fig. 6.32 show a solid ossification, roughly triangular in shape, arising from the radial tuberosity with its apex directed proximally and anteriorly. The interior of the lesion is hyperintense on T2w MRI, and edema-like signal is noted in proximity to the lesion. The lesion is hypointense on T1w images. A fat-suppressed image after IV contrast administration (▶ Fig. 6.32 **m**) shows marked enhancement within the lesion and its surroundings.

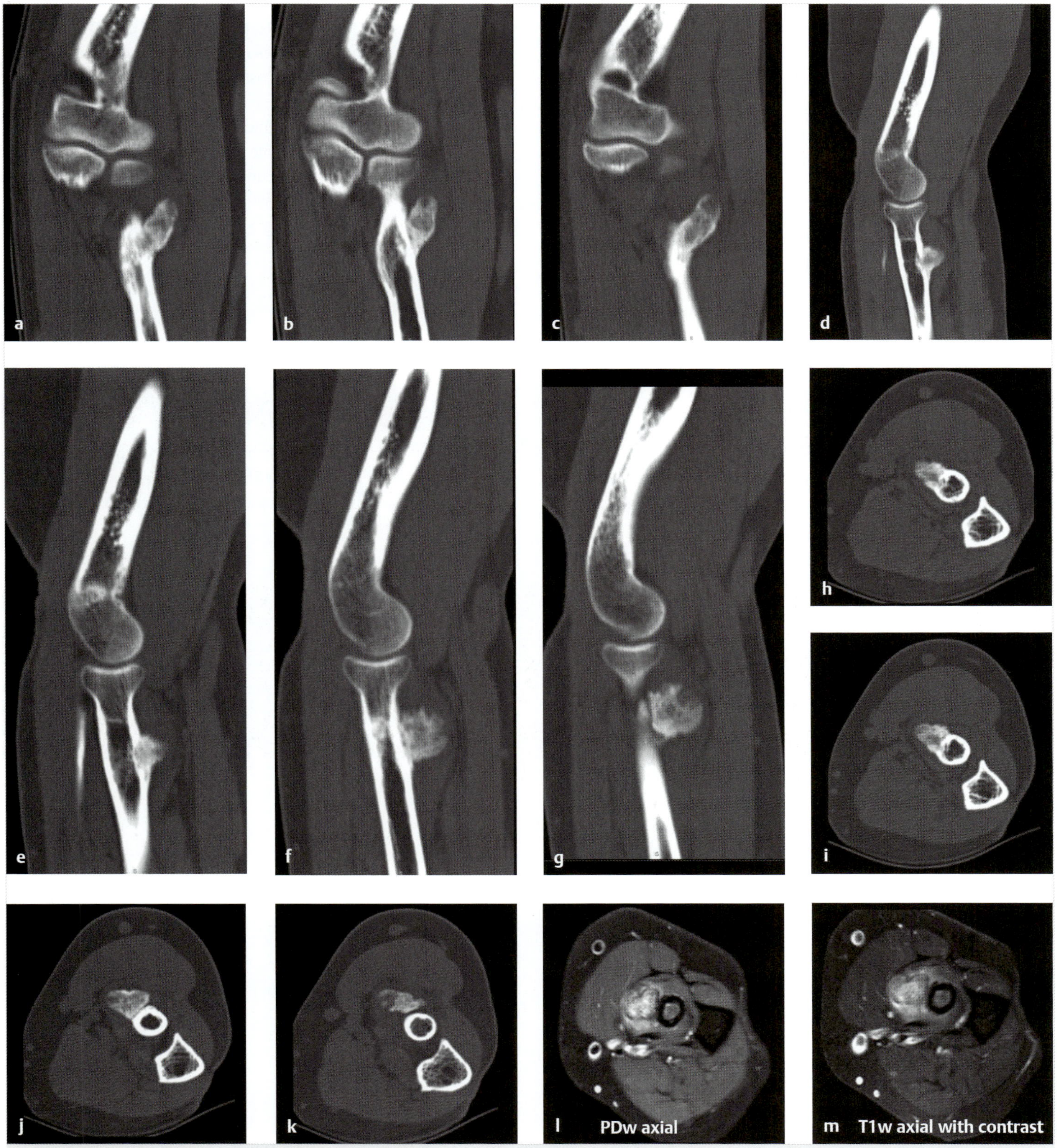

Fig. 6.32 a–m Juxtacortical osteosarcoma?

Location

The lesion arises anatomically from the radial tuberosity and is aligned in the direction of muscular traction from the biceps brachii.

Pathoanatomic Background of the Findings

The contrast enhancement shows that the solid ossified lesion must still have a florid soft-tissue component both in the interior of the lesion and in its surroundings. The location and principal alignment of the lesion strongly suggest a relationship to the insertion of the biceps brachii tendon.

Assignment to a Possible Basic Entity

▸ **Normal variant or malformation?** No. While prominence and widening of the radial tuberosity may occur as a normal variant in response to mechanical loads,[17] a solid exophytic ossification does not occur as a normal variant in or on the radial tuberosity.

▸ **Trauma?** Quite possible. The patient is right-handed and works in a carpentry shop, so her right arm is subjected to greater mechanical loads. Thus a calcifying tendinitis may have developed at the biceps tendon attachment (see above under Location). But the strong enhancement of the lesion and its surroundings would be more consistent with heterotopic ossification or myositis ossificans traumatica resulting from one or more traumatic events (see also Case 29, Case 30, Case 63, Case 64, and Case 156).

▸ **Tumor or tumorlike lesion?** A juxtacortical (paraosseous) or even periosteal osteosarcoma would be possible based on the ossification pattern. But this diagnosis is not supported by the absence of a well-defined cap of nonossified tumor matrix—clearly demonstrable by MRI and is usually seen with these tumors. With an osteochondroma, we should see an open medullary cavity forming a definite communication between the radius and exophytic growth.

Synopsis and Discussion

The above considerations narrow the differential diagnosis to two main possibilities:

1. A reactive trauma-induced process, either
   - an acute inflammatory calcifying tendinitis (enthesiopathy), or
   - a still-florid myositis ossificans traumatica caused by one or more traumatic events
2. Paraosseous osteosarcoma

The radial tuberosity is an unusual location for all three entities. Trauma-induced enthesiopathies more commonly occur on the proximal humerus (see Case 102, Case 103, and Case 104) and femur (see Case 75) and in numerous entheses on the pelvis. Sites of predilection for paraosseous osteosarcoma are the femur, tibia, and humerus.

Given the prior history of high occupational stresses on the patient's right arm, it is reasonable to diagnose a trauma-induced reactive process. But since a *conclusive* diagnosis could not be made from the clinical or radiologic findings, an open excisional biopsy was performed, yielding a histologic diagnosis of calcifying tendinitis.

Final Diagnosis

Reactive ossifying process on the radial tuberosity caused by calcifying tendinitis.

Comments

With a heavily ossified exophytic process developing on bone, the differential diagnosis should always include extraosseous osteosarcoma even if the lesion is located at an enthesis.

Case 114 (▶ Fig. 6.33)

Case description

- Referring physician: radiologist.
- Prior history and clinical question: A 12-year-old boy suffered a fall, and his left wrist was x-rayed the following day to exclude a fracture. The radiograph showed a rounded osteolytic lesion in the distal radial diametaphysis, which was tentatively classified as plasma cell osteomyelitis or a Brodie abscess. The boy was clinically healthy and reported no local complaints involving the distal left wrist. Question: Should the lesion be investigated by biopsy?

Radiologic Findings

Radiographs (▶ Fig. 6.33 **a, b**) show a rounded osteolytic area with a sclerotic margin (Lodwick grade IA) in the distal radial diametaphysis. A lucent band of approximately the same diameter runs from the osteolytic lesion to the distal epiphyseal plate. It has very faint sclerotic margins with a tram-track appearance. The distal ends of the radial metaphysis and especially the ulnar metaphysis appear very dense, and the growth plates appear to be slightly widened. The lesion appears on CT (▶ Fig. 6.33 **c**) as a soft-tissue mass that has (measured) attenuation values of cartilage.

Location

The most interesting aspect of the changes from a location standpoint is the connection between the diaphyseal lesion and the distal metaphysis, which shows increased density.

Pathoanatomic Background of the Findings

As stated above, a connection exists between the diaphyseal lesion and the markedly dense distal metaphysis. When we note that the interior of the diaphyseal lesion is isoattenuating to cartilage, it is conceivable that growth cartilage may have migrated or been displaced toward the diaphysis during longitudinal bone growth as a result of mechanical stress. This is suggested by the dense trabeculae structures in the distal metaphyses and the apparent widening of the growth plates of the radius and ulna.

Assignment to a Possible Basic Entity

▶ **Normal variant or malformation?** This question is appropriate, since we are dealing with an asymptomatic finding in a growing child. But there is no known precedent for an osteolytic area in the distal radial metadiaphysis, increased metaphyseal density, and slightly widened growth plates occurring as a normal variant.

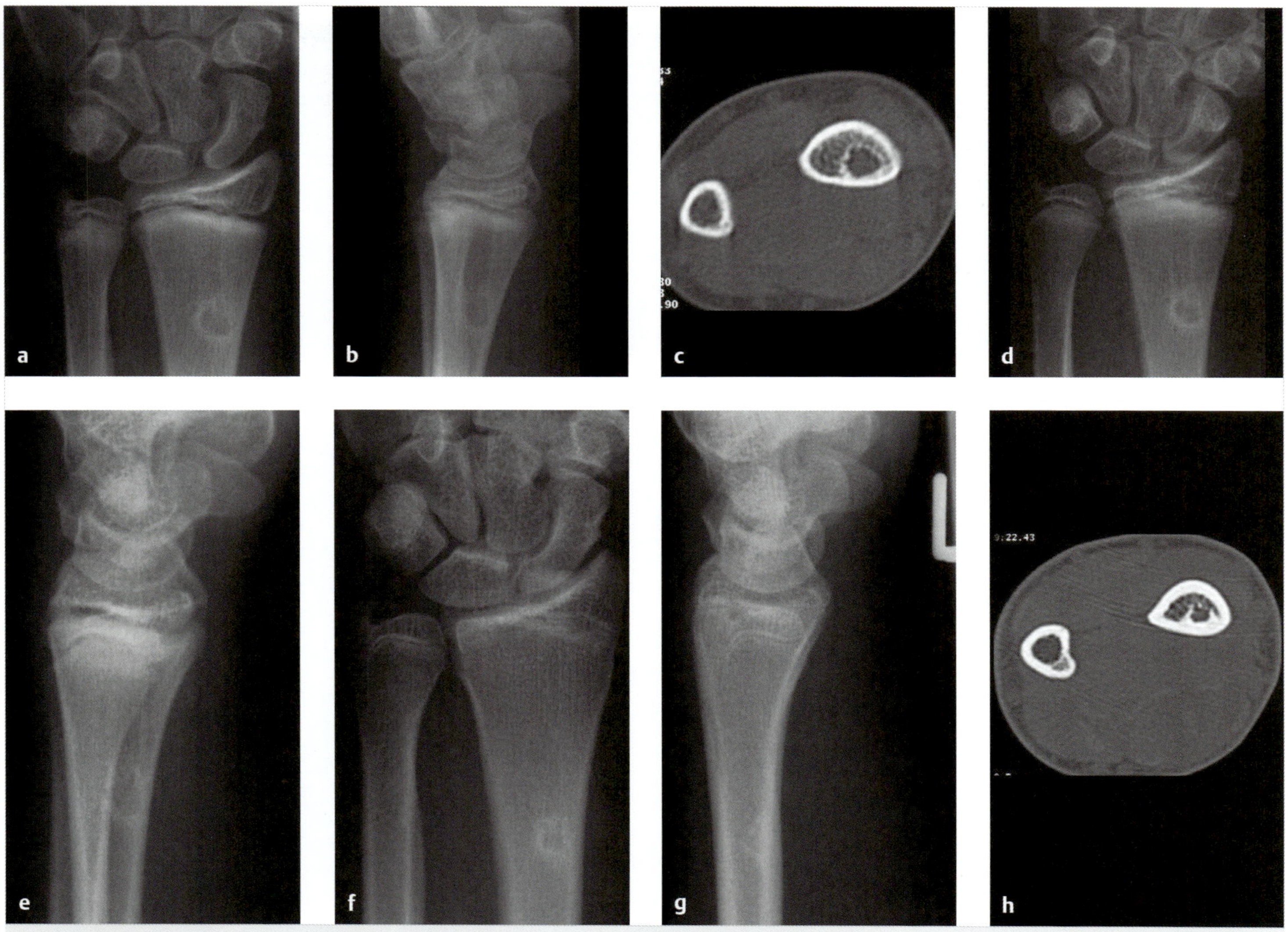

Fig. 6.33 Brodie abscess or plasma cell osteomyelitis? The images were acquired in June 1998 (a–c), in October 1998 (d, e), and in June 2001 (f–h).

► **Trauma?** To answer this question, which had not yet been raised, we interviewed the boy and his parents. We learned that he was an avid goalkeeper in soccer matches, and that the games were often very rough. The parents confirmed that their son would often appear "roughed up" after returning home from a game. Also, he would frequently throw himself to the ground with outstretched hands when trying to block a shot. He stated that several weeks earlier an opponent had stepped on the flexor side of his right hand with a soccer shoe, leaving spike imprints that were visible for days. This history is strongly suggestive of a trauma- or stress-induced process.

► **Inflammation?** No. The boy had no local or systemic signs of inflammation either before or after radiologic documentation.

► **Tumor?** No, the unusual geometry of the changes is not consistent with a tumor.

Synopsis and Discussion

When the lesion was interpreted elsewhere as a primary chronic inflammatory process, the special prior history and absence of complaints were not taken into account. Radiographs were obtained to exclude an acute fracture, so the changes were purely an incidental finding.

How can the finding, which we interpret as stress-related, be explained? Chronic stress on growth plates leads to widening of the plates and a reactive increase in the density of the adjacent metaphyseal cancellous bone. To date, this phenomenon has been most commonly observed in the growth plates about the knee (see also Case 152). Chinese authors[45] published one study on stress-induced changes in the distal growth plates of the forearms. The study involved adolescent gymnasts at a Chinese opera school, who danced daily on their hands. As in our case, imaging of the wrists showed widening and irregularities of the growth plates and increased density of the adjacent metaphyseal cancellous bone on both sides. The authors attribute the physeal widening to a thickening of the growth cartilage, which shows increased proliferation at sites of stress-induced resorptive changes in the bone.

A radiograph of the contralateral side in our case showed the same changes in the growth plates and adjacent metaphyses. As mentioned above, the more proximal lesion in our case is explained by the displacement of physeal cartilage, whose pathogenesis may be as follows: Chronic stress or even a single event may press or seed physeal cartilage into the zone of provisional calcification. If the cartilage is not resorbed there, the heterotopic cartilage tissue may extend into the diaphysis during growth; it "migrates" toward the diaphysis. Since growth cartilage can continue to proliferate, regardless of its anatomic location, it may conceivably form a kind of column similar to that in enchondromatosis (see Case 115). In contrast to enchondromatosis, however, the lesion becomes "fused" to the diaphysis as shown by the follow-up images in ► Fig. 6.33 **d–h**. A follow-up radiograph (not pictured here) was taken when the boy was 17 years old, 2 years after the image in ► Fig. 6.33 **g**, and the radiologist stated that the bone changes had resolved completely. Even by age 15 years (► Fig. 6.33 **g**) the growth plates were closed and the metaphyseal densities had been resorbed.

Diagnosis

Stress-induced displacement of epiphyseal plate cartilage in the radius.

Comments

Unusual radiologic findings that are difficult to classify can be solved in most cases by eliciting (or re-eliciting) a detailed history.

Case 115 (▶ Fig. 6.34)

Case description

- Referring physician: orthopedist.
- Prior history and clinical question: The right forearm of a 9-year-old boy was x-rayed after a bicycle fall. The radiographs showed an unusual fluted pattern in the distal radial diametaphysis. The orthopedist wanted to know the cause. Clinically the boy had only a slight bowing of the distal radius toward the palmar side, which his mother had known about for some time. The boy had no functional abnormalities of the wrist or forearm.

Radiologic Findings

Radiographs show elongated, fluted or columnlike lucencies with slightly sclerotic margins in the distal radial diametaphysis (▶ Fig. 6.34 **a, b**). The bone contour appears "roughened" on the ulnar side. At the proximal end of the changes, the radial shaft is slightly bowed toward the palmar side. Bone development in the carpus appears normal for age. Four rounded structures in the radius show very high signal intensity on axial T2w MRI (▶ Fig. 6.34 **c**). They partially extend beyond the cortical bone.

Location

The column-shaped structures are closely related to the growth plate.

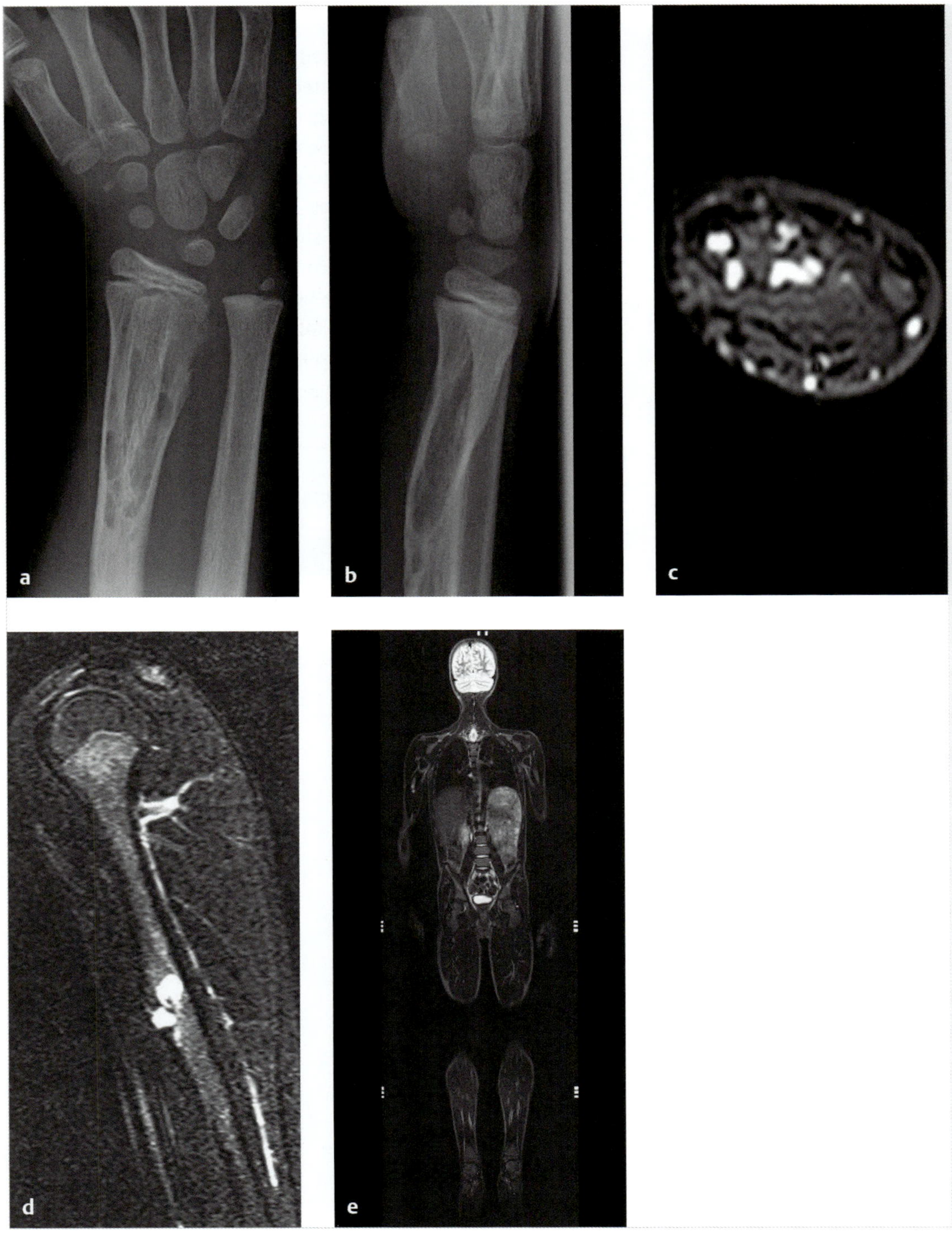

Fig. 6.34 a–e Normal variant?

Pathoanatomic Background of the Findings

The column-shaped structures are cartilage columns. This imaging term is used only in connection with enchondromatosis and is pathognomonic for that condition along with other lesions such as expansile enchondromas. The signal intensity is also suggestive of cartilage. Unfortunately, the sagittal and cortical images were blurry and cannot be presented here. The typical MRI appearance of the cartilage columns is illustrated in ▶ Fig. 6.41 **m, n** of Case 120. The roughness on the ulnar side of the radius represents the edge of the subperiosteal cartilage column (see also Case 105). The axial MR image in ▶ Fig. 6.34 **c** shows that other cartilage columns also extend to the bone surface.

Assignment to a Possible Basic Entity

▶ **Normal variant or malformation?** This question is justified by the incidental nature of the finding, but there is no known precedent for a normal variant of this kind. The question of how the changes are classified as dysplasia is addressed below.

▶ **Trauma?** No, the boy had no history of chronic trauma or any previous single injury to the right forearm. It is obvious that the changes cannot stem from acute trauma.

▶ **Inflammation?** No clinical manifestations.

▶ **Tumor?** No, this is not consistent with the striking geometry of the cartilage columns.

Synopsis and Discussion

As explained under Pathoanatomic Background of the Findings, there is only one plausible diagnosis for the radiologic findings, namely enchondromatosis. This is a bone dysplasia (dyschondroplasia) caused by the heterotopic proliferation of epiphyseal chondroblasts. This process interferes with enchondromatous ossification, leading to changes that include shortening and deformation of the affected bone, usually on one side (Ollier disease). The proliferating cartilage masses are located mainly in the metaphysis, from which they may spread to the diaphysis. As in our case, it is not uncommon to find sites of subperiosteal and juxtacortical cartilage proliferation as in periosteal chondromas.

There are various forms of enchondromatosis that differ in their genetics, pattern of spread, clinical presentation, and radiologic findings. Here we shall mention only the Ollier type, which is usually characterized by predominant unilateral involvement of the lower limbs, and Maffucci syndrome, marked by a combination of multiple chondromas and soft-tissue hemangiomas. In both subtypes the probability of malignant transformation of one of the chondromas is extremely high, at more than 60%. These patients should therefore be followed clinically and radiologically (preferably by whole-body MRI) at a maximum of 2-year intervals. The disease is manifested in infancy and childhood by deformities and longitudinal growth disturbances. Some cases present initially with a relatively large, symptomatic enchondroma or periosteal chondroma (see Case 105), and enchondromatosis develops only over a period of years. These children should be closely followed clinically and radiologically due to the high rate of malignant transformation.[18] As mentioned above and illustrated in Case 120, the radiology of Ollier disease is marked by osteolytic lesions with or without matrix ossification (depending on the "maturation stage" of the tumor) and by cartilage columns, which are pathognomonic for the disease. They are depicted most convincingly in water-sensitive MRI sequences. Malignant transformation of one of the lesions is usually signaled by lesion enlargement over a short period of time, accompanied by pain.

In our case we ordered whole-body MRI, which revealed an additional lesion in the middle of the right humeral diaphysis (▶ Fig. 6.34 **d, e**). The boy is currently followed at 2-year intervals by whole-body MRI.

Final Diagnosis

Enchondromatosis in the right upper limb (humerus, radius).

Comments
Cartilage columns are pathognomonic for enchondromatosis.

6.3 Hands (Bone and Joint Diseases)

Case 116 (▶ Fig. 6.35)

Case description

- Referring physician: hand surgeon.
- Prior history and clinical question: A 5-year-old child presented with unusual radiologic changes in the metaphyses of the hand skeleton. The child manifested growth retardation and slight bowing of the arms.

Radiologic Findings

Radiographs of the hands and feet (▶ Fig. 6.35 **a–c**) show deep cupping of the metaphyses with normally shaped epiphyses. Irregular cartilaginous calcifications are visible within the depressions. The shafts of the small tubular bones appear shortened. The metaphyseal contours about the knee and elbow joints (▶ Fig. 6.35 **d, e**) appear somewhat irregular but do not show as much cupping as in the hands and feet. The spine appears normal (▶ Fig. 6.35 **f, g**). Overall, the bones appear slightly more radiolucent than normal.

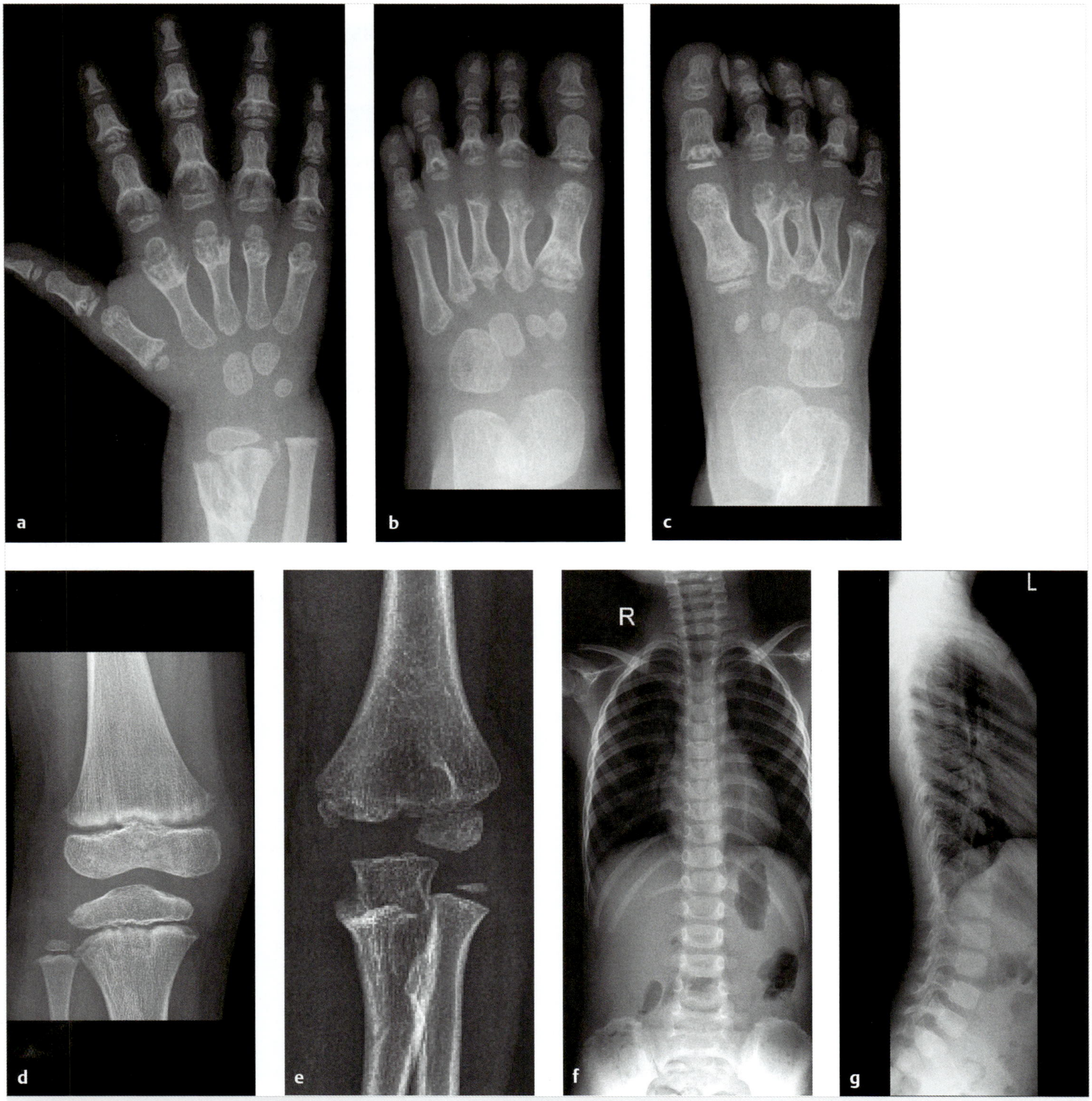

Fig. 6.35 a–g Rickets or dysplasia?

Location

The pathologic changes described above are confined entirely to the metaphyses, most notably in the hands and feet.

Pathoanatomic Background of the Findings

The changes, limited to the metaphyses, are actually consistent only with skeletal dysplasia based on a chondrocyte defect in the growth plates, resulting in underdeveloped metaphyses.

Assignment to a Possible Basic Entity

▸ **Normal variant or malformation?** Based on the considerations above, we are compelled to classify the changes as a developmental abnormality or dysplasia.

Synopsis and Discussion

Once the changes have been classified as a disorder of skeletal development with maldeveloped metaphyses, it is an easy matter to find the disease in a catalog of bone dysplasias. Spranger et al[37] described the condition as the "Jansen type of metaphyseal dysplasia." It is based on mutations of the *PTHR1* gene, which is located on chromosome 3p22-p22.1. The mutations lead to the constitutive, ligand-independent activation of the G-protein-coupled receptor for the parathyroid hormone-related protein in pre-hypertrophic chondrocytes of the growth plate. This in turn delays the differentiation of the chondrocytes, leading to a disturbance of bone formation. The principal radiologic changes in children are as follows:

- Variable degree of osteopenia (as in our case)
- Rickets-like metaphyseal cupping, which may be extreme in early school-age children (as in our case)
- Cortical erosions and increased subperiosteal bone (absent in our case)
- Calvarial changes (density and structure; unknown in our patient because skull radiographs were not obtained)

Even severe rickets would not cause such deep defects in the metaphyses of the hands and feet.

Final Diagnosis

Jansen type of metaphyseal dysplasia.

Comments

Using an established radiologic hallmark and consulting reference atlases can pave the way to a correct diagnosis.

Case 117 (▶ Fig. 6.36)

Case description

- *Prior history and clinical question:* This case was diagnosed and furnished to use by Dr. C. T. Muth of Cottbus, Germany. It involves a grotesque but painless hypertrophy of the third finger of the left hand in a 73-year-old man, allowing us to dispense with our usual descriptions and deductions. The radiograph of the left hand was obtained after an injury (▶ Fig. 6.36).

Traditionally, the pathogenesis of *macrodystrophia lipomatosa* is related to the hypertrophy of all mesodermal tissues, but with a dominant fat component, caused by the lipomatosis of a nerve (fibrolipomatous hamartoma). The affected nerve undergoes a "sausagelike" enlargement due to the abnormal proliferation of fibrofatty tissue.[46,47] The median nerve and its branches or the plantar nerves are most commonly affected. The lipomatosis of the nerve apparently leads to a localized macrodactyly characterized by the hypertrophy of one or more bones and subcutaneous fat in the hand or foot. This hypertrophy is also known as *localized gigantism*. In very care cases, even large nerves such as the sciatic nerve may be involved.

Based on more recent observations, the dominant fibrolipomatous tissue is found in association with arteriovenous fistulas or circumscribed, hypertrophic vascular structures (arterial, venous, lymphatic). Since macrodystrophia lipomatosa is also thought to be associated with neurofibromatosis type I, it is reasonable to ask whether it may be a subtype of the phacomatoses. One member of this group is *proteus syndrome*, a hamartoneoplastic syndrome involving all three germ layers. This extremely rare disease is characterized by the following symptoms:

- Localized gigantism of the hands and/or feet
- Nevi
- Hemihypertrophy due to overgrowth of a long tubular bone
- Subcutaneous tumors (lipomas, lymphangiomas, hemangiomas)
- Macrocephaly

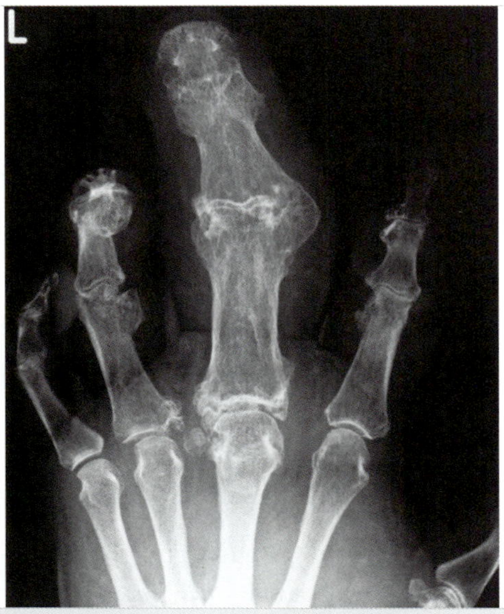

Fig. 6.36 Gigantism of the middle finger. Cause?

- Cranial hyperostosis
- Pulmonary and renal anomalies

The disease apparently results from a (somatic) mosaicism. We have seen two cases in which the dominant features were gigantic fat hypertrophy and vascular anomalies (venous malformations, arteriovenous malformations) with hemihypertrophy. One of the cases is published in Freyschmidt (2008).[13] Based on current understanding, proteus syndrome is classified among the PTEN hamartoma tumor syndromes (PTEN = phosphate and tensin homolog, deleted on chromosome 10).[48]

Reportedly, ultrasound and MRI can unequivocally demonstrate the changes of macrodystrophia lipomatosa.[46,47] Ultrasound shows a diffusely enlarged nerve with alternating hyperechoic (fatty) and hypoechoic bands (nerve bundles) that have a cablelike appearance. MRI shows a similar pattern of longitudinal cylindrical areas of low to intermediate signal intensity (nerve bundles) surrounded by fatty tissue in a diffusely thickened nerve. Patients with macrodactyly also have increased fatty tissue content in the fingers. A proportionate degree of bony hypertrophy is present, as in our case. When cylindrical or serpiginous structures are seen on MRI or CT, we would also consider vascular malformations and try to visualize them with contrast medium. In our case the faint serpiginous structures visible in the soft tissues of the third finger may well represent abnormal vessels.

Final Diagnosis

Macrodystrophia lipomatosa with gigantism of the left third finger.

Comments

Localized gigantism of one finger or toe or multiple fingers or toes should raise suspicion of a hamartoneoplastic syndrome.

Case 118 (► Fig. 6.37)

Case description

- Referring physician: hand surgeon.
- Prior history and clinical question: A 41-year-old woman presented with recurrent pain in her left hand, predominantly on the extensor side. The symptoms were interpreted as tenosynovitis caused by accessory ossicles or heterotopic ossifications. Based on the MRI findings, the surgeon asked if a different diagnosis should be considered.

Radiologic Findings

Three well-differentiated bony elements are visible on the dorsal side of the distal row of carpal bones, and a fourth is located deep in the carpal tunnel (► Fig. 6.37 **a–d**; arrows in c, d). These small bony elements are surrounded by thick soft-tissue structures that are isointense to articular cartilage on the T1-image (f) and on the water-sensitive MR sequences (► Fig. 6.37 **e, g**). The second through fourth extensor tendons are significantly displaced.

Location

The epicenter of the osseous and soft-tissue changes appears to be located in the scaphoid.

Pathoanatomic Background of the Findings

It is likely that the "supernumerary" bony elements have something to do with the surrounding thick soft-tissue structures. They may have originated from them. This is also suggested by their differentiated structure with cancellous bone, medullary cavities, and surrounding cortex, resembling the head of an osteochondroma.

Assignment to a Possible Basic Entity

► **Normal variant or malformation?** The presence of thick, surrounding cartilaginous structures in itself suggests that the supernumerary bony elements are not accessory bones. The same reasoning would rule out heterotopic ossifications. If we follow the line of reasoning under Pathoanatomic Background of the Findings, they may actually represent osteochondromas, although they cannot have originated in the usual way from heterotopic physeal cartilage but from an epiphysis (dysplasia epiphysealis). It is helpful to note that an "irregular" bone such as the scaphoid does not have a classic epiphysis like that found in tubular bones. Instead, the bone itself constitutes an epiphysis consisting of an ossification center surrounded by an acrophysis and covered by articular cartilage. Acrophysis (synonym: spherical growth plate) is a term applied to all other normal growth plates that do not conform to the classic anatomy of an epiphyseal plate. An acrophysis is composed of cartilage cells that are arranged in different zones, as in an ordinary epiphyseal plate:

- Zone of resting cartilage
- Zone of proliferation
- Zone of cartilage column formation
- Zone of hypertrophy
- Zone of provisional calcification

► **Trauma?** No trauma history.

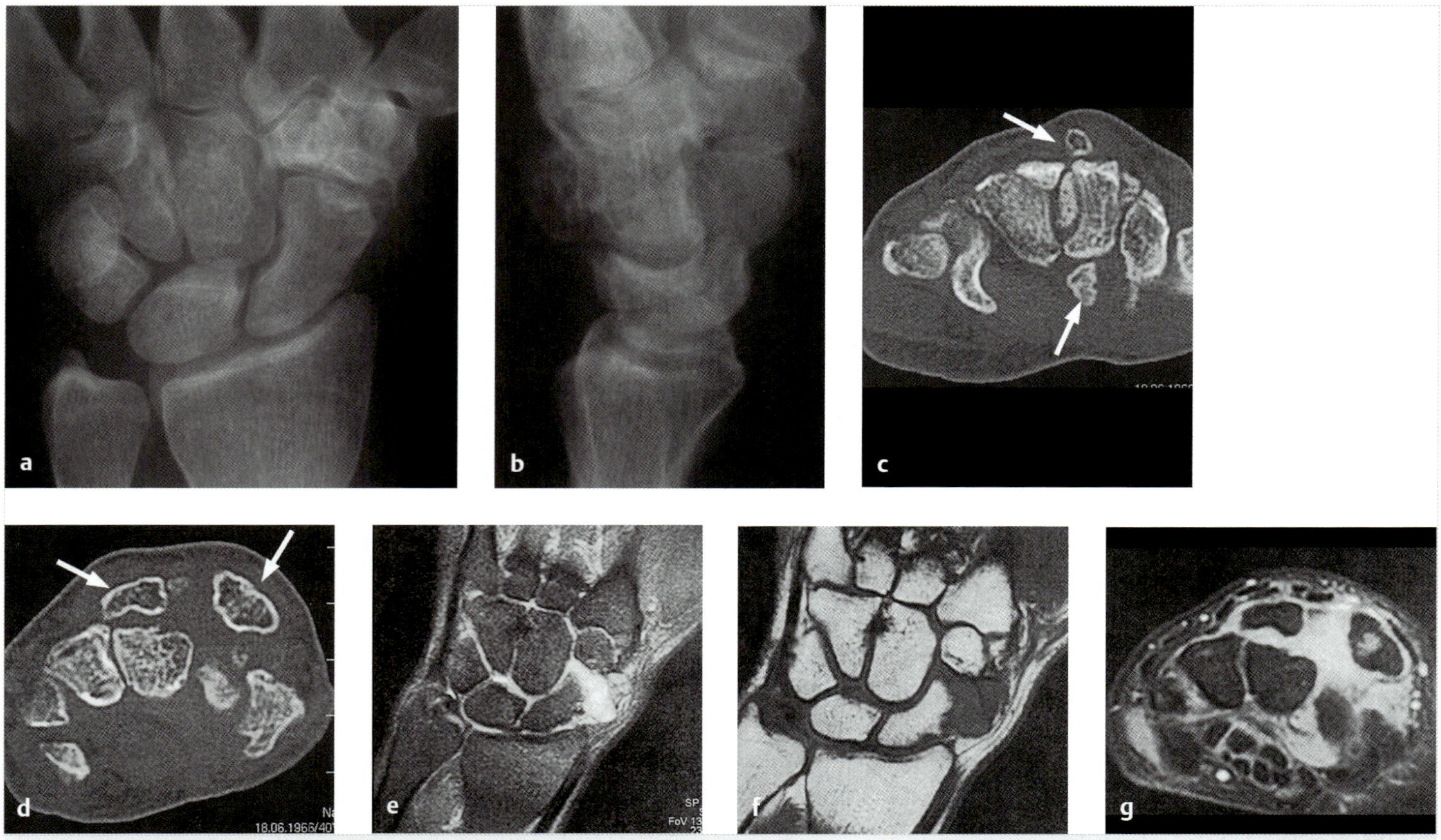

Fig. 6.37 a–g Accessory ossicles or heterotopic ossification?

▶ **Tumor?** No. A cartilage-forming tumor or tumorlike lesion (e. g., synovial chondromatosis, extraskeletal chondrosarcoma) has a more inhomogeneous cartilaginous ossification pattern. In our case we are dealing with very mature bony elements that appear to have been present for a long time.

Synopsis and Discussion

All of the above considerations lead us to epiphyseal osteochondromas, known also as dysplasia epiphysealis or Trevor disease. It may be considered a variant of osteochondroma. This very rare disease more commonly affects the lower limb than the upper limb and is typically unilateral. Cartilage proliferation is usually confined to the medial or lateral side of the affected limb (hemimelic)—in our case the radial side of the carpus. There is also a localized (monostotic) form, a classic form in which more than one bone segment is affected, and a generalized form involving the whole limb. The localized form most commonly affects the bones of the hindfoot or distal tibia, while the classic hemimelic form affects more than one, but not all, epiphyses within a lower limb, most commonly about the knee and ankle joints.

Areas of cartilage proliferation consist of a lobulated mass with a cartilage cap, which develops from the ossified epiphyseal center. Because the scaphoid bone often consists of two growth centers or possibly more, multiple osteochondromas may develop. Conventional radiographs show a well-differentiated bony element that is either located some distance from the associated bone or is adherent to it. The key feature is the surrounding cartilage mantle, which is best demonstrated by MRI. Enchondral ossification may give rise to very dense bone (see ▶ Fig. 6.38). If the tendon sheaths are displaced, as in our case, tenosynovitis may develop causing the patient to become symptomatic.

▶ Fig. 6.38 illustrates another case of Trevor disease, also originating from the scaphoid. In this case, a 5-year-old girl, the osteochondroma has developed in a distal and dorsal direction and is attached to the original scaphoid. Portions of the lesion show extremely dense ossification.

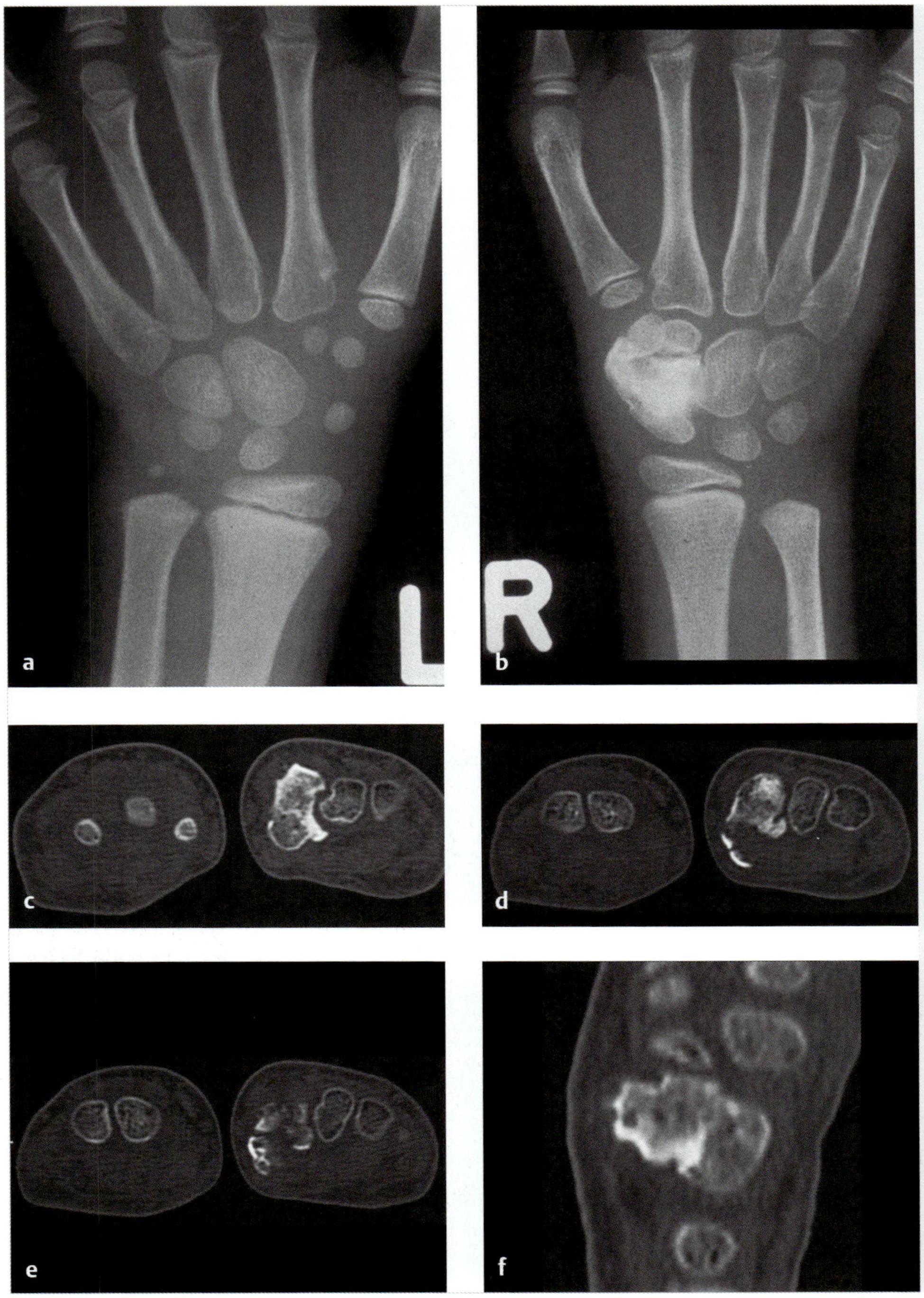

Fig. 6.38 a–f Dysplasia epiphysealis hemimelica originating from the scaphoid in a 5-year-old girl.

Final Diagnosis

Dysplasia epiphysealis hemimelica (Trevor disease) originating from the scaphoid bone.

Comments

Large, differentiated supernumerary, bony elements surrounded by a cartilage mass suggest epiphyseal osteochondroma formation in Trevor disease.

Case 119 (▶ Fig. 6.39)

Case description

- Referring physician: surgeon.
- Prior history and clinical question: A 32-year-old woman complained of recurrent pain in the bones of her hands and feet. The patient claimed to have experienced increasing forgetfulness and occasional loss of orientation in the past 2 years.

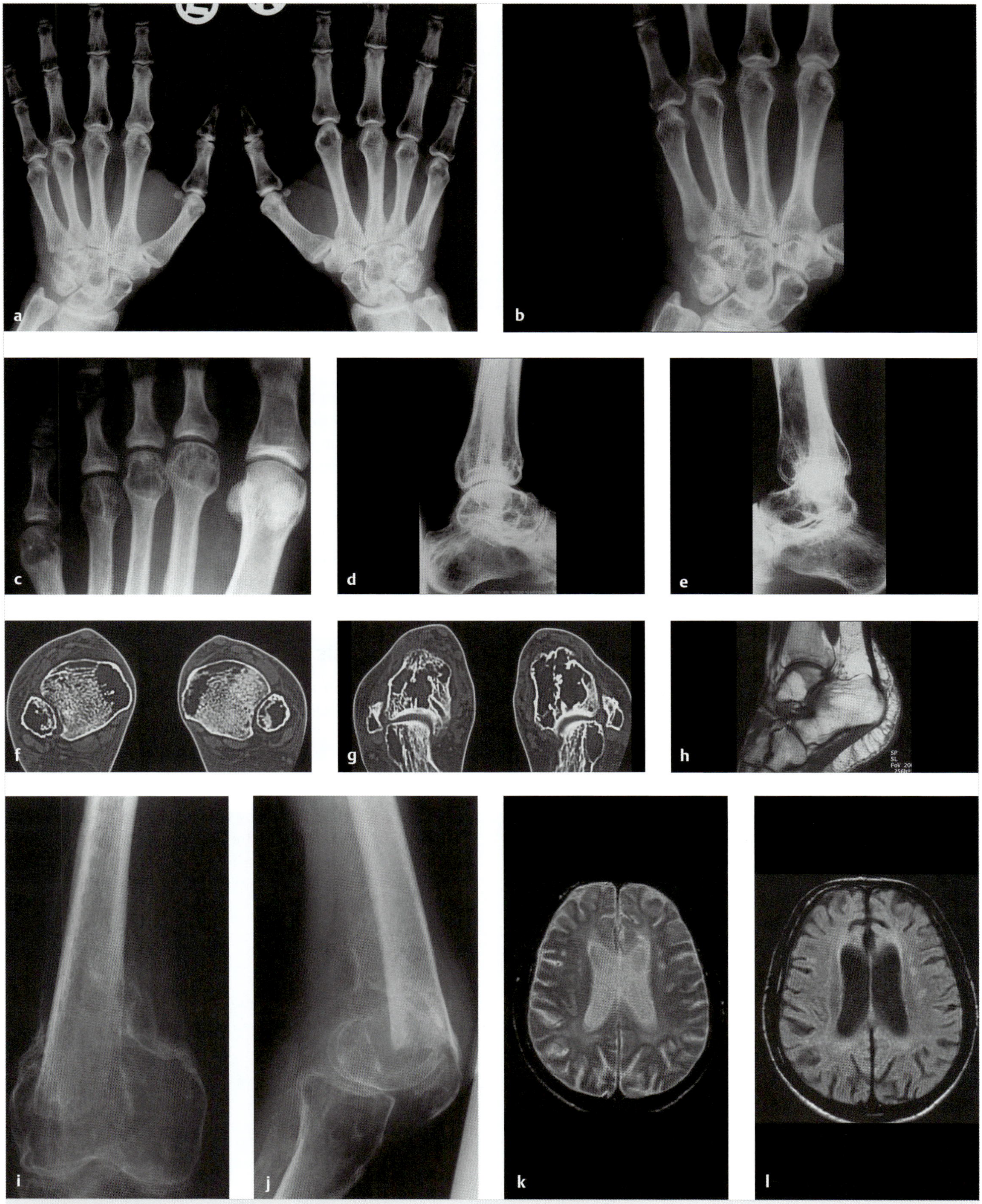

Fig. 6.39 a–l "Cystic" systemic disease or enchondromatosis?

Radiologic Findings

On the plain radiographs, loss of trabecular structure is noted in both carpi, in the metacarpal heads, and in the bases of the proximal phalanges, creating a "cystic" appearance (▶ Fig. 6.39 **a, b**). The metatarsal heads exhibit similar changes (▶ Fig. 6.39 **c**). Lateral radiographs of the ankle joints (▶ Fig. 6.39 **d, e**) show an extreme loss of trabecular structure in all imaged bones, with areas of severe cortical thinning. The CT scans in ▶ Fig. 6.39 **f, g** show fatty tissue in the lucent zones. Attenuation measurements in scans with a soft-tissue window showed attenuation values of –20 to –70 HU. On the T1w MR image in ▶ Fig. 6.39 **h**, the areas showing loss of trabeculation are isointense to fat. Sectional images of the hands yielded similar findings.

Location

The abnormal lucencies in the imaged bone segments are confined to the intraosseous space.

Pathoanatomic Background of the Findings

The "cystic" changes noted in the cancellous bone can be explained by fat replacement. Changes of this kind are found only in *polycystic lipomembranous osteodysplasia.* This term encompasses the cardinal symptoms described by the patient:
- (Pseudo)cystic changes
- Fatty tissue
- Multifocal bone dysplasia

Assignment to a Possible Basic Entity

▶ **Normal variant or malformation?** Yes, in the sense of a developmental disorder. As there is no realistic differential diagnosis for the findings acquired with various modalities (multifocal fat replacement), there is no need to consider other possible categories.

Synopsis and Discussion

The present case of polycystic lipomembranous osteodysplasia could be diagnosed noninvasively by imaging studies alone. CT and MRI were instrumental in proving the fatty nature of the "polycystic" changes.

Polycystic lipomembranous osteodysplasia is generally associated with sclerosing leukoencephalopathy. This combination is called *Nasu–Hakola disease (polycystic lipomembranous osteodysplasia with sclerosing leukoencephalopathy)* after the authors who first described it. Defined in very general terms, the disease is a "congenital disorder of fatty tissue marked by changes in the bone and central nervous system." As described above, the pathoanatomic background of the bone changes is a multifocal replacement of normal cancellous bone by fatty tissue. Interspersed among the otherwise normal fat lobules are membranes composed of mucopolysaccharides and lipoproteins that are PAS-positive (PAS = periodic acid-Schiff reaction). Typically, the changes develop symmetrically in the limb bones, especially in the hands and feet but later in the epimetaphyses of the long tubular bones. The sclerosing leukoencephalopathy is marked by a general atrophy and sclerosis of the white matter, particularly in the frontal lobes. Microscopy reveals general diffuse astrogliosis and demyelination. The disease is hereditary and is ascribed to a mutation of the *DAP-12* gene.[49] A possible link between the osseous and cerebral changes is beyond our present scope, but further details may be found in Freyschmidt (2008).[13]

Based on our own experience with nine cases, and in agreement with the approximately 200 cases published in the literature,[50] symptoms begin at approximately 20 years of age with pain following minor trauma or a greater stress to the affected bones. Pathologic fractures develop by about 30 years of age, with associated onset of neuropsychiatric symptoms that resemble Alzheimer disease. This eventually progresses to frank dementia, and epileptic seizures occur. Most patients die at approximately 50 years of age.

Our patient and her two brothers with the same disease, whom we were able to follow for many years, also developed increasing neuropsychiatric symptoms. Brain MRI in our patient (▶ Fig. 6.39 **k, l**) showed significant white matter atrophy with ventricular dilatation and diffuse foci of demyelination, which accounted for the clinical symptoms. The skeletal changes progressed at a relatively rapid rate in all three siblings. One brother, for whom we have complete radiologic documentation, developed grotesque fractures of the long bones (▶ Fig. 6.39 **i, j**) with eventual pathologic fractures in the pelvis and spine.

Final Diagnosis

Polycystic lipomembranous osteodysplasia with sclerosing leukoencephalopathy (Nasu–Hakola disease).

Comments

Symmetrical cystlike lucencies in the bones of the hands and feet should be investigated further by sectional imaging to determine whether they contain fat. If so, the patient may have polycystic lipomembranous osteodysplasia.

Case 120 (▸ Fig. 6.40)

Case description

- Referring physician: hand surgeon.
- Prior history and clinical question: A 24-year-old man complained of occasional pain in the left hand. The ulnar head was slightly prominent dorsally and was too far proximal, apparently because the ulna was too short. The surgeon wanted to know the cause of the osteolytic changes in the third and fourth fingers.

Radiologic Findings

Osteolytic lesions, some expansile (e.g., in the third metacarpal head), are noted in the distal half of the third and fourth metacarpals and associated phalanges (▸ Fig. 6.40 **a, b**). When the films were viewed with a magnifier, fine calcifications were visible in some of the lesions. The third finger is slightly too long, and the ulnar head on the left side is too far proximal. The distal radial articular surface is sharply sloped toward the ulnar side. The bones of the right hand appear normal.

Location

The pathologic findings are confined to the bones of the left hand.

Pathoanatomic Background of the Findings

When we consider the finding in the distal left radial and ulnar epiphysis, which may be termed a pseudo-Madelung deformity, plus the slightly elongated third finger of the left hand, and the fact that the osteolytic changes are confined to the left hand, we may classify the osteolytic changes in the third and fourth fingers generally as bone dysplasia with foci of cartilage proliferation.

Assignment to a Possible Basic Entity

▸ **Normal variant or malformation?** Yes, see Pathoanatomic Background of the Findings and Synopsis and Discussion.

▸ **Tumor or tumorlike lesions?** The osteolytic lesions are caused by enchondromas, as indicated by the fine intralesional calcifications. The enchondromas in the ulnar base of the proximal phalanx and in the proximal half of the middle phalanx of the middle finger on the ulnar side are more protuberant than at other sites (enchondroma protuberans). Other possible causes of osteolytic changes in the third and fourth fingers such as granulomas in sarcoidosis, brown tumors of hyperparathyroidism, or gouty tophi do not fit into the above context (unilateral occurrence, signs of dysplasia).

Synopsis and Discussion

The dysplastic changes in the bones of the left hand combined with enchondromas are consistent with the Ollier type of enchondromatosis. The WHO classification of bone tumors[15] defines Ollier disease as:

"A developmental disorder caused by a failure of normal enchondral ossification. Furthermore, there is production of cartilaginous masses (enchondromas) in the metaphyses and adjacent regions of the shafts and flat bones, with varying degrees of bone deformity. There is predominant unilateral involvement. The multiple enchondromas appear in childhood and there is widespread skeletal involvement."

Enchondromatoses do not constitute a uniform group of diseases due to their varied clinical, genetic, and radiologic features. Six different types are distinguished, of which only the Ollier type (unilateral involvement predominantly of the lower limb) and Maffucci syndrome (combines the features of Ollier disease with soft-tissue hemangiomas) are mentioned here. The diseases are

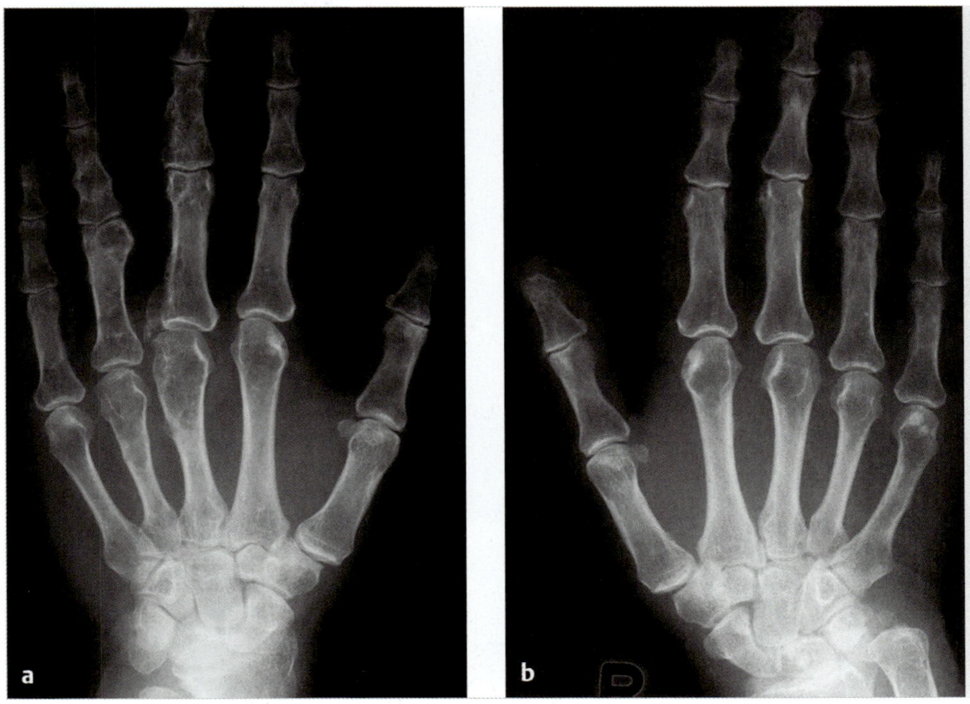

Fig. 6.40 a, b What caused the "cysts" in the third and fourth fingers?

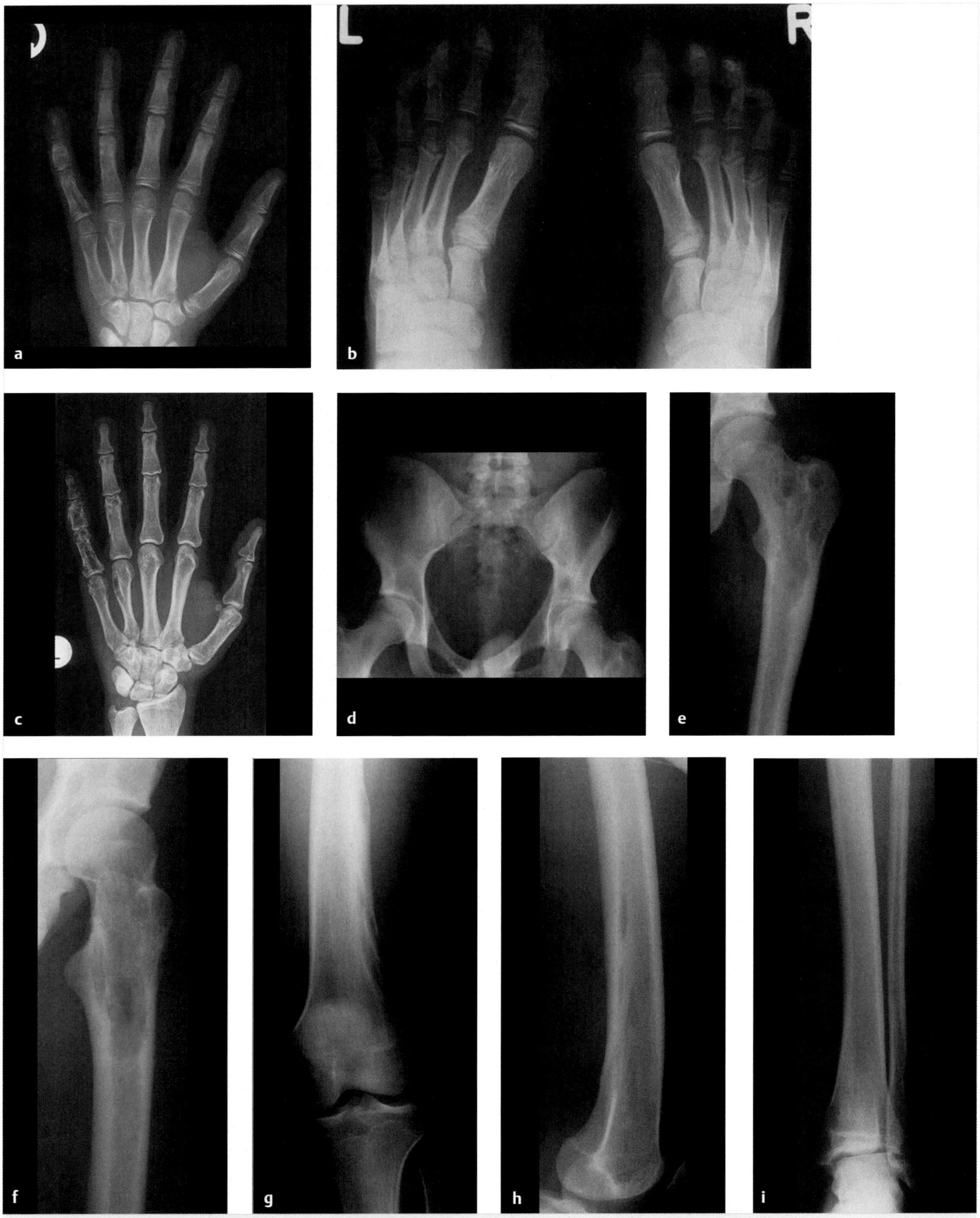

Fig. 6.41 Classic enchondromatosis. The Images were obtained in 1993 (a, b) and in 2004 (c–q).

generally manifested in early childhood by external deformities and longitudinal growth disturbance. With involvement of the upper limb, the ulna is often shortened relative to the radius, leading to a pseudo-Madelung deformity, as in the present case.

Our own experience with more than 30 cases indicates that enchondromatosis may begin with large, solitary, clinically symptomatic enchondromas and periosteal chondromas, with additional cartilaginous tumors developing much later on the same side of

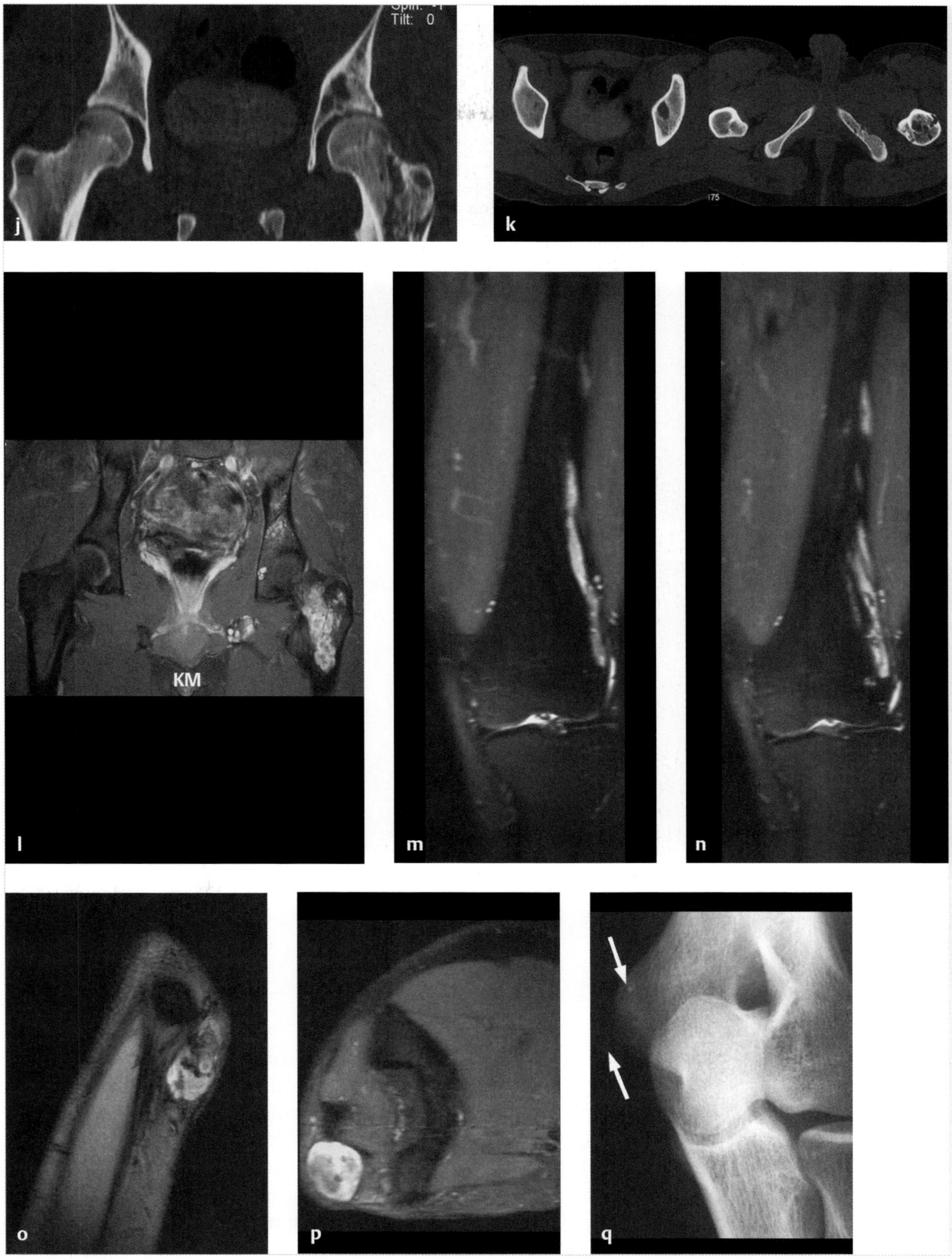

Fig. 6.41 Continued.

the body. This is significant in that enchondromatoses have an approximately 60% rate of malignant transformation, even at an early age, and therefore patients require life-long clinical and radiologic follow-ups (whole-body MRI every 2 years). Enchondromatosis is not only associated with enchondromas (as the name implies) but also with periosteal chondromas, which are otherwise very rare (see Case 105). Columnar zones of cartilage proliferation appear radiographically as lucent streaks, bands, grooves, or helical lucencies with sclerotic margins in the metadiaphyses (see Case 115). T1w MRI depicts them as linear hypointensities or signal voids which "light up" on T2w images (▸ Fig. 6.41 **m, n**).

▸ Fig. 6.41 presents the case of an initially 10-year-old boy with a classic form of enchondromatosis, whom we were able to follow for 11 years. The most striking radiographic findings at age 10 were columnar lucencies in the fourth and fifth fingers and in the proximal phalanx of the big toe on the left side (▸ Fig. 6.41 **a, b**). Eleven years later (▸ Fig. 6.41 **c**) the skeletal changes in the hand were significantly larger. At that time disseminated osteolytic lesions were found in the left acetabulum (▸ Fig. 6.411 **d, j–l**), left proximal femur (▸ Fig. 6.41 **e, f**), distal femoral shaft (▸ Fig. 6.41 **g, h**), and left distal fibular shaft. The cartilaginous nature of the changes is clearly appreciated on MRI (▸ Fig. 6.41 **l–n**). This par-

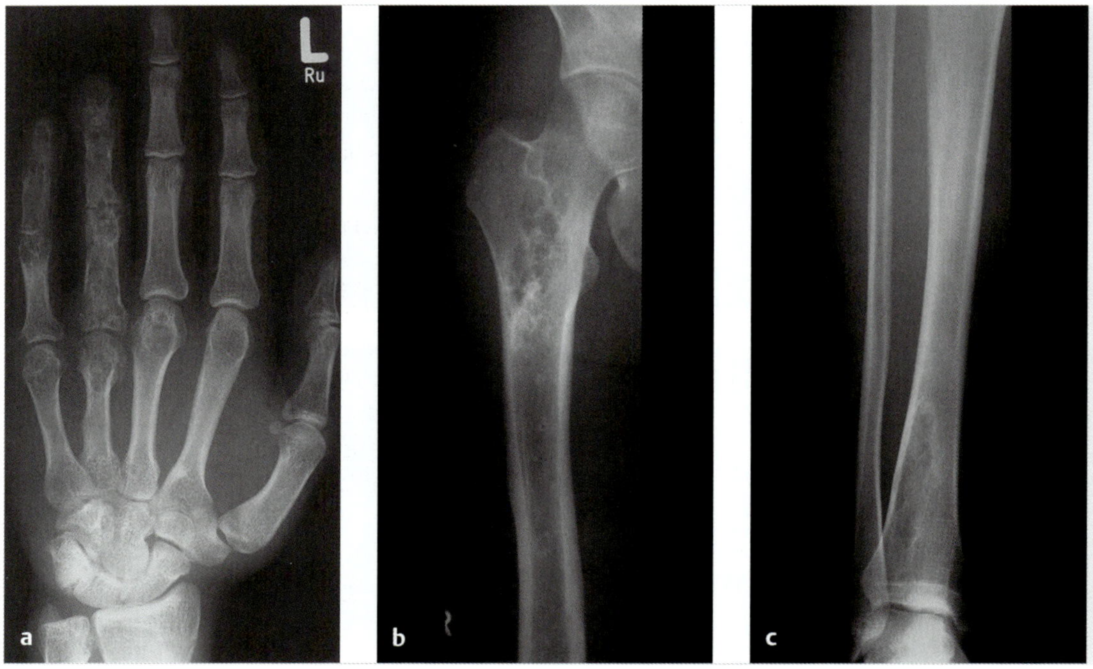

Fig. 6.42 a–c Unusual bilateral enchondromatosis in a 31-year-old man.

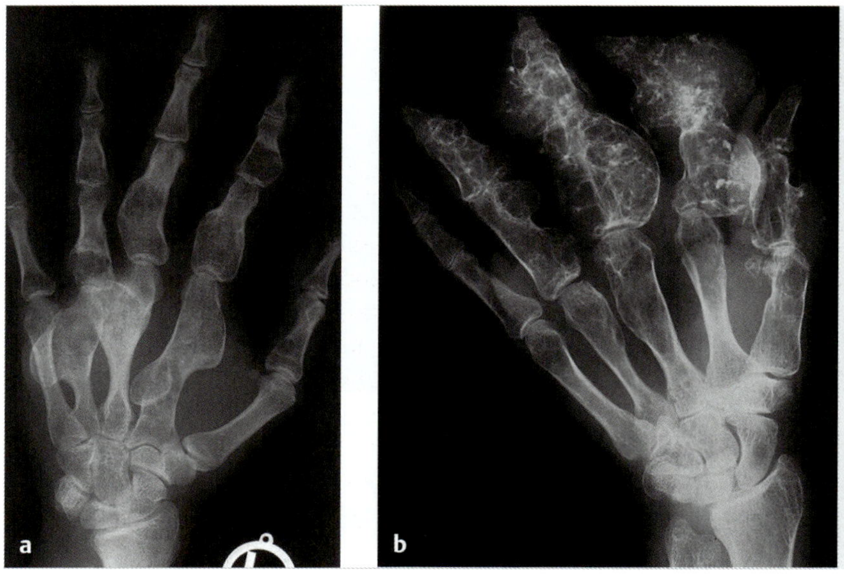

Fig. 6.43 a, b Enchondromatosis in two additional patients.

ticularly applies to the cartilage columns in the left, lateral distal femoral shaft (▶ Fig. 6.41 **m, n**). Four small phleboliths (arrows in ▶ Fig. 6.41 q) located within a hemangioma (▶ Fig. 6.41 **o, p**) are seen just above the level of the olecranon and projected over the ulnar epicondyle. These findings were definitive for Maffucci syndrome. Because the enchondromas in the left proximal femur looked particularly aggressive, we obtained several percutaneous CT-guided biopsies at those sites, all of which indicated pure enchondroma with no malignant elements. Since then the young man has presented for 2-year MRI follow-ups, which have shown no significant progression of the changes.

▶ Fig. 6.42 presents another case of enchondromatosis in a 31-year-old man. An unusual feature of this case is the extensive "crossover" skeletal changes involving the left hand and the right lower limb. They appear to be very aggressive in the hand, where the radiograph shows cortical perforations in the affected phalanges. Note that the cartilaginous ossifications in the right femur extend far into the shaft.

▶ Fig. 6.43 shows additional cases of enchondromatosis with grotesque skeletal changes in the hands: a 30-year-old man (▶ Fig. 6.43 **a**); an incidental finding in a man over the age of 60 (▶ Fig. 6.43 **b**). It is noteworthy that cartilage masses have perforated into the soft tissues, especially about the middle phalanges. If the patient had reported pain and lesion enlargement at those sites, malignant transformation to chondrosarcoma would have been very likely.

Final Diagnosis

Enchondromatosis in the left hand.

Comments

Multiple osteolytic lesions, possibly with expansile features, combined with dysplastic changes and cartilaginous calcifications with unilateral involvement are almost always pathognomonic for enchondromatosis.

Case 121 (▶ Fig. 6.44)

Case description

- *Referring physicians:* hand surgeon and rheumatologist.
- *Prior history and clinical question:* A 57-year-old woman had a long history of pain in her hands. The second proximal interphalangeal joint of her left hand was completely ankylosed, and she reported incipient stiffness of the third and fourth proximal interphalangeal joints. She also described swelling of the affected joints. Physical examination revealed nodular swellings on the sides of all proximal and distal interphalangeal joints. She claimed that her mother had had similar symptoms, which had been diagnosed as gout. The referring physicians were confused by the marked osteolytic areas below the trochleae of the second and third proximal phalanges of the right hand.

Radiologic Findings

The radiographs (▶ Fig. 6.44) show joint space narrowing in all distal interphalangeal joints of both hands. Subchondral sclerosis is noted at the bases of the distal phalanges, especially on the left side, and marginal osteophytes are faintly visible. Severe destructive changes are noted in all proximal interphalangeal joints of both hands, accompanied by marginal proliferation, subchondral sclerosis, and osteophytes, creating a bird's-wing appearance along the bases of some of the middle phalanges (especially the third finger of the left hand). "Cystic" lucencies are visible around the proximal interphalangeal joints of the right hand. One particularly large osteolytic lesion is located below the trochlea of the third proximal phalanx and extends far into the shaft. The second proximal interphalangeal joint of the left hand is completely ankylosed, and incipient ankylosis is noted in the third and fourth proximal interphalangeal joints of the left hand and the second proximal interphalangeal joint of the right hand. Joint space narrowing and subchondral sclerosis have also developed in the scapho-trapezio-trapezoid (STT) joints.

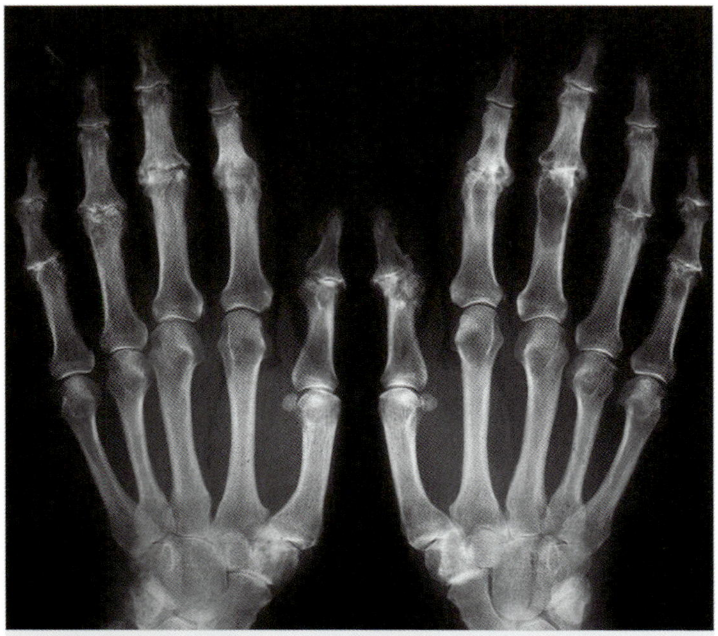

Fig. 6.44 Gout?

Location

The changes described above involve the proximal and distal interphalangeal joints and STT joints. The remaining carpal and metatarsophalangeal joints appear normal.

Pathoanatomic Background of the Findings

The key finding is cartilage loss, which has led to instability of the affected joints and reactive changes in response to further loading, such as subchondral sclerosis, marginal osteophytes, and subchondral cysts or geodes. As there are no signs of an inflammatory process originating from the synovial membrane, such as juxta-articular osteoporosis and classic erosions, we are dealing with a chondroarthropathy, that is, a disease process arising from damaged cartilage.

Assignment to a Possible Basic Entity

▶ **Normal variant or malformation?** No.

▶ **Trauma?** No trauma history.

▶ **Inflammation?** As noted above, there are no signs of an inflammatory articular process.

▶ **Tumor or tumorlike lesion?** This question relates mainly to the large osteolytic lesion in the proximal phalanx of the third right finger. Large, solitary osteolytic lesions in the hand most often represent harmless enchondromas. When we consider that the osteolytic lesion in this case does not have the lobular scalloping or enchondral cartilaginous bone formation typical of an enchondroma, and that it may be considered just the largest of many smaller osteolytic foci around the proximal interphalangeal joints, enchondroma becomes a less likely diagnosis. Another possibility would be a large gouty tophus, which also may extend far into the diaphysis, but the patient did not give a prior history of gout attacks.

Synopsis and Discussion

The above considerations on a primary process arising from the articular cartilage leaves only one plausible diagnosis, namely polyarticular osteoarthritis of the Bouchard and Heberden type. The clinical course and radiologic findings point to a relatively aggressive type of *polyarticular osteoarthritis*, the *destructive or erosive (inflammatory) form*. According to the standard literature, this form is particularly common in women of 50 to 60 years of age and appears to have an hereditary predisposition. It takes an aggressive clinical course marked by severe pain and swelling of the affected joints. The radiologic changes are rather pronounced and are characterized by severe destructive and erosive joint changes (without juxta-articular osteoporosis), early ankylosis, and large subchondral cysts that may extend far into the diaphysis and resemble gouty tophi (▶ Fig. 6.45). Among our own patients, the destructive form of polyarticular osteoarthritis has predominantly affected males over 40 years of age. It accounts for approximately 5% of all cases of polyarticular osteoarthritis.

To aid in the differential diagnosis of "cystic" skeletal lesions in the hand, ▶ Fig. 6.45 illustrates a case of gouty arthritis that was

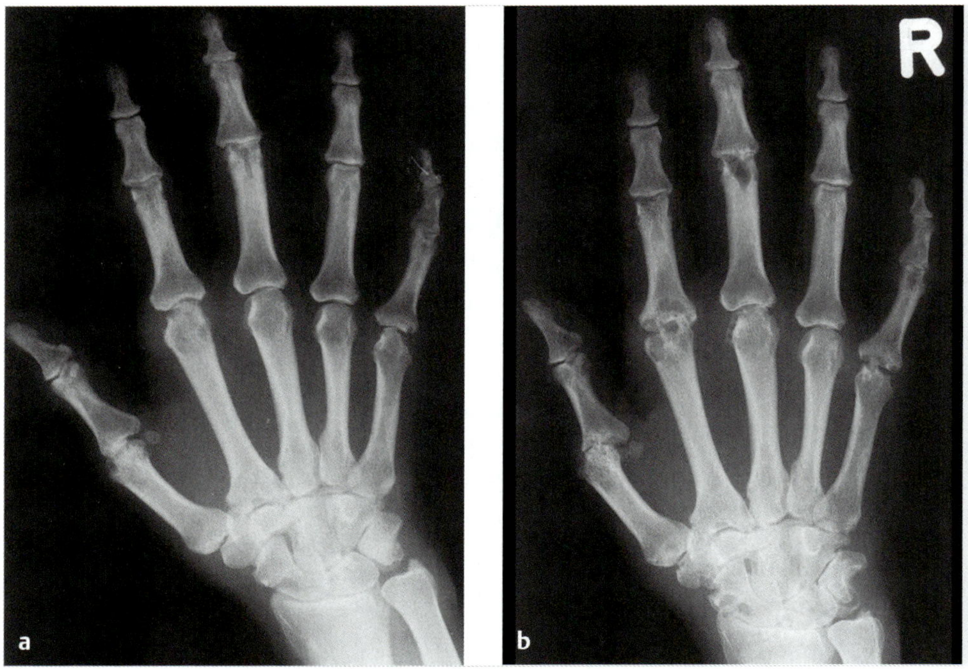

Fig. 6.45 a, b Gouty arthritis followed for 1 year.

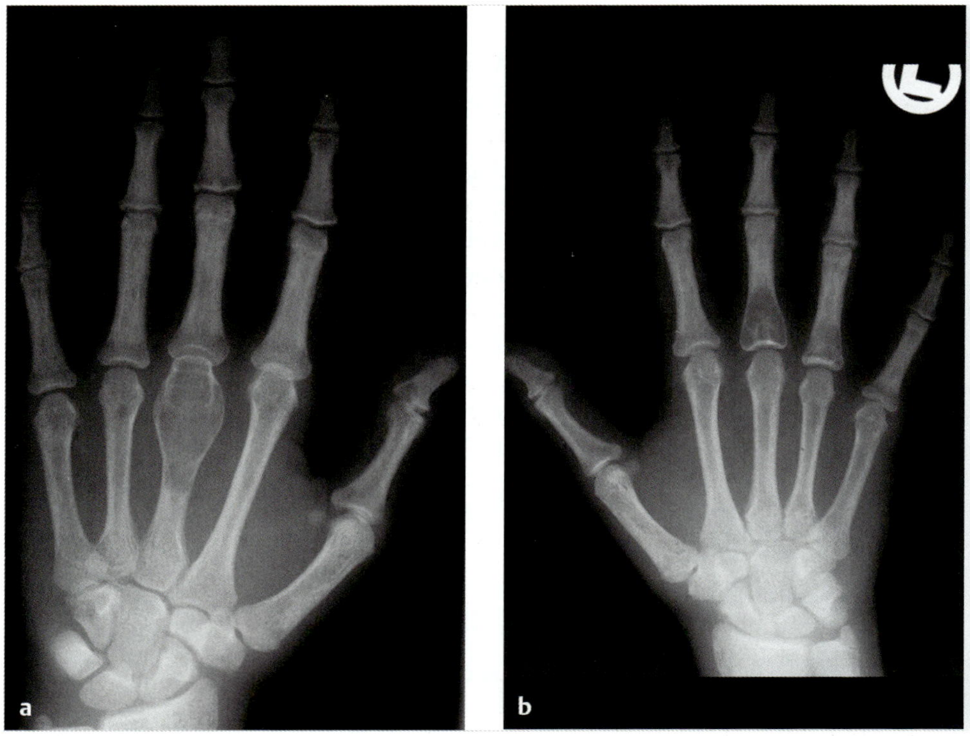

Fig. 6.46 a, b Brown tumors of hyperparathyroidism.

followed for 1 year. The "cysts" in this case represent gouty tophi. Clinically, the patient was plagued by attacks of gout and had very high uric acid levels. The destructive process also involves the radiocarpal joint, intercarpal joints, and metacarpophalangeal joints and has a very different distribution pattern than osteoarthritis.

The differential diagnosis of "cystic" skeletal lesions in the hand also includes *brown tumors of hyperparathyroidism.* ▶ Fig. 6.46 shows a patient with renal osteopathy and secondary hyperparathyroidism with large brown tumors in the third metacarpal of the left hand and third proximal phalanx of the right hand. The key to this diagnosis lies in the marked structural and density changes throughout the bones of the hands. Note the overconstricted shafts of the middle phalanges due to subperiosteal resorption and the erosion of the terminal tufts.

Final Diagnosis

Erosive or destructive osteoarthritis of the hands.

Comments

Marked osteoarthritic changes in the hands may be associated with unusually large subchondral cysts or geodes.

Case 122 (▶ Fig. 6.47)

Case description

- Referring physician: rheumatologist.
- Prior history and clinical question: A 46-year-old woman had moderate pain in her hands and feet accompanied by general malaise. When questioned, she told us that some time ago she had had a fever accompanied by painful, red, firm, nodular skin eruptions on the extensor side of both thighs. Her family doctor diagnosed her condition as panniculitis but did not consult with a dermatologist. Reddish-brown hyperpigmented patches were still visible on her thighs. A rheumatologist ordered radiographs to investigate the pain in her hands and feet, but could not explain the destructive changes detected in the bones of the hands and feet. In any case, the rheumatologist stated that neither the radiographs nor clinical findings were suggestive of a rheumatoid disorder. The patient did not mention her skin lesions to the rheumatologist.

Radiologic Findings

Radiographs of the hands (▶ Fig. 6.47 **a, b**) show the following:

- Sclerotic changes in the second through fourth distal phalanges of the left hand and second through fifth distal phalanges of the right hand
- Severe narrowing (mutilation) of the fifth middle and distal phalanges of the left hand and the distal phalanx of the right thumb
- Narrowing of the shafts of the fourth proximal phalanges on both sides and mid-shaft constriction of the proximal phalanx of each index finger
- Osteolytic lesions in the base of the fourth proximal phalanx of each hand, the base of the proximal phalanx of the left thumb, both ends of the proximal phalanx of the right thumb, and in the third metacarpal head of the left hand

Radiographs of the feet (▶ Fig. 6.47 **c, d**):

- Gross mutilating changes, most pronounced in the distal phalanges of the left foot
- Gross destruction of the interphalangeal joint of the left big toe
- Concomitant destruction of the interphalangeal joint of the right big toe
- Osteolytic lesions in the base of the proximal phalanx of the each big toe
- Erosions and osteolytic lesions in the metatarsal heads of both big toes
- Narrowing of almost all proximal phalanges, especially on the left side

Location

Changes are evident in almost all the imaged bones of the hands and feet. There is no obvious "rule" regarding a possible distribution pattern. The mutilating changes in several small tubular bones in the hands and feet and the mutilating changes in the distal phalanges of the feet most likely originated from the periosteal side or from the surrounding soft tissues. The osteolytic lesions, however, apparently resulted from an intramedullary process on the intraosseous side. Moreover the synovial membrane, especially of the metatarsophalangeal joints, must have incited the destructive changes in the affected bones.

Pathoanatomic Background of the Findings

The pronounced changes must be based on an underlying process which has a component associated with abnormal sclerosis and bone destruction, and which takes place in and around the altered bones and in the synovial membrane of the first metatarsophalangeal joints. This suggests a diffuse granulomatous process that causes sclerosis in some bones, osteolysis in others, and subperiosteal cortical resorption in yet others while also involving the synovial membrane. In Europe, a process with such variegated features is known to occur only with sarcoidosis.

Assignment to a Possible Basic Entity

Assignment of the process to a basic entity was accomplished under Pathoanatomic Background of the Findings above.

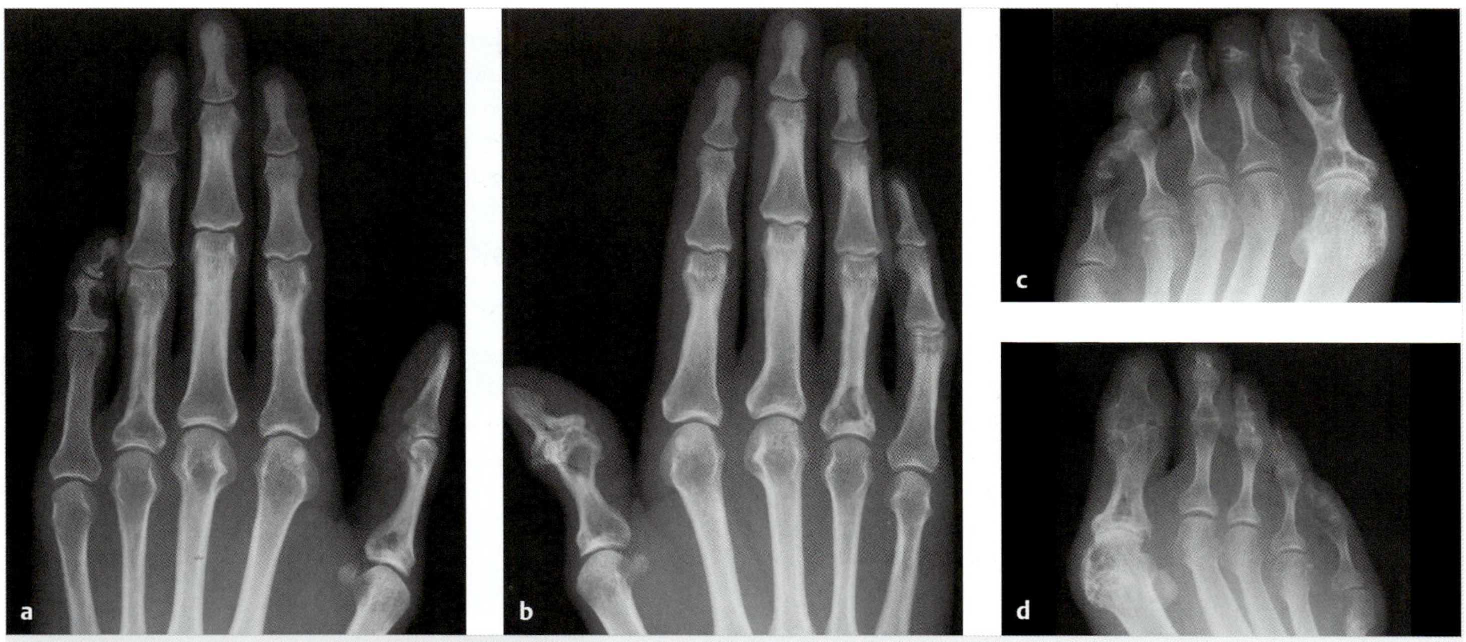

Fig. 6.47 a–d "Cysts" and mutilating changes in the bones of the hands and feet. Cause?

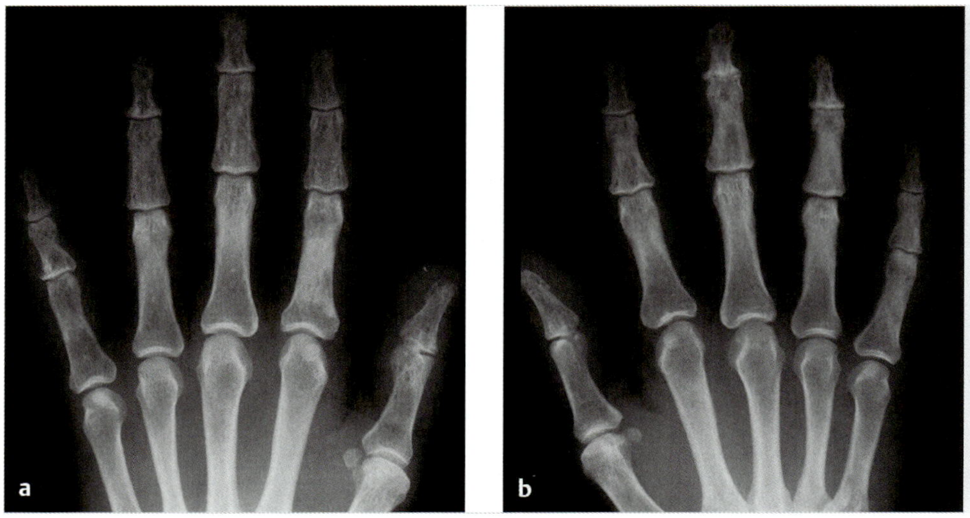

Fig. 6.48 a, b Sarcoidosis involving the bones of the hand in a different patient.

Synopsis and Discussion

The diversity of radiologic changes found in the bones of the hands and feet is very typical of skeletal involvement by sarcoidosis. This diagnosis is further supported by the cutaneous manifestations that could be interpreted as *erythema nodosum*, which the patient described in response to our specific questions. As a final proof, we obtained a chest radiograph which definitely showed stage II sarcoidosis (bilateral hilar lymphadenopathy with interstitial changes in the lung parenchyma).

The pathogenesis of the skeletal lesions in the hands and feet is explained as follows: When noncaseating epithelioid cell granulomas collect in the bone marrow, they may cause a perigranulomatous spongiolysis while also inciting a reactive sclerosis in the surrounding cancellous bone. When deposited in the periosteum, the granulomas cause a subperiosteal resorption that may narrow or even mutilate the affected tubular bone and may also induce various forms of periosteal bone formation (frayed, spiculated). Occurrence in the synovial membrane may incite the development of an acute, subacute, or chronic synovitis or arthritis.

The spectrum of conventional radiographic changes ranges from permeative lesions in the cortex (▶ Fig. 6.48) due to haversian canal involvement and "punched out" lesions in the cancellous bone to subperiosteal resorption and sclerotic changes. Especially in the bones of the hand, the following changes may be found either in isolation or in various combinations:

- Polyostotic form, known formerly as osteitis multiplex cystoides. This form is characterized by punched-out lesions in the epimetaphyseal portions of the phalanges and metacarpals (▶ Fig. 6.47 **a, b**) and in the metatarsals.
- A lacy reticular pattern initially in the epimetaphysis and later spreading to the whole bone (▶ Fig. 6.48).
- Mutilating late form characterized by gross destructive changes, especially in the distal phalanges. The changes resemble those in neuropathic acro-osteolysis, like that found in scleroderma or leprosy—small finger of the left hand (▶ Fig. 6.47 **a**); distal phalanges of the left foot (▶ Fig. 6.47 **c**).
- Patchy sclerosis of the cancellous bone—distal phalanges of the hands (▶ Fig. 6.47 **a, b**).
- Subperiosteal bone resorption with narrowing of the small tubular bones—second and fourth proximal phalanges of both hands; proximal phalanx of the right index finger (▶ Fig. 6.47 **a, b**).
- Periosteal and subperiosteal erosions with frayed or spiculated margins of the small tubular bones, similar to the findings in hyperparathyroidism.
- Erosions of joints (▶ Fig. 6.47 **c, d**).

▶ Fig. 6.48 illustrates involvement of the hand skeleton by sarcoidosis with permeative bone destruction in another patient.

Final Diagnosis

Sarcoidosis involving the bones of the hands and feet.

Comments

A "variegated" pattern of variable bone destruction and osteosclerotic lesions in the bones of the hands and feet should raise immediate suspicion of skeletal sarcoidosis.

Case 123 (▸ Fig. 6.49)

Case description

- Referring physician: rheumatologist.
- Prior history and clinical question: A 37-year-old woman presented with diffuse joint pains. She did not have morning stiffness. Rheumatoid serology was negative. Various radiographic views of the hands and feet and all the large joints showed erosions and other destructive joint changes that "did not quite fit" with rheumatoid or psoriatic arthritis, a connective-tissue disease, osteoarthritis, or chondrocalcinosis. This case did not fulfill the American Rheumatism Association (ARA) criteria for rheumatoid arthritis.

Radiologic Findings

Radiographs of the left fingers and wrist (▸ Fig. 6.49 **a, b**) show erosions in all the carpal bones, radius, and second and fourth metacarpophalangeal joints along with gross destructive changes in all interphalangeal joints, involving a combination of marginal erosion and central contour destruction. Similar findings are noted in the bones of the foot (▸ Fig. 6.49 **d**) and in the shoulder, elbow, hip, knee, and ankle joints. There is no evidence of juxta-articular osteoporosis or reactive-reparative processes.

Location

The erosive and destructive changes are located in large and small joints that have a synovial membrane.

Pathoanatomic Background of the Findings

The erosive and destructive changes in all of the imaged synovial joints point to a proliferative synovial process, but one that does not have a significant diffuse inflammatory component due to the absence of demonstrable osteoporosis. This pattern is consistent only with granulomatous changes like those found in very rare multicentric reticulohistiocytosis or in sarcoidosis.

Assignment to a Possible Basic Entity

▸ **Inflammation?** No, there are no significant clinical or radiologic signs (soft-tissue swelling, juxta-articular osteoporosis) of a diffuse inflammatory destructive process that could account for the very pronounced erosive and destructive changes.

▸ **Systemic granulomatous disease?** Yes. Inspection of the patient's skin revealed a papular skin eruption consisting of firm, yellowish- or brownish-red to flesh-colored papules that were painless, nonpruritic, and were clustered around the affected joints.

Synopsis and Discussion

The skin changes (arrows in ▸ Fig. 6.49 **c**) and radiologic findings are consistent with *multicentric reticulohistiocytosis*. This diagnosis was confirmed by dermal histology. The key to the correct presumptive radiologic diagnosis of this rare erosive–destructive joint disease lies in noting the absence of associated osteoporosis. This can distinguish the disease from rheumatoid arthritis, the most common inflammatory erosive–destructive joint disease

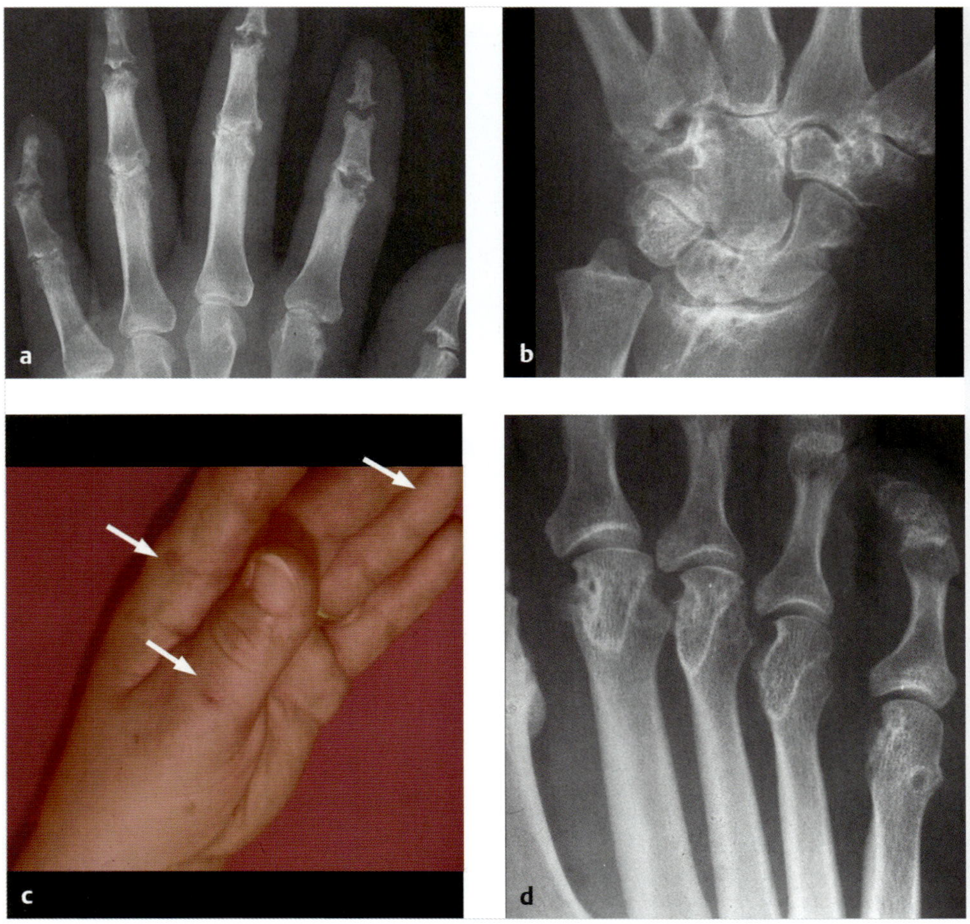

Fig. 6.49 a–d Rheumatoid arthritis?

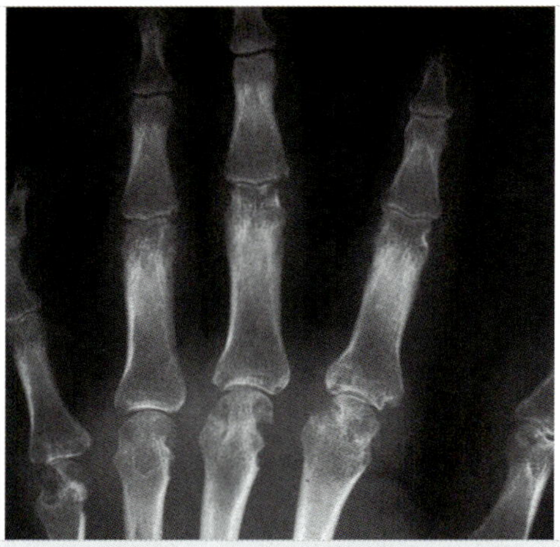

Fig. 6.50 Erosive changes in classic rheumatoid arthritis.

(see ▶ Fig. 6.50 in case presented below), which is almost always associated with osteoporosis. The next diagnostic step is to look at the patient's skin and request a dermatology consult for histologic confirmation.

We believe that multicentric reticulohistiocytosis only appears to be rare because radiologists and rheumatologists do not consider it, as a look at our collection shows. But the radiologist or rheumatologist should become suspicious when faced with a systemic erosive–destructive joint disease that has no clinical signs of inflammation and no associated osteoporosis. He or she should also notice, as in our case, that the metacarpophalangeal joints are less affected than the interphalangeal joints—a pattern that does not fit rheumatoid arthritis. If the dermatologist correctly identifies the skin lesions but does not consider a possible underlying systemic disease, the diagnosis of multicentric reticulohistiocytosis often remains obscure.

The disease is based on the formation of granulomas composed of atypical, bizarre-shaped histiocytes with a finely granular cytoplasm as well as multinucleated giant cells with a foamy-looking, partly vacuolated cytoplasm. These different histologic components have given rise to various synonyms:

- Lipoid dermatoarthritis
- Giant cell histiocytomatosis
- Reticulohistiocytic granulomas
- Giant cell reticulohistiocytosis
- Lipoid rheumatism

Multicentric reticulohistiocytosis is a multisystemic disease, meaning that granulomas may be found in the skin, subcutaneous tissue, synovial membranes, mucous membranes, in the bone, heart, kidneys, and lungs.

The disease is thought to have a female preponderance. The average age at initial diagnosis is 40 years. The joints of the hands and feet are sites of predilection (70–80% of cases). Patients suffer clinically from spontaneous and exercise-related joint pain. The joints may be swollen; local warmth is absent due to the lack of an inflammatory component. The disease has a more favorable prognosis than rheumatoid arthritis, although it may cause gross joint destruction. Spontaneous remission may occur in 6 to 8 years. The dermatologic and radiologic aspects of the disease are explored more fully in the monograph by Freyschmidt and Freyschmidt (1996).[19]

For comparison, ▶ Fig. 6.50 illustrates a case of *classic rheumatoid arthritis* of the hand with gross erosions predominantly affecting the metacarpal heads and with significant associated osteoporosis.

Final Diagnosis

Multicentric reticulohistiocytosis.

Comments

Multicentric reticulohistiocytosis is the main differential diagnosis for erosive polyarticular joint disease not associated with osteoporosis.

Case 124 (▶ Fig. 6.51)

Case description

- *Referral:* parents of the patient.
- *Prior history and clinical question:* A 3-year-old boy had firm, painless swellings on his left index finger.

Radiologic Findings

The dorsopalmar radiograph (▶ Fig. 6.51 **a**) shows an elliptical lesion with sclerotic margins in the medullary cavity of the proximal phalanx. The lateral radiograph (▶ Fig. 6.51 **b**) identifies this lesion as an extraosseous, slightly sclerotic dorsal mass. A similar lesion is present on the radial side of the middle phalanx. The intraosseous portion of each lesion appears as a faint calcification in the lateral view (▶ Fig. 6.51 **b**).

Location

Both lesions have extra- and intraosseous components.

Pathoanatomic Background of the Findings

The intraosseous portion of both lesions shows subtle calcification, best appreciated in the lateral view. This may result from reactive and reparative calcification or bone formation or from the ossification of a fibrous, cartilaginous, or bony matrix. The images do not show a possible cause of reactive bone formation, however, so the more likely cause is matrix ossification. Thus, there are two foci in the proximal and middle phalanges of the index finger which have an intra- and extraosseous component and exhibit matrix calcification. The faint extraosseous calcification on the proximal phalanx (▶ Fig. 6.51 **b**) may be a calcified shell of periosteal new bone. Since the remaining structures in the finger appear normal, we are dealing with two painless tumorous lesions.

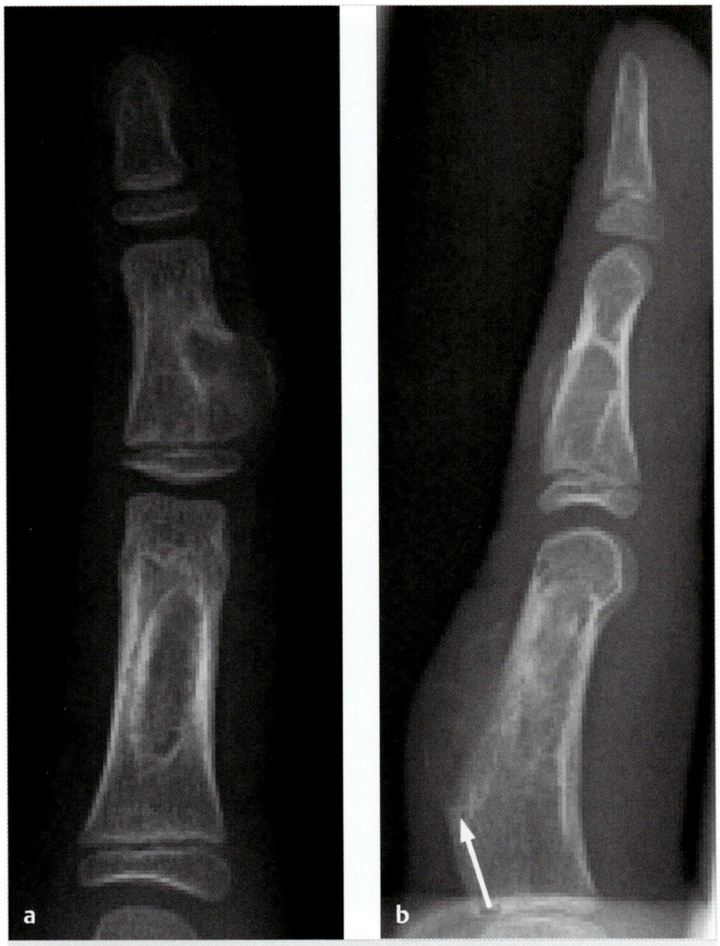

Fig. 6.51 a, b Unexplained "cystic" lesions in the left index finger.

Assignment to a Possible Basic Entity

▶ **Normal variant or malformation?** There are no known precedents for normal variants in this form. Nor is there evidence of skeletal dysplasia anywhere else in the hand.

▶ **Trauma?** While the index finger, like all the fingers, is subject to varying degrees of trauma in daily life (see Case 125), trauma could not explain lesions with an intra- and extraosseous component in the proximal and middle phalanges of the index finger. The boy did not have a known prior history of a single traumatic event.

▶ **Inflammation?** No clinical manifestations.

▶ **Tumor or tumorlike lesion?** Yes. The most common skeletal tumors in the hand are chondromas (ca. 60% of all cases). If we add clinically asymptomatic and undetected cases, the true figure is probably higher than 80%. On the other hand, at least 60% of all chondromas occur in the hand. The matrix calcifications found in both lesions are fully consistent with chondromas. There are enchondromas, occurring predominantly in small and thin bones, which grow exophytically due to the limited space available inside the bone. This type of lesion is called enchondroma protuberans. Its multifocal occurrence in the hand would fit the pattern of benign cartilage-forming tumors, as multiple enchondromas often occur in the hand even in patients who do not have enchondromatosis. By contrast, bone-forming tumors (osteoid osteoma, osteoblastoma) generally occur as solitary lesions, and the majority are painful.

Synopsis and Discussion

The above line of reasoning supports a diagnosis of two protuberant *enchondromas*. The sclerotic margin seen in the frontal view of the lesion (▶ Fig. 6.51 **a**) is explained mainly by reactive buttressing processes in the cortex at the lesion edge, where the tumor protrudes from the cortex. The lateral view shows a corresponding small bone spur or raised margin at that location (arrow in ▶ Fig. 6.51 **b**). The tumor is surrounded by a periosteal bony shell, which is clearly visible over the extraosseous tumor component in the lateral view. The differential diagnosis might include a sessile osteochondroma, but in that case the cortex of the bone at the base of the lesion would be continuous with the tumor cortex. Moreover, osteochondromas do not have an intraosseous component and are extremely rare in the bones of the hand. In summary, the following data support a diagnosis of two enchondroma protuberans in our case:

- Clinical presentation of firm, painless nodules on both affected bones

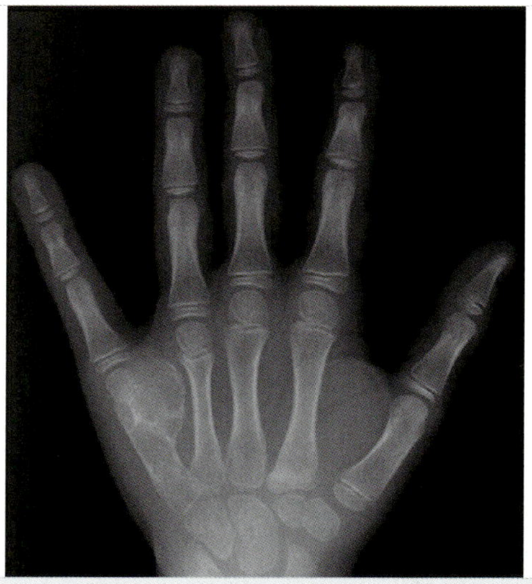

Fig. 6.52 Enchondroma protuberans in the fifth metacarpal of an 11-year-old boy.

- Occurrence in the hand, which is a site of predilection for enchondromas
- Radiographs showing both intra- and extraosseous tumor components
- Multifocal occurrence, since two or more enchondromas are not unusual in the bones of the hand

The child should still be followed up for the next 10 years, however, due to the potential for the development of enchondromatosis (see Case 120).

▶ Fig. 6.52 demonstrates an enchondroma protuberans located in the fifth metacarpal of an 11-year-old boy. This lesion was palpable and was associated with mild pain.

▶ Fig. 6.53 illustrates a *grade I chondrosarcoma* in the proximal phalanx of the middle finger of a symptomatic 72-year-old man. While chondrosarcomas are rare in the bones of the hand, occurring chiefly in the axial skeleton and proximal long tubular bones, the large extraosseous component in this case (arrows) and the lateral cortical destruction suggest a malignant, bone-forming tumor.

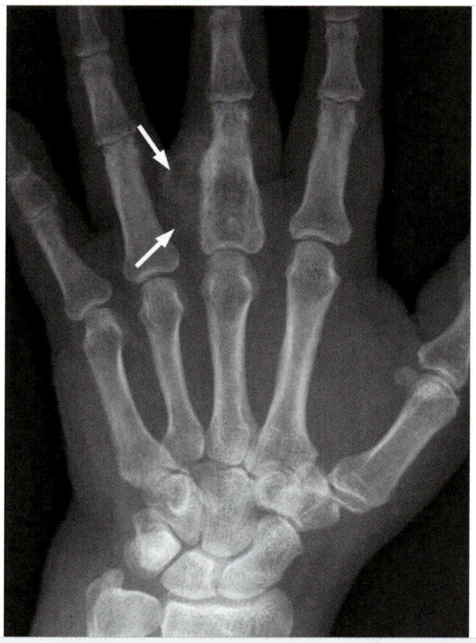

Fig. 6.53 Grade I chondrosarcoma in the proximal phalanx of the middle finger of a 72-year-old man.

Final Diagnosis

Enchondroma protuberans in the proximal and middle phalanges of the left index finger.

Comments

Skeletal masses in the hand that have intra- and extraosseous components are suggestive of enchondroma protuberans.

Case 125 (▶ Fig. 6.54)

Case description

- Referring physician: radiologist.
- Prior history and clinical question: A 44-year-old man had a painful swelling on the palmar side of his left thumb. He claimed to have suffered a crushing injury of the thumb approximately 5 months earlier and since then had noticed an increasing firm swelling.

Radiologic Findings

The lateral radiograph demonstrates a solid ossification on the palmar side of the proximal phalanx of the thumb. Its central portion has a firm, stalklike attachment to the cortex while a space is visible between its more distal portion and the cortex. Its proximal portion has a more streaky appearance (▶ Fig. 6.54 **a**). The CT scans in ▶ Fig. 6.54 **c–k** demonstrate the spatial relationships of the lesion. The cortex on the palmar side appears fully intact with no perforations. The CT scans clearly show that the

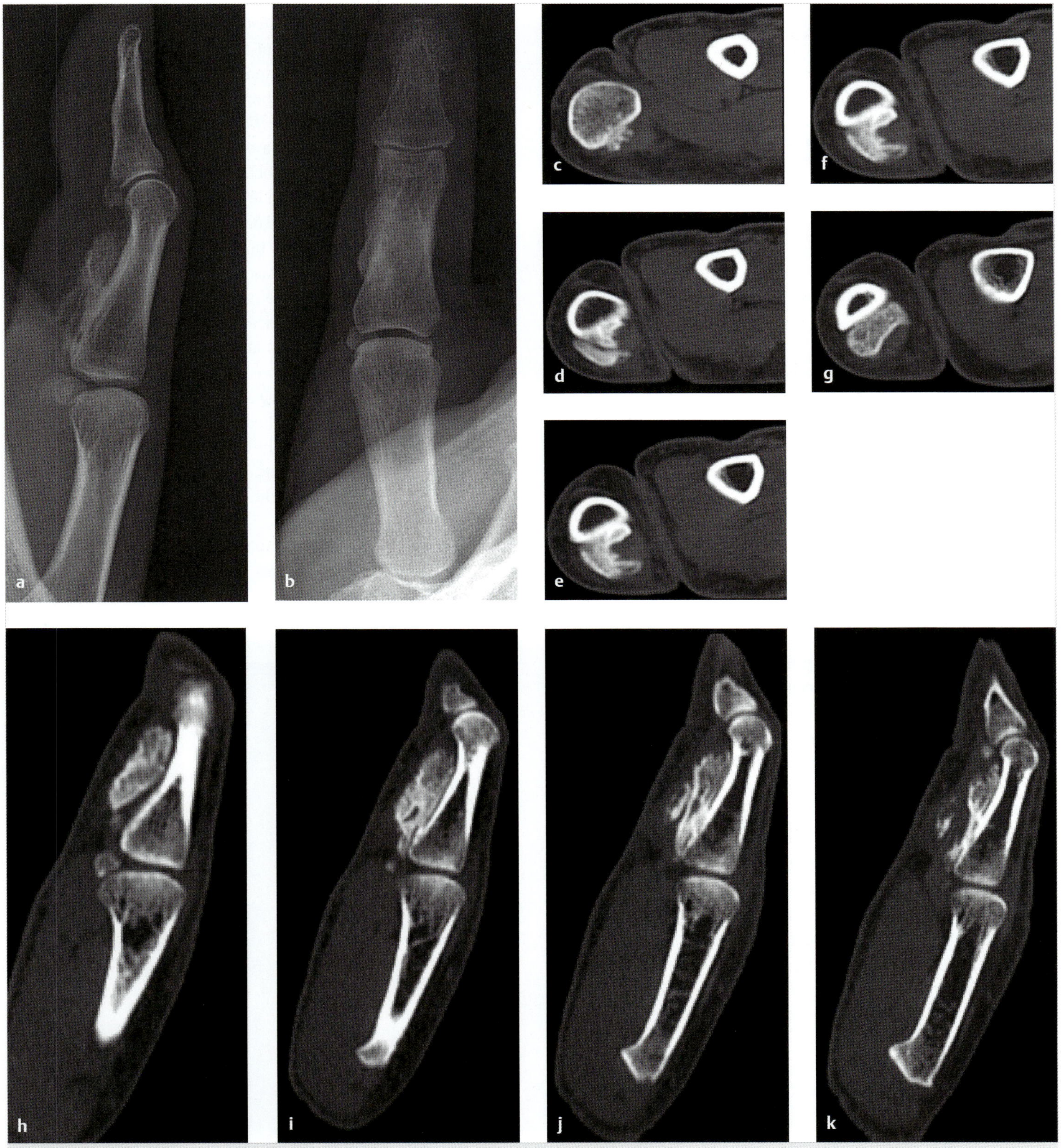

Fig. 6.54 **a–k** Osteochondroma?

ossification is denser externally than internally and thus has a kind of cortex.

Pathoanatomic Background of the Findings

From a pathoanatomic standpoint, the bony excrescence could have either of the following causes:

- Heterotopic, myositis ossificans–like reactive bone formation
- Ossification arising from an osteoid tumor matrix, as with a paraosseous or periosteal osteosarcoma

The fact that the ossification is denser externally than internally suggests reactive bone formation. With a paraosseous or periosteal osteosarcoma, the tumor ossification is denser near the bone than at its periphery because its central portion is older and therefore "more mature."

Assignment to a Possible Basic Entity

► **Trauma?** Yes, the patient sustained a crushing injury to the thumb some time ago. This caused a subperiosteal and extraperiosteal hemorrhage, from which a myositis ossificans–like lesion eventually developed.

► **Inflammation?** The marked soft-tissue swelling of the thumb does have inflammatory features, but with a reactive cause.

► **Tumor?** A paraosseous or periosteal osteosarcoma cannot be excluded, although the radiologic ossification pattern is not consistent with that diagnosis (see Pathoanatomic Background of the Findings).

Synopsis and Discussion

Ossification processes on the small, tubular bones of the hands, especially the phalanges, are almost always reactive when the cortex is intact, since osteosarcomas are extremely rare in the hand. The most common diagnoses are *florid reactive periostitis* when the ossification is confined to the periosteum or a *"Nora lesion"* when the bony mass projects into the soft tissues. The Nora lesion is named after the physician who first described this paraosseous ossification and is also known histologically as *bizarre parosteal osteochondromatous proliferation* (BPOP). The presence of a fine cartilaginous cap distinguishes this lesion histologically from florid reactive periostitis. Today it is generally accepted that florid reactive periostitis corresponds to the initial stage of a reactive proliferative periosteal process on a finger bone, while BPOP represents a more mature stage with greater bone and cartilage proliferation. The symptoms vary accordingly. Florid reactive periostitis causes severe pain and swelling that appears inflammatory. Nora lesion is associated with less pain and a firm swelling that does not have inflammatory features. The process may develop to an even later stage called *turret exostosis*. In principle, this entity falls under the heading of heterotopic ossification or myositis ossificans owing to its trizonal structure, which is always demonstrable by imaging to some degree (see Case 156). The similar clinical presentation with inflammatory-type swelling supports this view. The main problem with these proliferative periosteal processes lies less in their radiologic features, which are quite typical, than in the potential for histologic confusion with osteosarcoma, especially the paraosseous form. This is due to the proliferating fibroblasts with mitotic figures (but without definite anaplasia) and the variable proportions of osteoid, bone, and cartilage. Much experience in histology is required to make a correct diagnosis, and it is important for the radiologist to be specific. The same applies to treatment: The risk of recurrence declines as the lesions mature, so surgery should be delayed as long as possible. Hence the radiologist and hand surgeon must keep their nerve and elicit a second opinion if necessary. In our case the lesion was surgically removed, and our diagnosis of a Nora lesion was confirmed. A full year after the operation the patient was free of complaints.

► Fig. 6.55 and ► Fig. 6.56 illustrate two more cases of a Nora lesion. Both patients were school-age children, and both had a recent history of trauma. The case in ► Fig. 6.55 closely resembles the case in ► Fig. 6.54 in its radiographic features, while the case in ► Fig. 6.56 looks more like *florid reactive periostitis*, which ► Fig. 6.57 illustrates in a classic form. Because the case in ► Fig. 6.56 showed greater osteochondral differentiation histologically, it was classified as a Nora lesion.

Finally, we illustrate an unusual case of an osteochondroma-like Nora lesion in the finger of a child (► Fig. 6.58 **a–c**). The hyperostotic process in this case grew from the distal end of the proximal phalanx of the small finger. The CT scan in ► Fig. 6.58 **b** demonstrates an apparent open communication between the exostotic process and the affected bone, simulating an osteochondroma. But we believe that the cortex under the hyperostotic process is very atrophic, so that open communication is only simulated. The shell-like ossification around the lesion corresponds to the peripheral ossification, well known from myositis ossificans. Otherwise the absence of unequivocal cancellous bone in the lesion is an argument against osteochondroma.

A detailed discussion of the problems associated with proliferative processes in the phalanges can be found in Freyschmidt (2008)[13] and Freyschmidt et al. (2010).[18]

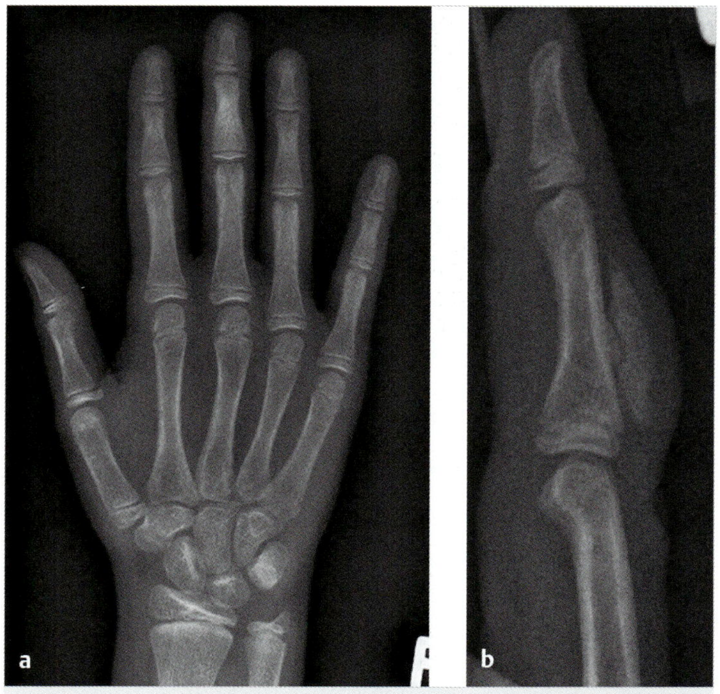

Fig. 6.55 a, b Nora lesion in a school-age child.

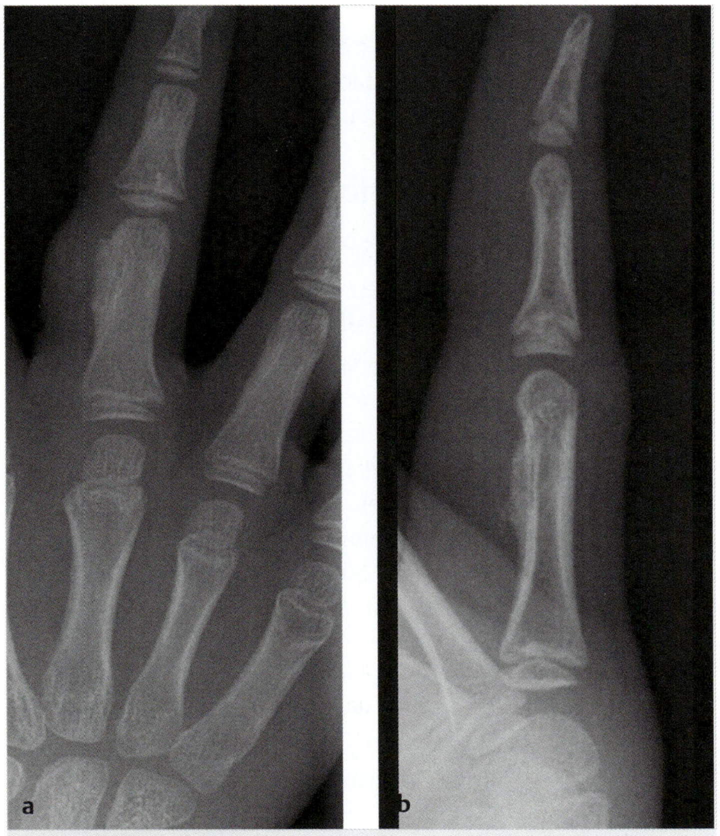

Fig. 6.56 a, b Nora lesion that resembles florid reactive periostitis.

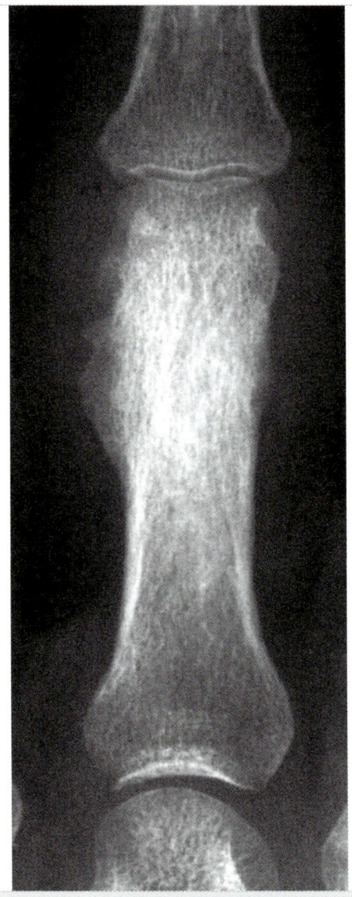

Fig. 6.57 Classic appearance of florid reactive periostitis.

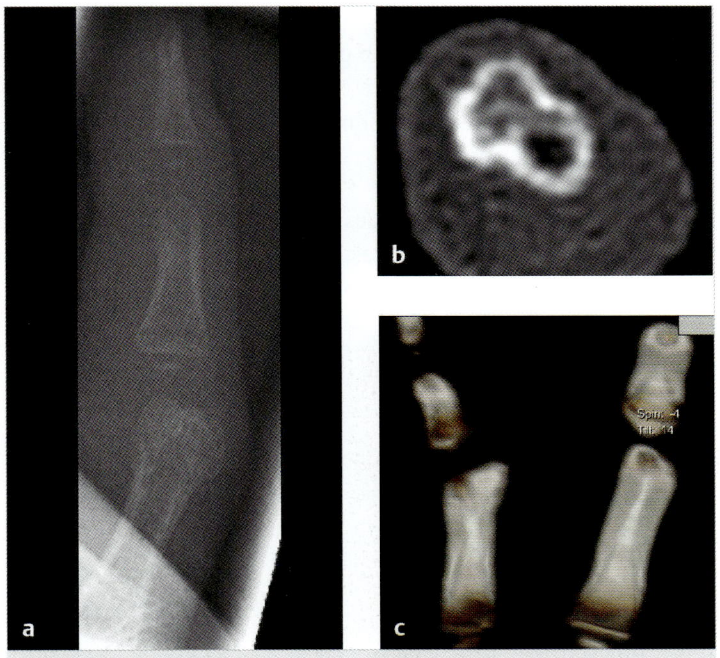

Fig. 6.58 a–c Osteochondroma or Nora lesion?

Final Diagnosis

Nora lesion (BPOP) on the proximal phalanx of the thumb.

Comments

Ossified processes in the periosteum and adjacent phalangeal bone with an intact cortex are generally one of two conditions: florid reactive periostitis or a Nora lesion.

Case 126 (▶ Fig. 6.59)

Case description

- Referring physician: pulmonologist.
- Prior history and clinical question: A 42-year-old man had severe pain and swelling in his hands and feet. Clubbing of the fingers was noted on physical examination. The patient was in a pulmonary clinic for the treatment of adenocarcinoma in the right lung. The clinical manifestations led the pulmonologist to suspect a paraneoplastic syndrome, but he was confused by the radiographic findings (especially in the hands) and asked whether the changes were metastatic to the lung cancer.

Radiologic Findings

Extensive periosteal new bone formation is visible along the third metacarpal of the left hand (▶ Fig. 6.59 **a, b**) and the fourth and fifth metacarpals of the right hand (▶ Fig. 6.59 **c, d**). The distal, ulnar margins of the two right metacarpals have a somewhat rough or shaggy appearance, although the ossifications as a whole appear to be continuous. The underlying cortical structures show variable thinning but are intact. Somewhat patchy areas of marked osteoporosis are noted in the phalanges. Significant swelling of the digital soft tissues is difficult to see in these reproductions.

Pathoanatomic Background of the Findings

Multiple foci of periosteal new bone formation on the hands and feet with clubbing of the fingers occur mainly as trophic phenomena as in a variety of lung diseases (cancer, bronchiectasis) or in inflammatory bowel diseases (e.g., Crohn disease). It is believed that certain cells involved in the pulmonary disease process produce mediators (e.g., platelet-derived growth factor and vascular endothelial growth factor), which can stimulate periosteal proliferation and subsequent bone formation via hyperperfusion, for example, but also digital clubbing and general nonspecific joint inflammation with associated osteoporosis. Interestingly, these phenomena may regress spontaneously with resolution of the underlying disease or following surgical vagotomy.

Assignment to a Possible Basic Entity

The essentials of this process are covered in the section above.

Synopsis and Discussion

Multifocal periosteal new bone formation like that described in the present case is also known as *hypertrophic osteoarthropathy*. It occurs in association with numerous inflammatory, suppurative, fibrotic, neoplastic (paraneoplastic syndrome), pulmonary, pleural and mediastinal diseases, and occasional gastrointestinal diseases. The periosteal new bone formation most commonly involves the bones of the hands and feet, forearm and lower leg, and less commonly the femur and humerus. The periosteal new bone envelops the diaphyses like a cuff that tapers toward the metaphyses, sparing the epiphyses. The outer surface of the periosteal new bone is rough and resembles tree bark.

Hypertrophic osteoarthropathy has a broad radiologic spectrum. Five patterns are distinguished:

- Solid ossifications with smooth outer margins that are separated from the underlying cortex by a small space, as in our case
- Onion-skin–like ossifications with longitudinal striations
- Radial striate or stellate pattern of sporadically occurring periosteal new bone
- Predominantly solid, sleevelike periosteal new bone with undulating outer margins
- Fusion of the periosteal new bone with the cortex, with resultant cortical thickening

The differential diagnosis includes acquired polyostotic periosteal new bone formation like that resulting from bone perfusion disorders, rheumatic diseases, intoxications (fluorosis, retinoids,

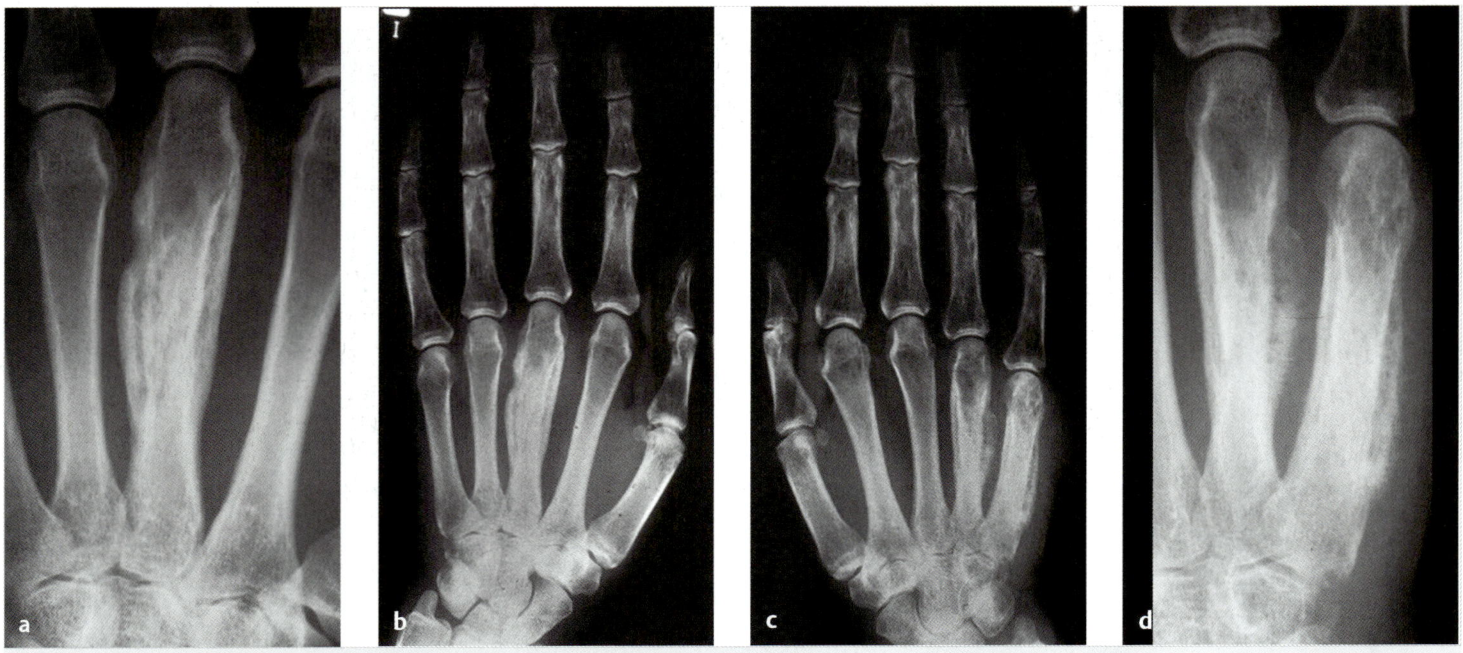

Fig. 6.59 a–d Patient with lung cancer. Metastases?

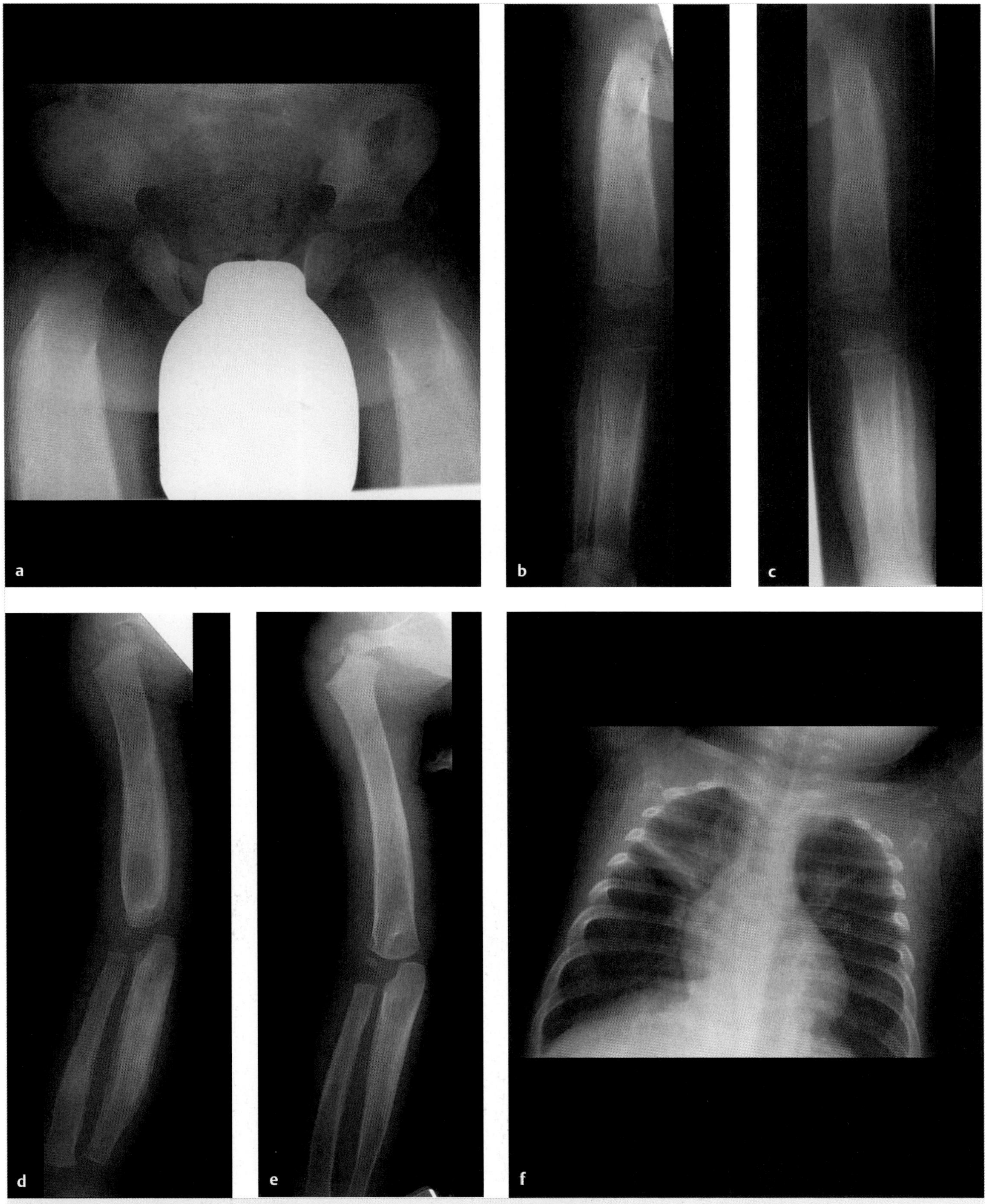

Fig. 6.60 Periosteal new bone formation in an infant with pulmonary infiltrates. Radiographs were taken in October 2000 (a–d) and in June 2001 (e, f).

prostaglandins, etc.), infectious diseases (especially viral), and EMO syndrome (exophthalmos, myxedema, osteopathy). Further details are beyond our scope, and a correct assignment can be made only within the clinical context. Congenital forms of multifocal periosteal new bone formation are very rare and are found in pachydermoperiostotis, hereditary palmoplantar keratosis, etc.

► Fig. 6.60 presents the case of a 3½-month-old infant with fever and limb swelling. Pulmonary infiltrates (► Fig. 6.60 **f**) developed at various sites over a 7-month period. Skeletal radiographs showed grotesque, cufflike periosteal new bone along the diaphyses of the upper and lower long bones (► Fig. 6.60 **a–c**), which regressed quickly after clearing of the pulmonary infiltrates (► Fig. 6.60 **d, e**). The differential diagnosis of the initial periosteal new bone included *infantile cortical hyperostosis (Caffey disease).* However, the periosteal new bone in this disease will be found chiefly on the mandible, clavicles, and ulnae and less commonly on the long tubular bones, pelvis, and lateral rib segments. We also considered another rare polyostotic form of periosteal new bone formation, namely *chronic recurrent multifocal periostitis,* which has a reputed predilection for the lower limbs. Little has been published on this condition to date, however, especially regarding its differentiation from Caffey disease.

Final Diagnosis

Pulmonary hypertrophic osteoarthropathy in a lung cancer patient.

Comments

Patients with clinically symptomatic, multifocal, solid periosteal new bone formation should be investigated for an underlying pulmonary, pleural, mediastinal, or gastrointestinal cause.

Case 127 (▶ Fig. 6.61)

Case description

- Referring physician: pathologist.
- Prior history and clinical question: A 37-year-old man presented with severe pain and swelling of the right hand.

Radiologic Findings

Initial MR images show a pathologic soft-tissue process, especially pronounced in the dorsal carpus, with an inhomogeneous intermediate signal intensity on T1w images (▶ Fig. 6.61 **a**) and patchy inhomogeneous signal intensity in a water-sensitive sequence (▶ Fig. 6.61 **b**). A proliferative synovial process was considered. As the condition could not be further specified, we ordered a subsequent CT examination (▶ Fig. 6.61 **c–i**) which showed fine, rounded, calcified bodies diffusely embedded in the soft-tissue process. Sites of adjacent carpal bone erosion were also observed (▶ Fig. 6.61 **e, f, h**). The small calcified or ossified bodies were most numerous dorsally but were also present on the palmar side (▶ Fig. 6.61 **e, f**).

Location

The proliferative soft-tissue process and the calcified bodies embedded in it are localized to the synovial membrane.

Pathoanatomic Background of the Findings

A proliferative soft-tissue process arising from the synovial membrane is combined with small, embedded calcified bodies. This pattern exists in synovial osteochondromatosis but may also occur in chondrocalcinosis if the calcium pyrophosphate crystals or other crystalline calcium compounds (in the case of secondary chondrocalcinosis, as in gout) form aggregated deposits (▶ Fig. 6.62, see below).

Assignment to a Possible Basic Entity

The basic entity has already been identified, so there is no need for further consideration of this issue.

Synopsis and Discussion

The radiologic diagnosis of *synovial osteochondromatosis* was confirmed histologically, and we also learned that it was a recurrence. Surprisingly, the pathologist also described a primary chondrocalcinosis (calcium pyrophosphate deposition disease, CPPD). It was not radiologically apparent because incipient ossification of the small chondromas was indistinguishable from the aggregated crystal deposits. Moreover, this case did not show the destructive changes in the proximal row of carpal bones with scapholunate dissociation that are characteristic of chondrocalcinosis. The nature of synovial osteochondromatosis was described earlier in Case 72.

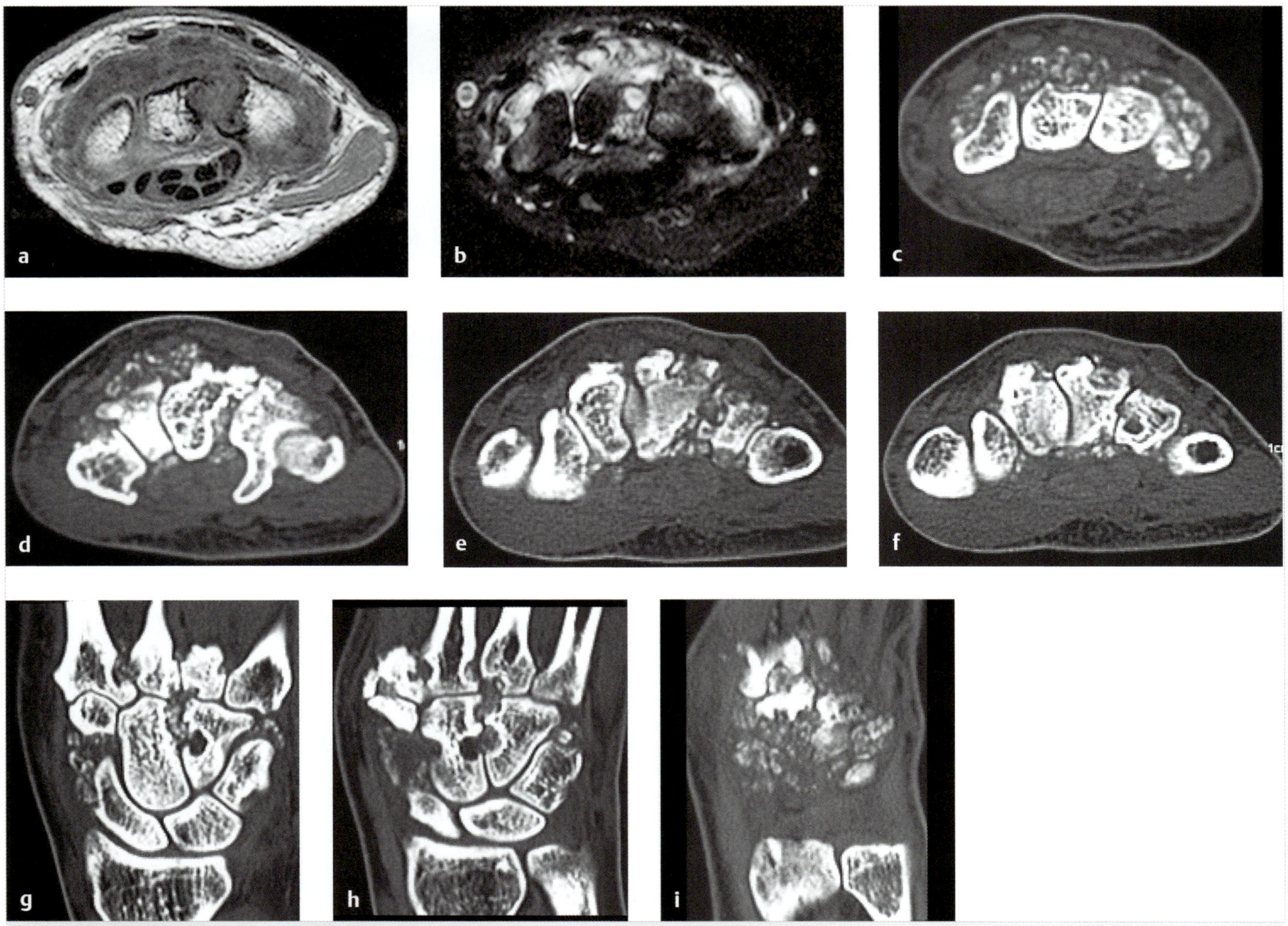

Fig. 6.61 a–i Proliferative synovial process?

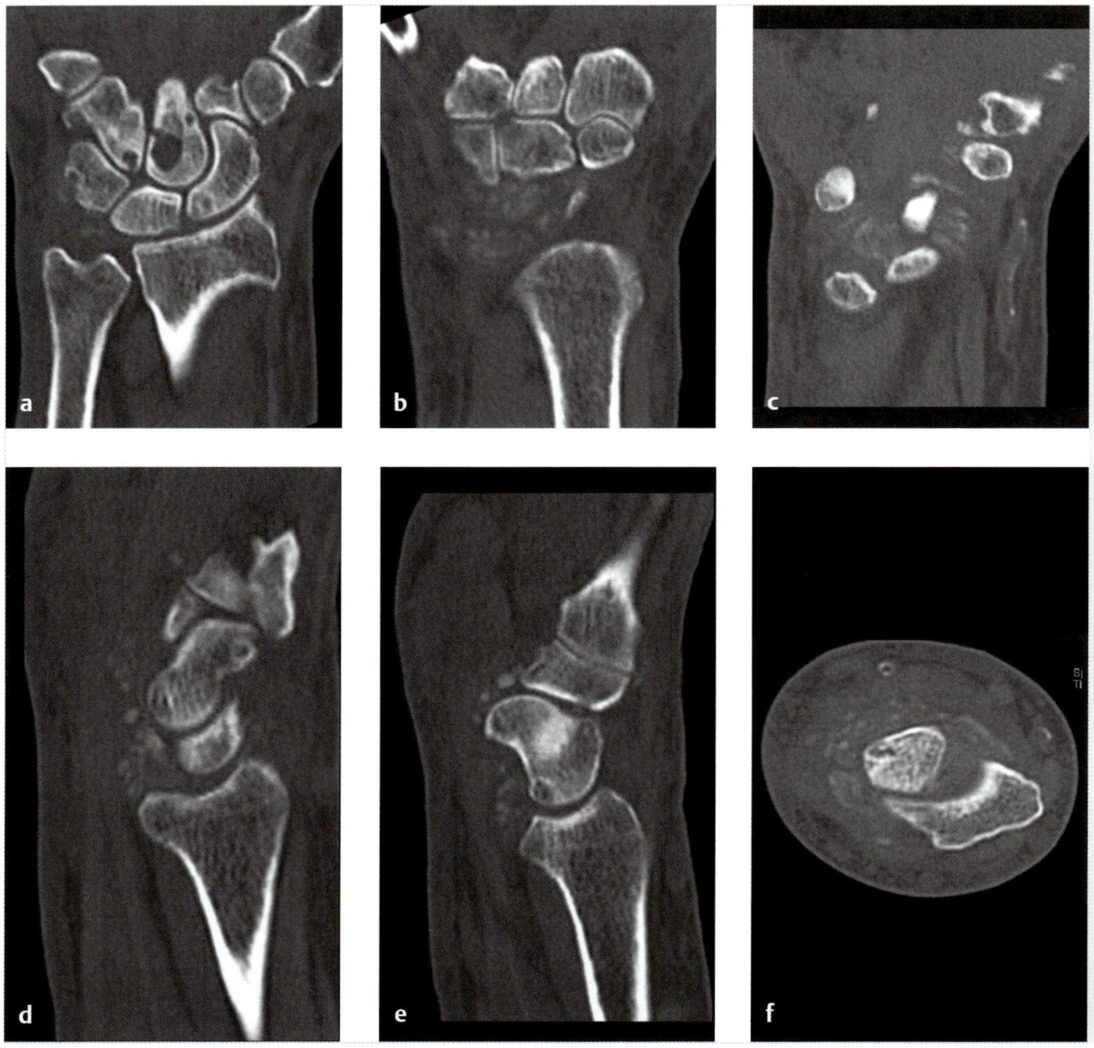

Fig. 6.62 a–f For comparison: carpal involvement by gout in a 70-year-old man.

As an aid to differential diagnosis, ▶ Fig. 6.62 shows the case of a 70-year-old man with known severe gout, who consulted a rheumatologist for a swollen, extremely painful left wrist. The CT images showed small, rounded calcifications accompanied by predominantly flaky aggregates with attenuation values much lower than those of chondromas in articular chondromatosis. Pathoanatomically, they consist of synovial tophi.

Comments

A soft-tissue mass that arises from the synovial membrane and contains small, well-defined calcified or ossified bodies is suggestive of synovial osteochondromatosis. Histologic differentiation is required from malignant transformation of synovial osteochondromatosis.

Final Diagnosis

Synovial osteochondromatosis and CPPD in the carpus.

7 Lower Limb

7.1 Equivocal MRI Findings

Case 128 (▶ Fig. 7.1)

Case description

- Referring physician: radiologist.
- Prior history and clinical question: A 25-year-old woman sustained a twisting injury and was referred for MRI of the right knee joint. Signal anomalies were noted chiefly in the distal femoral metadiaphysis, raising a broad range of diagnostic possibilities.

Radiologic Findings

On T1-weighted (T1w) MRI, the imaged portions of the femur and tibia show scattered spots of relatively low signal intensity (▶ Fig. 7.1 **a, b**), which appear bright in the water-sensitive sequence (▶ Fig. 7.1 **c**). The spots enhance after intravenous (IV) contrast administration (▶ Fig. 7.1 **d**). Similar changes were found on the contralateral side.

Location

All the findings are located in the medullary cavity of the diametaphysis while sparing the epiphyses.

Pathoanatomic Background of the Findings

The foci must have a moderately high proton density and must have a sufficient vascular supply based on their enhancement characteristics. They could be aggregates of normal but heterotopic bone marrow cells, or myeloproliferative lesions such as mastocytosis or malignant lymphoma.

Assignment to a Possible Basic Entity

▶ **Normal variant or malformation?** Possibly. Islands of bone marrow in medullary cavities containing mostly fatty marrow may occur in the long bones of healthy individuals, especially women. Some persons, currently healthy, may also have a prior history of one or more episodes of significant blood loss or heavy menstruation.

▶ **Inflammation?** No clinical manifestations.

▶ **Tumor or tumorlike lesion?** Yes, in principle, such as localized non-Hodgkin lymphoma, plasmacytoma, etc.

Synopsis and Discussion

Since the lesions were detected incidentally during knee MRI in a clinically healthy young woman, the spotty areas of altered signal intensity in the medullary cavity should be classified as an incidental finding or normal variant. This is even more likely when the same changes are found on the opposite side. The referring physician should be told, however, that a clinical examination (liver, spleen, and lymph nodes) and blood count are necessary to exclude an incipient hematologic disease. There is no need, however, to alarm the patient or referring physician.

Finally, it should be mentioned that islands of bone marrow in fat-containing diametaphyseal segments of long bones may not only form in the setting of increased hematopoiesis, for whatever reason, but may also occur physiologically during the conversion of red bone marrow to fatty marrow at about 20 years of age and then disappear completely by about 24 years of age. Apparently this process does not occur in some individuals, however, with the result that islands of bone marrow are still detectable for years or even for life.

Final Diagnosis

Islands of red marrow detected incidentally in the distal femoral metadiaphyses.

Comments

Islands of altered MRI signal intensity (hypointense on T1w images, hyperintense on T2w and STIR images, enhancing after contrast administration) in the distal femoral metadiaphysis should be considered a normal variant in otherwise healthy individuals.

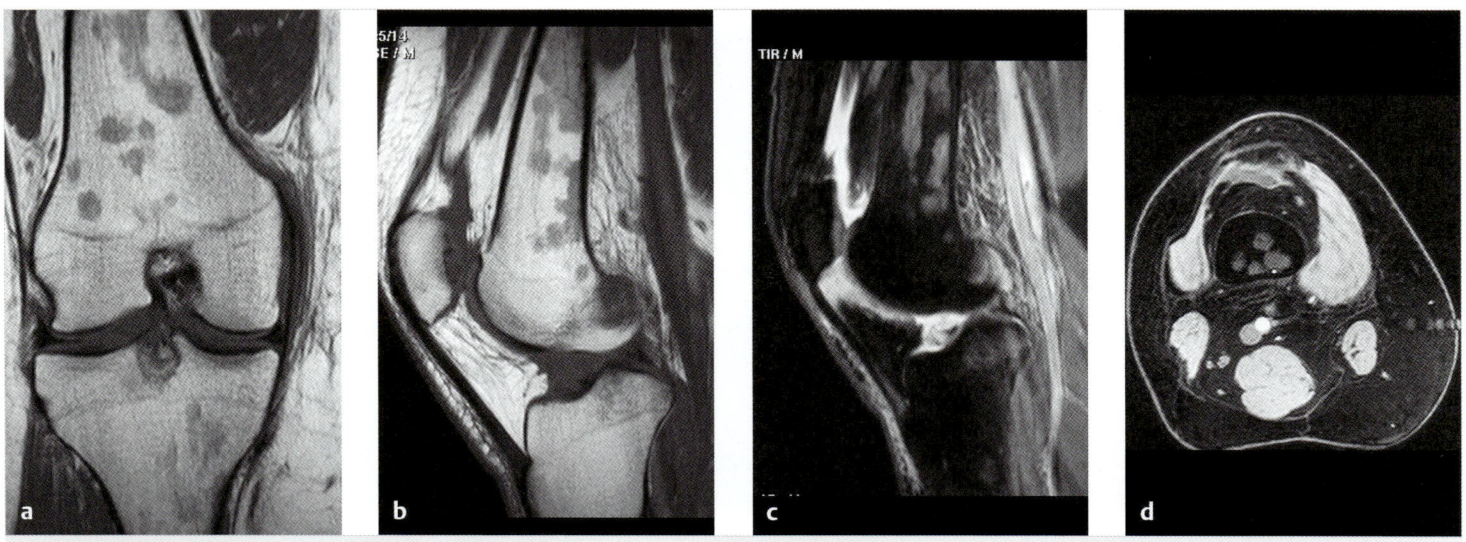

Fig. 7.1 a–d Infiltrates in the medullary cavity?

Case 129 (▶ Fig. 7.2)

Case description

- *Referral:* parents of the patient.
- *Prior history and clinical question:* A 6-year-old girl complained of exercise-related pain in her left proximal femur. Her parents stated that she also had several episodes of fever (about 38°C) in recent weeks. MRI of the left thigh raised suspicion of an eosinophilic granuloma or another tumor “that could not be ruled out.” Repeat scans 2 weeks later showed no change, and biopsy was recommended. A radiograph (▶ Fig. 7.2 **b**) taken at the time of initial MRI appeared normal.

Radiologic Findings

Both initial MRI (▶ Fig. 7.2 **a**) and the follow-up series (▶ Fig. 7.2 **c, d**) demonstrate a predominantly medial area of edema-like signal in the middle third of the left femoral shaft. A linear hyperintensity is visible along the medial cortex.

Location

The above MRI findings are arranged eccentrically about the medial side of the femoral cortex, so the cortex may be their epicenter. This suggests that the process does not originate from the bone marrow or medullary cavity (compare with Case 130).

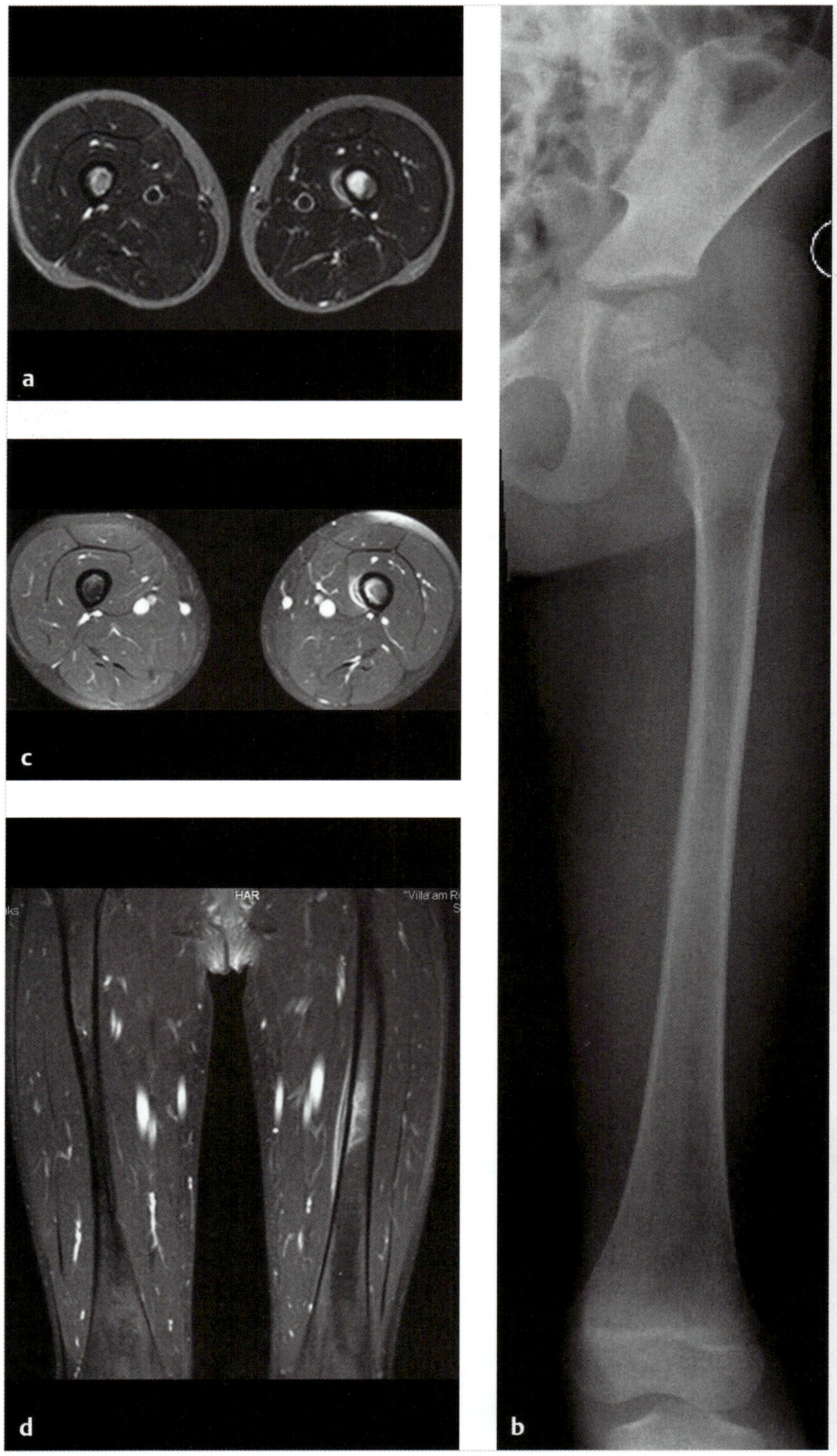

Fig. 7.2 Ewing sarcoma? Images **c,d** were obtained two weeks later

Pathoanatomic Background of the Findings

As noted under Location, a primary process arising from the medullary cavity (Ewing sarcoma, eosinophilic granuloma, osteomyelitis) appears unlikely. Edema-like signal changes with a cortical epicenter may have a traumatic etiology.

Assignment to a Possible Basic Entity

▸ **Normal variant or malformation?** No, we are dealing with a pathologic MRI finding which explains the clinical symptoms.

▸ **Trauma?** Very possible, but two things would be needed to prove a traumatic cause:
- A more detailed history
- A supplemental CT examination for direct visualization of the bone and of a fine fracture line that may not have been visualized by MRI

When we elicited a more detailed history, we learned that the girl was very active in tennis, ballet, and horse riding. Low-dose CT confined to the region of interest revealed a fracture line running obliquely through the cortex (arrows in ▸ Fig. 7.3).

▸ **Inflammation?** The febrile episodes described by the parents could suggest an atypical, primary chronic osteomyelitis. But osteomyelitis would not produce eccentric medullary changes and would not be distributed along the periosteum.

▸ **Tumor or tumorlike lesion?** This diagnosis does not fit the eccentric pattern of the signal intensity changes with an apparent epicenter in the cortex (see Case 130). A tumor would cause cortical destruction noticeable over a 2-week period. Episodes of low-grade fever (38°C) in a 6-year-old child would not qualify as a "B symptom" suggestive of malignancy.

Synopsis and Discussion

The detection of an oblique fracture line in the medial cortex accompanied by a solid periosteal reaction on CT (arrows in ▸ Fig. 7.3) confirms a stress fracture at a typical site in the femur. Biopsy is unnecessary. The fracture should be managed by non-weight-bearing for at least 2–3 weeks, followed by graded resumption of weight bearing at 3–4 kg/week on crutches. This is necessary to allow for complete fracture healing. The girl should wait at least 6 months before a careful return to sports, leaving ballet dancing to last. We always recommend swimming and bicycle ergometry for maintaining physical fitness. Patients should also learn to interpret any future pain as a warning sign that the bone has not yet adapted to a certain stress level and that a stress fracture may develop if exercise is continued.

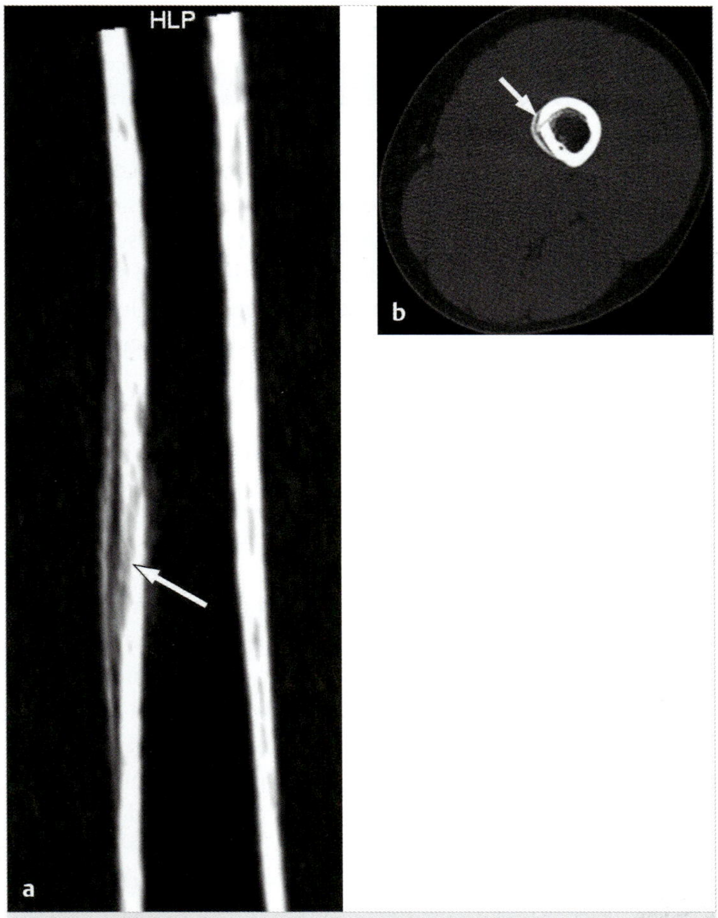

Fig. 7.3 a, b CT scans were obtained (3 weeks later, in comparison to a,b) for further investigation of the MRI findings shown in ▸ Fig. 7.2.

Final Diagnosis

Classic stress fracture in the medial cortex of the left femoral shaft.

Comments

Before eccentric edema-like signal in a tubular bone of the lower limb is interpreted as a tumor, a stress reaction should be confirmed or excluded. A detailed history is essential for this purpose. If plain radiographs are negative, low-dose CT should be used to detect or exclude a fracture line.

Case 130 (▸ Fig. 7.4)

Case description

- Referring physician: pediatric surgeon.
- Prior history and clinical question: A 10-year-old boy complained of increasing, non–exercise-related pain in his upper left thigh. The boy was an active soccer player and his symptoms, present for several weeks, had been attributed to that activity. MRI was finally performed, demonstrating a lesion in the proximal left femur that could not be positively identified.

Radiologic Findings

The radiograph (▸ Fig. 7.4 **a**) shows very slight cortical thickening in the proximal third of the femoral diaphysis. The coronal MR images after IV contrast administration (▸ Fig. 7.4 **b, c**) demonstrate a lesion in the medullary cavity, whose proximal portions display a lobular structure. On both sides of the bone is a linear hyperintensity relating to the periosteum or its immediate surroundings. The axial images (▸ Fig. 7.4 **d, e**) show that the hyperintensity encircles the bone. The intraosseous lesion shows intense peripheral enhancement after contrast injection (▸ Fig. 7.4 **d, e**). Markedly increased signal intensity is also noted in the medullary cavity proximal and distal to the main lesion (▸ Fig. 7.4 **c**). CT scans of the affected region (representative axial scan in ▸ Fig. 7.4 f) show small calcific densities in the medullary cavity.

Location

Unlike the previous case (Case 129), the epicenter of the changes is at the center of the medullary cavity.

Pathoanatomic Background of the Findings

The medullary cavity of the femur appears to contain a solid (enhancing) process with a partially calcified or ossified matrix. Cortical thickening shows that the intramedullary process is interacting with the cortex.

Assignment to a Possible Basic Entity

▸ **Normal variant or malformation?** No known precedent. Also, the finding appears to be the cause of the clinical complaints.

▸ **Trauma?** This question is justified in the young, avid soccer player, but imaging has shown no evidence of a stress fracture or other injury (see Case 129). Moreover, the boy's complaints are non–exercise-related!

▸ **Inflammation?** No clinical manifestations. With such an extensive process, the boy would have fever and other systemic signs.

▸ **Tumor?** Yes, see under Pathoanatomic Background of the Findings.

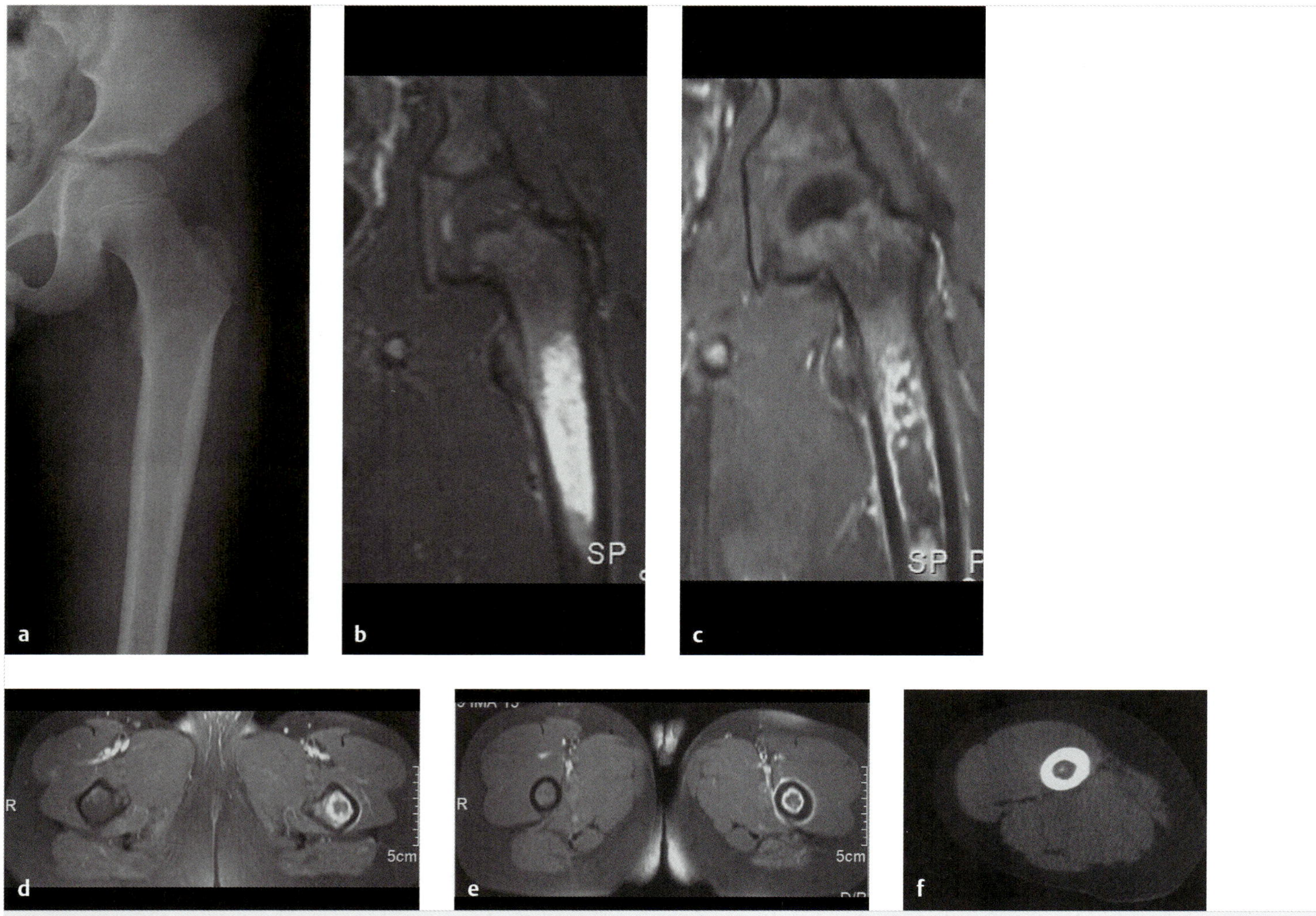

Fig. 7.4 a–f Bone marrow infarction?

Synopsis and Discussion

Considering the lobular lesion structure demonstrated by MRI and the matrix ossification detected by CT, the most likely diagnosis is a cartilage-forming tumor. But since the tumor had already caused cortical thickening and had produced both an extraosseous and an incipient intraosseous edema-like signal, we believed the tumor to be a *primary chondrosarcoma*, even though that entity would not ordinarily be diagnosed in such a young patient. At the time of diagnosis, moreover, the boy had no signs of enchondromatosis indicating a high chondrosarcoma risk (see also Case 120). The diagnostic criteria for grade I chondrosarcoma (atypical cartilaginous tumor) are reviewed in Case 108.

We then considered how to proceed further. The usual course of action would have been an en bloc resection, but the parents refused. Finally, a compromise was reached and a biopsy was performed, although everyone knew that it might not yield a representative sample. Histology showed a "cartilaginous tumor with no atypias or invasive features, consistent with enchondroma." Focal reactive periosteal new bone formation was interpreted as evidence of an active process. At that point it was necessary to proceed with open tumor removal by curettage, as the size of the lesion and age of the patient indicated a relatively high risk of later malignant transformation. Surprisingly, the curettage specimen showed "a fragment of a frankly destructive tumor component that had infiltrated local trabeculae and had disrupted and destroyed the local bone." This was recognized as a typical and unmistakable feature of grade I chondrosarcoma. The case was discussed with several other experienced bone pathologists, who confirmed the diagnosis of grade I chondrosarcoma. No additional surgical steps followed; the treating physician reports that the boy is still free of disease.

Only about 2 to 8% of grade I chondrosarcomas are diagnosed at age 10 years, and we presume that the young patient will eventually develop enchondromatosis. Consequently he should present for regular whole-body MRI follow-ups every 2 years (see also Case 120).

Final Diagnosis

Grade I chondrosarcoma (atypical cartilaginous tumor) in the proximal femoral shaft, possibly an early feature of enchondromatosis.

Comments

Biopsies of large cartilage-forming tumors are unreliable.

Case 131 (▶ Fig. 7.5)

Case description

- *Referring physicians:* pathologist and orthopedist.
- *Prior history and clinical question:* A 20-year-old man had a 6-month history of non–exercise-related pain in his right lower thigh and knee. The pain was responsive to NSAIDs but did not go away. MRI demonstrated a "lesion in the medullary cavity," which the radiologist interpreted as paraosseous osteosarcoma. Radiographs or CT scans were not obtained. Biopsy revealed nonspecific new bone formation with no evidence of osteosarcoma. What does the patient have?

Radiologic Findings

The water-sensitive MRI sequences (▶ Fig. 7.5 **a–c**) show wispy hyperintensities in the distal femoral metaphysis. ▶ Fig. 7.5 **c** additionally shows partial destruction of the anterior cortex and a paraosseous mass along the anterior side of the bone. The mass shows inhomogeneous high signal intensity, similar to the hyperintensities in the medullary cavity, and enhances slightly after IV contrast injection (not pictured here).

Location

The findings appear to have their epicenter in the anterior cortex.

Pathoanatomic Background of the Findings

No specific conclusions can be drawn from the MR images, except that some pathologic process is occurring in the anterior cortex. We shall make no attempt to assign the findings to a particular entity.

Synopsis and Discussion

Four months later we ordered CT scans, which clearly demonstrated a typical, centrally calcified nidus in the anterior cortex (▶ Fig. 7.6 **b**). The scan in ▶ Fig. 7.6 **a** still shows the defect from the previous excisional biopsy. This case clearly demonstrates that the nidus of an osteoid osteoma cannot (yet) be positively identified by MRI, especially when the nidus is very small. (The essential features of osteoid osteoma and its diagnosis are reviewed in Case 74. This is consistent with reports in the international literature. Our own collection includes many osteoid osteomas that did have a nidus identifiable by MRI, but there are many others in which a nidus was detectable only by CT or when a SPECT bone scan was added. In this case the nidus was removed percutaneously under CT guidance. The patient was immediately free of complaints and was also freed from the burden of having an osteosarcoma.

Final Diagnosis

Cortical osteoid osteoma in the anterior femoral diaphysis.

Comments

Any MRI finding suspicious for a bone tumor should be investigated further by CT before an invasive procedure is performed.

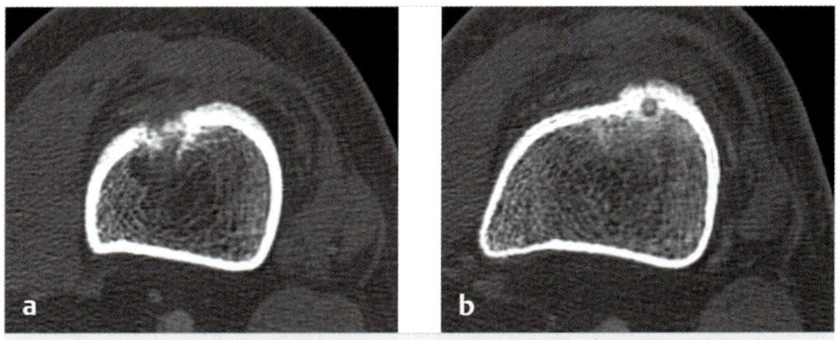

Fig. 7.6 a, b CT scans of the lesion shown in ▶ Fig. 7.5 (4 months later).

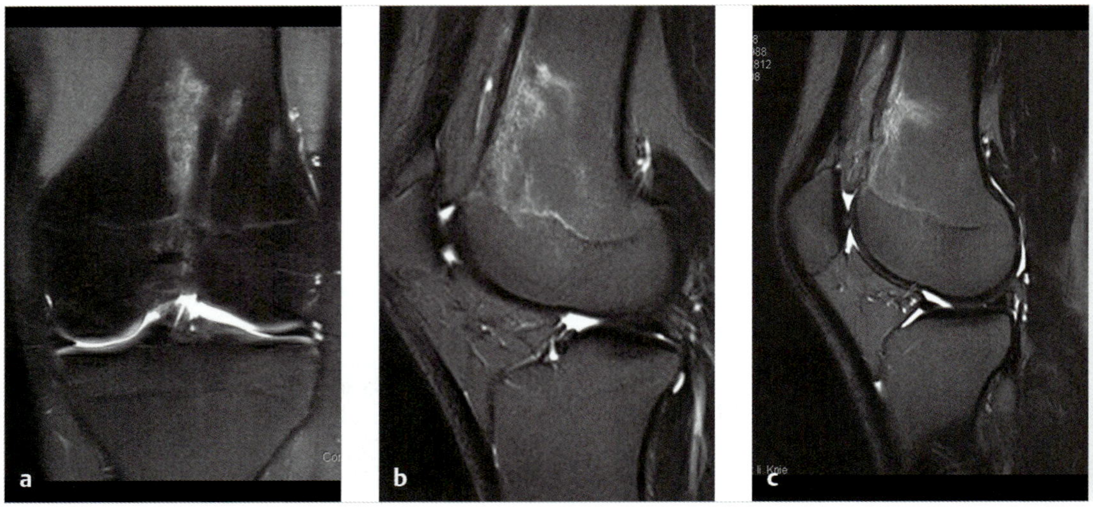

Fig. 7.5 a–c Osteosarcoma?

7.2 Predominantly Osteolytic Changes

Case 132 (▶ Fig. 7.7)

Case description

- Referring physician: pediatric surgeon.
- Prior history and clinical question: A 9-year-old boy felt pain in the left groin area after playing soccer. He had previously been free of complaints. The pediatric surgeon suspected a bone cyst and asked if his diagnosis was correct.

Radiologic Findings

Radiographs (▶ Fig. 7.7 **a, b**) demonstrate a large osteolytic area in the left femoral neck extending into the intertrochanteric region and corresponding to Lodwick grade IA. The axial projection shows that the osteolytic area is expansile with a trabeculated appearance. The T2w image demonstrates water signal intensity throughout the osteolytic area (▶ Fig. 7.7 **c**), which shows peripheral enhancement after IV contrast injection (▶ Fig. 7.7 **d**). The axial image in ▶ Fig. 7.7 **e** displays a fluid level or sedimentation.

Location

The lesion is intraosseous and occupies the entire femoral neck from the epiphyseal plate to the intertrochanteric region.

Pathoanatomic Background of the Findings

The fluid level and strictly peripheral enhancement of the lesion indicate a fluid-filled cystic process. The enhancing rim could represent the wall of a unicameral bone cyst. The fluid level also indicates intracystic hemorrhage with subsequent sedimentation of corpuscular elements. The trabecular pattern visible in the axial radiograph is caused by ridgelike bony prominences which, like the concentric expansion, are typical of a unicameral bone cyst.

Assignment to a Possible Basic Entity

The lesion was assigned to a basic entity under Pathoanatomic Background of the Findings, as there is no other reasonable possibility.

Synopsis and Discussion

The osteolytic lesion in the left femoral neck and intertrochanteric region corresponds to a unicameral bone cyst. Since the patient is a child, the bone cyst is also described as "juvenile." Below we shall review the key radiologic and clinical findings that are characteristic of a juvenile bone cyst:

- *Age of the patient and location:* Approximately 70 to 80% of all cases are detected in the first or second decade of life. They almost exclusively involve the metadiaphyseal region of a long bone (ca. 51% in the proximal humerus, 30% in the proximal femur).

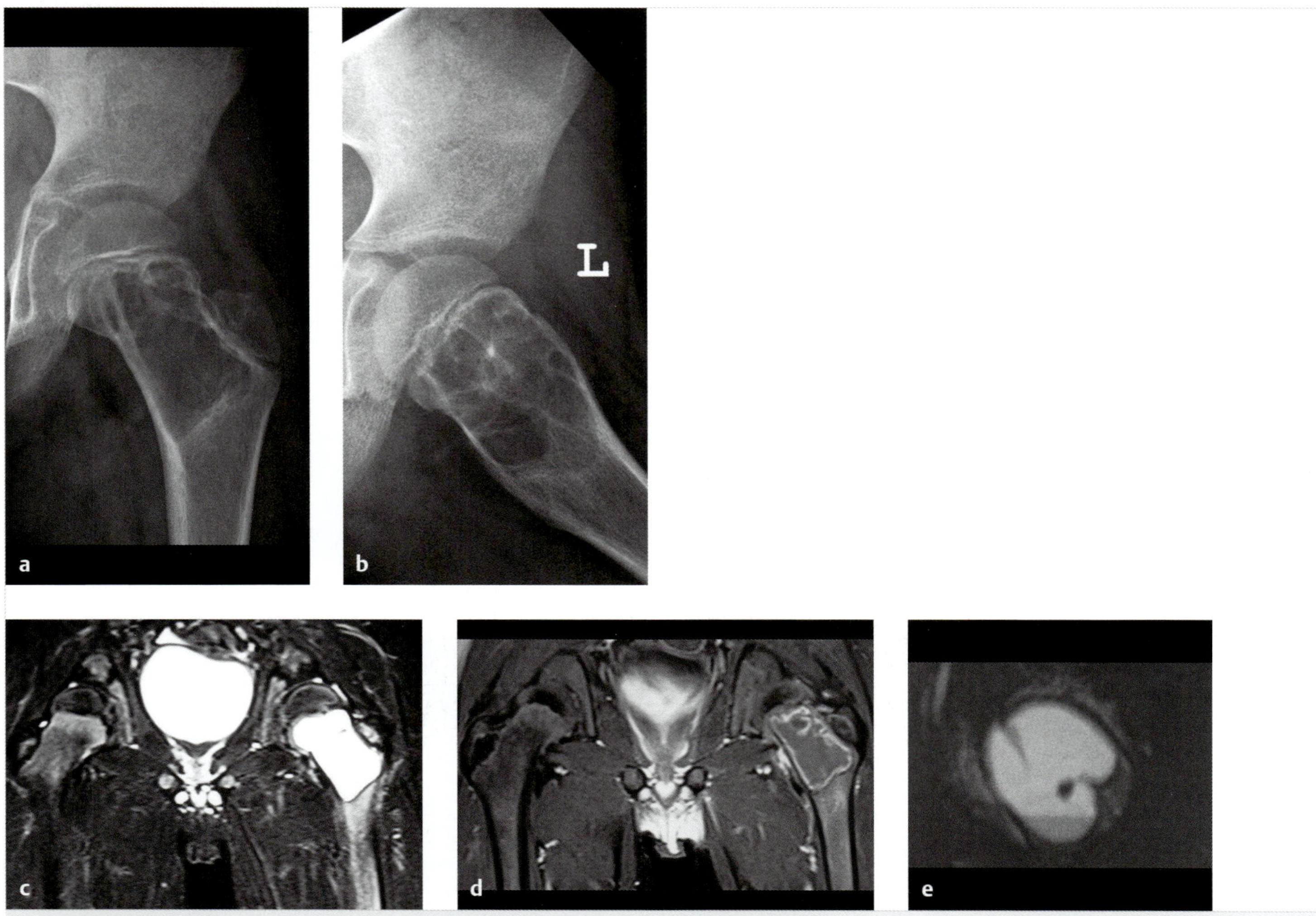

Fig. 7.7 a–e Juvenile bone cyst?

- *Clinical presentation:* Patients with a juvenile bone cyst typically have an extremely short history. Except in cases with a spontaneous fracture or, more commonly, a fissure fracture, the patients are free of complaints.
- *Radiology:*
  - Detection of fluid contents, most clearly manifested by a fluid level and by enhancement confined to a peripheral rim. The rim enhancement occurs in the cyst wall, which is pathognomonic for histologists; without it, they cannot make a confident diagnosis of juvenile bone cyst. The wall is composed of a thin membrane of dense fibrous tissue that is partially hyalinized and generally hypocellular. The cyst wall appears grossly as a fibrous membrane, 1 mm in thickness and of a grayish-white color. It is no wonder that many percutaneous biopsies are inconclusive, as it is largely a matter of chance whether the needle samples the cyst wall. In any case, percutaneous biopsies are unnecessary in most cases because a confident diagnosis can be made from radiologic findings.
  - *The "fallen fragment" sign:* A minor injury displaces a bone fragment from the thinnest site into the lesion. There it descends through the cyst fluid to the most dependent part of the lesion, often appearing radiographically as a "fallen fragment" when imaged in a tangential projection. In our case it was not visualized as this would have required either a positioned view with a clear projection of the lowest part of the cyst or a CT scan at that level. But this was unnecessary since the MRI findings were conclusive. In principle, however, a radiograph showing a more or less expansile lesion of Lodwick grade IA–IB in the metadiaphysis of a long bone with a "fallen fragment" sign provides adequate grounds for diagnosing a unicameral bone cyst. ▶ Fig. 7.8 illustrates another case of a juvenile bone cyst, located this time in the humerus and displaying two "fallen fragments" (arrows).

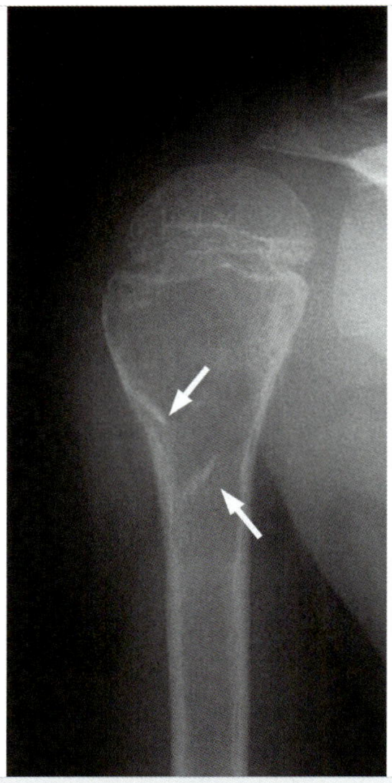

Fig. 7.8 "Fallen fragment" sign of a juvenile bone cyst.

Final Diagnosis

Juvenile bone cyst in the femoral neck and intertrochanteric region.

Comments

The detection of a cyst wall by contrast-enhanced MRI and/or a fallen fragment in a Lodwick grade IA–IB lesion in the metadiaphysis of a long bone is pathognomonic for a juvenile bone cyst.

Case 133 (▶ Fig. 7.9)

Case description

- *Referral:* self-referral by the patient.
- *Prior history and clinical question:* A 40-year-old man was found incidentally to have an osteolytic lesion in the inter- and subtrochanteric region of the left femur in 1996. Radiographs were repeated 5 years later and showed practically no change. The patient asked us if there was a risk of instability and wanted to have a definitive diagnosis.

Radiologic Findings

Radiographs demonstrate a Lodwick grade IB osteolytic lesion with a trabecular structure in the left intertrochanteric region (▶ Fig. 7.9 **a–c**). The lesion is not expansile. The whole-body bone scan (▶ Fig. 7.9 **d**) shows slightly increased uptake in the left intertrochanteric region. T1w MRI and CT scans (▶ Fig. 7.9 **e–i**) show that the lesion consists of at least four components, one of which is definitely fat.

Location

The lesion is located precisely in the intertrochanteric (metadiaphyseal) region and is confined to the medullary cavity.

Pathoanatomic Background of the Findings

The aforementioned multicomponent structure makes classification of the lesion difficult. The absence of complaints and lack of change over a 5-year period suggest a benign process. This is also indicated by the substantial fatty component. Water-sensitive and contrast-enhanced MRI sequences (not pictured here) suggested that the other components consisted of connective tissue, a myxomatous component, and ossified tissue.

Assignment to a Possible Basic Entity

▶ **Normal variant or malformation?** No, at least no known precedent—unlike the lesion in Case 73, which was definitely open to that interpretation.

▶ **Trauma?** No specific history, either for a single acute trauma or for chronic repetitive trauma.

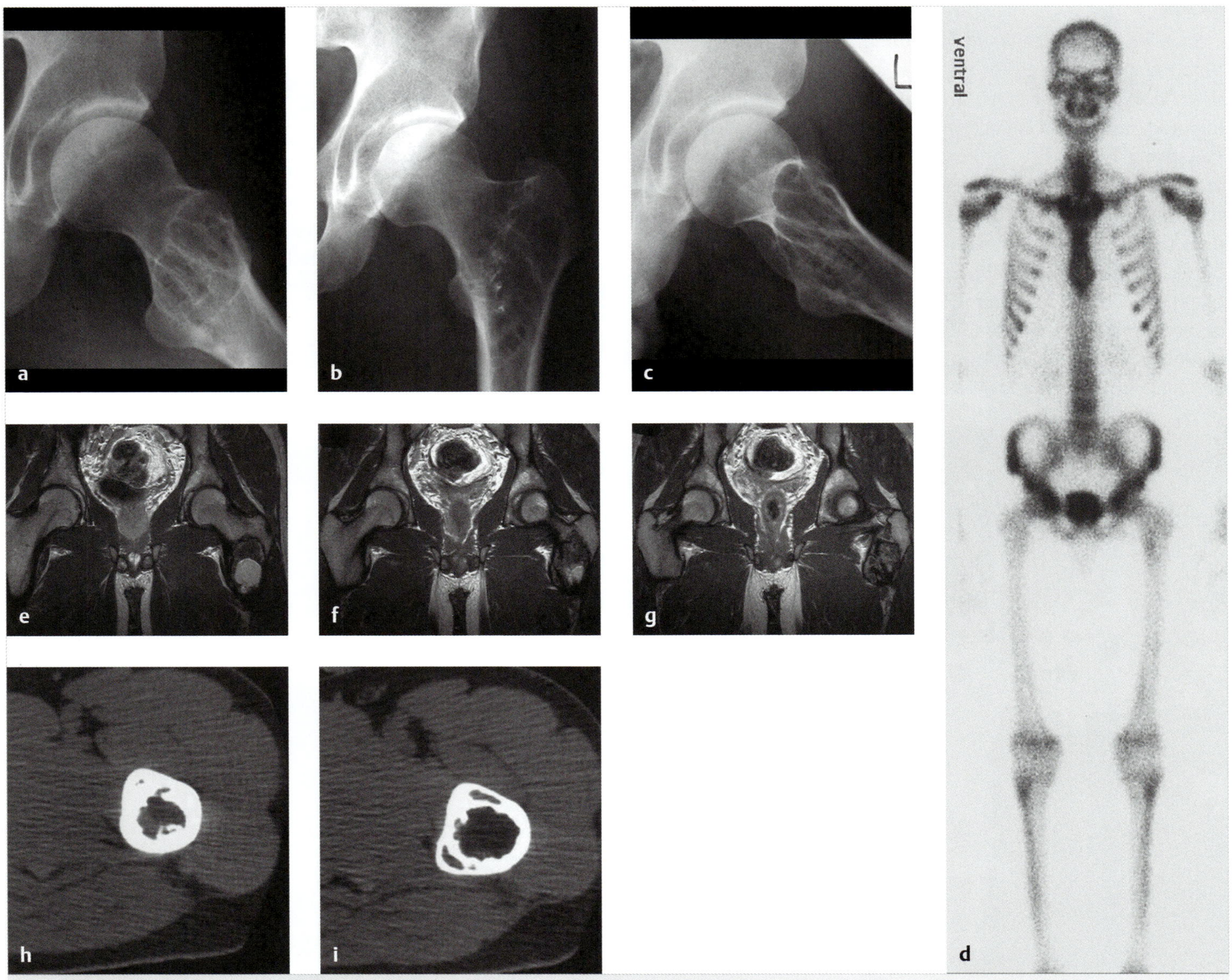

Fig. 7.9 Indeterminate osteolytic lesion: Does it compromise stability? Images a and b were acquired in 1996, images c–i in 2001.

▸ **Inflammation?** No clinical manifestations, and the detection of fat does not support a diagnosis of osteomyelitis, at least an active form. The history shows no evidence of a reactive inflammatory process.

▸ **Tumor or tumorlike lesion?** Yes, see details under Synopsis and Discussion.

Synopsis and Discussion

A lesion replacing normal cancellous bone in the left intertrochanteric region was detected incidentally. It is very difficult to reconcile its four components when assigning it to a particular entity. Lesions of this kind may develop from pre-existing benign entities due to regressive processes such as circumscribed necrosis with liquefaction and later fatty infiltration (replacement by fat) or degenerative myxomatous changes. When such lesions occur in the intertrochanteric region, the pre-existing entity may well be fibrous dysplasia, since that area is a site of predilection for fibrous dysplasia in the femur. Another possible precursor lesion is benign fibrous histiocytoma, or even an intraosseous lipoma with heavy regressive changes, although this would require a dominant fatty component (see ▸ Fig. 4.42 in Case 73). A final candidate is an old bone cyst, although the femoral neck would be a more typical site of occurrence for that lesion (see Case 132).

Such lesions are relatively common incidental findings in daily practice, and the need for biopsy is a question that is often addressed. We advise against it. It will not yield a definitive histologic diagnosis, since a large specimen will contain multiple components, analogous to the imaging pattern, and the pathologist will be unable to establish a single entity. This would require a molecular pathology test (in a non–acid-decalcified specimen) to detect the *GNAS-1* gene mutation that would prove fibrous dysplasia. All of the potential precursor entities listed above consist of only two, three, or at most four components, one of which may be predominant. This dominant component makes them easier to classify histologically and radiologically, as illustrated by woven bone with a ground-glass pattern in fibrous dysplasia, connective tissue in a benign fibrous histiocytoma, or fatty tissue in a lipoma.

Kransdorf et al (1999)[51] and Heim-Hall and Williams (2004)[52] coined the somewhat cumbersome term "liposclerosing myxofibrous tumor" in an attempt to describe the many components of fibro-osseous lesions with a predilection for the intertrochanteric region. Among the 39 cases reviewed by Kransdorf et al, four patients showed evidence of sarcomatous transformation, and all four were symptomatic. We feel that patients who are asymptomatic do not require biopsy or curettage ("leave me alone" or "don't touch me" lesion) or even continual radiologic follow-ups, although it may be very helpful to obtain an initial bone scan showing little or no tracer uptake. We also recommend use of the well-established term "fibro-osseous lesion." A detailed discussion of this lesion can be found in Freyschmidt et al (2010).[18]

As far as stability issues are concerned, the sectional images in particular show in our patient that the lesion did not cause significant bone destruction. This fact, plus the associated buttressing effect, should preclude the risk of a spontaneous fracture.

Final Diagnosis

Fibro-osseous lesion detected incidentally in the left intertrochanteric region; no need for biopsy.

Comments

If sectional imaging reveals at least three different tissue components in a lesion detected incidentally in the intertrochanteric region, the most likely diagnosis is a fibro-osseous lesion. Diagnostic confidence is further increased by a bone scan showing little or no tracer uptake in the affected region.

Case 134 (▶ Fig. 7.10)

Case description

- Referring physician: family doctor.
- Prior history and clinical question: A 44-year-old woman had a long history of pain in both thighs, with associated equivocal radiologic changes. A biopsy of the right femur was inconclusive.

Radiologic Findings

Radiographs demonstrate fine vermiform or serpiginous cortical lucencies in both femurs (only the right side is shown in ▶ Fig. 7.10 **a, b**). The changes were still very subtle in the 1999 radiograph (▶ Fig. 7.10 **a**) and are much more pronounced by 2004 (▶ Fig. 7.10 **b**). The larger defect in the proximal diaphysis is from a biopsy 6 months earlier. The T2w MR image in ▶ Fig. 7.10 **c** shows linear and focal hyperintensities along the area of the radiographic abnormality. MR angiography (MRA) (▶ Fig. 7.10 **d**)

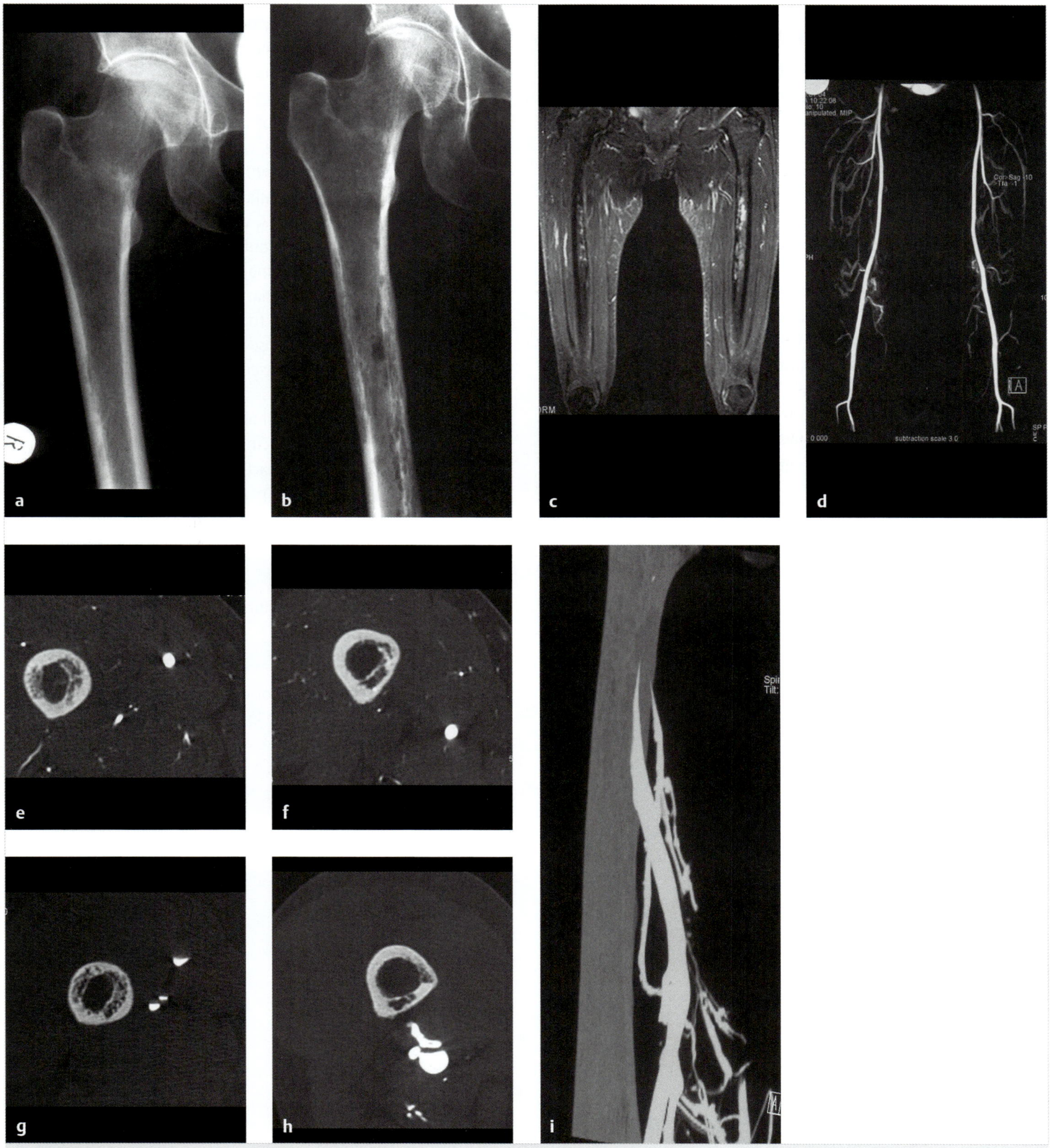

Fig. 7.10 Small- and round-cell tumor with a moth-eaten pattern? The first image shown was obtained in 1999 (a), and all others in 2004 (b–i).

and digital subtraction angiography (DSA) of the femoral arteries did not add useful information.

Location

The imaging abnormalities are limited to the cortical bone on both sides.

Pathoanatomic Background of the Findings

The radiographic and MRI findings are easily identified as vascular structures. They represent "vascular prints."

Assignment to a Possible Basic Entity

► **Normal variant or malformation?** No, this interpretation is not supported by the progression of findings over a 5-year period.

► **Trauma?** No trauma history.

► **Inflammation?** No clinical manifestations of inflammation or a reactive inflammatory process such as psoriasis.

► **Tumor or tumorlike lesion?** Because we are dealing with vascular structures, only two causal entities could be considered: a vascular malformation or angiomatosis. To resolve this question, we performed direct CT venography of the lower limb (► Fig. 7.10 **e–i**) with contrast injection into a dorsal pedal vein and a tourniquet on the upper thigh. Contrary to our expectations, this did not opacify any venous plexuses in the cavities of the cortical bone. This excluded a venous malformation but did not exclude a lymphatic malformation.

Synopsis and Discussion

Based on the radiologic findings and a re-evaluation of the histologic findings, we diagnosed the condition as cystic angiomatosis. The patient was treated with thalidomide, an inhibitor of vascular proliferation and angioneogenesis, which was followed by rapid improvement of symptoms. Unfortunately, we could not persuade the patient to consent to follow-up.

Key information on cystic angiomatosis is presented in Case 33 and Case 34. Here, we shall note again below that in dealing with vascular pathology, it is important to distinguish between vascular malformations on the one hand and vascular neoplasms on the other.

A vascular malformation may be arteriovenous with a fistula (high flow), purely venous (slow flow), lymphatic (slow flow), or a complex form. The first two types in bone can be differentiated by various current imaging techniques (MRA, DSA, CT angiography, CT venography). Lymphatic vascular malformations can be identified only histologically. With neoplastic vascular lesions, a distinction is made between malignant and benign tumors.

Hemangiomatosis is classified as a benign lesion. It is also called "angiomatosis" or, in the case of lytic lesions, "cystic hemangiomatosis." It is defined as the occurrence of multiple hemangiomas in bone and/or soft tissues, all with the same clinical, radiologic, and histologic characteristics. While simple hemangiomas of the skin or bone generally occur in infancy and childhood and regress spontaneously with puberty, it is our experience that hemangiomas usually do not become symptomatic until adulthood. They may resolve spontaneously or may be progressive, (see Case 33). Occurrence in adulthood and the potential for progression is a feature they share with vascular malformations. This raises the question of whether at least some observed cases of hemangiomatosis are vascular malformations. This is suggested in immunohistochemical studies by Bruder et al (2009),[33] who found that vascular malformations of bone had a proliferation rate of less than 1%, were GLUT1-negative, and minimally WT1-positive, which would not be consistent with neoplasms. If we consider that hemangiomas can be difficult to distinguish from vascular malformations by conventional histologic methods, there is good reason to doubt the histologic diagnoses of some benign vascular lesions, and it would be better to base the final diagnosis on radiologic criteria including the presence or absence of flow characteristics.

In our case, we exhausted all available radiologic options (see under Radiologic Findings), placing special emphasis on direct CT venography, which helped to exclude a venous intraosseous vascular malformation. In the case of a malformation, we would have performed a vascular occlusion by interventional radiology.

Final Diagnosis

Cystic angiomatosis in both femurs.

Comments

The description of serpiginous or vermiform lucencies forming vascular prints in a bone should immediately suggest a hemangioma or vascular malformation, which can often be differentiated by radiologic means.

Case 135 (▶ Fig. 7.11)

Case description

- *Referral:* self-referral by the patient.
- *Prior history and clinical question:* A 43-year-old man underwent MRI for the investigation of suspected meniscal symptoms, and a lesion was detected incidentally in the distal metaphysis of the right femur. When neither a diagnosis nor prognosis was forthcoming, the patient asked for our opinion.

Radiologic Findings

The radiographs in ▶ Fig. 7.11 **a, b** demonstrate an osteolytic lesion in the lateral side of the distal femoral metaphysis, corresponding to Lodwick grade IA. A latticework of sclerotic trabeculations is visible within the lesion. In the T1w images (▶ Fig. 7.11 **c, d**), the lesion has high signal intensity and is isointense to the infrapatellar fat pad. The signal intensity in the fat-suppressed image (▶ Fig. 7.11 **e**) approximately equals that of subcutaneous fat. To obtain more information on the osseous structures, we ordered CT scans (▶ Fig. 7.11 **f, g**) which not only confirmed the fatty content of the lesion but also supplied two possible explanation for the lattice of sclerotic trabeculations, viz. (1) irregular ossifications, probably woven bone, arising from the tumor margin, or (2) residual cancellous trabeculae that were not resorbed by the tumor.

Location

The lesion is entirely intraosseous, located within the distal femoral metaphysis.

Pathoanatomic Background of the Findings

The lesion is composed mainly of fat and bony elements, which may be interpreted as residues of incomplete trabecular resorption by the tumor, may be metaplastic in nature, or may represent a buttressing process.

Assignment to a Possible Basic Entity

▶ **Normal variant or malformation?** By its nature, an incidental finding usually raises the possibility of a normal variant. In cases of disuse osteoporosis due to prolonged inactivity, fat may accumulate in the enlarged medullary cavity, but this should occur in the epiphysis and not in an eccentric pattern as in our case.

▶ **Trauma or inflammation?** There is no clinical evidence for either of these basic entities.

▶ **Tumor or tumorlike lesion?** Yes, based on the structure of the lesion, which has replaced normal osseous structures. The preponderance of fat suggests a lipoma (see Synopsis and Discussion).

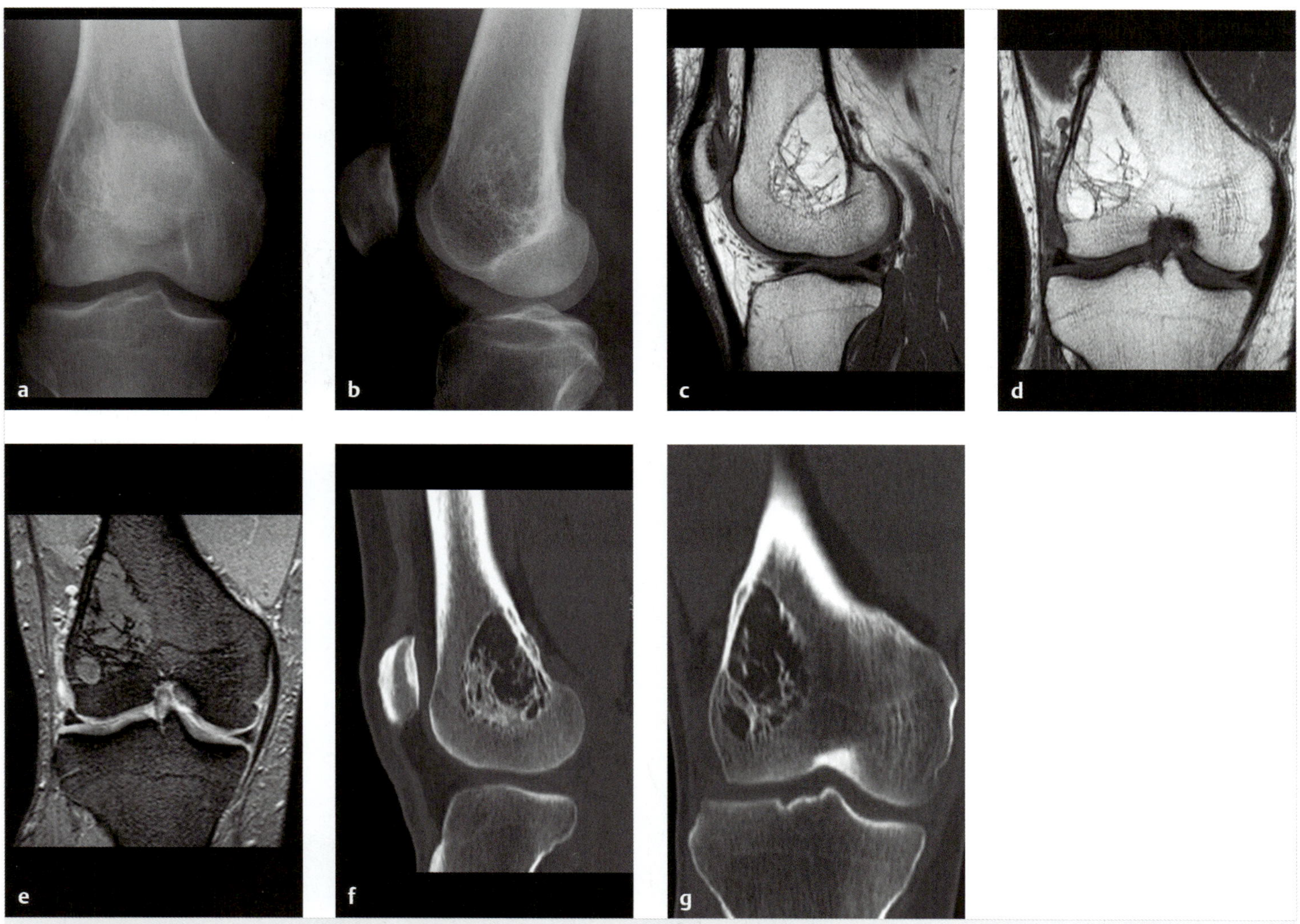

Fig. 7.11 a–g Incidental finding, but what is it?

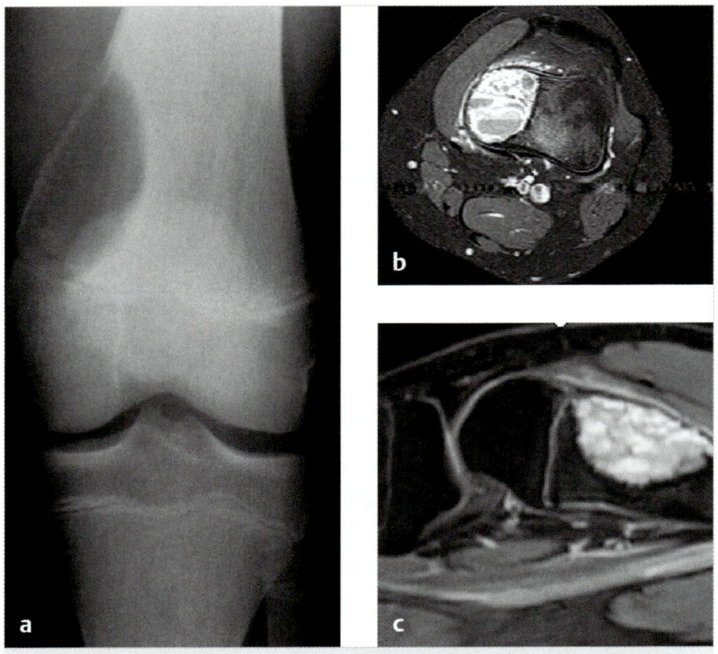

Fig. 7.12 a–c Aneurysmal bone cyst in the distal femoral metaphysis of a 14-year-old girl.

Synopsis and Discussion

Because fat is predominant in the Lodwick grade IA lesion, it should be interpreted as an intraosseous lipoma. According to the WHO definition,[15] "lipoma of bone is a benign neoplasm of adipocytes that arises within the medullary cavity, cortex, or on the surface of bone." Many authors question whether lipomas are true neoplasms, suggesting that they more closely resemble a hamartoma. They may also result from the fatty transformation of old fibrous dysplasia, old bone cysts that have healed with fatty replacement, or even giant cell tumors that have resolved by fatty transformation (see also Case 133). A diagnosis of lipoma should always be made cautiously when dealing with large intraosseous collections of fatty tissue in regions that physiologically have a high fat content, such as the femoral neck (see Case 73) or the body of the calcaneus. Larger lipomas, in particular, may undergo regressive changes over time, the most common of which is central fat infarction. If the necrotic area calcifies (necrotic fat is a calcium scavenger) or undergoes dystrophic ossification, a radiograph or CT scan will demonstrate a calcific nidus (e.g., in the calcaneus). Most intraosseous lipomas that we diagnose do not require histologic evaluation if their principal component is fat, since CT or MRI can identify fat with very high confidence. Because lipomas generally grow very slowly and have already been present for years when detected (Lodwick grade IA!), they do not pose a risk of spontaneous fracture.

For comparison, ▶ Fig. 7.12 shows the case of a 14-year-old girl with a clinically symptomatic (painful) *aneurysmal bone cyst* in the medial portion of the distal femoral metaphysis. It bears a superficial resemblance to lipoma. The osteolytic lesion is classified as Lodwick grade IB (▶ Fig. 7.12 **a**), indicating a faster growth rate than lipoma. While lipoma stimulates a marked buttressing effect with cortical thickening over the lesion, the cortex over the aneurysmal bone cyst is very thin and "bulging." An aneurysmal bone cyst cannot be diagnosed from radiographs alone, so MRI was added to detect a dominant fluid level (▶ Fig. 7.12 **c**) and marked enhancement of the stroma (▶ Fig. 7.12 **b**), consisting of ridges or septa (see Case 45). This is pathognomonic for an aneurysmal bone cyst.

Final Diagnosis

Intraosseous lipoma detected incidentally in the medial portion of the distal femoral metaphysis.

Comments

Incidentally detected tumors composed mainly of fat according to CT or MRI measurements should be classified as lipomas and left alone.

Case 136 (▶ Fig. 7.13)

Case description

- Referring physician: orthopedist.
- Prior history and clinical question: A 64-year-old man complaining of intermittent pain in both knees was referred for knee arthroscopy. Previous MRI had shown signs of a tumor arising from the synovial membrane in each knee joint. More details on the history are presented below.

Radiologic Findings

A plain radiograph shows osteolytic areas in the distal femoral epiphysis and opposing tibial epiphysis (▶ Fig. 7.13 **a**). A contralateral radiograph (not pictured here) showed almost identical findings on the opposite side. T1w MRI (▶ Fig. 7.13 **b**) clearly demonstrates a hypointense process that originates from the joint space and has spread into the adjacent bones and paraosseous sites over the epicondyles. The postcontrast image in ▶ Fig. 7.13 **c** shows marked enhancement of the thickened synovial membrane, which is permeated by hypointense streaks. This finding, too, was mirrored on the opposite side.

Location

Anatomically, the pathologic changes are localized to the synovial membrane, from which they have spread to involve the adjacent bones.

Pathoanatomic Background of the Findings

The radiologic changes indicate a solid process that most likely originates from the synovial membrane and has caused bone destruction. The bilateral occurrence suggests a systemic condition. It is also possible, however, that the process has spread to the joint from the bone or from the joint to the bone.

Assignment to a Possible Basic Entity

▶ **Inflammation?** We may be dealing with an inflammatory synovial process in both knee joints, but in that case we would expect to find an effusion.

▶ **Tumor or tumorlike lesion?** The extensive bone destruction might well result from a tumor or tumorlike lesion of the synovial membrane, in which case the hypointense streaks could represent intralesional hemorrhages with iron deposition. Synovial proliferation with iron deposits is typical of pigmented villonodular synovitis (PVNS), also known as tenosynovial giant cell tumor.

Synopsis and Discussion

Although the bilateral occurrence of the lesions was not consistent with PVNS, we did offer the latter as our initial diagnosis and requested histologic confirmation. At arthroscopy, the orthopedist encountered grayish-white masses which he, as an experienced arthroscopist, immediately identified as sodium urate deposits. Subsequent determination of the uric acid level yielded an abnormal value. We then re-examined the patient with CT (▶ Fig. 7.14). The bone-window and especially the soft-tissue window views revealed masses containing sodium urate crystals. It should be added that the intraosseous soft-tissue masses are not necessarily gouty synovial structures that invaded the bone but are more likely intraosseous tophi, which may also invade the joint. If we had considered that possibility, PVNS would have been an unlikely diagnosis. This case clearly illustrates the fact that *gout* is rarely if ever considered in the diagnosis of proliferative synovial processes accompanied by osteolytic lesions. We should have considered this diagnosis at once, since the very fact that the knee changes were bilateral suggested a systemic condition rather than a tumorlike process such as PVNS. This fact was noted during our deliberations, but still no one thought of gout!

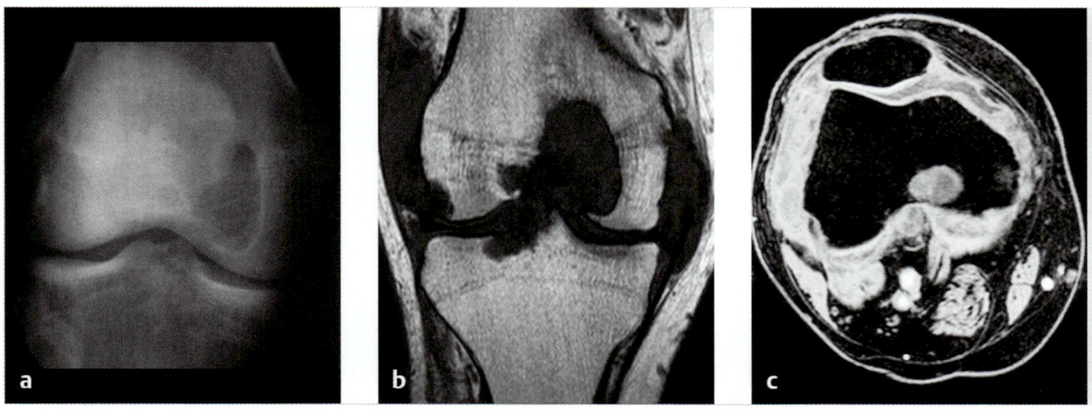

Fig. 7.13 a–c Pigmented villonodular synovitis?

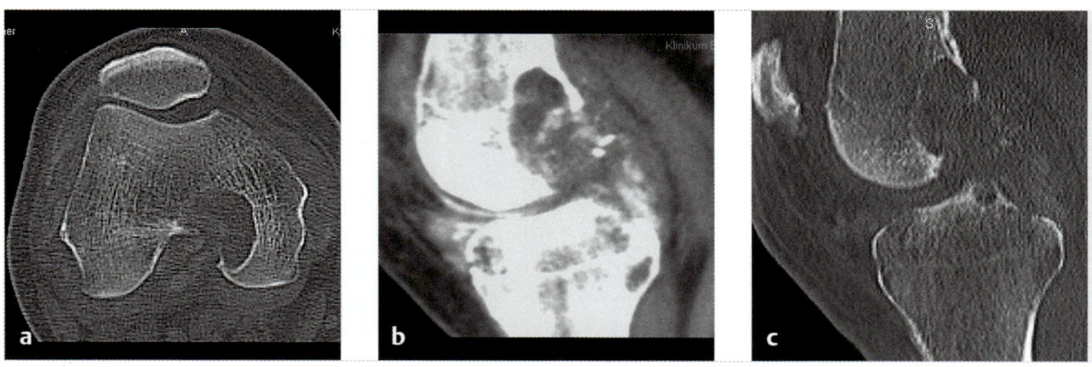

Fig. 7.14 a–c CT scans supplementing the images in ▶ Fig. 7.13.

This underscores the importance of the old adage, "When in doubt, think of gout" (see also Case 41).

▶ Fig. 7.15 shows the case of a 78-year-old man who experienced nonspecific bilateral knee pain, especially when dancing. This case, fully elucidated, was furnished to us by Dr. H. Fauster of Leoben District Hospital in Austria. The radiographs (▶ Fig. 7.15 **a, b**) led the orthopedist to suspect osteochondritis dissecans, except that an osteochondral fragment could not be found. This prompted the radiologist to perform MRI (▶ Fig. 7.15 **c–f**), which showed a hypointense mass in the subchondral bone defect. A hyperintense, enhancing membranelike structure, apparently granulation tissue, was found at the junction with unchanged bone. All these findings weigh against a diagnosis of osteochondritis dissecans but were not specific for any other entity, and our colleague ordered supplemental CT scans (▶ Fig. 7.15 **g–i**). The scans revealed calcified structures within the lesion and in the thickened synovial membrane, which were diagnostic of gout. Sediment from aspirated joint fluid had a uric acid concentration of 5.4 mg/dL! Normal joint fluid does not contain uric acid sediment.

Final Diagnosis

Large gouty tophi in juxta-articular portions of the femur and tibia on both sides.

Comments

"When in doubt, think of gout."

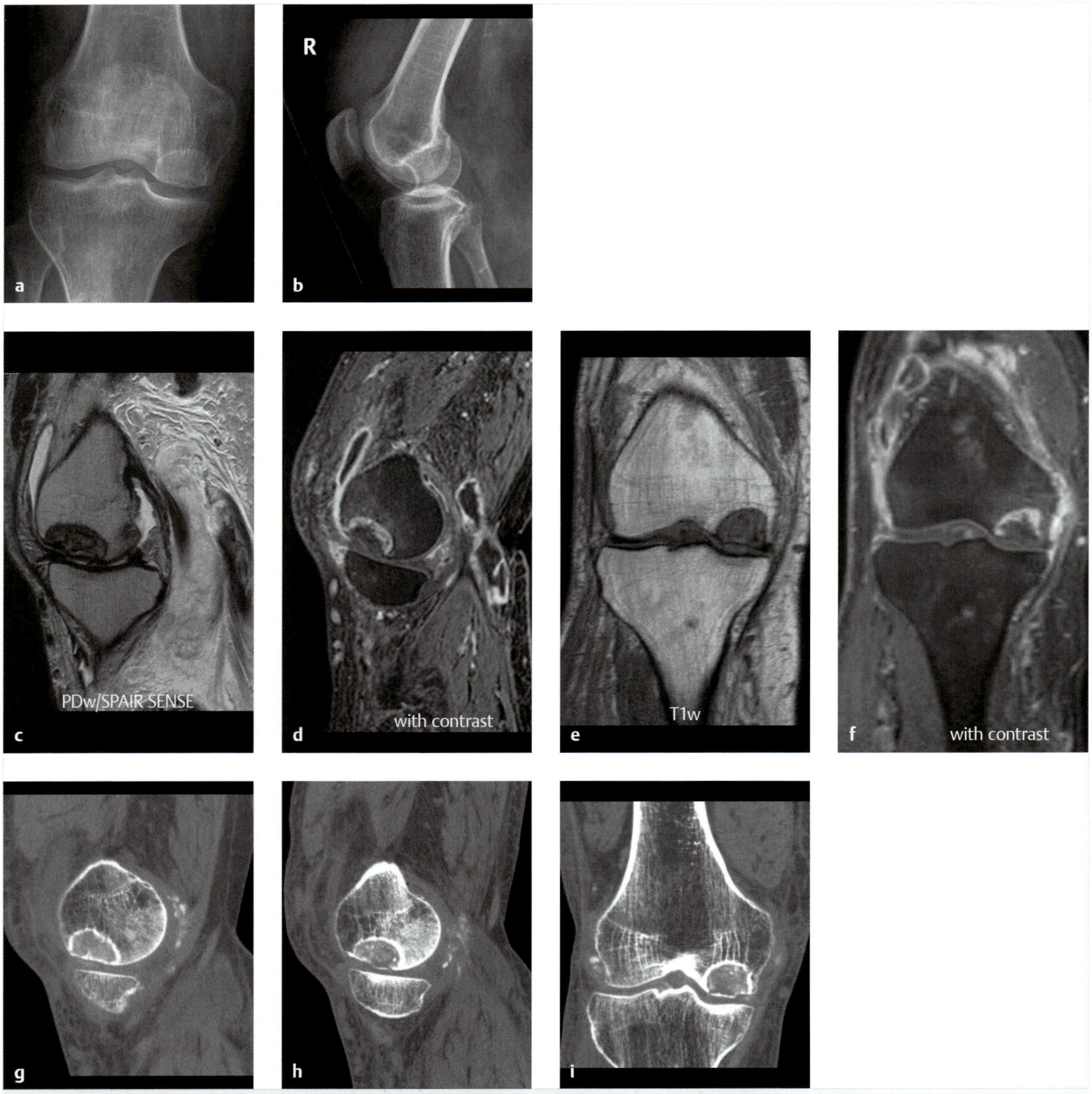

Fig. 7.15 a–i Gout in a 78-year-old man, equivocal on radiographs and MRI, finally diagnosed by CT.

Case 137 (▶ Fig. 7.16)

Case description

- *Referring physicians:* orthopedist and trauma surgeon.
- *Prior history and clinical question:* An 18-year-old female came to the emergency room with acute left knee pain.

Radiologic Findings

Radiographs of the left knee (▶ Fig. 7.16 **a-c**) show gross osteolytic changes in the femur, tibia, and patella. The osteolytic areas show coarse "trabeculations." On closer scrutiny, we find that the surrounding cancellous bone shows a porous or coarse trabecular structure. The orthopedist and trauma surgeon suspected a spontaneous fracture of the distal femur as the cause of the acute pain and proposed surgical intervention (curettage and reconstruction with methylmethacrylate cement). The working diagnosis was a giant cell tumor. The radiologist on call suspected oligo-ostotic fibrous dysplasia because the interior of the lesions had a ground-glass appearance. He obtained a full-length, standing anteroposterior (AP) radiograph (▶ Fig. 7.16 **d**), which surprisingly showed similar changes on the contralateral side. Osteolytic lesions were additionally found in the left tibial shaft and distal portions of the fibula. The original images (not these reproductions) showed more lesions in the middle third of the right femoral shaft (long segmental osteolysis with very thin residual medial cortex) and above the left acetabulum. Overall, the cortex on all portions of the femur and tibia was too thin for an 18-year-old.

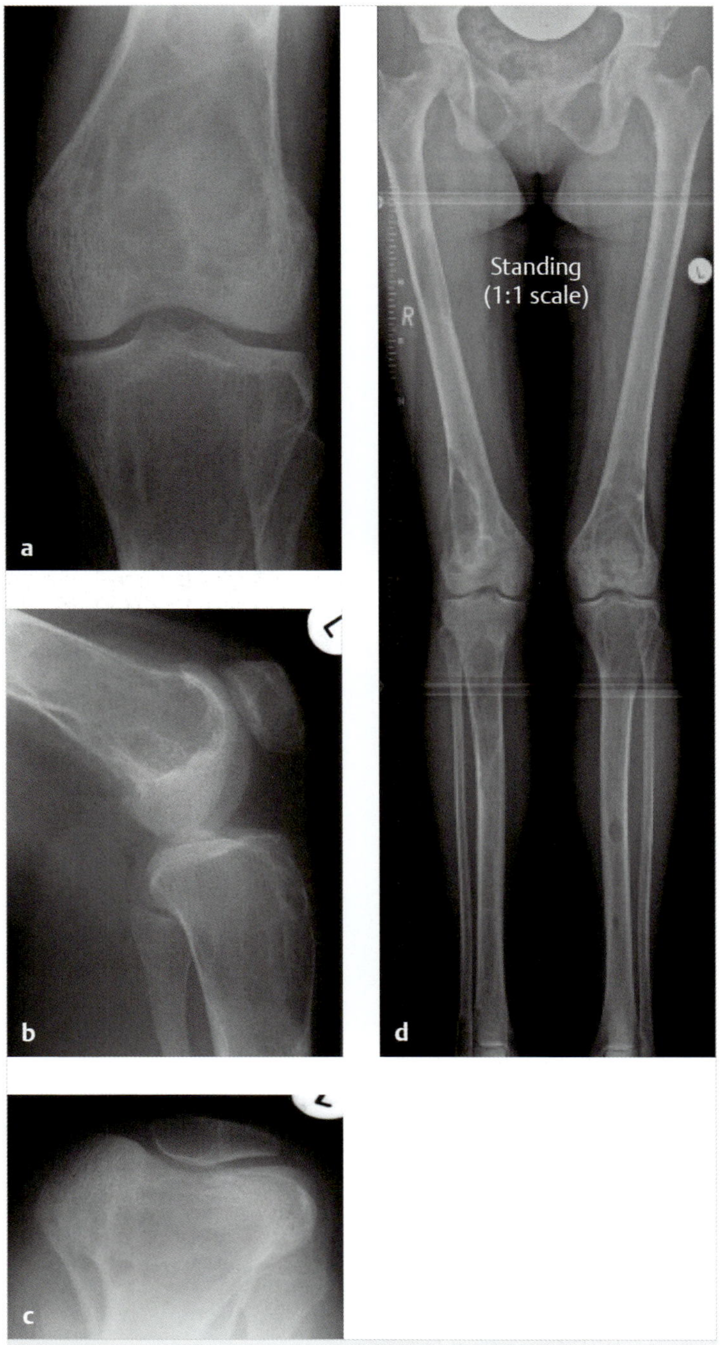

Fig. 7.16 a–d Fibrous dysplasia or giant cell tumor?

Location

The above changes appear to involve all portions of the imaged bones.

Pathoanatomic Background of the Findings

We are dealing with a generalized process that causes bone resorption and has produced relatively large osteolytic areas. The only disease that causes changes of this description is hyperparathyroidism. We feel that any attempt to assign the changes to a different entity would be unrealistic.

Synopsis and Discussion

The osteolytic areas represent brown tumors of primary hyperparathyroidism—"primary" because the patient had no renal disease or other signs that might indicate secondary hyperparathyroidism (e.g., osteomalacia). Her parathormone level, at 122 pmol/L, was extremely high (normal = 1.5–6.0 pmol/L). Her serum calcium was 5.5 mmol/L (normal = 2.20–2.65 mmol/L). Parathyroid ultrasound detected a mass measuring 2.9 cm × 2.6 cm × 1.6 cm, consistent with parathyroid adenoma. The surgical specimen weighed 9.3 g. The unusual feature of this case was that the patient had no other signs of primary hyperparathyroidism such as cardiac arrhythmia, ECG abnormalities due to hypercalcemia, etc. Unfortunately, we have no information on any subjective symptoms such as depression, which are a frequent clue to primary hyperparathyroidism if the internist or psychiatrist considers that diagnosis and orders a serum calcium test.

Generally speaking, a diagnosis of primary hyperparathyroidism is not often considered because the disease is thought to be rare, but that is not true: it is the second most common metabolic bone disease after osteoporosis, with an estimated incidence of 21–25 cases per 100,000 population per year. Older women are most commonly affected, although the disease may occur at any age. According to our endocrinologist, one case of primary hyperparathyroidism is seen each week at a maximum care hospital.

Early detection of the disease is essential because longstanding cases may develop a potentially fatal hypercalcemia syndrome as well as irreversible vascular damage that includes the coronary arteries. The radiologist should consider this disease whenever the following changes are noted on radiographs (see also Case 15 and Case 111):

- Very dense bone in the early stage of the disease due to the initial anabolic effect of parathormone (which is why that hormone is used in the treatment of osteoporosis).
- Coarsening of the original trabecular pattern due to the mineralization of woven bone. This is most apparent in the metaphyses of the long bones, as in our case.
- Cortical tunneling or striations and subperiosteal resorption, especially at entheses.
- Osteolytic lesions, which correspond to brown tumors.

The radiographic test region is the hand (see ▶ Fig. 3.29 in Case 15), as the above changes are usually manifested initially in the hand skeleton (see Freyschmidt 2008 for a detailed discussion).[13]

Final Diagnosis

Brown tumors of primary hyperparathyroidism.

Comments

When one or more osteolytic lesions are found, hyperparathyroidism is suggested by a coarse trabecular pattern, cortical tunneling, and adjacent areas of subperiosteal resorption.

Case 138 (▶ Fig. 7.17)

Case description

- Referring physician: orthopedist.
- Prior history and clinical question: A 16-year-old boy complained of exercise-related knee pain. Three years earlier he had been diagnosed with Sinding–Larsen–Johansson syndrome, which was managed conservatively. Radiographs of the knee (▶ Fig. 7.17 **a–c**) showed an osteolytic lesion in the superolateral quadrant of the patella (arrows). This prompted further investigation by MRI, with equivocal findings (tumor? deep osteochondral lesion?).

Radiologic Findings

Radiographs show an osteolytic lesion with a sclerotic rim in the superolateral quadrant of the patella. They also demonstrate a dysplastic femoropatellar articulation with a Wiberg type III patella (▶ Fig. 7.17 **a–c**). The MR images (▶ Fig. 7.17 **d–g**) prove that the patellar articular cartilage extends at least partially into the patellar defect, meaning that the defect is partially lined by articular cartilage. Finally, a cartilage anomaly (▶ Fig. 7.17 **e**) and a Baker cyst (▶ Fig. 7.17 **d**) are recognizable.

Location

The bony patellar defect, which is partially lined by cartilage, is located precisely in the region where "dorsal patellar defects" occur.

Pathoanatomic Background of the Findings

The cartilage lining of the patellar defect suggests that the defect has been present for some time. Because the patient is only 16 years old, it is reasonable to assume that the defect developed during the boy's growth period.

Assignment to a Possible Basic Entity

▶ **Normal variant or malformation?** Yes. The finding on the "plain radiograph" corresponds to what is called a *dorsal patellar defect*. This lesion is present in approximately 1% of individuals in the second or third decade of life.[17,53] The etiology of the defect is unclear; it probably represents an ossification disturbance. This is supported by the finding that the articular cartilage over and within the defect is intact; it may even be thicker. Moreover, the defects tend to regress spontaneously leaving a sclerotic rim. Van Holsbeeck et al (1987)[54] also discuss a possible association with ossification disturbances (bipartite or multipartite patella). They

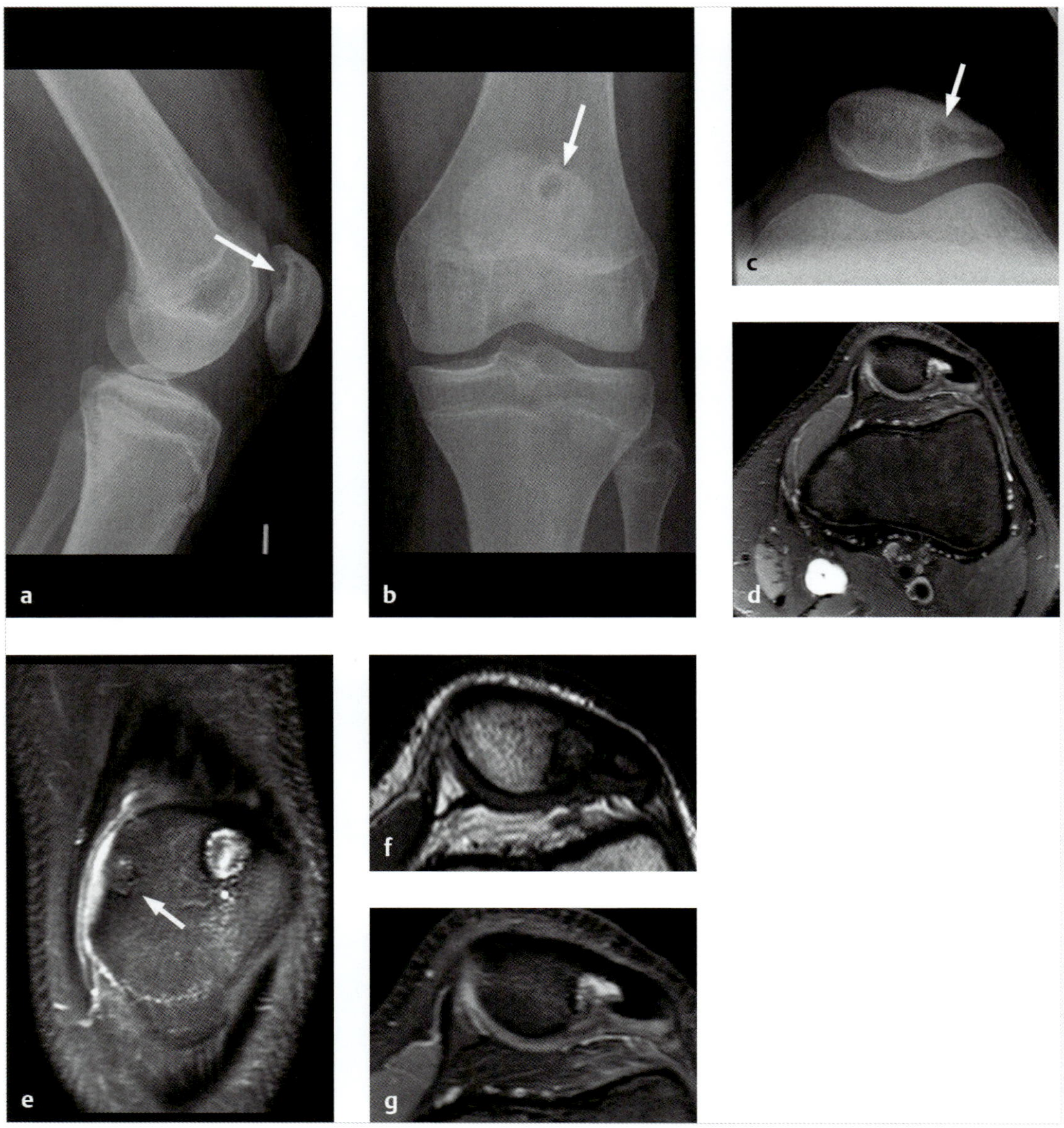

Fig. 7.17 a–g Osteochondritis dissecans?

suggest among others that the initial lesion may be a traction lesion at the insertion of the vastus lateralis muscle rather than an ulceration of articular cartilage.

► **Trauma?** The defect is not the result of a "recent" trauma. But as noted above, it may be a result of earlier chronic trauma.

► **Inflammation?** No clinical manifestations.

► **Tumor?** No. Why would the articular cartilage fit so precisely into a tumor-related defect?

► **Degenerative change?** One possibility would be osteochondritis dissecans, but an osteochondral fragment is not visible on any of the MR images. We would also expect to find articular fluid within the osteochondritis defect. In most cases of osteochondritis dissecans, edema-like signal is observed about the lesion; it is not detectable in the present case.

Synopsis and Discussion

The principal arguments for a *normal variant* were discussed above. The boy has a prior history of patellar complaints 3 years earlier. MRI at that time showed the patellar defect initially; a large arthrocele detected in the region of a "Baker cyst" by current MRI was not found in the earlier examination and could be implicated as the cause of the current complaints. A Baker cyst generally develops following an inflammatory (synovitic) articular process.

It is conceivable that a traction effect at the insertion of the vastus lateralis due to overuse promoted the development of the defect, if the latter is interpreted as an ossification disturbance. This is consistent with the prior history of Sinding–Larsen–Johansson syndrome, which often is a catch-all diagnosis.

The boy's nonspecific complaints might also be attributed to a *cartilage ulcer* at a more medial site (arrow in ► Fig. 7.17 **e**), which we have not explicitly documented here.

As far as the complaints are concerned, it should be kept in mind that normal variants are not always harmless and may become symptomatic if they interfere with physiologic processes.

We do not know if the increased signal intensity at the base of the defect has any significance. It could account for unexplained patellar symptoms or joint fluid at the base of the pit, where the cartilage is perhaps absent or extremely thin. This cannot be determined from the images, however.

Ultimately, the exact cause of the clinical complaints is uncertain, and it is reasonable to consider whether arthroscopy might advance the diagnosis.

Preliminary Diagnosis

Dorsal patellar defect as a normal variant, cartilage ulcer at a more medial site, arthrocele in the form of a Baker cyst.

Comments

Anomalies of bone should always suggest a normal variant, especially in younger patients, and may be responsible for clinical symptoms.

Case 139 (▶ Fig. 7.18)

Case description

- Referring physician: orthopedist.
- Prior history and clinical question: A 48-year-old man underwent MRI for investigation of unexplained knee pain, which showed a suspicious finding in the adjacent tibia. This prompted a further work-up that included radiographs and CT. The changes were interpreted as fibrous dysplasia or possibly a cartilage-forming tumor. The orthopedist requested our opinion before proceeding with biopsy.

Radiologic Findings

Fusiform expansion is noted radiographically in the middle third of the tibial diaphysis, and the cortex in that area appears slightly thinned (▶ Fig. 7.18 **a, b**). This finding may also be described as an expansile lesion with a bony shell. Ground-glass densities, some with a streaky appearance, are visible throughout the imaged portion of the tibial shaft. This is particularly evident on CT scans (▶ Fig. 7.18 **c, g–i**). The ground-glass densities are outlined by fine sclerotic margins. Basically there are three consecutive lesions that dominate the CT images. They have very high signal intensity in the STIR sequence (▶ Fig. 7.18 **f**) but are inhomogeneous, containing small areas isointense to fluid. In the axial T1w image in ▶ Fig. 7.18 **d**, one lesion is isointense to muscle. It shows only slight enhancement after IV contrast administration (▶ Fig. 7.18 **e**).

Location

All the described changes are intraosseous.

Pathoanatomic Background of the Findings

The three lesions in the medullary cavity of the tibia are solid masses with associated cortical thinning, which is most pronounced in the middle third of the diaphysis. The unmistakable ground-glass pattern on CT, signifying woven bone, combined with a mass effect immediately evokes a familiar engram: ground-glass pattern → woven bone → fibrous dysplasia. This eliminates the need to consider other possible entities.

The small areas of water signal intensity on MRI (▶ Fig. 7.18 **f**) probably represent circumscribed areas of necrosis with liquefaction.

Synopsis and Discussion

In summary, the following findings prove the diagnosis of fibrous dysplasia and exclude a cartilage-forming tumor:

- Incidental finding
- Expansile lesion with a bony shell but no scalloping typical of a cartilaginous tumor (caused by the advancement of growing cartilage lobules toward the inner cortical surface)
- Ground-glass pattern in the tumorlike lesions
- No lobular pattern in water-sensitive MRI, which would be typical of a cartilaginous tumor (see Case 108), and no septal enhancement

The findings are so typical that there is no need for biopsy. Other cases of fibrous dysplasia are illustrated in Case 4, Case 7, Case 20, and Case 36. An expert in bone tumor radiology could certainly diagnose fibrous dysplasia from MRI alone, but the signal characteristics are highly variable from case to case and within a given lesion because fibrous dysplasia may undergo a dynamic process with various stages of maturation and degeneration. We have not yet identified a consistent MRI feature of fibrous dysplasia that is as reliable as a ground-glass pattern on plain radiographs and CT scans.

As an aid to differential diagnosis, ▶ Fig. 7.19 **a** illustrates *unicameral bone cyst* in a 15-year-old boy who felt pain in his right tibia after a minor injury. The radiograph shows an elongated Lodwick grade IB lesion that appears "empty," lacking the mineralized matrix found in the case above. The lesion has water signal intensity in the T2w MR image (▶ Fig. 7.19 **b**), while the postcontrast fat-suppressed image in ▶ Fig. 7.19 **c** shows an enhancing cyst wall (see also Case 132 and ▶ Fig. 7.25 in Case 143).

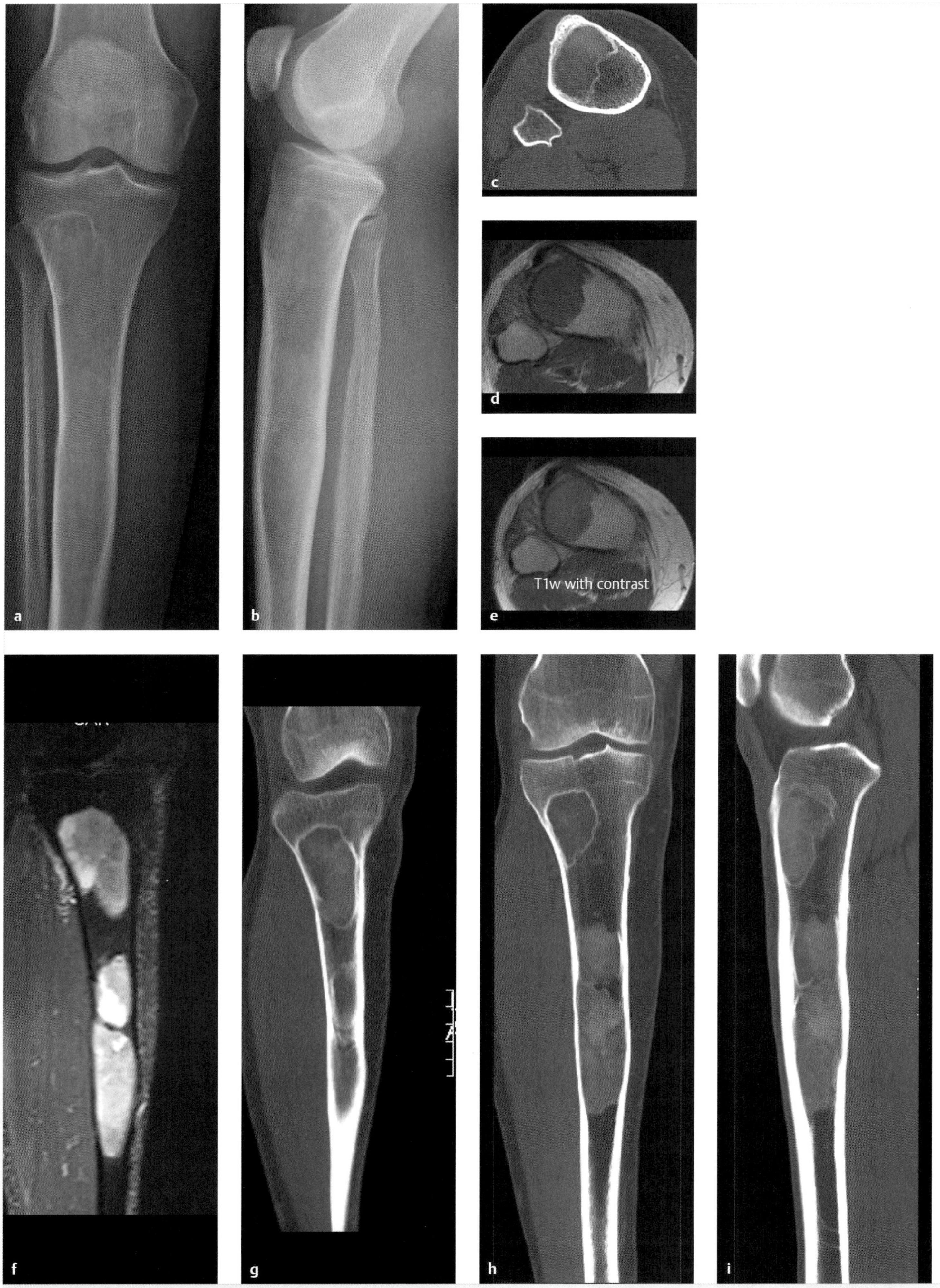

Fig. 7.18 a–i Cartilage-forming tumor? Biopsy?

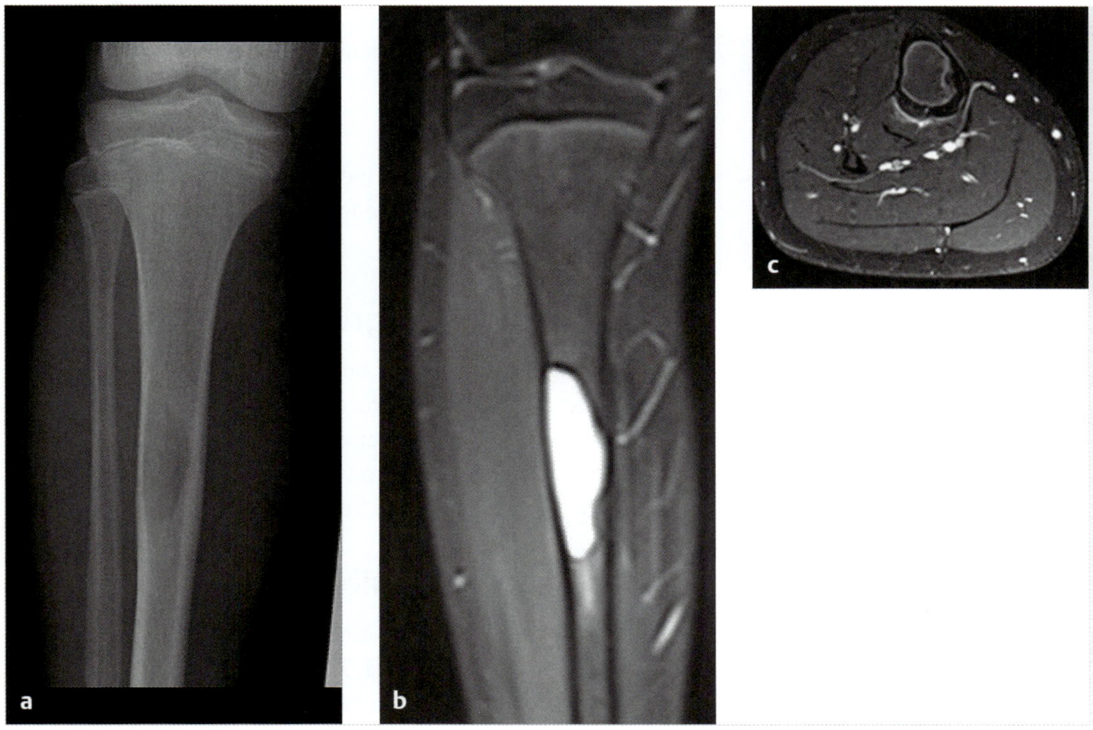

Fig. 7.19 a–c Unicameral bone cyst in a 15-year-old boy.

Final Diagnosis

Elongated area of fibrous dysplasia in the right tibia, classified as a “leave me alone” or “don’t touch me” lesion.

Comments

A ground-glass pattern on radiographs and/or CT enables us to classify an expansile lesion as fibrous dysplasia. There is still no pathognomonic sign for fibrous dysplasia on MRI.

Case 140 (▶ Fig. 7.20)

Case description

- Referring physician: rheumatologist.
- Prior history and clinical question: A 58-year-old man had experienced increasing left knee pain for years. Arthroscopic findings were deemed normal for age. MRI showed nonspecific edema-like signal in the upper tibia. A radiograph showed an unspecified lucency in the anterior tibial epimetaphysis (▶ Fig. 7.20 **a**), and subsequent CT revealed “nonspecific structural changes” in the upper tibia (▶ Fig. 7.20 **c**). Finally, scintigraphy with technetium 99m-labeled anti-granulocyte antibodies was performed after initial standard Tc bone scan (▶ Fig. 7.20 **b**). The Tc scan showed intense uptake in the upper tibia, while the antibody scan was only weakly positive. Even so, the differential diagnosis at that time consisted of osteomyelitis versus a bone tumor (e. g., non-Hodgkin lymphoma). To resolve the issue, an open biopsy was taken from the tibial tuberosity. The pathologist found neither a tumor nor a granulocytic inflammation but did find “pagetoid” bone remodeling. Because the patient had a normal alkaline phosphatase level, a diagnosis of Paget disease was ruled out. Other laboratory parameters were within normal limits. We were asked for our opinion.

Radiologic Findings

The lateral radiograph (▶ Fig. 7.20 **a**) shows increased lucency in the anterior tibial epimetaphysis as mentioned above. The AP radiograph (not pictured here) showed no abnormalities. Whole-body bone scintigraphy (▶ Fig. 7.20 **b**) shows intense tracer uptake in the epiphysis on delayed images. The uptake tapers into the anterior and lateral metaphysis in a geometric *wedge-shaped* pattern. Early-phase images (not pictured here) showed increased blood flow in the affected region. The bony structures in the upper tibia have a rarefied appearance on CT scans (▶ Fig. 7.20 **c**), with a coarsening of the “residual” structures. The tibial tuberosity also shows marked involvement by the remodeling process.

Location

The key radiologic findings are located in the proximal tibial epiphysis and form a V-shaped “wedge” that tapers into the anterior metaphysis.

Pathoanatomic Background of the Findings

We are dealing with an active bony process (bone scan) that is apparently destroying or transforming the bone. The location in the epimetaphysis and the distal wedge-shaped pattern of tracer uptake should evoke the engram for Paget disease (osteitis deformans). But beware of hasty conclusions!

Assignment to a Possible Basic Entity

▶ **Normal variant or malformation?** No. The increased lucency in the anterior upper tibia (▶ Fig. 7.20 **a**), which may be a normal variant in older individuals, should be considered pathologic due to the abnormal bone scan. This also applies to the coarsening and rarefaction of the trabecular pattern on CT.

▶ **Trauma?** No. The patient does not have a known trauma history sufficient to cause pagetoid bone changes.

▶ **Inflammation?**

- Not in the form of *osteomyelitis*, given the absence of bone destruction, sequestration, and periosteal reaction. Moreover, the clinical manifestations do not fit osteomyelitis, and the antibody scan is negative.
- Not in the form of *reactive osteitis* due to psoriasis, for example, because we do not see the pattern of concomitant bone destruction and reactive-reparative bone proliferation, especially at the periosteal level (see Case 145).

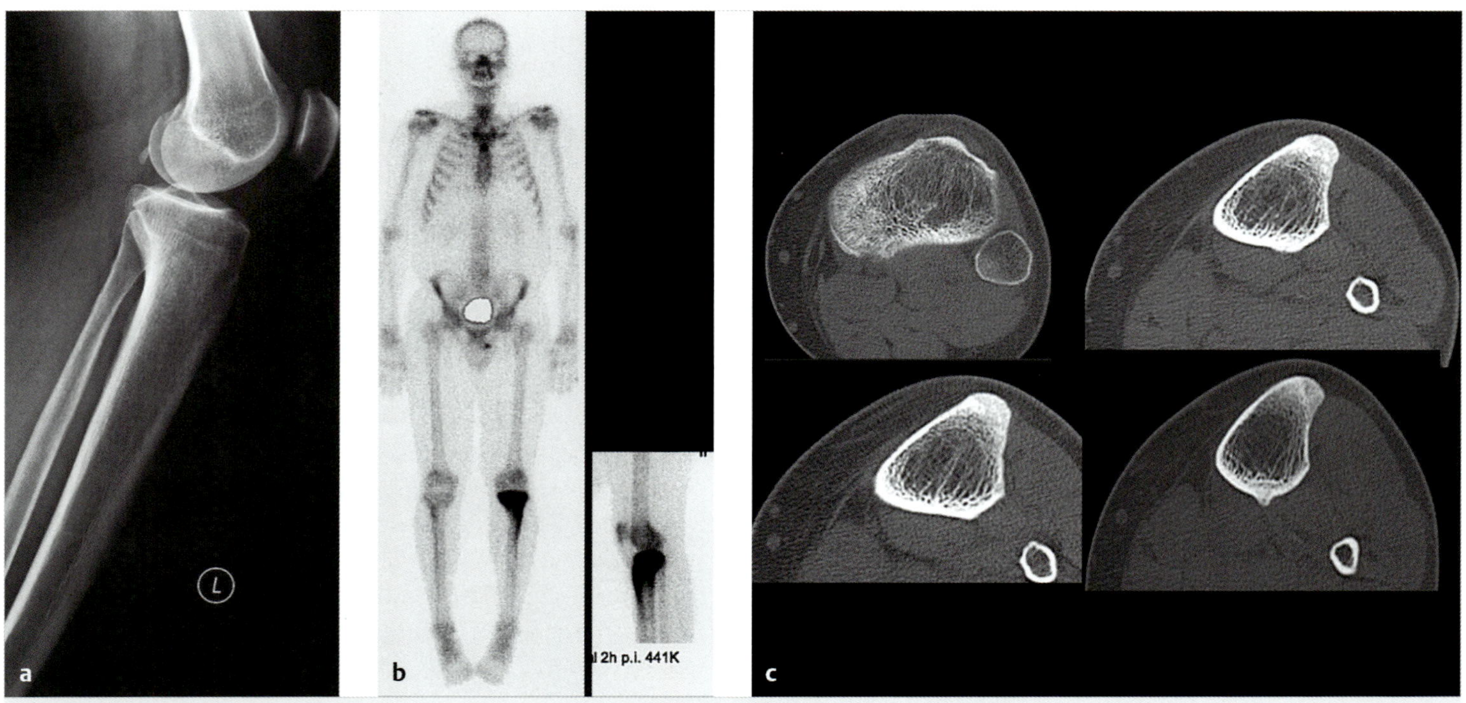

Fig. 7.20 a–c Osteomyelitis or tumor? Is another biopsy necessary?

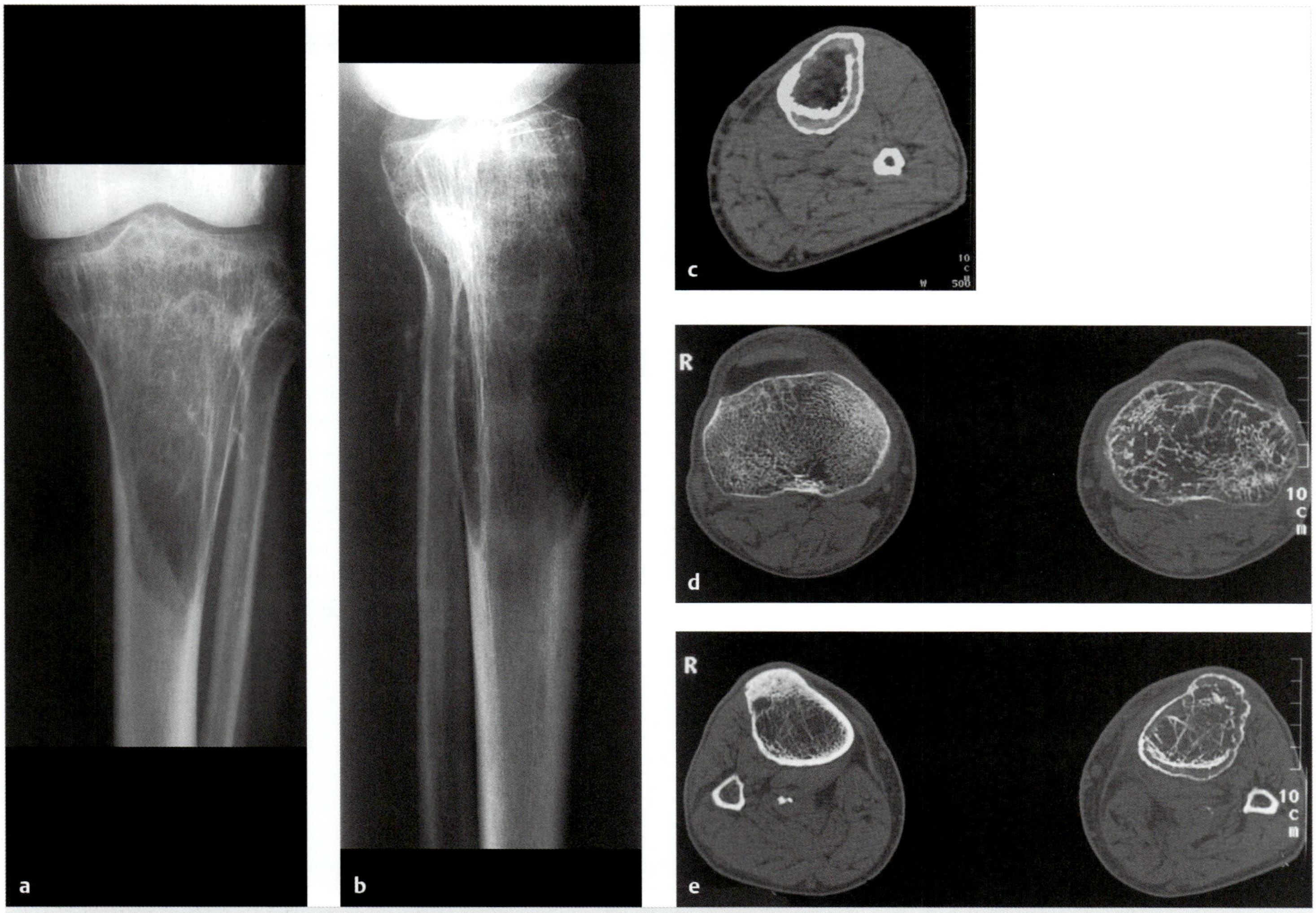

Fig. 7.21 a–e Paget disease of the proximal tibia in an elderly patient.

- In the form of *Paget disease*, yes. This disease involves uncontrolled bone resorption by stimulated osteoclasts and its replacement by primitive woven bone. This accounts for the increased lucency in the active phase of the disease and the coarsening of the "residual" trabeculae (▶ Fig. 7.20 **a, c**). The extreme tracer uptake on both early and delayed bone scans is also consistent with Paget disease, because increased tracer uptake in a bone segment is always a function of increased blood flow and increased bone turnover. Moreover, the disease begins almost exclusively in the epiphysis and then spreads to the metadiaphysis at an estimated rate of approximately 1 cm/year. The resorption front advances like a "drill head," creating a typical wedge-shaped pattern on bone scans (▶ Fig. 7.20 **a, b**). In the present case, the wedge is located in the tibial tuberosity.

▶ **Tumor?** No. A primary bone tumor would have caused geographic or moth-eaten destruction (osteolysis) of cancellous and/or cortical bone and might even have produced a calcified matrix. The bone scan is not consistent with osteoid osteoma (no double-density sign), and CT did not detect a nidus.

▶ **Degenerative change?** No, for what would have degenerated? The adjacent knee joint shows no clinical or radiologic signs of osteoarthritis.

Synopsis and Discussion

The following findings support a diagnosis of Paget disease:

- Age of the patient
- Location in the epimetaphysis of the tibia (a site of predilection)
- Plain radiographic and CT findings
- Highly specific bone scan
- Histologic description of findings was available, although a histologic evaluation is by no means conclusive in Paget disease

In at least 90 to 95% of cases, the diagnosis can be made from imaging findings alone. There are two findings that *might* argue against a diagnosis of Paget disease:

- *Normal serum alkaline phosphatase:* If the affected bone volume is small, the number of osteoblasts expressing alkaline phosphatase may be too low to cause a measurable elevation of alkaline phosphatase levels in the blood. Thus, the rise in alkaline phosphatase level correlates with the burden of osteoblastic activity. Moreover, an individual's level may vary considerably within the general normal range. This means that if a healthy patient normally has a low individual level, that level may be elevated as a result of disease but still fall within the generally normal range. (In the present case, incidentally, a follow-up at 8 months showed a definite elevation.)

- *Presence of pain:* Most cases of Paget disease are asymptomatic and are detected incidentally. Some cases are symptomatic, however. This may result from a low individual pain tolerance and/or increased regional blood flow in the active stage with increased prostaglandin production.

▶ Fig. 7.21 **a–e** illustrates another case of Paget disease of the proximal tibia in the lytic stage. The elderly patient noticed occasional slight local warmth and a prickling sensation in the proximal tibia, which also felt slightly warm to the touch. The proximal epimetaphysis shows almost a complete loss of normal cancellous bone structures, and only a few (new/old?) coarse trabeculae are visible (▶ Fig. 7.21 **a, b, d**). The osteolytic lesion tapers distally to a wedge shape (▶ Fig. 7.21 **a, b**) corresponding to the resorption front, which is a highly specific sign of Paget disease (see third point under Inflammation? above). The cortex is greatly thinned laterally and posteriorly. Axial scans of the diaphyseal portions of the lesion show a target pattern (▶ Fig. 7.21 **c, e**) with two outer rings formed by the split cortex and an inner zone formed by the fatty and intact medullary cavity. If further progression is not stopped by bisphosphonate therapy, the process will spread to the distal epiphysis over the next two decades, accompanied by "saber shin" bowing of the tibia. We assume that the disease began approximately 15 years earlier in the subchondral bone (see also Case 107). The patient's alkaline phosphatase level was elevated to four times normal.

Final Diagnosis

Paget disease (lytic stage) in the upper tibia, symptomatic and requiring bisphosphonate therapy.

Comments

What can we learn from this case? The diagnosis of Paget disease, which had been considered based on histologic findings, was deemed unlikely due to the normal alkaline phosphatase level, although it is known that many diseases do not always have a full "textbook" presentation. Bone scans showing a highly specific V-shaped configuration of the resorption front were disregarded, the pathoanatomic background was not reviewed, and scant attention was given to the remodeling processes depicted by radiographs and CT. On a more positive note: good results come from experience, and experience comes from bad results. The patient was finally placed on bisphosphonate therapy for 1 year and is free of complaints.

Case 141 (▶ Fig. 7.22)

Case description

- Referring physician: orthopedist.
- Prior history and clinical question: A 26-year-old woman underwent MRI for investigation of unexplained knee pain. The images showed a lesion in the proximal tibial metadiaphysis that was difficult to classify. Biopsy?

Radiologic Findings

The T2w image (▶ Fig. 7.22 **a**) shows a very hyperintense lesion with serpiginous margins located at a lateral, eccentric site in the proximal tibia. Fat-suppressed images after IV contrast administration (▶ Fig. 7.22 **b, c**) show intense rim enhancement with faint evidence of central septal enhancement. The cortex is thinned where it abuts the lesion. Supplemental CT images (▶ Fig. 7.22 **d–f**) reveal fine central calcifications. A striking feature is the undulating erosion, or scalloping, of the posterolateral cortex. The depth of the erosions is approximately one-half the normal cortical thickness.

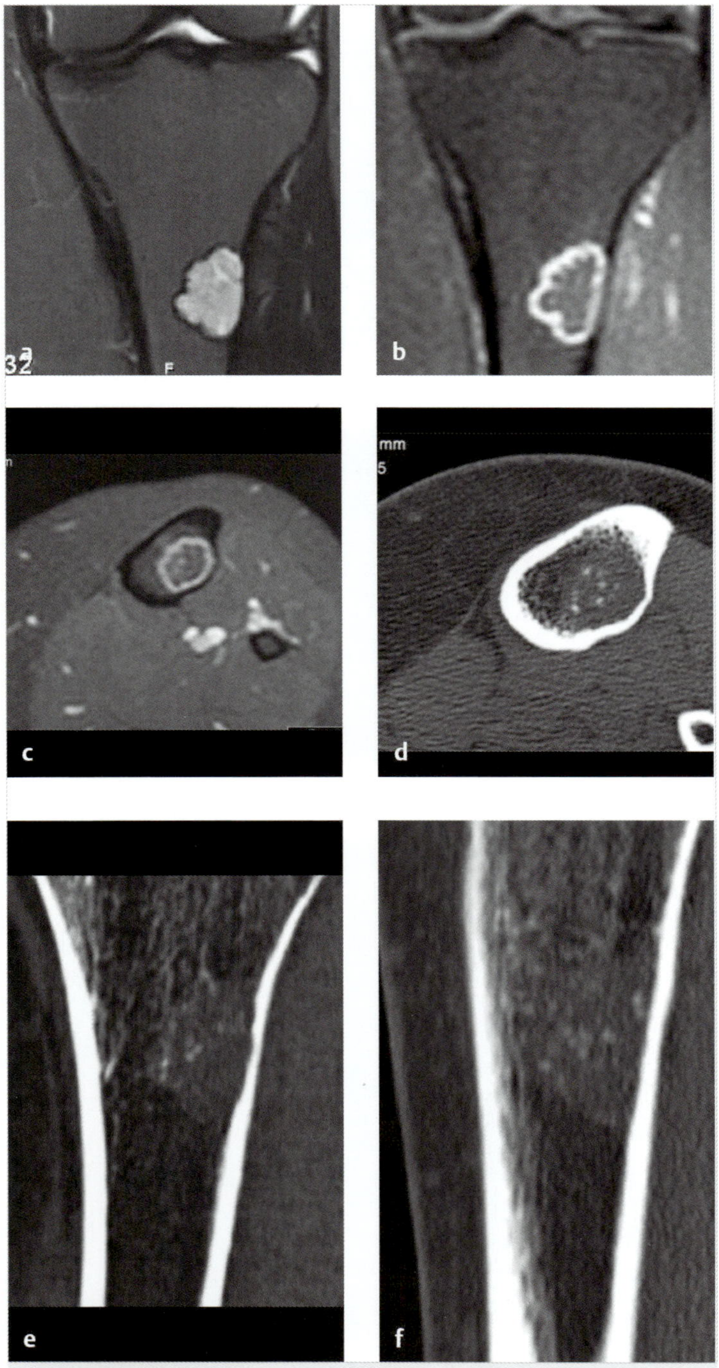

Fig. 7.22 a–f Tumor? Should it be biopsied?

Location

The lesion is located at an eccentric site in the proximal tibial diametaphysis.

Pathoanatomic Background of the Findings

The images show a solid mass lesion that has replaced the normal cancellous bone. The lobular structure of the lesion, indicated by its serpiginous margins and relatively high signal intensity, plus the septal enhancement and small calcific densities at the center, indicate a cartilage-forming tumor with active resorption of the adjacent compact bone.

Assignment to a Possible Basic Entity

▶ **Normal variant or malformation?** No. The lesion was detected incidentally, but a normal variant has no known precedent at this location. The active state of the lesion (good blood flow, cortical bone resorption without an enosseous or periosteal reaction) is also inconsistent with a normal variant.

▶ **Trauma?** No trauma history.

▶ **Inflammation?** No. There were no clinical signs of inflammation, and the lesion was detected incidentally.

▶ **Tumor?** Yes. The key criteria for a tumor were described under Pathoanatomic Background of the Findings above.

Synopsis and Discussion

The tumor has a cartilaginous origin and was detected incidentally. It corresponds to a typical enchondroma. It shows no definite radiologic signs of a malignant cartilaginous tumor such as:

- Extensive cortical destruction (more than two-thirds of the cortical thickness over a significant length of bone), also called scalloping. The scalloping in our case was limited to one-half the normal cortical thickness. This also indicates absence of a paraosseous tumor component.
- Significant bone expansion, cortical thickening, and/or periosteal reaction.
- Large lesion with a longitudinal dimension greater than 10 cm. (The lesion in our case was ca. 3.5 cm long.)
- Intense inhomogeneous and/or septal enhancement on post-contrast MRI.

The diagnostic criteria for chondrosarcoma are also listed in Case 108.

Unlike tumors located at the center of the medullary cavity, eccentrically located cartilage-forming tumors in long bones tend to cause scalloping where they abut the cortex.[55] This is fairly self-evident and implies that cortical erosion with these lesions is a less critical issue.

Since none of the radiologic criteria for grade I chondrosarcoma (atypical cartilaginous tumor) are fulfilled, the lesion does not require biopsy or even surgical removal from an oncologic standpoint. It is reasonable to expect that the tumor will gradually mature and ossify over time, developing into what is called a "calcifying enchondroma." A follow-up should be scheduled at 2–3 years. If the tumor has not enlarged by that time, there is no need for additional follow-ups as long as the patient is free of complaints. This strategy should be carefully discussed with the patient. She should be told that in the very unusual event of malignant transformation in 20–30 years' time, the tumor will generally be a low-grade chondrosarcoma, which has a very good prognosis and requires only local surgical treatment. On the other hand, there would be no objection to having an experienced orthopedic surgeon remove the initial tumor by curettage, thus relieving the patient of any future problems.

Final Diagnosis

Active enchondroma growing at an eccentric site in the tibial medullary cavity.

Comments

Eccentric enchondromas in the medullary cavity tend to erode the adjacent cortex. This does not signify a malignant process.

Case 142 (▸ Fig. 7.23)

Case description

- Referring physician: orthopedist.
- Prior history and clinical question: A 16-year-old girl presented with an 8-week history of pain in her right thigh.

Radiologic Findings

An AP radiograph (▸ Fig. 7.23 **a**) shows subtle, moth-eaten osteolytic lesions (arrows) in the distal right tibial diametaphysis, classified as Lodwick grade III. A faint but continuous periosteal reaction is noted at the level of the lesions. Our colleague requested further investigation. The female patient did not present until 4 weeks later, by which time her pain had intensified and there was a palpable swelling on the medial side of her leg. The radiograph taken at that time (▸ Fig. 7.23 **b**) shows a massive increase in purely osteolytic bone destruction. The smaller osteolytic lesions have coalesced to a geographic area of bone destruction corresponding to Lodwick grade II. An overlying onion-skin periosteal reaction is present on the medial side.

Location

The osteolytic changes are located in the medullary cavity of the distal tibial diametaphysis and apparently have an extraosseous component, as indicated by the periosteal reaction.

Pathoanatomic Background of the Findings

The Lodwick grades of the lesion (initially grade III, later grade II) and the absence of any surrounding reactive sclerosis indicate a fast-growing process. This is also evidenced by the evolution of the periosteal reaction from a solid layer or shell to a lamellated pattern.

Assignment to a Possible Basic Entity

▸ **Trauma?** No trauma history.

▸ **Inflammation?** Possible from an imaging standpoint, since osteomyelitis may start with a moth-eaten pattern and then coalesce to a geographic lesion. Inflammation does not fit the clinical presentation, however. The lesion is so aggressive that the patient should have pronounced clinical symptoms (fever, periosteal abscess, etc.).

▸ **Tumor or tumorlike lesion?** Yes. The Lodwick grades signal a fast-growing process whose clinical features suggest a malignant tumor—either non-Hodgkin lymphoma or sarcoma. All we need for a more specific diagnosis is sectional imaging that can look inside the lesion. We next recommended CT (sectional imaging with x-rays!) to demonstrate any radiation-absorbing components in the lesion, that is, a mineralized matrix; this is problematic with MRI. The CT images (▸ Fig. 7.23 **c, d**) did show fine, unstructured calcifications within the lesion (arrow in ▸ Fig. 7.23 **c**). The cortex is perforated, and the onion-skin periosteal bone formation, a sign of discontinuous tumor growth, involves a good two-thirds of the bone circumference. This made the diagnosis clear: osteosarcoma. The tumor extent defined by subsequent staging MRI (▸ Fig. 7.23 **e**) roughly coincided with the CT findings.

Synopsis and Discussion

There can be no doubt about the diagnosis of osteolytic osteosarcoma, even if biopsy fails to give initial confirmation (in which case it should be repeated). The evidence for osteosarcoma is as follows:

- Age of the patient
- Tumor location (about 20% of all osteosarcomas occur in the tibial diametaphysis)

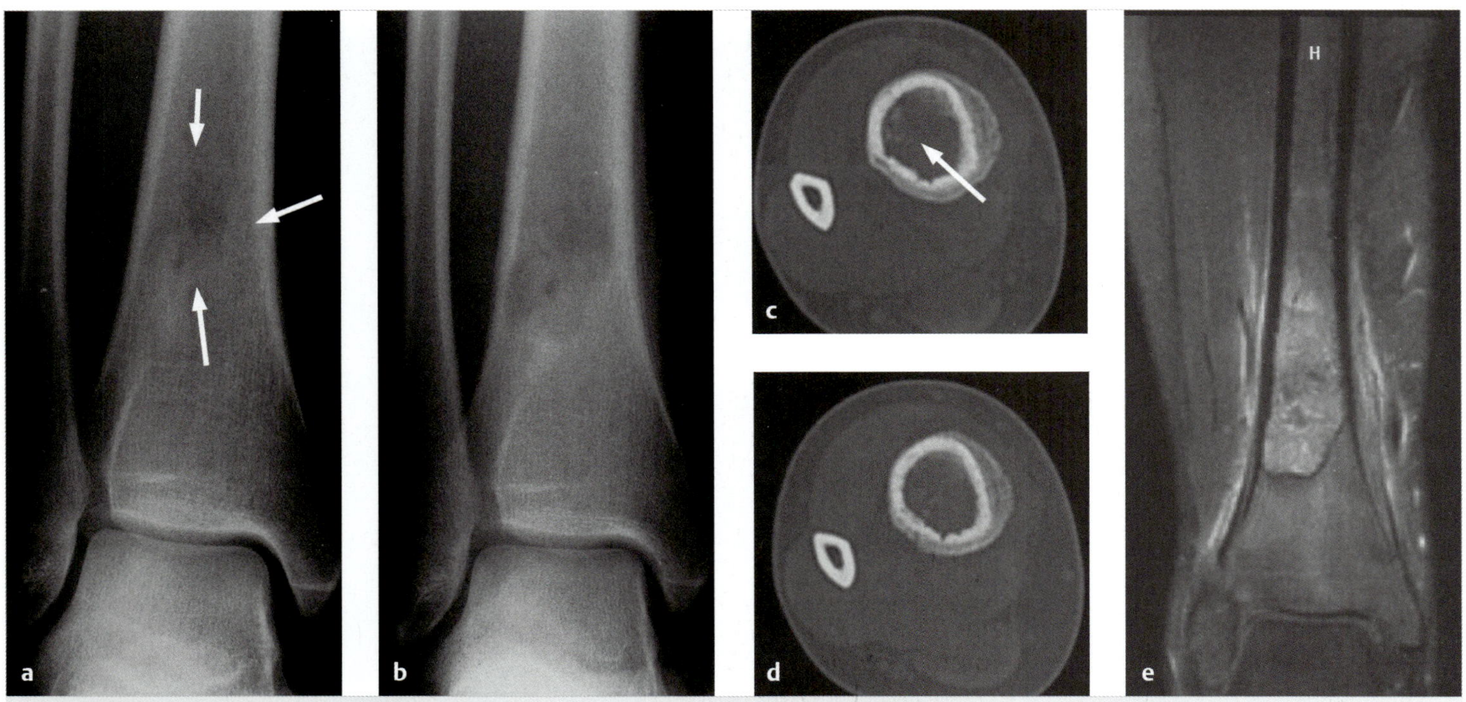

Fig. 7.23 Osteomyelitis? The images were obtained on April 1, 2003 (a), May 6, 2003 (b), and on May 14, 2003 (c–e).

- Pattern of destruction (Lodwick grades II and III, onion-skin periosteal bone formation)
- Mineralized matrix (does not support a diagnosis of non-Hodgkin lymphoma)

This diagnosis was confirmed histologically, but only after review by an expert reference pathologist.

The above critical remarks on histology do not mean that biopsy is redundant. It is the gold standard and will remain so, perhaps for the next 10 years. But when a radiologist is sure of the diagnosis, he or she should defend it and note the possibility of an inadequate specimen (sampling error) or lack of experience on the part of the pathologist, who may be highly specialized in a different area.

Final Diagnosis

Osteolytic osteosarcoma of the distal tibial diametaphysis.

Comments

An aggressive pattern of destruction (Lodwick grade II and III) on radiographs combined with a focal, coherent, but unstructured mineralized matrix in a long bone of a young patient is pathognomonic for osteosarcoma.

Case 143 (▶ Fig. 7.24)

Case description

- Referring physician: radiologist.
- Prior history and clinical question: A 15-year-old boy felt pain in his left tibia following a rough soccer match, prompting the radiographs in ▶ Fig. 7.24. The surgeon did not know what to make of these findings and proposed a biopsy followed by curettage, as he feared a spontaneous fracture. The radiologist at the same hospital interpreted the finding as a harmless, nonossifying fibroma of bone and requested "administrative assistance" to spare the boy unnecessary surgery.

Radiologic Findings

The radiographs (▶ Fig. 7.24 **a**, **b**) demonstrate an eccentric, relatively elongated, multicentric osteolytic lesion of Lodwick grade IA in the lateral portion of the left distal tibial diametaphysis. Each of the lucencies has rounded sclerotic margins. The pattern could also be described as resembling a "sack of tennis balls" or a bunch of grapes. The posterolateral cortex is thinned and expanded. Otherwise the surrounding bone appears normal.

Location

The lesion is located eccentrically in the distal metadiaphysis. It is clearly related to the tibial cortex.

Pathoanatomic Background of the Findings

The lesion appears to be loculated. The chambers are probably not closed compartments but peripheral septa-like bony prominences on the walls of the lesion. In considering how so many figures could appear on a plain radiograph, it should be noted that radiographic patterns often result purely from the summation effect of superimposed structures. The close topographic relationship to the cortex raises the question of whether the lesion may have originated from the metaphyseal cortex.

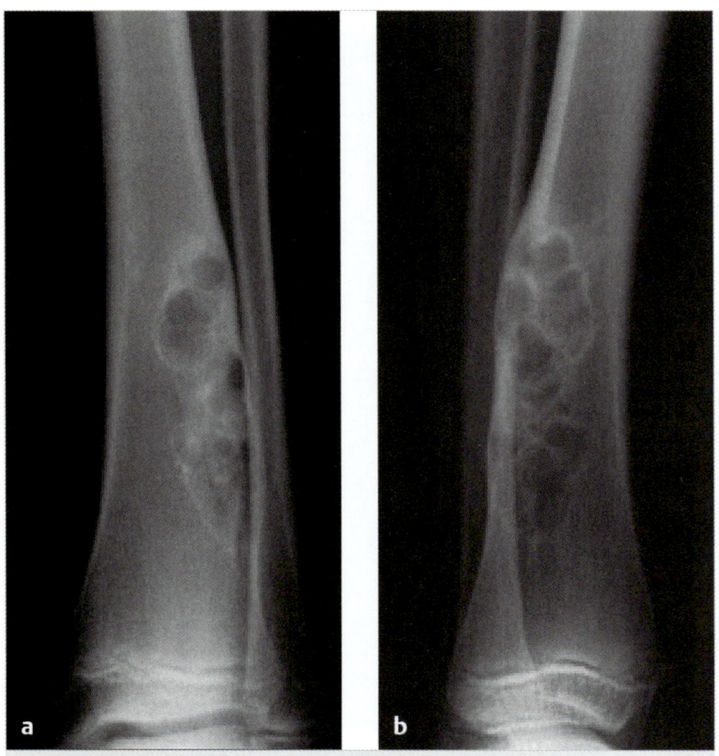

Fig. 7.24 a, b Is biopsy necessary?

Assignment to a Possible Basic Entity

▶ **Normal variant or malformation?** Possibly, if a nonossifying fibroma of bone is considered a normal variant. (Nonossifying fibroma is detected incidentally in ca. 5–7% of all knee examinations at an outpatient trauma center.)

▶ **Inflammation?** Even a previous episode of osteomyelitis would not leave this kind of radiographic pattern. Old osteomyelitis usually presents with sclerotic foci.

▶ **Tumor or tumorlike lesion?** Yes, our earlier discussions "let the cat out of the bag." We are dealing with a classic nonossifying fibroma of bone (or more correctly, a *fibrous metaphyseal defect in the stage of a nonossifying fibroma*).

Synopsis and Discussion

All the criteria for a *nonossifying fibroma of bone*, which today we interpret more as an osseous stress reaction at the enthesis of a tubular bone, are fulfilled. They include:

- Incidental finding
- Definite relationship to the metaphyseal cortex on which the enthesis is located, either as a ligamentous, muscular, or capsular attachment
- Skeletal immaturity
- Lodwick grade IA lesion with a cluster-of-grapes configuration

For comparison, ▶ Fig. 7.25 illustrates a *simple juvenile bone cyst*. The 9-year-old boy felt pain in the medial side of his distal left tibia after trauma. The pain could be localized to a single point (see marker in ▶ Fig. 7.25 **b**). The radiograph in ▶ Fig. 7.25 **a** shows an elongated osteolytic lesion in the distal medial tibial metadiaphysis corresponding to Lodwick grade IA. The medial cortex is thinned and slightly expanded. The arrow points to a

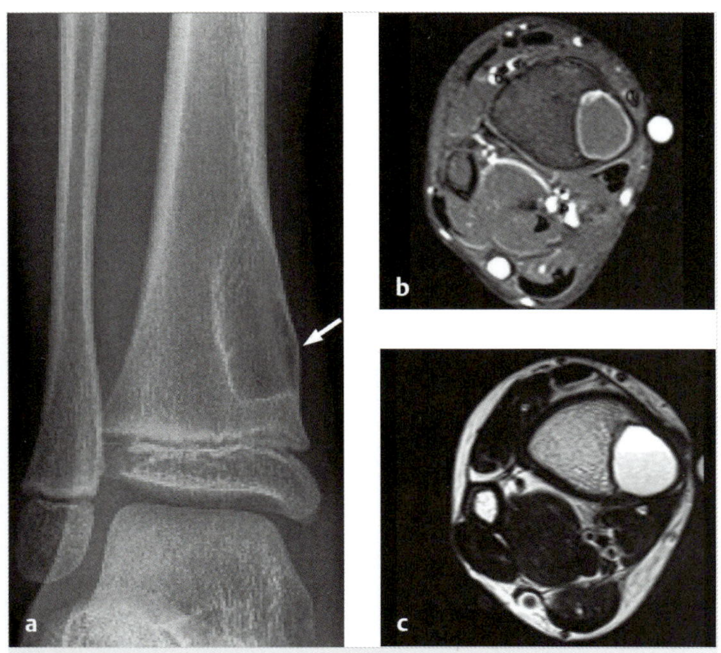

Fig. 7.25 a–c Simple juvenile bone cyst in a 9-year-old boy.

fine fracture line. The differential diagnosis included an atypical, nonossifying fibroma of bone (because of its relation to the cortex) and a juvenile bone cyst (unicameral lesion). But the eccentric location of the lesion was not typical of a juvenile bone cyst. Contrast-enhanced MRI (▶ Fig. 7.25 **b**) provided clarity by demonstrating the typical wall of a juvenile bone cyst (see Case 132). The fluid level in the axial image (▶ Fig. 7.25 **c**) confirmed the liquid content. Apparently the trauma caused the small cortical fissure fracture, which led to intracystic hemorrhage.

Final Diagnosis

Nonossifying fibroma in the distal posterolateral tibial metadiaphysis, a "don't touch me" lesion.

Comments

Incidental imaging findings should not be investigated routinely by biopsy just because their precise identity is unknown. An incidental lesion may consist of connective tissue and reparative bone, for example, which may also be mixed with giant cells. In many such cases the pathologist cannot supply a specific diagnosis and will turn to an experienced radiologist, or he may even interpret the histology as a giant cell tumor, etc.

7.3 Predominantly Osteosclerotic Changes

Case 144 (▶ Fig. 7.26)

Case description

- Referring physician: radiologist.
- Prior history and clinical question: A 19-year-old male complained of severe, non–exercise-related pain in the distal right thigh, also present at night and radiating to the knee. The region was warm to the touch. The patient did not have a trauma history. Unfortunately the first plain radiograph could not be located. A biopsy was taken from the distal medial surface of the femur without a presumptive diagnosis or suspicion. The pathologist could not classify the bone sample histologically and offered a vague diagnosis of "heterotopic ossification." Remarkably, however, he justified his diagnosis by the radiographic changes, which he considered typical of heterotopic ossification or myositis ossificans. The odyssey of the young man continued while his pain increased and was only moderately responsive to aspirin.

Radiologic Findings

First we reviewed the CT series, with the scans in ▶ Fig. 7.26 **a**, **c**, **e** shown here as representative images. They demonstrate an ossified mass abutting the medial diametaphyseal cortex of the distal femur. A narrow, spindle-shaped lucency is visible in the lower part of the lesion between the mass and the cortex. The lucency in turn contains a central linear ossification. The cortex beneath the spindle-shaped lucency is greatly thinned, and a cloudy sclerotic zone is visible in the underlying medullary cavity (arrows in ▶ Fig. 7.26 **a**). MRI (▶ Fig. 7.26 **b**) shows intramedullary and periosseous areas of edema-like signal.

Location

The epicenter of the lesion is definitely not located outside the bone, as in the case of heterotopic ossification. The lesion appears to be centered in the altered cortical bone.

Pathoanatomic Background of the Findings

The key question is whether the areas of new bone formation are tumor bone or result from reactive-reparative bone formation. Candidate lesions for tumor bone alone would be a periosteal or surface osteosarcoma. Tumor bone *plus* reactive bone formation may signify an osteoid osteoma, in which case the spindle-shaped lucency with internal ossification would be the nidus. The dense paraosseous and intracancellous bone formation would then be interpreted as a reactive process. A third realistic possibility would be a purely reactive process, such as enthesitic changes in a setting of psoriasis or pustulosis palmoplantaris (see Case 48, Case 82, and Case 145). From a pathoanatomic standpoint, we may exclude heterotopic ossification from the differential diagnosis for the reasons stated above.

Assignment to a Possible Basic Entity

▶ **Trauma?** The patient did not give a history of acute or chronic trauma.

▶ **Inflammation?** The possibility of a reactive inflammation was noted above, but the patient does not have cutaneous manifestations. The history does not support a septic inflammatory process with a central sequestrum, as the patient had no fever. Inflammatory markers were also normal. Osteo*myelitis* arising from the cortex also appears somewhat far-fetched.

▶ **Tumor or tumorlike lesion?** The two main candidates were noted above. But what was the next imaging study that could distinguish between osteosarcoma and osteoid osteoma before pro-

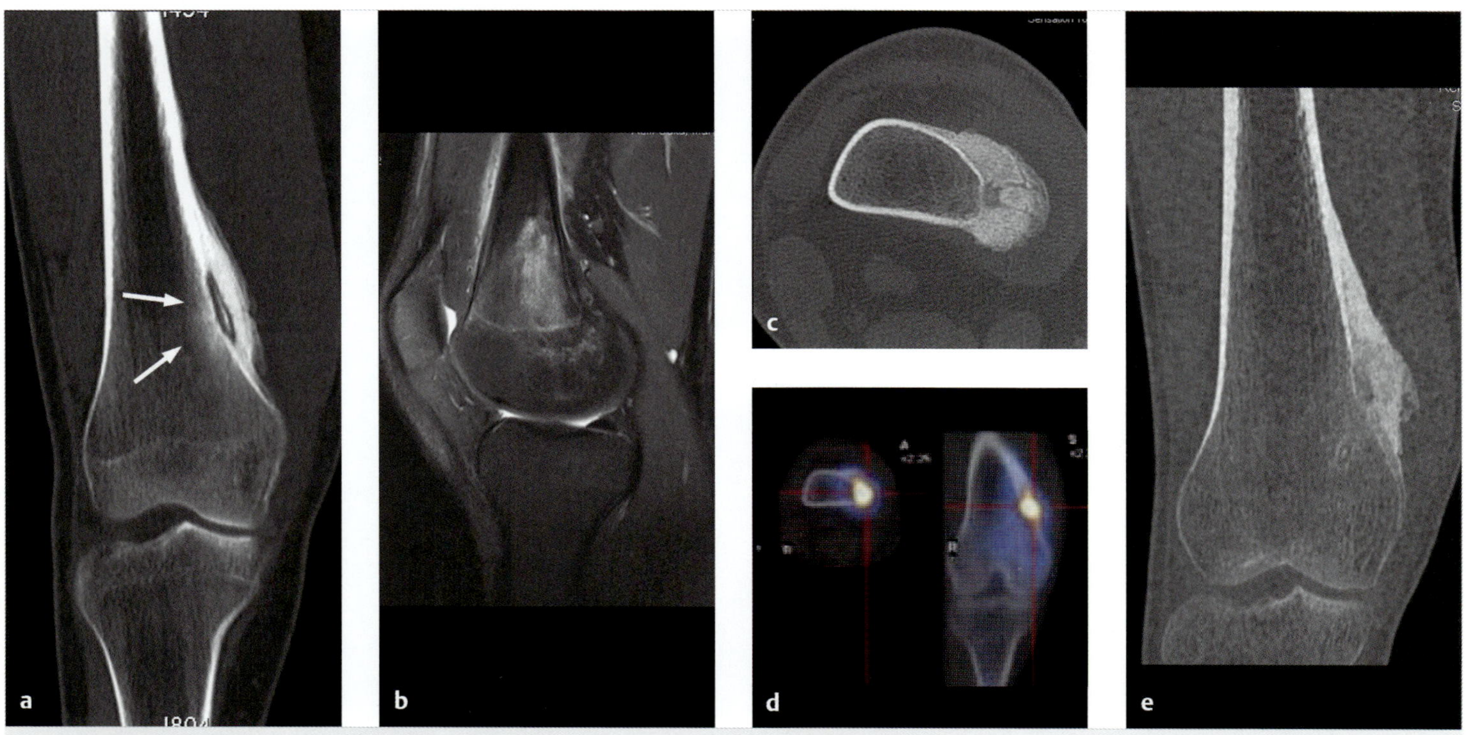

Fig. 7.26 a–e Heterotopic ossification?

ceeding with another biopsy? We chose the proven modality of bone scintigraphy (see also ▶ Fig. 4.44 **b** and ▶ Fig. 4.45 **c, d** in Case 74). Image fusion with CT (▶ Fig. 7.26 **d**) affords an impressive view of the double-density sign. The very bright center corresponds to the active nidus, while the surrounding activity is due to reactive new bone formation.

Synopsis and Discussion

The lesion is therefore identified as a *cortical osteoid osteoma*, which was subsequently enucleated under CT guidance and then confirmed histologically, although histology was not strictly necessary given the typical imaging findings. The patient was free of complaints on just the first day after surgery. This case clearly demonstrates where unprofessional image interpretation and a hasty blind biopsy may lead. The unusual feature of this osteoid osteoma is its spindle-shaped nidus, which is usually more round. But previous reports have been published on osteoid osteomas with a nidus up to 4 cm long.

As an aid to differential diagnosis, ▶ Fig. 7.27 shows an extensive *paraosseous grade I osteosarcoma* of the left distal femur in a 49-year-old man. The bone is encased by the densely ossified tumor masses (▶ Fig. 7.27 **a, b**). The underlying cortex is extremely thin and partly perforated on the medial side. The sectional images in ▶ Fig. 7.27 **c–f** show an intraosseous tumor component. This finding plus the cortical resorption and destruction are the principal arguments against an old subperiosteal hemorrhage culminating in myositis ossificans.

Final Diagnosis

Cortical osteoid osteoma with an unusual spindle-shaped nidus.

Comments

Bone scintigraphy is an underappreciated modality that can be very helpful when other imaging options have been exhausted. It indicates "where the action is."

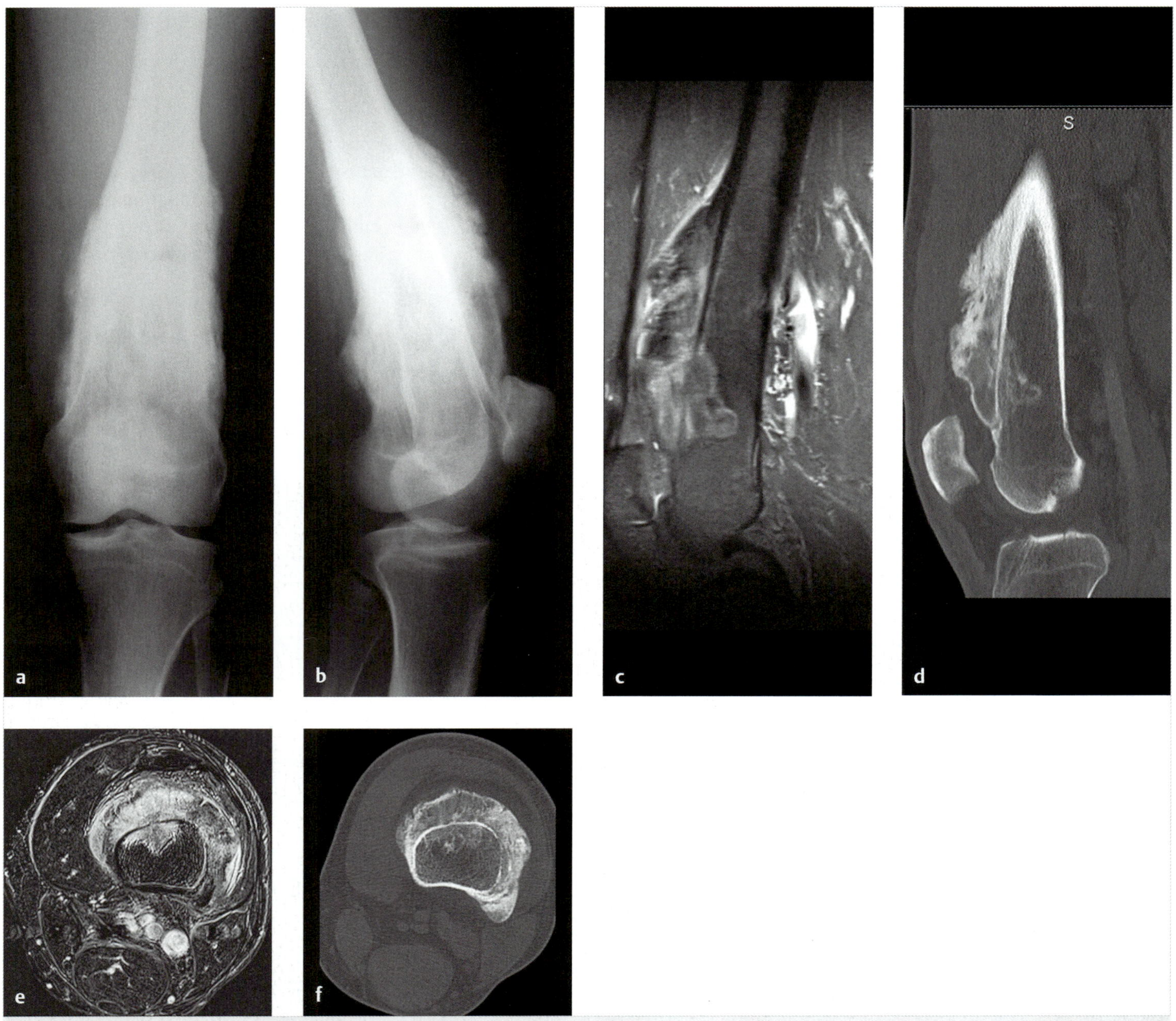

Fig. 7.27 a–f Paraosseous grade I osteosarcoma in a 49-year-old man.

Case 145 (▶ Fig. 7.28)

Case description

- Referring physician: radiologist.
- Prior history and clinical question: A 24-year-old man had an approximately 2-year history of pain in both knees but denied the occurrence of knee swelling at any time. He spent much of his time abroad. He had already undergone extensive rheumatologic and microbiologic tests, both domestically and abroad, but no specific disorder had yet been diagnosed. Water-sensitive MRI during the initial work-up (▶ Fig. 7.28 **f**) showed nonspecific increased signal intensity in juxta-articular portions of the femur and tibia, which were described only as "edema." Radiographs of both knees, particularly the right knee (▶ Fig. 7.28 **a, b**), showed sclerotic changes that could not be further classified. Whole-body bone scans (▶ Fig. 7.28 **c**) showed intense uptake in the right upper tibia and moderately increased uptake in both distal femoral diametaphyses (especially left anterior), mostly sparing the subchondral epiphyses. Consultation was requested, and we suggested CT as an adjunct to plain radiographs so that we could directly evaluate the surface and interior of the affected bones.

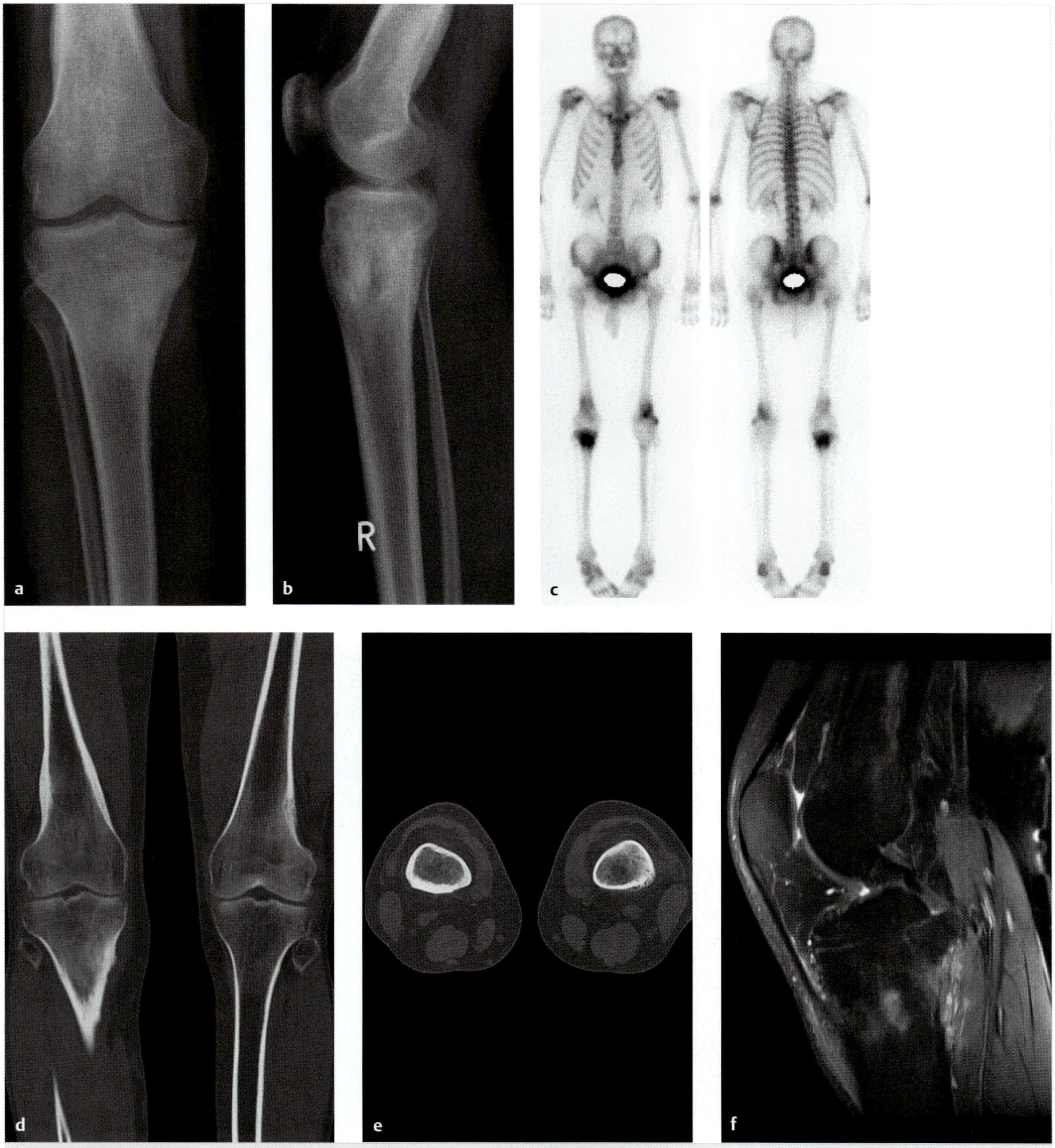

Fig. 7.28 a–f Chronic osteomyelitis?

Radiologic Findings

The findings on MRI, radiographs, and scintigraphy were described above. The CT images supplementing the radiographs (▶ Fig. 7.28 **d, e**) reveal sclerotic changes in the medullary cavities bordering the knee joint. The axial scans in particular (▶ Fig. 7.28 **e**) show that the productive sclerotic changes are accentuated on the cortical and periosteal sides and have led to marked thickening of the posterior cortex on the right side. Meanwhile, circumscribed destructive changes are noted in the posterior and posterolateral cortex on the left side.

Location

The above changes affect the diametaphyseal segments of the femur and tibia on both sides and involve both the cortical and cancellous bone, with relative sparing of the subchondral epiphyses.

Pathoanatomic Background of the Findings

The principal findings are as follows:

- Edema-like signal in the juxta-articular portions of the femur and tibia
- Active (bone scan!) sclerotic changes accompanied by some degree of cortical destruction
- Diffuse, bilateral medullary sclerosis

The bilateral occurrence of the changes suggests a systemic process that is associated with concomitant bone production and destruction at the attachment of the joint capsule and in the adjacent periosteum.

Assignment to a Possible Basic Entity

▶ **Normal variant or malformation?** No known precedents. Moreover, the patient is symptomatic and the imaging studies show signs of an active disease process.

▶ **Trauma?** No trauma history.

▶ **Inflammation?** Yes, but reactive in nature. This is evidenced by the bilateral occurrence of the findings, the edema-like signal, the positive bone scan, and the mixed destructive and proliferative changes. A bacterial inflammatory process is not consistent with the distribution pattern (diametaphyseal portions of the femur and tibia on both sides, sparing the joints and adjacent epiphyses).

▶ **Tumor or tumorlike lesion?** No, the bilateral occurrence in itself would not support this diagnosis.

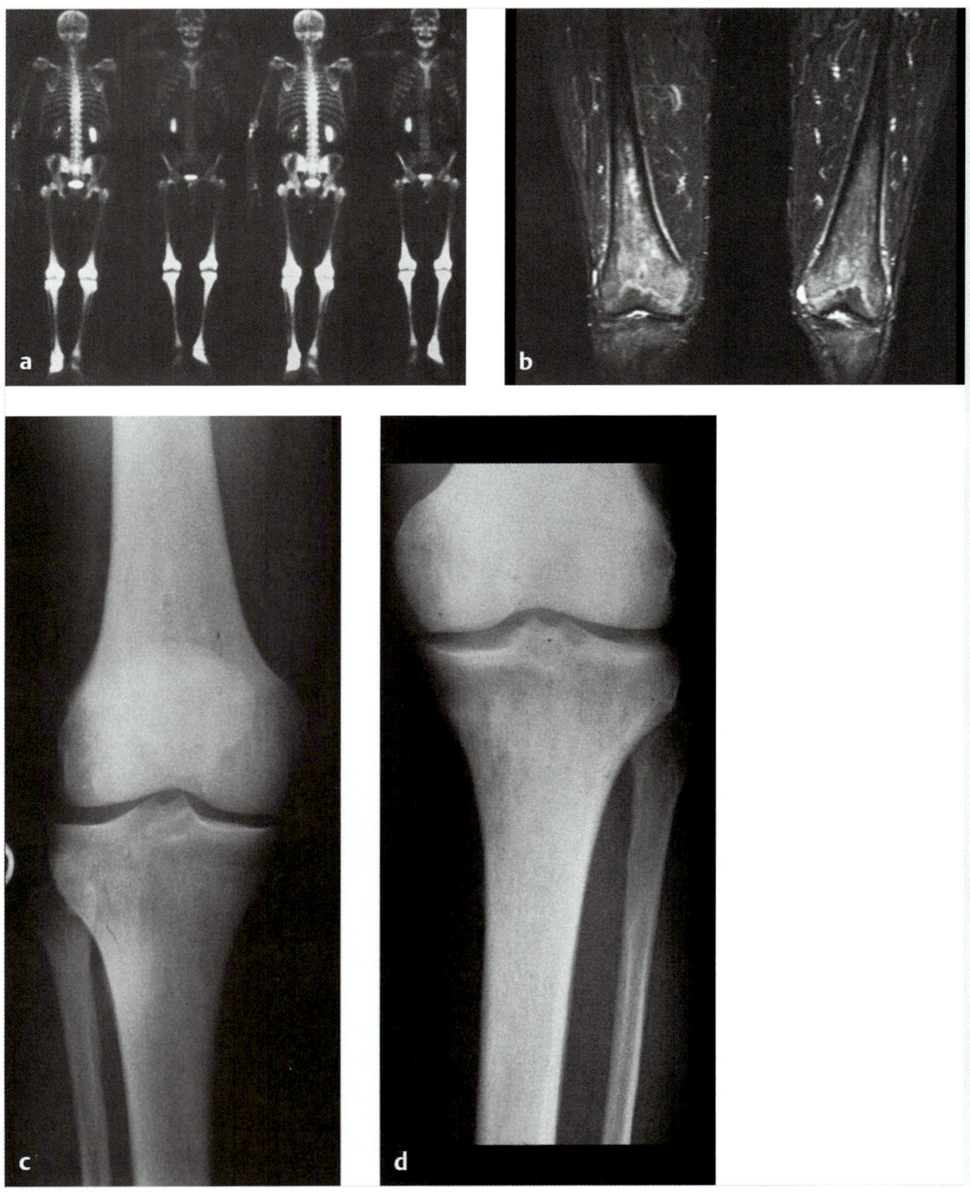

Fig. 7.29 a–d Lipoid granulomatosis in a 23-year-old man.

Synopsis and Discussion

Based on the above discussions, we are most likely dealing with a nonbacterial, reactive, systemic inflammatory process. The entheses—in this case the attachments of the knee joint capsule and the adjacent periosteum—are definite sites of predilection. This indicates a form of enthesitis, explaining why the changes are accentuated on the bone surface. At the same time, this does not exclude concomitant osteitis with an edematous component and sclerotic medullary changes; on the contrary, it makes such an interpretation quite likely. The distribution pattern and course are typical of the seronegative spondyloarthritides with or without involvement of the axial skeleton.

The patient's frequent trips abroad led us to consider Reiter syndrome, but subsequent examination by a dermatologist revealed very mild but histologically distinct psoriasis. Apparently the disease began at the sensitive entheses of the capsular and periosteal attachments to the bone, causing simultaneous bone destruction and proliferation at those sites and inciting an accompanying osteitis in the adjacent medullary cavities. A word about nomenclature: in rheumatology the disease would be called "psoriatic arthritis," although the patient did not have typical arthritis with joint effusion and swelling of the knee. Based on our current concepts, psoriasis-associated arthropathy with or without clinical effusion does not correspond to primary synovitis, like that occurring in rheumatoid arthritis, but to a nonspecific associated change that originates from the inflamed entheses. Consequently, we would avoid using the term "arthritis" for such changes and would rather name the disease in relation to its etiology, namely "psoriasis-associated enthesitis." Additional cases of "rheumatic" enthesitis are presented in Case 39, Case 40, Case 48, Case 49, and Case 97.

For comparison, ▶ Fig. 7.29 illustrates the case of a 23-year-old man with *lipoid granulomatosis (Erdheim–Chester disease)*. This is a systemic disease with obligatory skeletal involvement and frequently organ involvement (in 60% of cases). Affected medullary cavities and organs are infiltrated by histiocytes and multinucleated giant cells, and so this disease has parallels with Hand–Schüller–Christian disease. Nosologically, the disease is classified as a form of non–Langerhans-cell histiocytosis. The granulomatous changes in the bone marrow incite a reactive sclerosis, which is the radiologic hallmark. The medullary cavities about the knee joints are typically affected first, with possible additional involvement of the distal tibial metaphyses and regions about the hip joints. Later, the spine and skull base may also become involved. The typically diffuse or sometimes patchy sclerotic changes are confined to the medullary cavities (▶ Fig. 7.29 **c, d**). As in the case shown, there is an absence of periosteal new bone formation like that in psoriasis-associated enthesitis (▶ Fig. 7.28). The medullary cavities are hyperintense in water-sensitive sequences (▶ Fig. 7.29 **b**). Scintigraphic findings mirror the roentgen findings and are very specific, showing intense uptake about the knee joints (▶ Fig. 7.29 **a**) and in other epimetaphyseal areas that may be involved. Clinically, patients have bone pain only in pronounced cases, and symptoms arising from visceral involvement (e.g., retroperitoneum, heart, lungs, central nervous system, orbits, etc.) are usually dominant.[56–58]

Final Diagnosis

Psoriasis-associated enthesitis about both knee joints.

Comments

The decisive breakthrough to a clinically relevant diagnosis of psoriasis-associated enthesitis was accomplished by CT, which clearly demonstrated a mixture of bone destruction and bone proliferation at the entheses and their surroundings, which is very typical of this disease.

Case 146 (▶ Fig. 7.30)

Case description

- Referring physician: radiologist.
- Prior history and clinical question: A 41-year-old man had an approximately 7-month history of severe, non–exercise-related pain in the right knee, especially at night. He claimed that the knee had become increasingly swollen.

Radiologic Findings

A lateral radiograph of the right knee (▶ Fig. 7.30 **a**) demonstrates sclerosis in the upper tibia. MRI (STIR with fat suppression, ▶ Fig. 7.30 **b, c**) shows a large area of edema-like signal in the upper tibia and an intra-articular effusion. A small hyperintense focus (arrow in ▶ Fig. 7.30 **c**) is located medial to the midline beneath the anterior cortex. It appears on the supplemental CT scan (▶ Fig. 7.30 **d**) as a small osteolytic focus with central calcification (arrow).

Location

The small lesion is located in the subcortical upper tibia and is intra-articular, with an associated eccentric area of edema-like signal. Sclerosis is evident throughout the cancellous bone in the upper tibia (▶ Fig. 7.30 **d**).

Pathoanatomic Background of the Findings

It seems logical to relate the small lesion to the edema-like signal and sclerosis and consider it as the principal finding. The only lesion that is actually consistent with this set of findings is osteoid osteoma with associated edema and reactive sclerosis.

Assignment to a Possible Basic Entity

This assignment has already been made, and there is no reason to consider other possible entities.

Synopsis and Discussion

The history and imaging findings are so typical of osteoid osteoma that the patient was referred at once for CT-guided percutaneous enucleation. That procedure was successfully performed (postenucleation scan in ▶ Fig. 7.30 **e**) and the patient was completely free of complaints the following day.

This case again illustrates the distinctive features of osteoid osteoma:

- A small tumor with a big impact: The small size of the actual tumor, the nidus, is disproportionate to the extent of surrounding edema and sclerosis and the frequently severe pain, which is relieved by aspirin or NSAIDs in only about 60% of cases.
- The nidus is most clearly demonstrated by CT. A sure sign is central matrix calcification, which is visualized by MRI in many but not all cases.
- With an osteoid osteoma located in or near a joint, concomitant (sympathetic) effusion may be the dominant finding on MRI.

A somewhat unusual feature of this case is the age of the patient, since osteoid osteoma is rare after 40 years of age. Approximately 70% of cases occur in the first and second decades, around 20% in the third decade, and only about 10% in the fourth decade. In

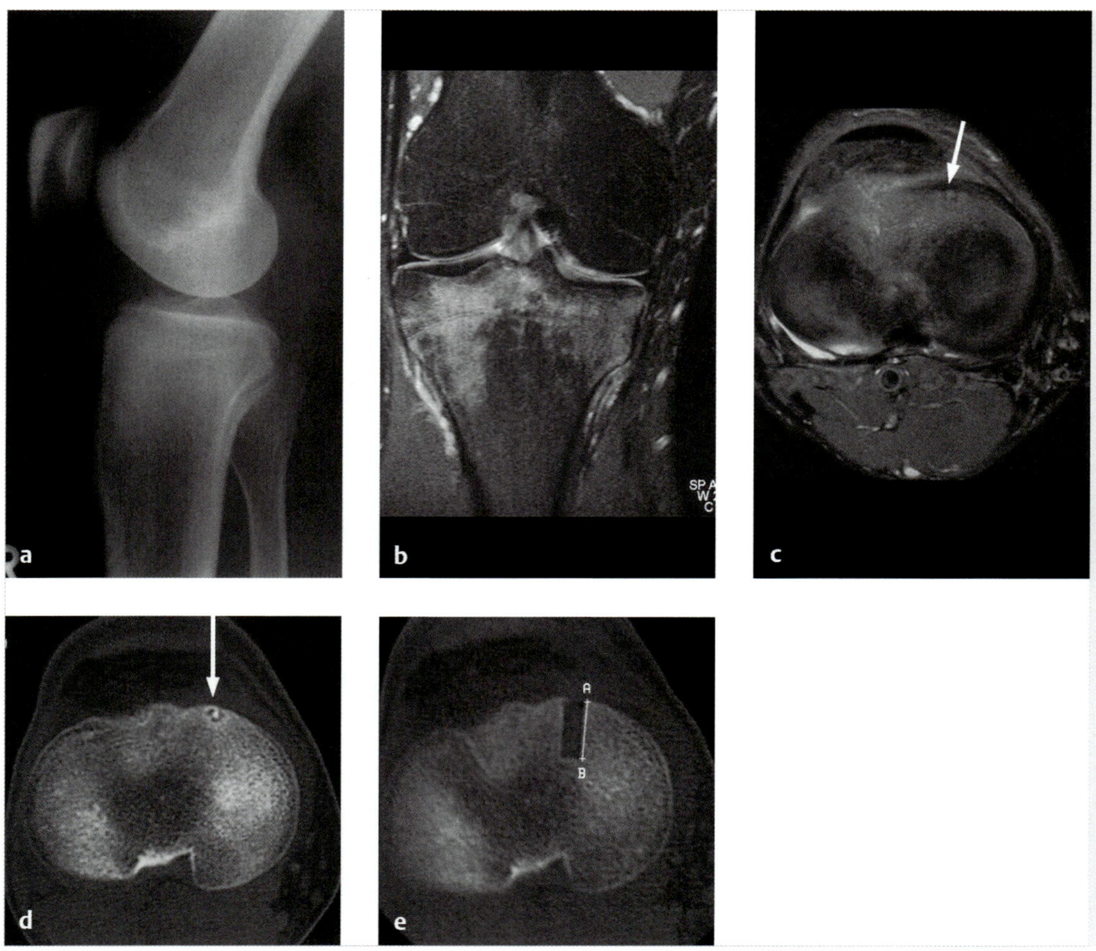

Fig. 7.30 a–e Chronic osteomyelitis?

recent years, however, we have repeatedly seen cases in which the tumor patient was in the fifth or sixth decade.

Neither this case nor the preceding one could be diagnosed on plain radiographs.

Final Diagnosis

Subcortical osteoid osteoma in the upper tibia.

Comments

Not infrequently, severe bone or joint pain in a young individual is caused by an osteoid osteoma, but this tumor may also occur in older patients.

Cases 147 and 148 (▶ Fig. 7.31 and ▶ Fig. 7.32)

These two cases are presented together for didactic reasons.

Case description

- Referring physician: radiologist.
- Prior history and clinical question:
  - Patient 1: A 48-year-old man had a 1-year history of exercise-related pain mainly in the right leg and more recently in the left leg. He claimed dysesthesias in the right leg and an occasional burning sensation plus local warmth. He denied any previous trauma. He was an active long-distance runner who ran 50 to 60 km per week.
  - Patient 2: A 15-year-old boy, very active athletically, complained of pain in his left lower leg, which was unrelated to exercise and worse at night. Clinically the area over the mid-tibia was warm to the touch.

Radiologic Findings

A lateral radiograph of the right tibia of patient 1 (▶ Fig. 7.31) shows massive fusiform thickening of the anterior cortex.

Radiographs of patient 2 (▶ Fig. 7.32) also show fusiform cortical thickening along the posterolateral circumference of the tibia.

Location

The hyperostotic tibial changes have a different location in each patient: anterior in the first, posterolateral in the second.

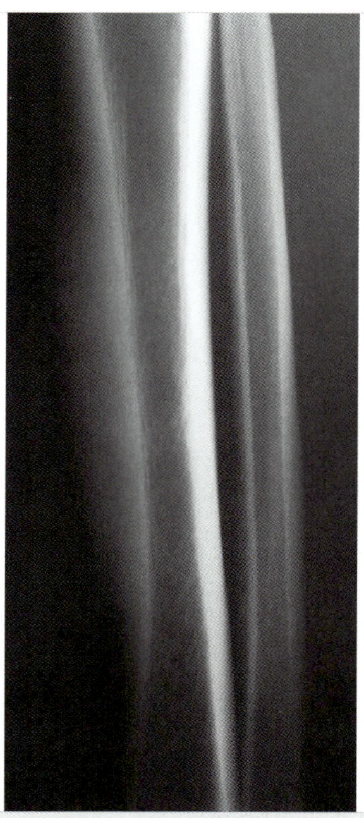

Fig. 7.31 Unexplained hyperostosis (patient 1).

Pathoanatomic Background of the Findings

It is reasonable to ask whether the solid cortical thickening has the same cause or a different cause in both cases. This question can be answered by reviewing the prior history of each patient:

- The most likely explanation in patient 1 is stress-induced hyperostosis.
- Given the age of patient 2, the location of the hyperostosis and the nocturnal pain, an inflammatory or neoplastic cause should also be considered.

This in turn suggests different imaging strategies for the further investigation of each case:

- Patient 1 should have a radiograph of the contralateral side, since hyperostosis should also be demonstrable on the left side if stress-induced hyperostosis is present.
- In patient 2, an effort should be made to “look inside” the hyperostosis and visualize a focus. This is best accomplished by sectional imaging.

Assignment to a Possible Basic Entity

▶ **Normal variant or malformation?** No. The radiologic changes in both cases are associated with definite clinical manifestations, apparently indicating a recent origin.

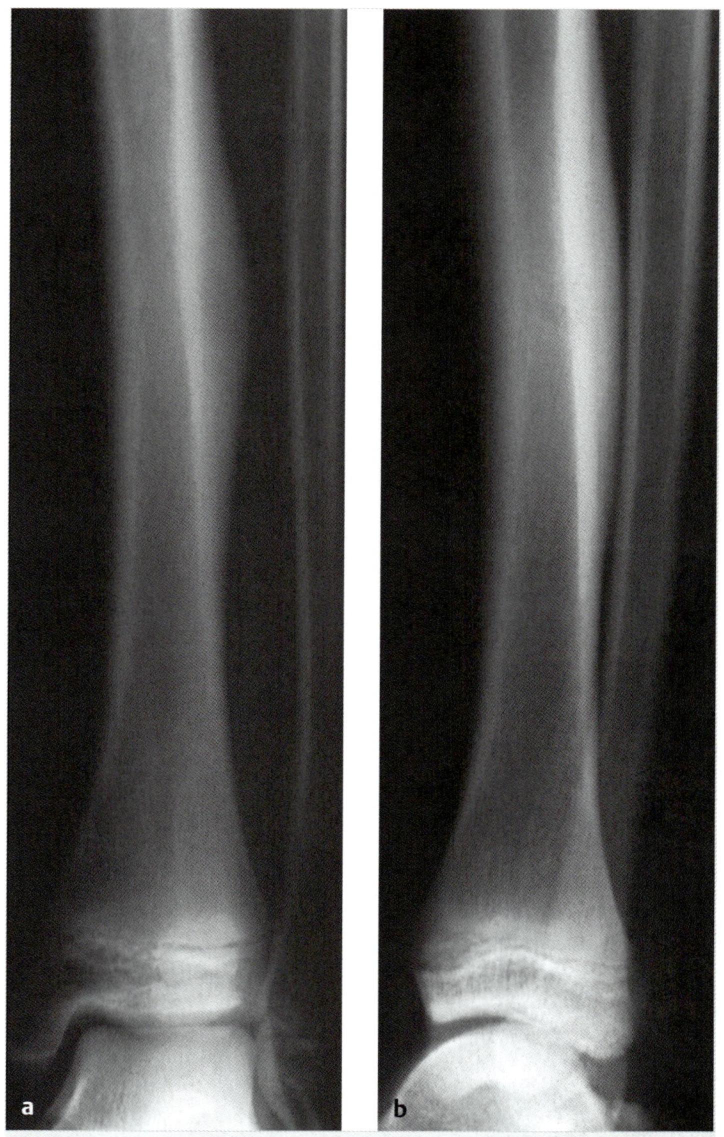

Fig. 7.32 a, b Unexplained hyperostosis (patient 2).

▶ **Trauma?** In patient 1: yes, his prior history as a long-distance runner implies an enormous sustained load on the anterior tibial margins. This is proven by the contralateral radiograph (▶ Fig. 7.33 **b**), which shows identical hyperostosis.

▶ **Inflammation?** In patient 2: no. The sectional images in ▶ Fig. 7.34 reveal a small cavity in the hyperostosis (marker in ▶ Fig. 7.34 **b**) and ossification within the cavity. This might be interpreted as a sequestrum in an abscess cavity, but the boy has no clinical symptoms of osteomyelitis (e.g., fever). Aside from this, the location of the proposed abscess cavity is implausible because it would imply cortical osteitis, which could result only from the external inoculation of an infectious organism through an open periosteal injury, for example.

▶ **Tumor?** For patient 2: yes. CT has "exposed" the typical nidus of an osteoid osteoma with central ossification. Osteoid osteoma is also consistent with the clinical presentation of non–exercise-related pain at night. In the representative MR image (▶ Fig. 7.34 **c**) the nidus appears as a faint, circumscribed hyperintensity within the hyperostosis. Its signal intensity is slightly higher than that of the tibial cortex, meaning that reactive new bone formation is still active. Marked edema-like signal is noted throughout the surrounding periosteal sleeve, which certainly contributes to the pain and local warmth felt at the mid-tibial level.

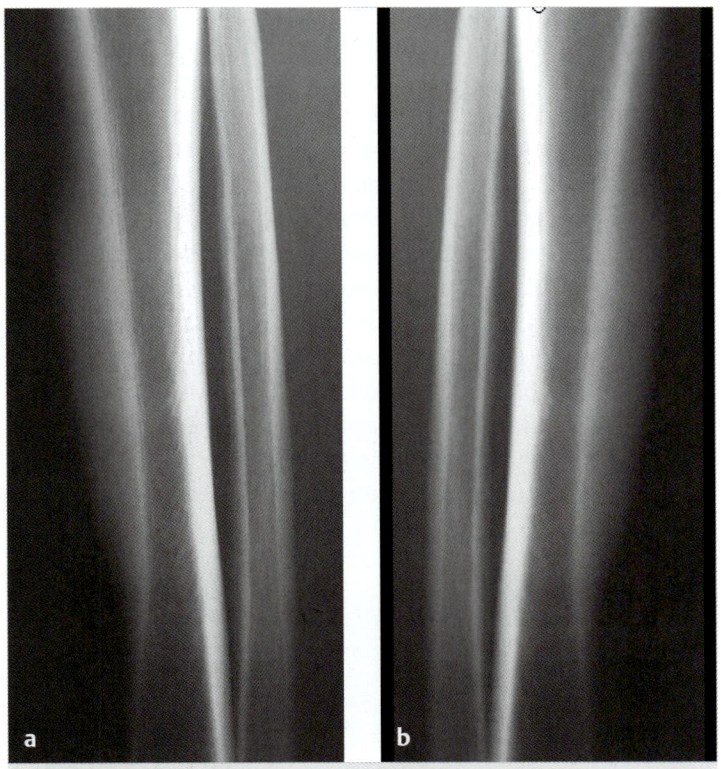

Fig. 7.33 a, b Radiographs of both sides in patient 1.

Synopsis and Discussion

The approach to correct classification of the tibial hyperostoses was based on the patients' histories and the supplemental imaging studies derived from those histories. In patient 1, a simple radiograph of the opposite side proved the presumptive diagnosis of stress-induced hyperostosis. In patient 2, supplemental CT was necessary to reveal the osteoid osteoma. It is also important to consider the different locations of the hyperostoses: The stress-induced case involved a typical site along the anterior tibial margin, whereas cortical osteoid osteoma does not have a known predilection for any particular side of the cortex, be it anterior, lateral, or posterior.

Of course, MRI could also have been performed in patient 1. It would probably have shown edema-like signal in the hyperostosis, adjacent medullary cavity, or adjacent anterolateral muscle consistent with an incomplete compartment syndrome. But this would not have had treatment consequences. As it is, the patient must discontinue jogging for the next 6 to 7 months and then, if he wishes, resume training in small steps according to pain tolerance. Our own observations have shown that stress-induced hyperostosis may well resolve when the affected bone is rested, and the complaints will subside as the bone regains its physiologic elasticity.

The diagnosis of stress fractures is illustrated in Case 129.

Final Diagnosis

- Patient 1: painful, stress-induced hyperostosis of the anterior tibial margin.
- Patient 2: osteoid osteoma with reactive new bone formation along the posterolateral aspect of the tibia.

Comments

Identical cortical hyperostoses on plain radiographs in different patients can be selectively investigated with simple techniques guided by each patient's history, age, and the location of the hyperostosis in the bone.

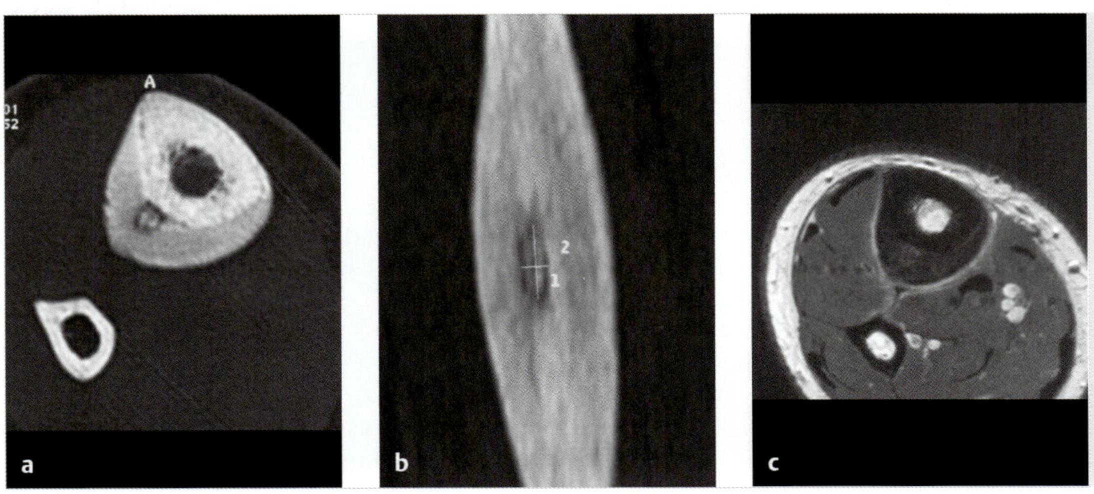

Fig. 7.34 a–c CT and MR slices of the tibia in patient 2.

Case 149 (▶ Fig. 7.35)

Case description

- Referring physician: rheumatologist.
- Prior history and clinical question: An 18-year-old man presented with signs of arthritis in the left ankle joint (swelling, local warmth, pain). We were asked to identify the cause.

Radiologic Findings

MRI of the affected ankle (▶ Fig. 7.35 **a**) shows definite edema-like signal in the talus and a joint effusion. Additional sequences and image planes did not add diagnostic information. We ordered a radiograph (▶ Fig. 7.35 **b**), which demonstrates sclerosis in the talus. The bone scan (▶ Fig. 7.35 **c**) shows very intense uptake in the talus.

Location

The MR images, radiograph, and bone scan show only an active pathologic process in the talus that cannot be further specified.

Pathoanatomic Background of the Findings

The sclerosis in the talus prompted us to look "behind the scenes," and CT was tailor-made for that purpose. The cancellous bone in the scans was obscured by diffuse sclerosis. At the center of the sclerotic area was a small lytic focus that was almost completely filled with a dense sclerotic figure (▶ Fig. 7.36). The small, centrally calcified or ossified focus in the talus, located just under its superior articular surface, apparently forms the epicenter of the process, that is, it is responsible for the sclerosis, the edema-like signal, and the intense uptake on the bone scan. The only lesion matching this description is osteoid osteoma. This diagnosis is also fully consistent with the patient's age.

Assignment to a Possible Basic Entity

It would be unrealistic to consider any other entity, as the clinical and radiologic findings are absolutely typical of osteoid osteoma (see also Case 74, Case 146, and Case 148).

Synopsis and Discussion

We present this case for two reasons:

- The patient was seen by a rheumatologist for painful monoarthritis. It was only natural for the rheumatologist to suspect a rheumatic disease (e.g., early ankylosing spondylitis, Lyme arthritis, etc.). He ordered MRI, which showed only an effusion in the ankle joint and edema-like signal in the talus. These could easily be interpreted as signs of arthritis. Ordinarily, the next study would be percutaneous aspiration of the joint for biochemical analysis of the effusion. In the present case, however, this procedure would not have yielded any useful information. The most likely presumptive diagnosis would have been nonspecific monoarthritis, prompting anti-inflammatory therapy that probably would have relieved the pain but would have been ineffective 2 weeks later due to persistent effusion.
- Starting the work-up with standard MRI of the left ankle and subtalar joints in this case masked the two essential features of osteoid osteoma: the nidus and surrounding sclerosis. If at least a simple lateral radiograph of the ankle joint had been obtained, the obvious sclerosis would have suggested the possibility of osteoid osteoma, and CT would then have been ordered to look for a nidus. As in other cases of osteoid osteoma included in this book (see also Case 74, Case 146, and Case 148), a specific MRI search for osteoid osteoma will detect the lesion in most but not all cases. But if this diagnosis is considered at all in a young man with monoarthritis, CT should be ordered as a practical matter to confirm the presence or absence of a nidus.

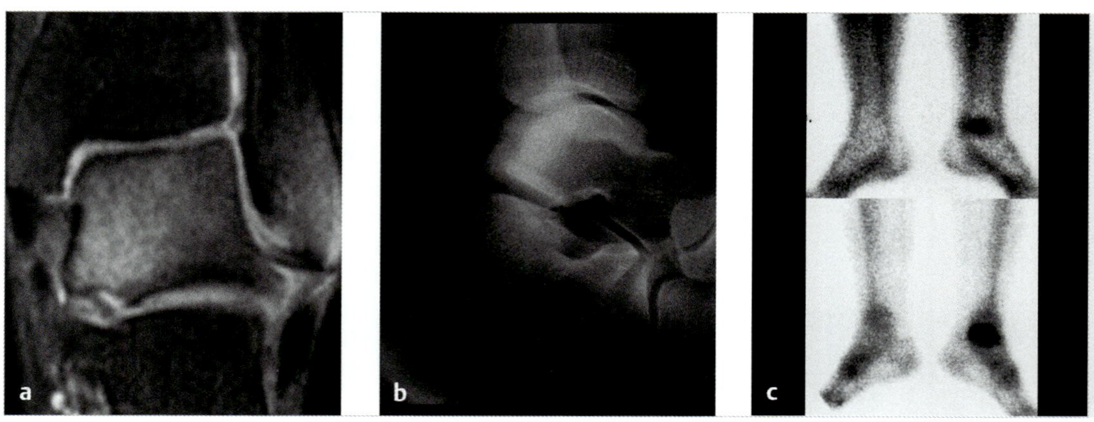

Fig. 7.35 a–c Arthritis with associated edema in the talus?

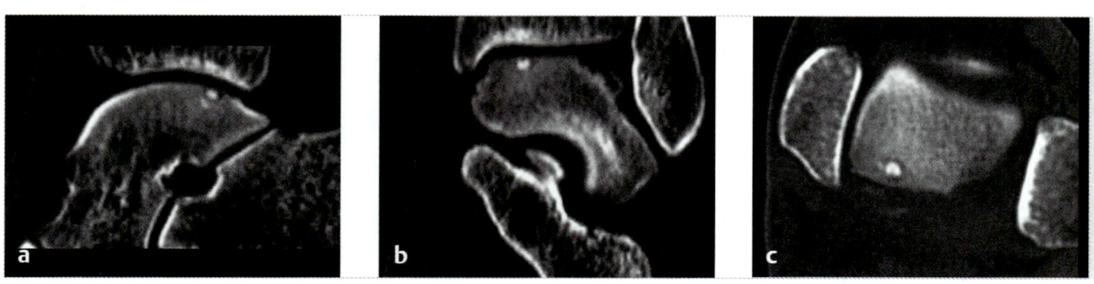

Fig. 7.36 a–c CT scans to supplement the findings in ▶ Fig. 7.35.

Final Diagnosis

Osteoid osteoma in the talus, located below the superior articular surface, with associated (sympathetic) arthritis.

Comments

During the investigation of monoarthritis in young patients, and especially in young males, it is important to consider the possibility of osteoid osteoma in the adjacent bone.

7.4 Changes with Mixed Features

Case 150 (▶ Fig. 7.37)

Case description

- Referring physician: orthopedist.
- Prior history and clinical question: A 10-year-old boy was kicked in the right knee while playing soccer. Afterward he complained of anteromedial knee pain and walked with a limp. He was an avid athlete and denied any previous joint complaints. Clinical examination 4 days later showed no external bruising and normal knee function. MRI was ordered "as a precaution."

Radiologic Findings

On the T1w images in ▶ Fig. 7.37 **a–c**, the bony portion of the lateral femoral condyle has a smaller volume posteriorly than the medial condyle, and the epiphyseal cartilage layer is very thick. The articular-sided border of the ossified lateral femoral condyle has a proximal convex outline and a somewhat jagged appearance. The water-sensitive images in ▶ Fig. 7.37 **d–h** show no evidence of edema-like signal in the lateral condyle. There is no visible bony element congruent with the apparent condylar defect.

Location

The apparent volume defect is located in the posterior bony portion of the lateral femoral condyle.

Pathoanatomic Background of the Findings

The ossification center of the distal femoral epiphysis (i.e., of the condyles) may have different medial and lateral calibers during growth and may present irregular contours. Asymmetries are not necessarily abnormal, therefore.

Assignment to a Possible Basic Entity

▶ **Normal variant or malformation?** Yes. As noted above, the medial and lateral portions of the ossification center of the distal femoral epiphysis may have different volumes during growth and may show corresponding volume changes in the overlying articular cartilage.[59] A normal variant is suggested by the negative history and by the absence of complaints at the time of clinical examination, with a normal gait and normal function tests. None of the MRI sequences shows any evidence of a pathologic process such as edema-like signal in the subchondral region of the medial femoral condyle.

Synopsis and Discussion

The apparent posterior depression in the ossification center of the lateral femoral condyle in this case prompted discussion about the possibility of osteochondritis dissecans. It was tempting, of course, to interpret the jagged bony depression as a defect due to osteonecrosis. But a matching fragment could not be found in the bone or in the adjacent joint. The cartilage overlying the depression does show compensatory thickening but otherwise appears completely healthy by MRI. There are no typical signs of

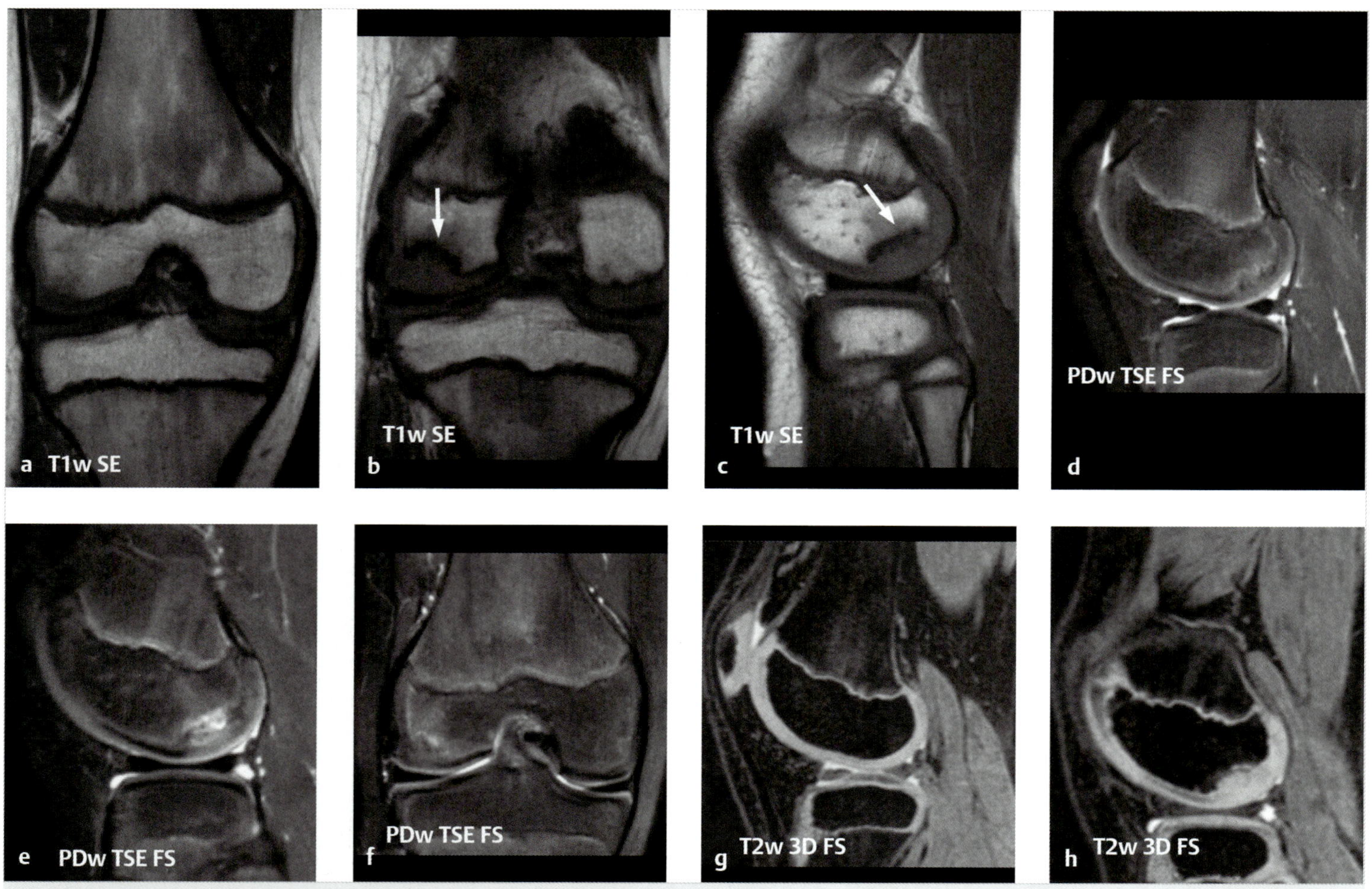

Fig. 7.37 a–h Osteochondritis dissecans?

osteochondritis dissecans such as edema-like signal in the adjacent bone or a hyperintense subchondral line or zone of demarcation. Moreover, the patient had no clinical manifestations and a negative prior history. By 1 year after initial imaging, the boy was completely free of complaints and was fully able to participate in sports. Since the advent of MRI in the diagnosis of osteochondritis dissecans, we have repeatedly observed similar findings that "resolved" over a period of months or years with no clinical sequelae.[17] Regardless of this, irregular contours and volume discrepancies between the medial and lateral portions of the distal ossification center, including multiple centers, are not unusual.

Final Diagnosis

Normal variant in the ossification of the distal lateral femoral epiphysis.

Comments

Variations in the volume and contours of ossification centers are likely to occur during skeletal growth. These normal variants require differentiation from osteonecrosis, especially osteochondritis dissecans.

Case 151 (▸ Fig. 7.38)

Case description

- *Referring physician:* pediatric orthopedist.
- *Prior history and clinical question:* A 1-year-old overweight child was found to have an increasing but painless varus deformity of the left knee and lower leg.

Radiologic Findings

Radiographs show a deep, medial depression with a sclerotic margin at the proximal meta-diaphyseal junction of the left tibia (▸ Fig. 7.38 **a**). The cortex distal to the depression is markedly thickened. Varus angulation of the tibia is also noted.

Location

The depression is located precisely at the insertion of the pes anserinus—the conjoined tendon of the sartorius, semitendinosus, and gracilis muscles.

Pathoanatomic Background of the Findings

The location of the depression at the pes anserinus insertion which is responsible for the varus deformity suggests that we are dealing with stress-induced bone resorption similar to a fibrous metaphyseal defect (e.g., at the insertion of the gastrocnemius heads).

Assignment to a Possible Basic Entity

▸ **Normal variant or malformation?** No, because we are dealing with an acquired, progressive change that became clinically apparent during the first year of life.

▸ **Trauma?** Yes. As mentioned above, the deformity was apparently a stress-induced change that developed when the somewhat overweight child learned to walk. The insertion of the pes anserinus is an enthesis, which appears to be very sensitive to overuse.

▸ **Inflammation?** No clinical manifestations.

▸ **Tumor or tumorlike lesion?** The concave defect could perhaps have been caused by an adjacent soft-tissue tumor. But the above considerations are more indicative of a stress-induced change that mimics a tumor and thus belongs in the category of tumorlike lesions.

Synopsis and Discussion

The stress-related defect in the medial tibial metaphysis is also known as *focal fibrocartilaginous dysplasia*. This term expresses the main histologic features of the lesion: the defect contains inactive fibrocytes and connective tissue with interspersed chondrocytes, which are elements of a fibrocartilaginous enthesis, except that the tissue is richer in collagen fibers and connective tissue than normal. The marked cortical thickening distal to the defect also suggests a stress-induced change. Similar to Blount disease (see ▸ Fig. 7.39), the dysplasia occurs in small children

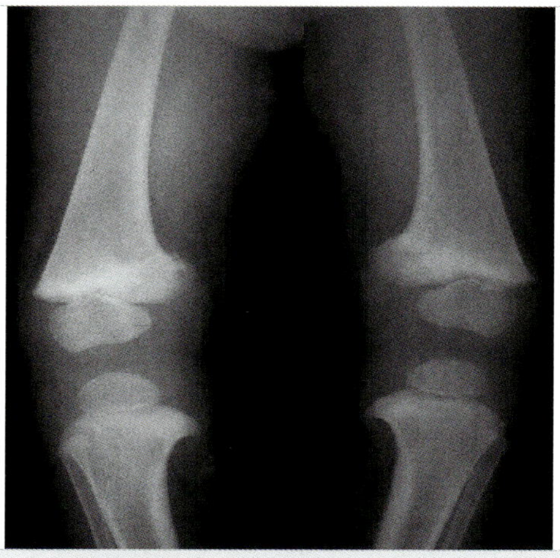

Fig. 7.39 Radiographic appearance of Blount disease.

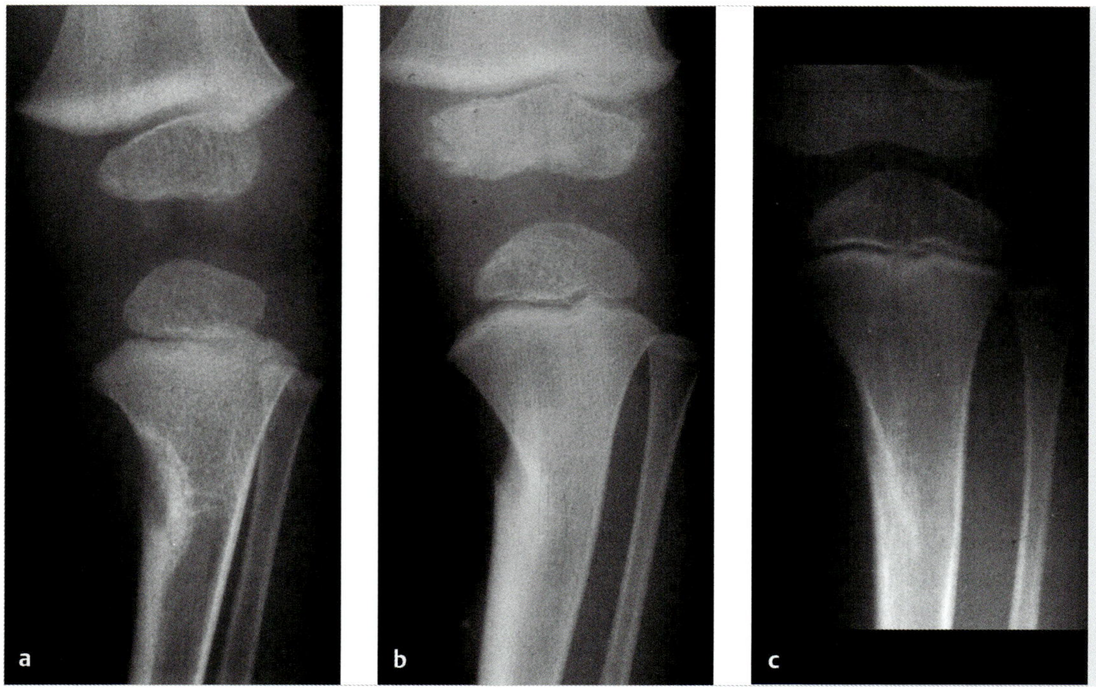

Fig. 7.38 Tumor? Images were taken in June 1997 (a), January 1999 (b), and in June 2000 (c).

learning to walk and apparently results from unaccustomed stress on the pes anserinus enthesis. Unlike Blount disease, it is typically associated with unilateral tibia vara. The stress-induced change resolves spontaneously over the next 2 to 3 years, as demonstrated by the follow-up images (▶ Fig. 7.38 **b, c**). Surgical correction and biopsy are both obsolete. As one would expect, MRI shows a mixed, predominantly hypointense signal pattern in the soft-tissue lesion.

▶ Fig. 7.39 illustrates a typical case of *Blount disease*, a growth disturbance characterized by bilateral varus bowing of the tibiae. It is observed in children and adolescents but, at least in the cases we have seen, appears to begin during the first year of life, affecting predominantly overweight children who learn to walk too early. Known also as "toddler's disease," it apparently results from a disturbance in the proliferation of growth cartilage in the medial proximal growth plates of the tibiae, leading to abnormal longitudinal growth on the medial side and varus bowing. Later, disturbances may also occur in the medial femoral growth plates. Unlike focal fibrocartilaginous dysplasia, the disease is progressive and does require surgical correction. A genetic predisposition is unknown. Radiographs typically show beaking of the medial tibial metaphyses with genu varum. In the case shown, similar changes are already apparent in the medial femoral metaphyses.

Final Diagnosis

Focal fibrocartilaginous dysplasia due to stress-induced enthesiopathy at the insertion of the pes anserinus.

Comments

The location of a lesion is often crucial for the correct interpretation of a radiologic abnormality.

Case 152 (▶ Fig. 7.40)

Case description

- Referring physician: radiologist.
- Prior history and clinical question: A 14-year-old boy presented with an extreme valgus deformity of the right knee with pain on weight-bearing. When we saw him, we elicited more details on his history and learned that he was a goalkeeper in his soccer team. When diving for a ball, he had a habit of landing on the ground with his right knee. He participated in soccer practice at least four times a week. A radiograph of the right knee joint showed extreme valgus deformity with maximum angulation at the growth plate, posterior slippage of the distal femoral epiphysis, and marked sclerotic changes about the lateral growth plate and over the bone surface. These sclerotic changes were considered suspicious for osteosarcoma.

Radiologic Findings

Radiographs of the right knee (▶ Fig. 7.40 **a, b**) show that the lateral portion of the femoral epiphysis is markedly diminished in height. There is abnormal widening of the growth plate laterally and posteriorly, and extensive sclerosis is noted about the plate. Ossifications are visible in the adjacent soft tissues, which CT (▶ Fig. 7.40 **d**) identifies as bone fragments. The posterior tilt of the epiphysis is best appreciated when compared with the contralateral side (▶ Fig. 7.40 **c**). The MR images (▶ Fig. 7.40 **e, f**) show a large area of edema-like signal in the distal femoral metaphysis. The sectional images most clearly define the massive extent of destruction and widening of the growth plate. Sagittal MRI (▶ Fig. 7.40 **f**) additionally shows a linear hypointense zone within the growth plate.

Location

The pathologic changes have their epicenter in the femoral growth plate.

Pathoanatomic Background of the Findings

The unusual changes in the growth plate and its surroundings are most likely a result of chronic trauma with necrosis and reactive sclerosis. The high signal intensity in the bone is probably due to accompanying osteitis.

Assignment to a Possible Basic Entity

▶ **Normal variant or malformation?** No, the changes first developed in association with abnormal stresses.

▶ **Trauma?** Yes. The deformities and structural changes are unquestionably related to the boy's habit of landing on his right knee when catching or deflecting the ball. Reliable signs of growth plate trauma are widening of the plate and surrounding sclerosis (see also Case 114). MRI shows signs of osteitis, which appears as increased signal intensity or a "bone bruise." The linear hypointensity in the growth plate (▶ Fig. 7.40 **f**) may be a slitlike discontinuity in the growth cartilage, probably due to necrosis or unresorbed bone debris.

▶ **Inflammation?** No clinical manifestations.

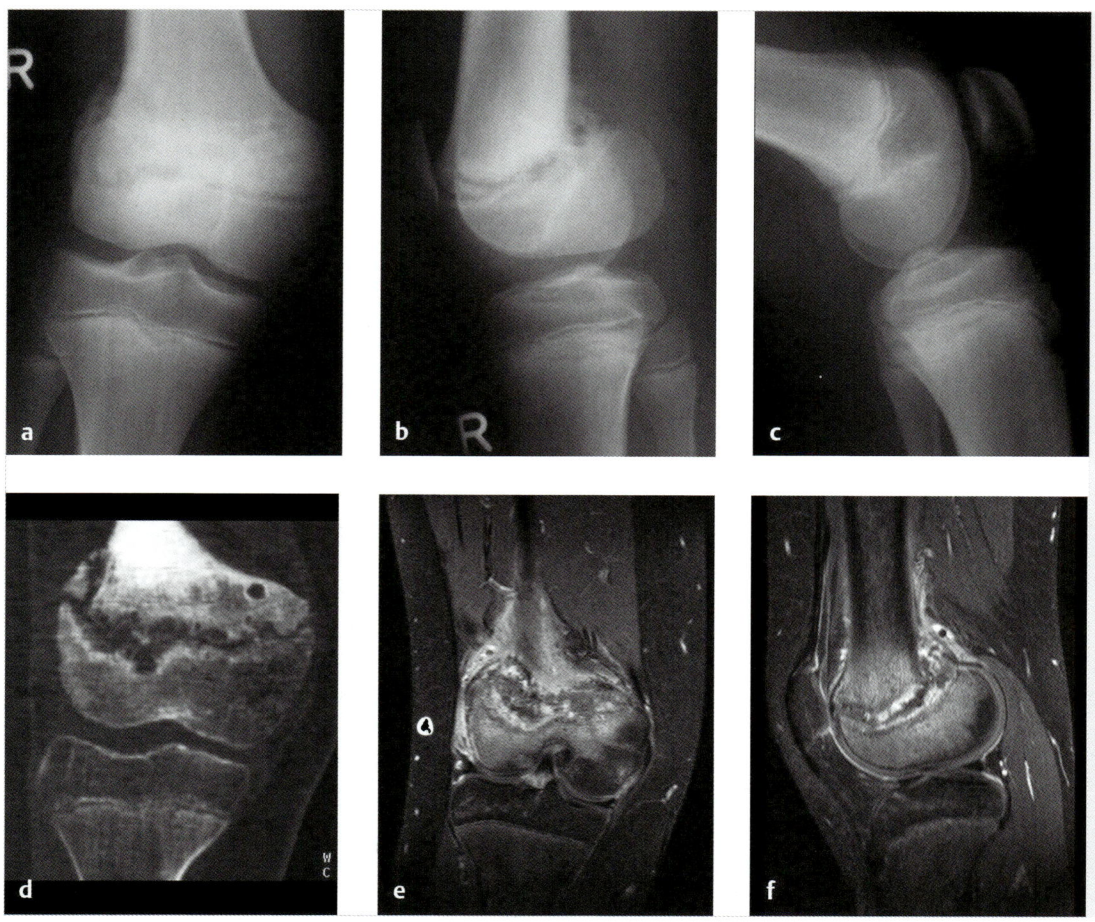

Fig. 7.40 a–f Osteosarcoma?

► **Tumor?** No, the sclerotic changes are reactive and do not represent the matrix ossification of osteosarcoma, for example. The paraosseous densities are bone fragments, as confirmed by CT. The epicenter of the changes is located in the growth plate, and there have been no previous reports of osteosarcoma originating at that location.

► **Necrosis?** It is certain that the changes include extensive foci of osteonecrosis, but they should be interpreted as epiphenomena.

Synopsis and Discussion

This case of severe growth plate destruction leading to loosening and displacement of the epiphysis due to repetitive trauma is very unusual. It is understandable, therefore, that its differential diagnosis would include a neoplastic process. In our view, the above arguments for traumatic destruction of the growth plate are so watertight that biopsy is unnecessary. Besides the typical imaging signs of growth plate destruction, the patient's history supplied the key to making a correct diagnosis.

An overview of growth-plate injuries in children and adolescents can be found in Frush and Lindenfeld[60] and Soprano and Fuchs.[61]

Final Diagnosis

Severe, stress-induced destruction of the distal femoral growth plate with displacement of the epiphysis, resulting from an unusual way of blocking kicks in soccer.

Comments

Widening of a growth plate combined with sclerosis of adjacent bone and displacement of the epiphysis are proof of primary damage to the growth plate. The most frequent cause of this damage is chronic repetitive trauma.

Case 153 (▶ Fig. 7.41)

Case description

- Referring physician: pediatrician.
- Prior history and clinical question: A 10-year-old boy presented with left knee pain, low-grade fever, and increased inflammatory markers in the blood.

Radiologic Findings

The radiographs show a destructive cancellous bone lesion, difficult to classify by Lodwick grade, located in the posterior portion of the proximal tibial metaphysis, in close proximity to the growth plate and more pronounced on the medial side. It has a moth-eaten appearance in the AP view, corresponding to Lodwick grade III (▶ Fig. 7.41 **a**), but it has a more IA appearance in the lateral view (▶ Fig. 7.41 **b**). The axial water-sensitive MR image in ▶ Fig. 7.41 **c** explains this discrepancy: The posterior string-of-beads hyperintensities, which correspond to the "holes" on the AP radiograph, occupy only about one-quarter of the sagittal diameter of the bone, so they are not dominant in the superimposed view. On the other hand, they occupy at least four-fifths of the transverse bone diameter in the frontal plane. This naturally has a much greater impact on the lateral superimposed view, which displays a complete geographic osteolytic lesion. Besides the destructive lesion, however, the radiographs also show areas of mild sclerosis. The MR image shows signs of joint effusion and slight involvement of paraosseous tissues. To narrow the differential diagnosis, additional MR images were obtained to look for more lesions. The coronal image in ▶ Fig. 7.41 **d** shows markedly increased signal intensity in the right inter- and subtrochanteric region, including the apophysis of the greater trochanter. A hyperintense ring is seen bordering the lower part of the apophyseal plate.

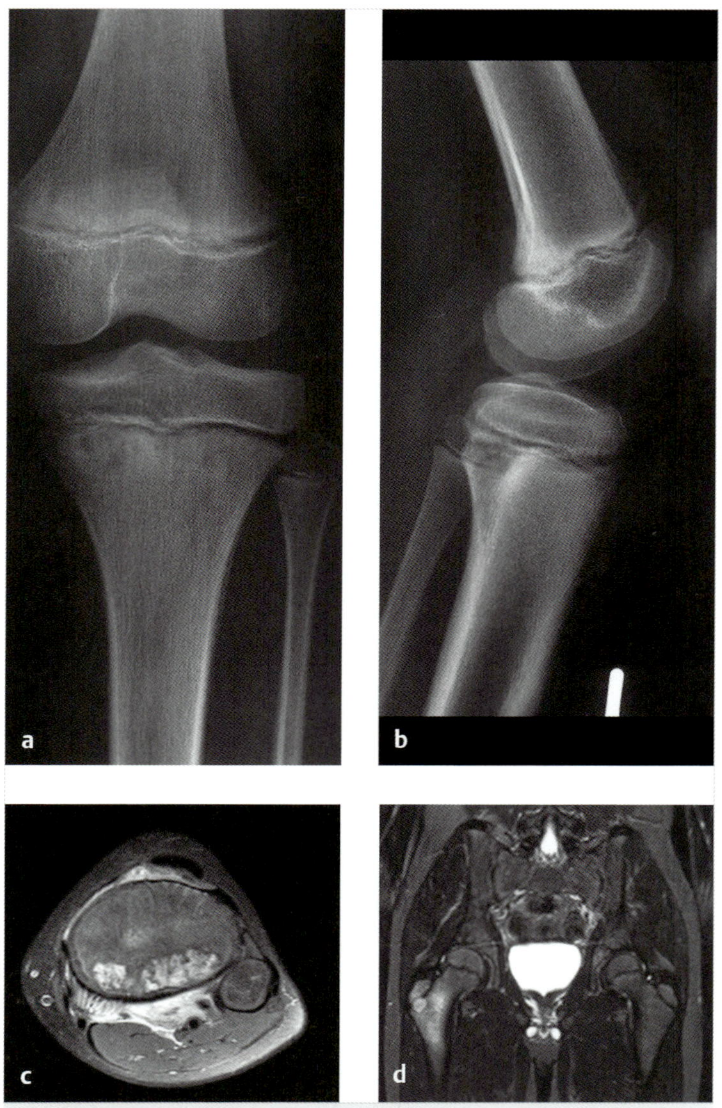

Fig. 7.41 a–d Osteomyelitis?

Location

The destructive process in the left tibia occupies an eccentric, posterior location in the proximal metaphysis. The hyperintensities in the right femur have an inter- and subtrochanteric location and also involve the apophysis. The hyperintense ring bordering the lower part of the apophyseal plate appears to be the epicenter of the lesion in the femur. Its signal intensity is similar to that in the tibia.

Pathoanatomic Background of the Findings

The radiographic destruction and sclerosis in the proximal tibial metaphysis and the abnormal signal intensities in the tibia and in the intertrochanteric region of the femur indicate two separate sites of a proton-rich process. The predominantly metaphyseal location of the foci is more consistent with an inflammatory process than a tumor (e.g., eosinophilic granuloma). The sclerosis associated with the destructive process is apparently reactive; this also fits with an inflammatory process.

Assignment to a Possible Basic Entity

▸ **Normal variant or malformation?** No, the imaging findings correlate with current clinical signs and symptoms (pain, fever, increased inflammatory markers).

▸ **Trauma?** No history of acute or chronic trauma.

▸ **Inflammation?** Yes. An inflammatory process is consistent with the clinical presentation (fever, etc.) and radiologic changes.

▸ **Tumor?** A tumor cannot be completely ruled out, perhaps an eosinophilic granuloma (Langerhans-cell histiocytosis). But this would not explain the metaphyseal location of both foci, which would be extremely unusual for eosinophilic granuloma. Also, that disease would not fit the clinical manifestations of this patient.

Synopsis and Discussion

All of the findings are most consistent with chronic nonbacterial osteomyelitis (CNO), which occurs predominantly in the metaphyses of the long tubular bones. ("CRMO" would be a misnomer in this case, as explained in Case 82). The findings suggestive of CNO are as follows:

- Fever, pain, increased inflammatory markers
- Metaphyseal location
- More than one focus

- Simultaneous bone destruction and reactive new bone formation on radiographs and a high proton density on MRI

As explained in Case 82, we classify this autoimmune disease as a rheumatic disorder, and more specifically as pustulous enthesio-osteitis (incorrectly termed "SAPHO") in patients who have clinical psoriasis or pustulosis palmoplantaris or a corresponding family history.

The child was treated with NSAIDs, resulting in rapid clinical and radiologic improvement.

Final Diagnosis

CNO with two foci (intertrochanteric region of the femur and proximal tibial metaphysis).

Comments

Multiple foci with a metaphyseal location that display mixed destructive and proliferative changes in a child or adolescent are always highly suspicious for CNO.

Case 154 (▶ Fig. 7.42)

Case description

- Referring physician: radiologist.
- Prior history and clinical question: A 13-year-old girl had increasing pain and swelling in her right lower leg. A sitting position appeared to aggravate her symptoms.

Radiologic Findings

The reformatted CT images in particular (▶ Fig. 7.42 **a, b**), as well as the axial scans (▶ Fig. 7.42 **d, f, g**), demonstrate marked vermiform or serpiginous lucencies with sclerotic margins in the tibia. These tracks are sometimes called "vascular or vessel prints" in radiology jargon. The MR images in ▶ Fig. 7.42 **c, e** show pathologic vascular structures in the bone, which correlate with the vascular prints.

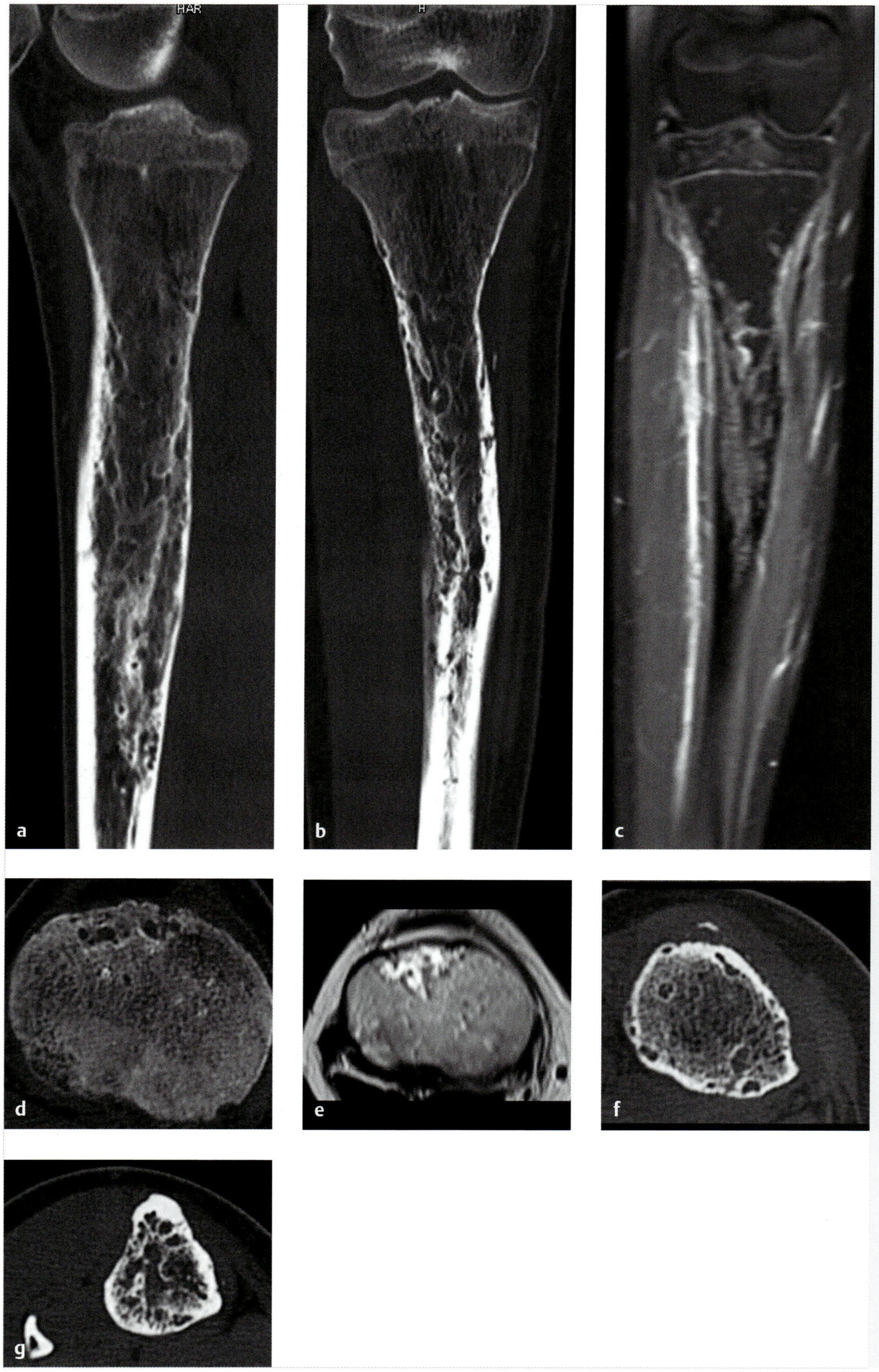

Fig. 7.42 a–g Was this done by a bark beetle?

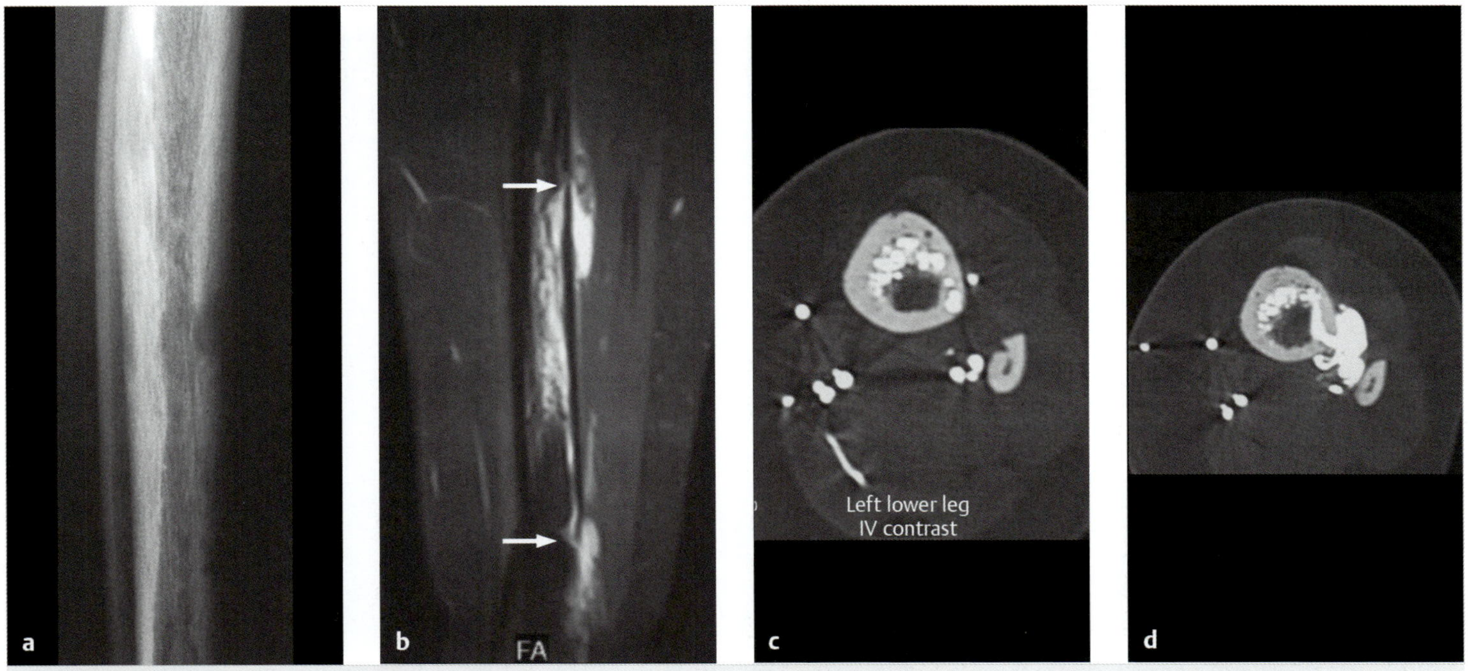

Fig. 7.43 a–d Venous malformation in a 14-year-old girl.

Pathoanatomic Background of the Findings

MRI proves that we are dealing with vessels in bony channels. They appear to be pathologic vessels, whose large caliber indicates a vascular malformation.

Assignment to a Possible Basic Entity

This step has already been completed. It remains to determine what kind of vascular malformation it is: arteriovenous, venous, or lymphatic? High flow or slow flow? Further angiographic studies identified the lesion as a venous malformation in the bone and adjacent soft tissues. This differs from Case 134, which involved angiomatosis, but is identical to the case in ▶ Fig. 7.43 below.

Synopsis and Discussion

Vascular malformations in bone and soft tissues require treatment because of their tendency for progressive enlargement. We recommend detailed venographic imaging to identify the feeding and draining vessels, which can provide access for sclerotherapy (see also the case in ▶ Fig. 7.43).

Vascular malformations require differentiation from *neoplastic vascular lesions* in the form of *hemangiomas*, as illustrated in Case 134. If treatment is indicated, these lesions are treated with angiogenesis inhibitors or by direct sclerotherapy. Hemangiomas usually present a fine honeycomb structure on plain radiographs and cause few if any complaints, even when the affected body region is in a dependent position. As a rule, only functional imaging tests can reliably distinguish a vascular malformation from a benign vascular neoplasm (hemangioma), as histologic differentiation is very problematic, see Case 134.

▶ Fig. 7.43 shows another venous malformation in the lower leg with pronounced extra- and intraosseous draining veins. The radiograph (▶ Fig. 7.43 **a**) demonstrates typical vascular prints, while MRI shows the large-caliber intra- and extraosseous veins, which communicate with one another proximally and distally through the cortex (arrows in ▶ Fig. 7.43 **b**). The distal drainage is clearly documented by CT venography (▶ Fig. 7.43 **c, d**). The 14-year-old girl had considerable pain in her left lower leg, especially in a dependent position. We gradually occluded the extra- and intraosseous draining vessels and the tortuous intraosseous venous channels, and afterward the patient was free of complaints. This case is fully documented in Freyschmidt (2008).[13]

As an aid to differential diagnosis, ▶ Fig. 7.44 shows a lesion that appears to have the classic imaging appearance of a *hemangioma*. The lesion was detected in the right tibia of a 21-year-old man, who complained of only mild pain in the affected region. But that was more of an incidental finding, since the main finding was in the left femoral shaft: a very painful stress fracture (see also the bone scan in ▶ Fig. 7.44 **c**). The patient was a jogger. The coarse trabecular structures in the proximal tibial shaft (▶ Fig. 7.44 **a, b**) were found to include fatty tissue (not shown here). Intravenous contrast produced honeycomb enhancement, especially in anterior and lateral peripheral areas in the cortex (▶ Fig. 7.44 **d–f**). This honeycomb pattern may represent capillary and venous vascular spaces that coalesce in the intensely enhancing areas and may include larger nutrient vessels. But it may also represent a venous malformation that is just developing in this patient. This would be consistent with the intense tracer uptake in the bone scan. Another argument against a hemangioma would be the observation that it is usually a congenital tumor that may regress by puberty, whereas malformations first develop and become symptomatic at that age. Since we felt that histologic evaluation would not yield significant information that would aid in treatment planning (see Case 134), we advised against biopsy. The final diagnosis will probably have to await follow-up: If clinical and radiologic progression occurs, the lesion is a malformation. If the lesion regresses and shows fatty infiltration, it was a hemangioma that was late to resolve.

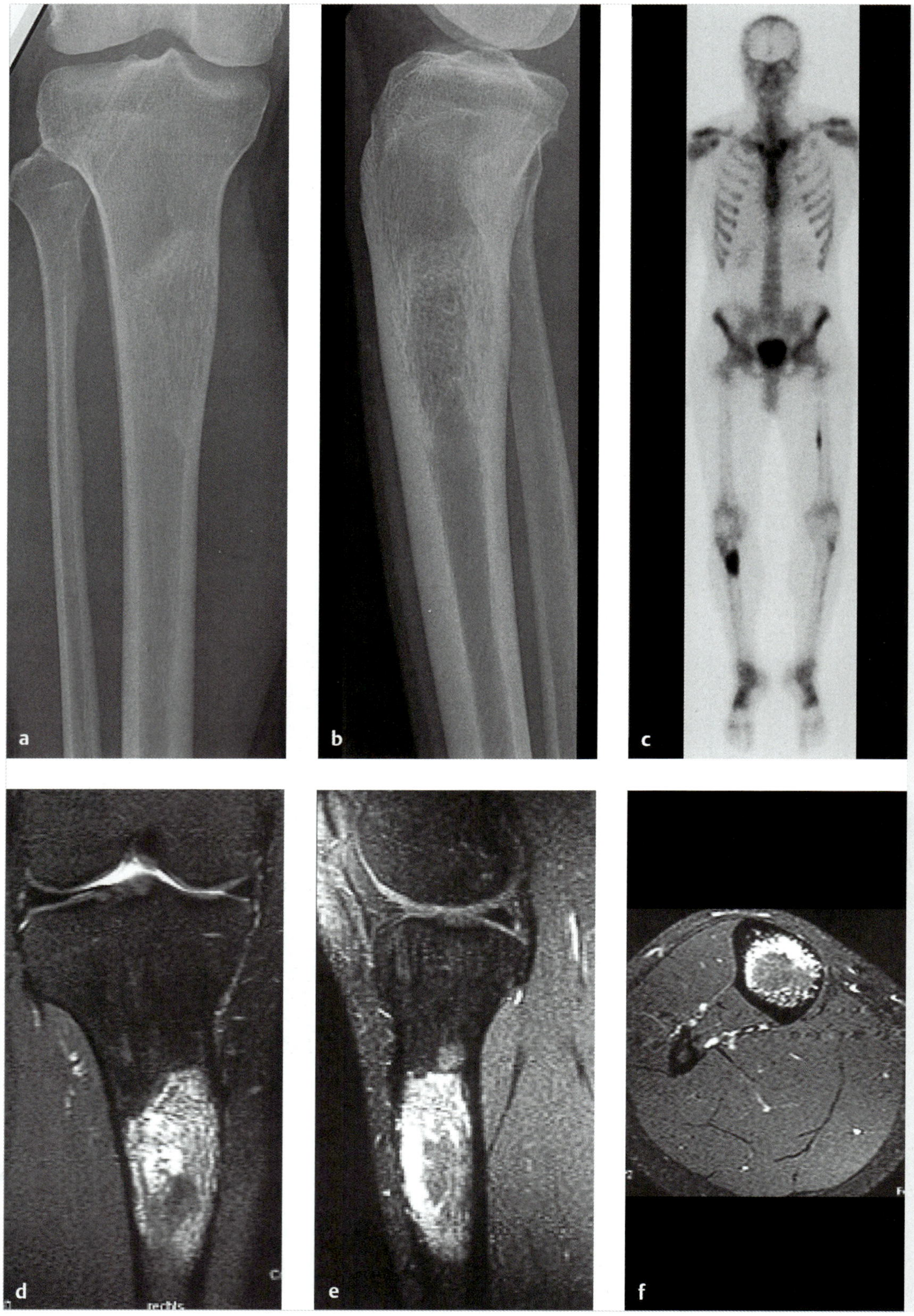

Fig. 7.44 a–f Vascular malformation or hemangioma?

Final Diagnosis

Intraosseous venous vascular malformation.

Comments

Vascular (vessel) prints are the imaging hallmark of a vascular anomaly located in or on the bone.

Case 155 (▶ Fig. 7.45)

Case description

- Referring physician: rheumatologist.
- Prior history and clinical question: A 62-year-old man had a history of recurrent ankle joint effusions, predominantly on the right side. He had been diagnosed with hemochromatosis 5 years earlier, and since then he had undergone three joint replacements. A suitable explanation could not be found for the MRI changes in the ankle joints.

Radiologic Findings

MRI demonstrates subchondral rounded figures in all the bones of the right ankle and subtalar joints. They have very high signal intensity on the STIR images (▶ Fig. 7.45 **a, b**) and low signal intensity on the T1w image (▶ Fig. 7.45 **c**). The figures are surrounded by moderate edema-like signal. Contralateral images (not shown here) revealed identical changes. Radiographs of the hands (▶ Fig. 7.45 **d, e**) show destructive changes in the radiocarpal joints with the scaphoid bones "burrowing into" the radial joint contours. Rounded lucencies are visible in the scaphoid bones. The triangular fibrocartilages are calcified. All the metacarpophalangeal joints show significant joint space narrowing with erosion of the metacarpal heads and smaller rounded, subchondral osteolytic areas. The distal and proximal interphalangeal joints appear normal. There is no evidence of juxta-articular osteoporosis.

Location

All of the pathologic findings noted above involve the subchondral region of the affected bones. The articular changes in the hand are confined to the radiocarpal and metacarpophalangeal joints, while the distal and proximal interphalangeal joints appear normal.

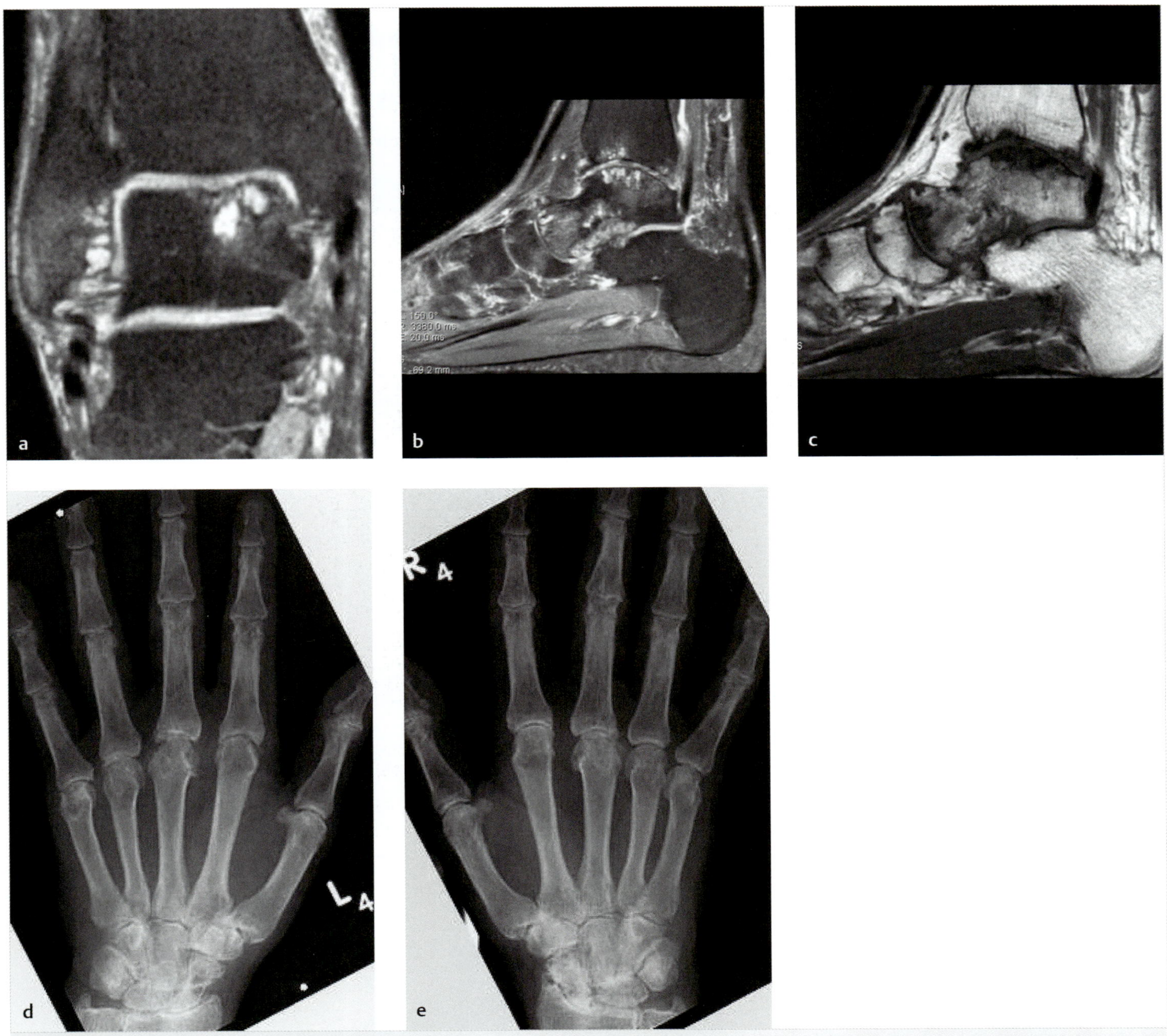

Fig. 7.45 a–e Unexplained signal changes in the tarsus.

Pathoanatomic Background of the Findings

The epicenters of the osseous changes (subchondral lucencies or osteolytic areas) are located in the joints, meaning that a systemic articular process is responsible for the subchondral changes. Considering the fact that there is no juxta-articular osteoporosis about the affected joints of the hands, we are probably dealing with an articular disease originating not from the synovial membrane but from the cartilage; hence it belongs to the group of chondroarthropathies. The erosions in the metacarpal heads may result from secondary involvement of the synovial membrane or breaking down of the subchondral bone.

Assignment to a Possible Basic Entity

Our discussions under Pathoanatomic Background of the Findings have already identified the underlying entity as a systemic chondroarthropathy.

Synopsis and Discussion

The MRI changes in the right ankle joint that caused confusion are actually typical of secondary chondrocalcinosis in a setting of hemochromatosis. The changes represent subchondral cysts, which probably developed from circumscribed necrosis. The edema-like signal surrounding the cysts may be reactive osteitis due to static insufficiency and/or synovitis. The MRI changes in the ankle joints and other large joints should be interpreted within the context of the very specific radiologic changes in the hands. There, the second and third metacarpophalangeal joints are predominantly affected and show joint space narrowing, subchondral cysts, as well as marginal defects, which probably result from wall fractures in marginal cysts or from secondary synovitis.

The subchondral plate may be disintegrated, causing the subchondral cancellous bone to acquire a "nibbled" appearance over time. This is clearly evident in ► Fig. 7.45 **d, e** and even in the T1w image in ► Fig. 7.45 **c**. All these changes eventually lead to the clinical and radiologic picture of osteoarthritis, accompanied by an erosive component.

The pathogenesis of hemochromatosis arthropathy is not yet fully understood. Iron or hemosiderin deposits probably have an irritating effect on the synovial membrane, resulting in hemosiderotic synovitis. Up to 30% of hemochromatosis cases are associated with secondary chondrocalcinosis, which can be explained by an altered ion balance in the synovial fluid due to the high local iron concentration, resulting in the deposition of calcium pyrophosphate and other calcium compounds. In turn, the secondary chondrocalcinosis can account for the severe, bilateral radiocarpal joint changes, which were also present in our patient. They result not only from the deposition of calcium pyrophosphate crystals in the cartilage, but also in the ligament attachments, especially between the scaphoid and lunate bones. This causes ligament laxity with scapholunate dissociation and rotary subluxation of the scaphoid. Stäbler (1992)[62] or Freyschmidt (2008)[13] may be consulted for details on the further course of the usually severe changes, which may even include "burrowing" of the scaphoid into the radius and scaphoid collapse.

Final Diagnosis

Typical articular involvement by hemochromatosis.

Comments

Articular changes in hemochromatosis are sometimes combined with secondary chondrocalcinotic changes, which add to the radiologic diversity of this rare disease.

7.5 Extraosseous Lesions

Case 156 (▶ Fig. 7.46)

Case description

- Referring physician: radiologist.
- Prior history and clinical question: A 24-year-old active soccer player presented approximately 6 months after being kicked in his left thigh. Afterward he had developed a hematoma followed by severe local pain and some local warmth. He stated that he returned to soccer after the symptoms subsided. When asked to give more details on his history in the light of imaging findings, he described a new impact trauma to the same site about 3 weeks earlier, followed by the same symptoms that occurred after the first injury. The radiologic differential diagnosis consisted of a periosteal osteosarcoma versus myositis ossificans (= heterotopic ossification).

Radiologic Findings

The sagittal reformatted CT image (▶ Fig. 7.46 **a**) shows a relatively homogeneous ossification approximately 6 to 7 cm long on the proximal femoral shaft. The lesion is directly applied to the anterolateral cortex in its proximal portion and spreads out distally, where it maintains a certain distance from the original cortex. The axial scans (▶ Fig. 7.46 **c, d**) show that the lesion is solid. It is bounded externally by a kind of cortex, while the interior contains bony structures that are not very differentiated. An incomplete fracture line is visible at the junction between the portion that abuts the femoral cortex and the portion that is separate. No destructive or erosive changes are visible anywhere in the cortex. Axial contrast-enhanced MRI (▶ Fig. 7.46 **b**) shows an intensely enhancing mass anterolateral to the femur, which has a central "core" corresponding to the ossified structure on CT. The mass around the core does not have a correlate on CT.

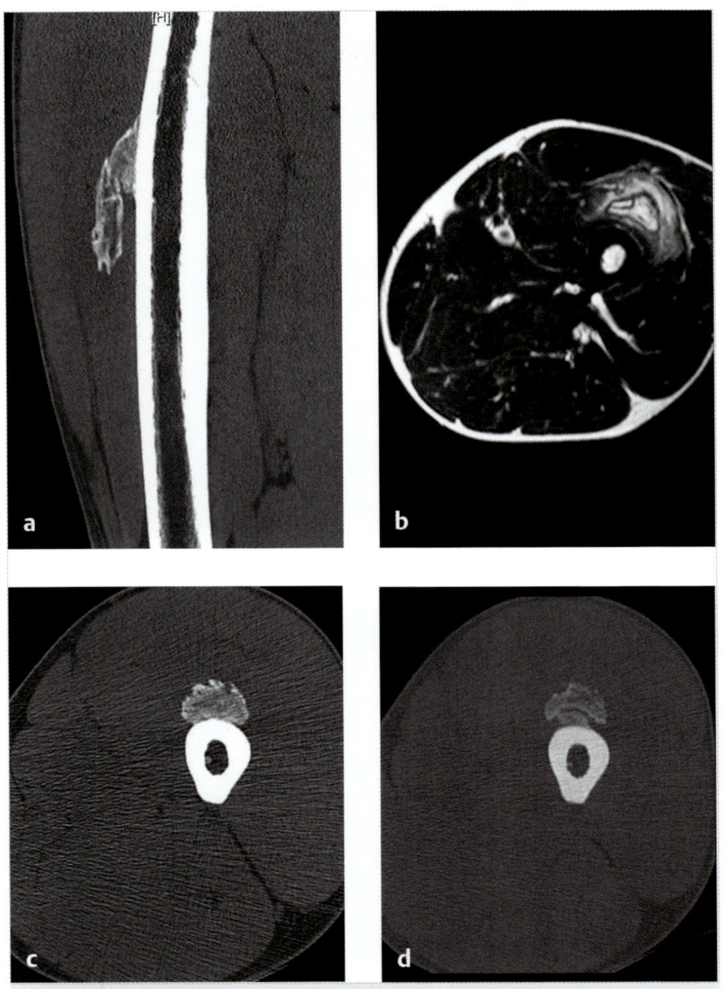

Fig. 7.46 a–d Periosteal osteosarcoma?

Location

The ossified mass is directly applied to the femoral cortex and projects into the adjacent soft tissues, so it is definitely paraosseous. A soft-tissue mass surrounds the ossification.

Pathoanatomic Background of the Findings

We must ask whether the ossified mass is the ossified tumor osteoid of a juxtacortical osteosarcoma (e.g., periosteal osteosarcoma) or whether it signifies myositis ossificans. The latter diagnosis is supported by the finding that the peripheral zone of the ossification is more solid than its center. A reverse trizonal structure is typical of periosteal osteosarcoma (see next paragraph), that is, the central ossifications that form first are denser than the peripheral ossifications. But what is the soft-tissue mass surrounding the ossification (▶ Fig. 7.46 **b**)? Is it tumor osteoid that has not yet ossified, or an area of myositis ossificans that is still fresh and well perfused?

Assignment to a Possible Basic Entity

Our discussions under Pathoanatomic Background of the Findings have limited the possible basic entities to a tumor or a reactive process, so there is no need to consider other possibilities.

First, it should be noted that solid ossifications occur in both periosteal osteosarcoma and myositis ossificans, but with a different pathogenesis. With periosteal osteosarcoma, it is the ossified tumor matrix; in myositis ossificans, it is a reactive process resulting from a traumatic hemorrhage, for example. It is believed that the traumatized tissue emits a signal that is generated by the cells of the injured tissue or by inflammatory cells that have infiltrated the injured area. This signal stimulates the formation of mesenchymal cells and their differentiation into fibroblasts and chondroblasts. Signal proteins such as bone morphogenetic protein (BMP) play a role in this process. As a rule, the resulting soft-tissue mass eventually develops into a highly vascularized pseudotumor with a characteristic trizonal structure:

- A center composed of immature, loose fibroblastic tissue that is easily confused with a spindle cell carcinoma or juxtacortical osteosarcoma due to its nuclear irregularities, mitoses, inflammatory round cells, and giant cells.
- An intermediate zone composed of metaplastic osteoid.
- An outer zone in which the newly formed bone matures to normal lamellar bone.

This structure is reflected in the radiographic, CT, and MRI appearance of myositis ossificans: unossified tissue is still present in the central zone while there is increasing ossification in the outer zones. In our case the ossification is already far advanced, although CT scans still show a lower central density and a higher peripheral density or even a mature cortex. As mentioned above, periosteal osteosarcoma has a reverse trizonal structure:

- "old" dense and mature bone at the center;
- less ossification at the periphery, or even an outer zone of pure tumor osteoid.

The problem in our case is the soft-tissue mass around the ossification demonstrated by MRI. In interpreting this finding, it is important to note that a cortex is present between the soft-tissue mass and the ossification, suggesting that the myositis ossificans developed in two stages. This coincides perfectly with the history of two traumatic events. The first part of the lesion, now ossified, formed after the first event, and the second part, still florid and well perfused, formed after the second event. Apparently the second injury caused the hook-shaped ossification to fracture at the base.

Synopsis and Discussion

The above considerations provide a solid clinical and radiologic basis for diagnosing myositis ossificans. There is no need for biopsy confirmation, which could even be misleading if the newer, immature portion of the mass were sampled. We also advised against surgical removal, as the risk of recurrence is very high for myositis ossificans that has not yet fully matured (see also Case 63, Case 113, and Case 125). It is better to wait until the newer portion of the lesion has also matured and is fully ossified. If the overall lesion is disabling to the patient at that time, it can be removed.

A three-phase bone scan may be helpful in evaluating the degree of maturation. A lesion at the florid stage still shows a high degree of perfusion. A fully mature lesion will show slightly increased uptake only in bone-phase images.

Final Diagnosis

Metachronous myositis ossificans (heterotopic ossification) on the femur.

Comments

The trizonal structure of the lesion is important in the radiologic differentiation of myositis ossificans from juxtacortical osteosarcoma.

Case 157 (▶ Fig. 7.47)

Case description

- Referring physician: radiologist.
- Prior history and clinical question: A 48-year-old man presented with a painful swelling in his right proximal lower leg. Ultrasound showed evidence of a liquid lesion but could not establish a cause, so the lesion was investigated further by MRI.

Radiologic Findings

The axial (▶ Fig. 7.47 **a**) and sagittal MR images (▶ Fig. 7.47 **b**) show a multiloculated or extremely tortuous (tubular) structure that appears to communicate with the tibiofibular joint (arrow in ▶ Fig. 7.47 **b**). The mass has a homogeneous signal of water intensity.

Location

The exact topography of the lesion is unclear from the images. In any case it is located between the proximal tibia and fibula and appears to follow the neurovascular sheath.

Pathoanatomic Background of the Findings

By its structure and signal intensity, the lesion may be an unusually large ganglion cyst arising from the anterior tibiofibular joint. Ganglion cysts of this kind may spread from the proximal anterior tibiofibular joint to the distal fibular nerve along the nerve sheath of the articular branch of the fibular nerve. A different route of spread has been discussed for intraneural ganglion cyst of the tibial nerve: The lesion spreads from the posteroinferior portion of the proximal tibiofibular joint and follows the articular branch on the posterior surface of the popliteus muscle, spreading from there along the posterior tibial nerve trunk by an intra- or epineural route. These lesions are called "intraneural ganglia" or "intraneural ganglion cysts."[63]

Since the lesion is already assigned to a basic entity, we need not consider other possibilities.

Synopsis and Discussion

The patient was referred to a plastic surgeon with the diagnosis of a fibular or tibial intraneural ganglion cyst, and operatively treated. The ganglion cyst was found in the proximal tibialis posterior compartment (fourth compartment of the lower leg) and was removed following fibular and tibial neurolysis, arteriolysis, venolysis, and tenolysis. The lesion was described grossly as an "opened cystic tissue mass 3.5 cm in diameter that was filled with gelatinous material." Microscopy identified degenerated tendon-sheath tissue as the cause of ganglion cyst formation. These findings indicate that the lesion was an extraneural ganglion cyst. Based on the imaging documentation, however, we still believe that the lesion was a fibular or tibial intraneural ganglion cyst owing to its tubular rather than globular structure, its course, and its communication with the proximal tibiofibular joint. If the lesion recurs, the joint connection should be closed at revision surgery, as was done by Spinner et al (2007)[63] in two patients with a recurrent tibial intraneural ganglion cyst.

Preliminary (Working) Diagnosis

Large intraneural ganglion cyst of the fibular or tibial nerve, though histology indicated an extraneural tendinous origin.

Comments

Intraneural ganglion cysts in the proximal thigh are rare. They should be considered when MRI shows a tubular structure of water signal intensity that communicates with the proximal tibiofibular joint.

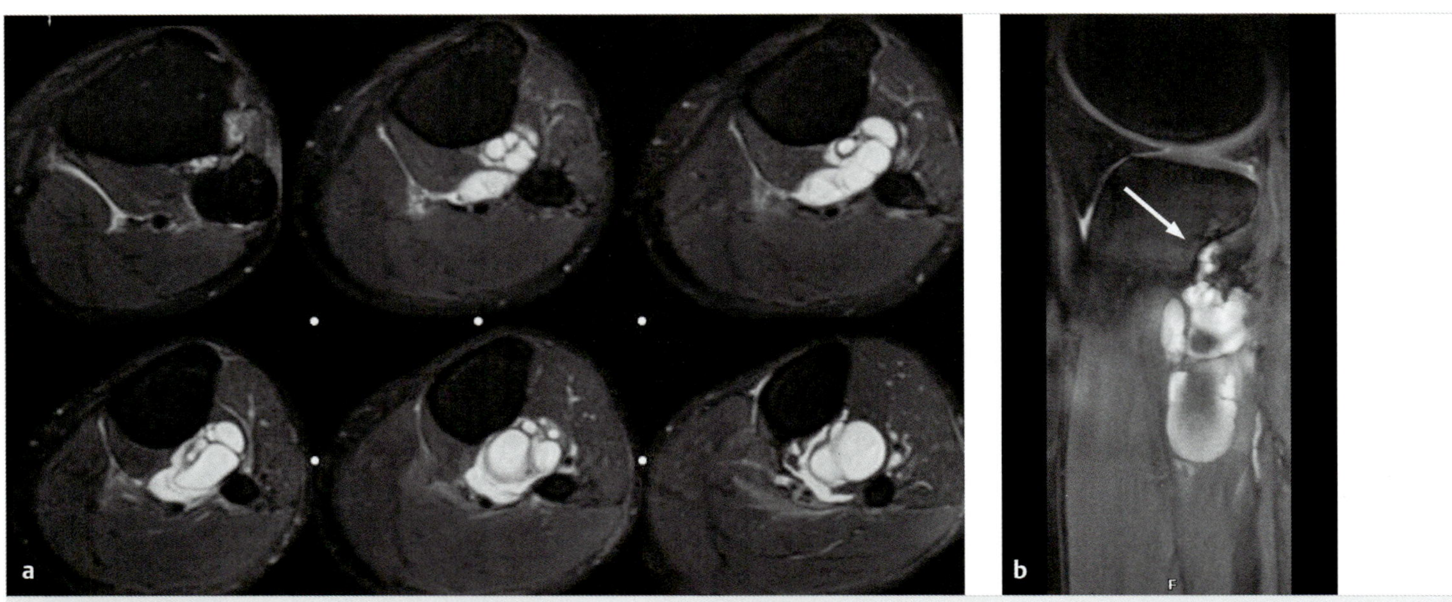

Fig. 7.47 a, b Unexplained "soft-tissue cysts": aneurysm?

Case 158 (▶ Fig. 7.48)

Case description

- Referring physician: radiologist.
- Prior history and clinical question: An 82-year-old woman complained of occasional pain and pressure sensation in her left lower leg. She was hospitalized for extensive inflammatory and ulcerative changes in that region. Radiographs showed a large, partially calcified mass, and biopsy was performed on the presumed calcified tumor. Histologic examination was inconclusive, and the case was referred for consultation.

Radiologic Findings

The postoperative radiographs (▶ Fig. 7.48 **a, b**) show an extensive, elongated, partially calcified mass projected over the tibia and fibula. The presence of a drain one day after open biopsy is also noted. The preoperative radiograph was unavailable, but we assume that it did not look much different from the postoperative film. The preoperative CT images (▶ Fig. 7.48 **d, e**) show a mass with predominantly shell-like calcifications located between the tibia and fibula. It has a heterogeneous interior density but is partially isointense to muscle and also contains fluid. Numerous clumps of calcification are visible within the lesion. In the MR image (▶ Fig. 7.48 **c**), the mass is mostly devoid of signal but contains focal hyperintensities of fluid signal intensity. The mass did not enhance after IV contrast administration.

Location

The mass is related anatomically to the tibialis anterior muscle.

Pathoanatomic Background of the Findings

Because the mass is located in the region of the tibialis anterior and appears to have replaced the muscle, it is reasonable to ask whether it represents a postnecrotic state with metaplastic and dystrophic calcifications or ossifications. To answer this question, we need more information on the patient's history since a muscle does not become necrotic without good cause. When questioned, the patient did report that she had sustained a tibial fracture more than 20 years ago. She also stated that complications arose, which we interpret as a compartment syndrome.

This gives us an apparent underlying entity, and we must consider that other possibilities are unrealistic.

Synopsis and Discussion

When we review the main features of this case—a large, inhomogeneous calcified mass with fluid-filled cavities that is located in the region of the tibialis anterior muscle and has replaced it—we must consider the possibility of antecedent trauma. Unless we had asked the patient specifically about a possible trauma history, this case would not have been solved, although a tumor with flocculent necrotic calcifications, for example, would have been unlikely on radiologic grounds alone. Why would a tumor of this size, such as soft-tissue sarcoma, conform to the boundaries of the tibialis anterior compartment and completely replace the muscle? The absence of IV contrast enhancement would also be unusual for a tumor.

The correct term for this lesion is *calcific myonecrosis*. This rare disease occurs almost exclusively in the lower limbs, is trauma-induced, and is usually mistaken for a tumor. It results from cystic degeneration of the muscle, giving rise to a painful, calcifying mass that is often detected many years after an injury (?) or may take many years (up to 65) to fully develop (?). This contrasts with myositis ossificans (see Case 156), which usually becomes symptomatic within 1 to 2 weeks after an injury. Patients with calcific myonecrosis often have a prior history of treatment for a compartment syndrome and/or a vascular lesion following the internal fixation of a fracture, for example, especially when a closed technique was used. Radiographs typically show plaquelike calcifications in the periphery of the mass with possible erosion of the adjacent bone. The mass contains fluid-filled spaces surrounded by a calcified pseudocapsule.[64,65] In our case the fluid component was less pronounced.

▶ Fig. 7.49 illustrates another case of calcific myonecrosis. The 47-year-old man had an infected left total hip replacement following a number of previous operations. The last operation revealed fluid-filled spaces but showed no definite signs of infection. An unusual feature of this case is that it involved all three compartments in the thigh, apparently because each of the previous operations had caused trauma leading to intracompartmental hemorrhage. In each case there were no radiologic or histologic signs of myositis ossificans.

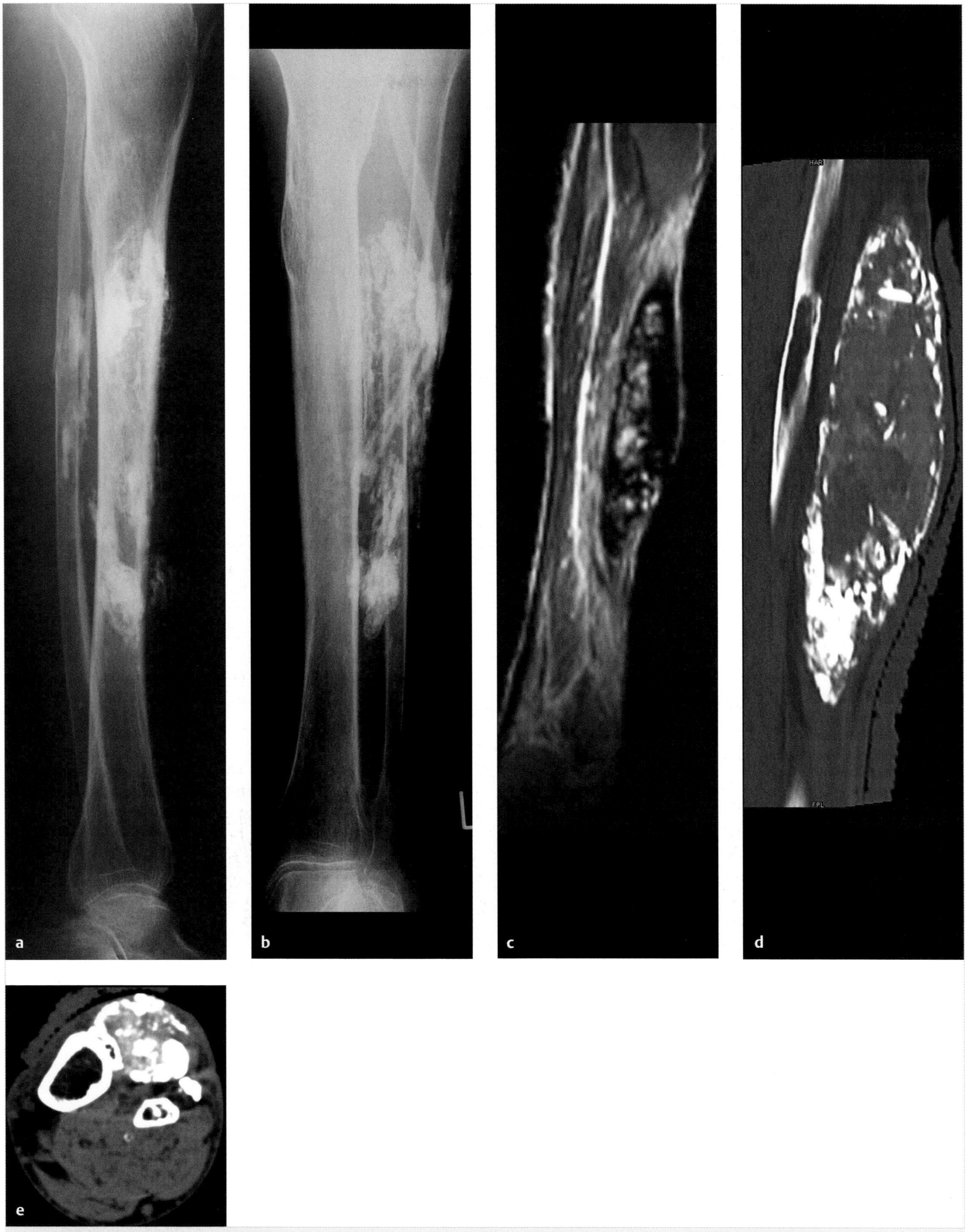

Fig. 7.48 a–e Calcified soft-tissue tumor?

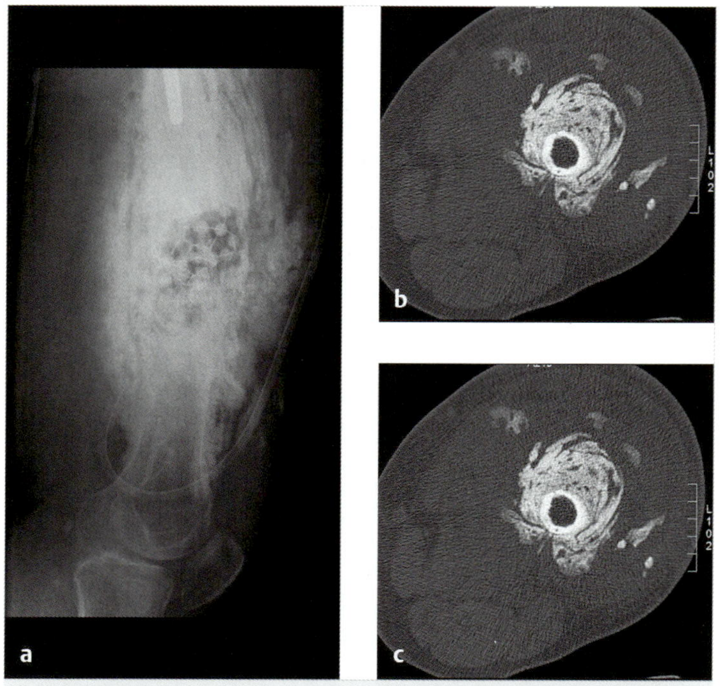

Fig. 7.49 a–c Calcific myonecrosis in the thigh of a 47-year-old man.

Final Diagnosis

Calcific myonecrosis involving the tibialis anterior muscle.

Comments

Calcified soft-tissue masses containing fluid areas in the lower limb which are localized to an anatomic compartment should not be interpreted as myositis ossificans but as calcific myonecrosis.

Bibliography

[1] Hach A, Freyschmidt J. Skelettszintigrafie, Kapitel 2.8: Mustererkennung. In: Stäbler A, Bandhrsg. Vol 1: Muskuloskelettales System. In: Freyschmidt J, ed. Handbuch Diagnostische Radiologie. Berlin: Springer; 2001: 72

[2] Jadvar H, Conti PS. Diagnostic utility of FDG PET in multiple myeloma. Skeletal Radiol 2002; 31: 690–694

[3] Dimopoulos M, Terpos E, Comenzo RL et al. IMWG. International myeloma working group consensus statement and guidelines regarding the current role of imaging techniques in the diagnosis and monitoring of multiple Myeloma. Leukemia 2009; 23: 1545–1556

[4] Liu T, Cheng T, Xu W, Yan WL, Liu J, Yang HL. A meta-analysis of 18FDG-PET, MRI and bone scintigraphy for diagnosis of bone metastases in patients with breast cancer. Skeletal Radiol 2011; 40: 523–531

[5] Aoki J, Watanabe H, Shinozaki T et al. FDG PET of primary benign and malignant bone tumors: standardized uptake value in 52 lesions. Radiology 2001; 219: 774–777

[6] Feldman F, van Heertum R, Manos C. 18FDG PET scanning of benign and malignant musculoskeletal lesions. Skeletal Radiol 2003; 32: 201–208

[7] Hawkins DS, Schuetze SM, Butrynski JE et al. [18F]Fluorodeoxyglucose positron emission tomography predicts outcome for Ewing sarcoma family of tumors. J Clin Oncol 2005; 23: 8828–8834

[8] Hawkins DS, Rajendran JG, Conrad EU III, Bruckner JD, Eary JF. Evaluation of chemotherapy response in pediatric bone sarcomas by [F-18]-fluorodeoxy-D-glucose positron emission tomography. Cancer 2002; 94: 3277–3284

[9] Gaston LL, Di Bella C, Slavin J, Hicks RJ, Choong PF. 18F-FDG PET response to neoadjuvant chemotherapy for Ewing sarcoma and osteosarcoma are different. Skeletal Radiol 2011; 40: 1007–1015

[10] Bredella MA, Essary B, Torriani M, Ouellette HA, Palmer WE. Use of FDG-PET in differentiating benign from malignant compression fractures. Skeletal Radiol 2008; 37: 405–413

[11] Shin DS, Shon OJ, Byun SJ, Choi JH, Chun KA, Cho IH. Differentiation between malignant and benign pathologic fractures with F-18-fluoro-2-deoxy-D-glucose positron emission tomography/computed tomography. Skeletal Radiol 2008; 37: 415–421

[12] Zanetti M, Bruder E, Romero J, Hodler J. Bone marrow edema pattern in osteoarthritic knees: correlation between MR imaging and histologic findings. Radiology 2000; 215: 835–840

[13] Freyschmidt J. Skeletterkrankungen. 3rd ed Berlin: Springer; 2008: 21, 453

[14] Freyschmidt J. Knochen(mark)ödem in der MRT - Befund oder nur Signal? Ein kurzer Blick hinter den Spiegel. Z Rheumatol 2012; 71: 8–11

[15] Fletcher CDM, Unni KK, Mertens F. World Health Organization classification of tumours. Pathology and genetics of tumours of soft tissue and bone. Lyon: IARC Press; 2002

[16] Garré C. Über besondere Formen der akuten infektiösen Osteomyelitis. Bruns Beitr Klin Chir 1893; 10: 241–298

[17] Brossmann J, Czerny C, Freyschmidt J. Freyschmidt's "Köhler/Zimmer." Grenzen des Normalen und Anfänge des Pathologischen in der Radiologie des kindlichen und erwachsenen Skeletts. 14th ed Stuttgart: Thieme; 2001

[18] Freyschmidt J, Ostertag H, Jundt G. Knochentumoren. 3rd ed Berlin: Springer; 2010

[19] Freyschmidt J, Freyschmidt G. Haut-, Schleimhaut- und Skeletterkrankungen —Skibo-Diseases. Berlin: Springer; 1996

[20] Hamers S, Freyschmidt J, Terwey B. Diagnostik tumorsimulierender intraossärer Arachnoidaldivertikel mittels flüssigkeitssensitiver MR-Sequenzen. Rofo 2000; 172: 850–852

[21] Dammert S, Krings T, Möller-Hartmann W. [Diagnosis of intraosseous epidermoid of the posterior part of the skull by the diffusion imaging] Rofo 2003; 175: 1272–1273

[22] Freyschmidt J. 'The vanished occiput'. Nephrol Dial Transplant 1999; 14: 499–500

[23] Freyschmidt J. Melorheostosis: a review of 23 cases. Eur Radiol 2001; 11: 474–479

[24] Mirra JM, Brien EW. Giant notochordal hamartoma of intraosseous origin: a newly reported benign entity to be distinguished from chordoma. Report of two cases. Skeletal Radiol 2001; 30: 698–709

[25] Yamaguchi T, Yamato M, Saotome K. First histologically confirmed case of a classic chordoma arising in a precursor benign notochordal lesion: differential diagnosis of benign and malignant notochordal lesions. Skeletal Radiol 2002; 31: 413–418

[26] Kyriakos M. Benign notochordal lesions of the axial skeleton: a review and current appraisal. Skeletal Radiol 2011; 40: 1141–1152

[27] Girodias JB, Azouz EM, Marton D. Intervertebral disk space calcification. A report of 51 children with a review of the literature. Pediatr Radiol 1991; 21: 541–546

[28] Gelineck J, Salomonsen M, Hviid C. Retropharyngeal tendinitis: radiographic and magnetic resonance imaging findings. Acta Radiol 2006; 47: 806–809

[29] Offiah CE, Hall E. Acute calcific tendinitis of the longus colli muscle: spectrum of CT appearances and anatomical correlation. Br J Radiol 2009; 82: e117–e121

[30] Jennin F, Bousson V, Parlier C, Jomaah N, Khanine V, Laredo JD. Bony sequestrum: a radiologic review. Skeletal Radiol 2011; 40: 963–975

[31] Frost HM. The biology of fracture healing. An overview for clinicians. Part II. Clin Orthop Relat Res 1989: 294–309

[32] Neumann A, Wuerfel J, Hunold P. [Wedge-shaped vertebra-an unusual complication of the pathomechanical cascade of ankylosing spondylitis-osteoporosis-vertebral body fraction] Rofo 2011; 183: 564–566

[33] Bruder E, Perez-Atayde AR, Jundt G et al. Vascular lesions of bone in children, adolescents, and young adults. A clinicopathologic reappraisal and application of the ISSVA classification. Virchows Arch 2009; 454: 161–179

[34] Sundaram M, Wolverson MK, Joist JH, Riaz MA, Rao BJ. Case report 133. Hemophilic pseudotumor of ilium and soft tissues. Skeletal Radiol 1981; 6: 54–57

[35] Batista GR, Rocha Oliveira PC, Alcantara FP, de Teles IG, Senna Najjar YJ, Kalil RK. Chronic diploic hematoma mimicking malignancy on imaging. Skeletal Radiol 2011; 40: 475–479

[36] Rossi F, Dragoni S. Acute avulsion fractures of the pelvis in adolescent competitive athletes: prevalence, location and sports distribution of 203 cases collected. Skeletal Radiol 2001; 30: 127–131

[37] Spranger JW, Brill PW, Poznanski A. Bone Dysplasias. 2nd ed. Munich: Oxford University Press; 2002

[38] Kim JA, Park JS, Jin W, Ryu K. Herniation pits in the femoral neck: a radiographic indicator of femoroacetabular impingement? Skeletal Radiol 2011; 40: 167–172

[39] Freyschmidt J. The apple core sign. Eur Radiol 2002; 12: 245–247

[40] Vande Berg BC, Malghem JJ, Lecouvet FE, Jamart J, Maldague BE. Idiopathic bone marrow edema lesions of the femoral head: predictive value of MR imaging findings. Radiology 1999; 212: 527–535

[41] Giordano A. Zwei familiäre Fälle von Ossifikation des "Ligamentum transversum scapulae superius." RöFo 1962; 96: 834–835

[42] Tshering Vogel DW, Steinbach LS, Hertel R, Bernhard J, Stauffer E, Anderson SE. Acromioclavicular joint cyst: nine cases of a pseudotumor of the shoulder. Skeletal Radiol 2005; 34: 260–265

[43] Craig EV. The geyser sign and torn rotator cuff: clinical significance and pathomechanics. Clin Orthop Relat Res 1984: 213–215

[44] Brien EW, Mirra JM, Kerr R. Benign and malignant cartilage tumors of bone and joint: their anatomic and theoretical basis with an emphasis on radiology, pathology and clinical biology. I. The intramedullary cartilage tumors. Skeletal Radiol 1997; 26: 325–353

[45] Shih C, Chang C-Y, Penn IW, Tiu CM, Chang T, Wu JJ. Chronically stressed wrists in adolescent gymnasts: MR imaging appearance. Radiology 1995; 195: 855–859

[46] Gupta SK, Sharma OP, Sharma SV, Sood B, Gupta S. Macrodystrophia lipomatosa: radiographic observations. Br J Radiol 1992; 65: 769–773

[47] Murphey MD, Carroll JF, Flemming DJ, Pope TL, Gannon FH, Kransdorf MJ. From the archives of the AFIP: benign musculoskeletal lipomatous lesions. Radiographics 2004; 24: 1433–1466

[48] Barletta JA, Bellizzi AM, Hornick JL. Immunohistochemical staining of thyroidectomy specimens for PTEN can aid in the identification of patients with Cowden syndrome. Am J Surg Pathol 2011; 35: 1505–1511

[49] Paloneva J, Kestilä M, Wu J et al. Loss-of-function mutations in TYROBP (DAP12) result in a presenile dementia with bone cysts. Nat Genet 2000; 25: 357–361

[50] Madry H, Prudlo J, Grgic A, Freyschmidt J. Nasu-Hakola disease (PLOSL): report of five cases and review of the literature. Clin Orthop Relat Res 2007; 454: 262–269

[51] Kransdorf MJ, Murphey MD, Sweet DE. Liposclerosing myxofibrous tumor: a radiologic-pathologic-distinct fibro-osseous lesion of bone with a marked predilection for the intertrochanteric region of the femur. Radiology 1999; 212: 693–698

[52] Heim-Hall JM, Williams RP. Liposclerosing myxofibrous tumour: a traumatized variant of fibrous dysplasia? Report of four cases and review of the literature. Histopathology 2004; 45: 369–376

[53] Tyler P, Datir A, Saifuddin A. Magnetic resonance imaging of anatomical variations in the knee. Part 2: miscellaneous. Skeletal Radiol 2010; 39: 1175–1186

[54] van Holsbeeck M, Vandamme B, Marchal G, Martens M, Victor J, Baert AL. Dorsal defect of the patella: concept of its origin and relationship with bipartite and multipartite patella. Skeletal Radiol 1987; 16: 304–311

[55] Bui KL, Ilaslan H, Bauer TW, Lietman SA, Joyce MJ, Sundaram M. Cortical scalloping and cortical penetration by small eccentric chondroid lesions in the long tubular bones: not a sign of malignancy? Skeletal Radiol 2009; 38: 791–796

[56] Brower AC, Worsham GF, Dudley AH. Erdheim-Chester disease: a distinct lipoidosis or part of the spectrum of histiocytosis? Radiology 1984; 151: 35–38

[57] Freyschmidt J, Ostertag H, Lang W. Case report 365: Erdheim-Chester disease. Skeletal Radiol 1986; 15: 316–322

[58] Veyssier-Belot C, Cacoub P, Caparros-Lefebvre D et al. Erdheim-Chester disease. Clinical and radiologic characteristics of 59 cases. Medicine (Baltimore) 1996; 75: 157–169

[59] Varich LJ, Laor T, Jaramillo D. Normal maturation of the distal femoral epiphyseal cartilage: age-related changes at MR imaging. Radiology 2000; 214: 705–709

[60] Frush TJ, Lindenfeld TN. Peri-epiphyseal and overuse injuries in adolescent athletes. Sports Health 2009; 1: 201–211

[61] Soprano JV, Fuchs SM. Common overuse injuries in the pediatric and adolescent athlete. Clin Pediatr Emerg Med 2007; 8: 7–14

[62] Stäbler A. [The pathophysiological etiological mechanism of destructive wrist joint arthropathy in pseudogout] Rofo 1992; 156: 73–76

[63] Spinner RJ, Mokhtarzadeh A, Schiefer TK, Krishnan KG, Kliot M, Amrami KK. The clinico-anatomic explanation for tibial intraneural ganglion cysts arising from the superior tibiofibular joint. Skeletal Radiol 2007; 36: 281–292

[64] Batz R, Sofka CM, Adler RS, Mintz DN, Dicarlo E. Dermatomyositis and calcific myonecrosis in the leg: ultrasound as an aid in management. Skeletal Radiol 2006; 35: 113–116

[65] Holobinko JN, Damron TA, Scerpella PR, Hojnowski L. Calcific myonecrosis: keys to early recognition. Skeletal Radiol 2003; 32: 35–40

[66] Masami M, Satoshi H. Images in Clinical Medicine. Crowned dens syndrome. N Engl. J. Med 2012; 367: e34

Index

D

E

F

G

H

I

J

K

L

P

R

S

T

U

V